Lower Extremity Joint Preservation

Mats Brittberg • Konrad Slynarski
Editors

Lower Extremity Joint Preservation

Techniques for Treating the Hip, Knee, and Ankle

Springer

Editors
Mats Brittberg
Kungsbacka Hospital, RHO
University of Gothenburg Kungsbacka
Hospital, RHO
Kungsbacka
Sweden

Konrad Slynarski
Słynarski Knee Clinic
Warsaw
Poland

ISBN 978-3-030-57381-2 ISBN 978-3-030-57382-9 (eBook)
https://doi.org/10.1007/978-3-030-57382-9

This Springer imprint is published by the registered company Springer Nature Switzerland AG
The registered company address is: Gewerbestrasse 11, 6330 Cham, Switzerland

Foreword

This book is a landmark contribution organized by orthopedic surgeons to put forth the newest technologies and techniques to optimize patient's skeletal outcomes. This is a landmark era because the orthopedic surgeons long referred to as "carpenters" who crafted mechanical solutions to skeletal problems have transformed into mixed media artists and cell biologists. The carpenters were seen to be cutting down huge limbs or delicately redirecting the ropes and pulleys to help the limbs carry load, swing a tennis racket, or pitch a ball. The carpenters still have their saws and hammers and their power tools for the really big jobs but enter the new age of orthobiologics and of cell-based therapies which changes the thinking, the approaches, and the successes.

Since the days of Aristotle, the ortho-docs have used the special sauce, the marrow, to add value to their reconstructions, so in a small way they were always into cell-based therapies. But now the marrow is used more wisely; the marrow and blood are fractionated and various components segregated from one another to more efficiently make use of one component's special capabilities while removing inhibitory or components which cause problems. Moreover, we now have a multitude of cell carriers, of containment barriers (membranes), and of enhancers for reconstruction of various skeletal tissues and a large array of biological solutions for orthopedic problems.

It was in the early 1990s that I introduced the concept that the bone marrow contained mesenchymal stem cells (MSCs). The concept that MSCs were multipotent stem cells in the marrow turns out to be wrong, but the current emphasis on the presence of osteogenic, chondrogenic, and adipogenic progenitors in the marrow explains how these three tissues can form from the marrow and why these three tissues can be found in the bone marrow. Availability of such distinctive progenitors explains the innate regenerative capacity of bones and the added value of the bone marrow to reconstructive surgeries. Indeed, we would now say that the physician's job is to devise strategies for maximizing the innate regenerative capacities of injured tissues. By using the principles of orthobiologics and cell-based therapies, the orthopedists of this era are experiencing greater surgical and medical successes by using these natural materials to augment reconstructive or reconditioned therapeutics. By unlocking some of the secrets of Mother Nature, by using some of her special sauces, and by training a new generation of orthopedists, more successful outcomes are being realized.

This book focuses on what's new and on how to better utilize what's old.

Arnold I. Caplan
Department of Biology, Skeletal Research Center
Case Western Reserve University
Cleveland, OH
USA

Preface

Joint homeostasis is when the articular joint is healthy and in equilibrium. When the joint is injured, we repair the intra- and peri-articular damaged structures. We try to restore the disturbed equilibrium. Injuries differ in their abilities to restore to near-normal stages. Age, gender and genetics are factors that influence the recovery as well as external factors such as obesity, smoking and metabolic diseases.

There are four 'R's in articular joint tissue engineering:

- Repair
- Restore
- Regenerate
- Rehabilitate

When we have more or less used one or more of the 'R's, the joint could be seen as preserved and it is then important to avoid future injuries and go from R to P, i.e. Prevention. Repeated injuries make a return to a normal or nearly normal state difficult. Increased knowledge is of the utmost importance about anatomy, trauma mechanisms and how one should repair the damaged structures back to a biomechanical situation restoring the homeostasis.

In this book, we have gathered a large number of experts on joint restoration and preservation, and they have all contributed their great knowledge to give you, the reader, updated information about joint preservation of the lower extremity.

Kungsbacka, Sweden — Mats Brittberg
Warsaw, Poland — Konrad Slynarski

Contents

Part I

Hip

Comprehensive Hip Preservation: Correction of Adult Hip Dysplasia and Repair of High-Grade Cartilage Injury

1

Graeme P. Whyte, David Bloom, Brian D. Giordano, and Thomas Youm

1.1 Introduction

Dysplasia of the hip results in coverage abnormality of the femoral head that is typically most prominent laterally and anteriorly. This malalignment is a leading cause of early joint failure, necessitating treatment with total hip arthroplasty when the cartilage injury becomes severe and diffuse [1]. Ganz et al. reported on a cohort or patients treated with a novel osteotomy about the acetabulum that was developed to correct the dysplastic deformity in skeletally mature individuals [2]. This periacetabular osteotomy frees the acetabulum in such a manner to allow normalization of coverage while at the same time preserving the posterior column completely along the posterior aspect. When performed prior to the development of high-grade diffuse chondral injury, it is the surgical treatment of choice for symptomatic adult hip dysplasia. Hip dysplasia that is not corrected is strongly associated with the development of osteoarthritis [3].

In those who have suffered associated injury to hip articular cartilage in the setting of hip dysplasia, there are options to repair chondral or osteochondral tissue at the time of alignment normalization. There are several cartilage repair techniques that may be performed arthroscopically either in a minimally invasive manner or in an open manner using a technique described by Ganz et al. to surgically dislocate the hip joint, with minimal risk of neurovascular injury [4]. There have been significant advancements in the treatment of high-grade injury to articular cartilage. Many techniques have been initially developed to treat injury in other joints, such as the knee, and are adaptable to the hip joint. These treatments include cell-based therapies, stem cell/signaling cell therapies, treatments using biologic scaffolds, and osteochondral grafting.

G. P. Whyte (✉)
New York Presbyterian Hospital, Weill Medical College, Cornell University, New York, NY, USA
e-mail: info@whytemd.com

NYU Langone Orthopedic Hospital, New York University School of Medicine, New York, NY, USA

D. Bloom · T. Youm
NYU Langone Orthopedic Hospital, New York University School of Medicine, New York, NY, USA
e-mail: David.Bloom@nyulangone.org; Thomas.Youm@nyumc.org

B. D. Giordano
University of Rochester Medical Center, Rochester, NY, USA
e-mail: Brian_Giordano@urmc.rochester.edu

1.2 Diagnostic Imaging in Adult Hip Dysplasia

Plain radiographs are the initial imaging modality of choice to evaluate alignment about the hip and in particular to evaluate coverage of the femoral head. Accurate measurements of several anatomic parameters about the hip help

M. Brittberg, K. Slynarski (eds.), *Lower Extremity Joint Preservation*,
https://doi.org/10.1007/978-3-030-57382-9_1

ensure that conditions such as hip dysplasia are identified.

Coverage is typically assessed laterally using the anteroposterior (AP) pelvis radiograph and anteriorly using the false-profile radiograph of the affected hip. Measurement of the lateral center-edge angle (LCEA), as described by Wiberg [5], is performed on the AP pelvis radiograph, while anterior coverage is evaluated using the anterior center-edge angle (ACEA), originally described by Lequesne [6], on the false-profile radiograph. Regarding the LCEA, a line is drawn representing the transverse pelvic axis, and then a perpendicular line is drawn to this through the center of the femoral head. The angle between this vertical line and a line drawn from the center of the femoral head to the edge of the condensed acetabular line is then drawn, resulting in the LCEA (Fig. 1.1a). When measuring the ACEA on the false-profile view, a vertical line is drawn through the center of the femoral head, followed by a line from the center of the head to the edge of the condensed acetabular line anteriorly (Fig. 1.1b). Importantly, for both of these measurements, the clinician must be sure to identify the edge of the condensed acetabular line which would correspond to the articulating coverage, as opposed to other points of bony prominence which are not articulating. Adherence to imaging protocols and measurement techniques are critically important, as there can be concern of inaccurate diagnosis of pathology related to femoral head coverage in cases of more subtle dysplasia or if standardized positioning protocols are not followed [7, 8]. Generally, an LCEA or ACEA measurement below 20° would indicate dysplasia, with borderline cases considered to be between 20° and 25°. Greater than 25° is considered within the normal range. It is important, however, to note that other factors play a role in symptomatic hip dysplasia in the adult, such as Ehlers-Danlos syndrome or other soft tissue considerations. Patients may have severe pain and dysfunction attributable to hip dysplasia even when measurements are described as "borderline" on radiographs.

The use of computed tomography (CT) imaging with three-dimensional reformatting is routinely of benefit to examine femoral head coverage (Fig. 1.1) and also to evaluate acetabular and femoral version abnormalities that may be contributing to the symptomatology in cases of hip dysplasia in the skeletally mature patient. Lateral coverage may be examined using the coronal center-edge angle (CCEA) and anterior coverage using the sagittal center-edge angle (SCEA) on CT. The diagnostician needs to be keenly aware that while the numerical values of the CCEA and SCEA are a helpful addition to the evaluation of coverage, these values do not directly correlate to the numerical values of LCEA and ACEA measured on plain radiographs. Femoral and acetabular version measurements are an important component to the diagnostic imaging evaluation of hip pathology. Biplanar plain radiography has been used for version measurement; however, these measurements typically lack the required accuracy and reproducibility. The preferable detailing of bony anatomy achievable with CT examination makes this the imaging of choice for acetabular and femoral version measurements. While MRI is frequently used to evaluate femoral version, there is not an exact correlation with CT measurements, perhaps related to the duration of the scan required for slices taken at the hip and knee and the potential for subtle patient movement of the lower extremity. When femoral or acetabular version analysis is used in the setting of planned operative correction, these values are preferably obtained using CT imaging.

MRI is another routinely used imaging modality used to evaluate hip pathology. There are a number of associated conditions that benefit from concurrent treatment in the setting of hip dysplasia. Labral tears are frequently encountered in the setting of adult hip dysplasia, and while it is not clear if all low-grade labral injuries benefit significantly from surgical treatment, many times the tear pattern involves a hypertrophic labrum that is significantly displaced and should be repaired. This associated injury is readily identified on MRI. Additionally, the condition of articular cartilage must be considered when treating hip dysplasia, as the prognosis is improved when

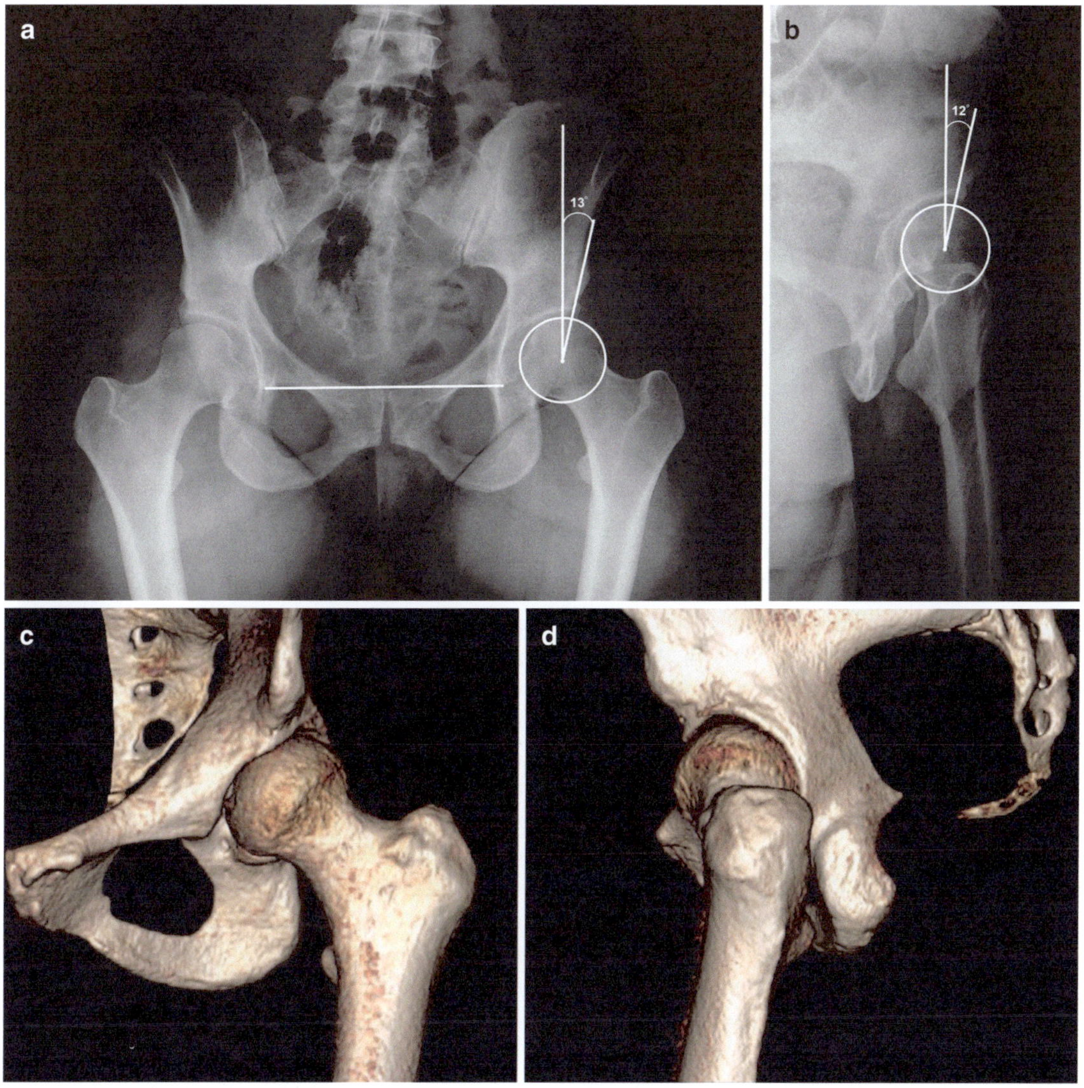

Fig. 1.1 Lateral center-edge angle (LCEA) measured for a left hip on the AP pelvis radiograph (**a**), anterior center-edge angle (ACEA) measured for a left hip on the false-profile radiograph (**b**); visualization of the left hip articulation using CT imaging with 3D reformatting in the coronal plane (**c**); visualization of the left hip articulation using CT imaging with 3D reformatting in the sagittal plane (**d**)

the alignment is corrected before significant articular cartilage injury develops. MRI may be used to examine both the articular cartilage and the underlying subchondral bone. Fast spin echo, T2-weighted, and proton density formats are often used. Recent developments in the field of delayed gadolinium-enhanced MRI of cartilage (dGEMERIC) and T2 relaxation time mapping have allowed for highly accurate evaluation of the status of articular cartilage.

1.3 Correction of Hip Dysplasia and Open Treatment of High-Grade Cartilage Injury

1.3.1 Periacetabular Osteotomy: Surgical Technique

The patient is positioned supine, and the lower extremity is draped appropriately to allow mobilization of the limb over the course of the procedure. General anesthesia is used and a Foley catheter is inserted prior to the procedure. Additionally, an epidural catheter may be placed to assist with postoperative pain management and to reduce blood requirements by enabling hypotensive anesthesia. Intraoperative blood salvage is used. A C-arm is used for fluoroscopy and is positioned perpendicular to the operative table on the contralateral side of surgery.

A curvilinear incision is made beginning superolateral to the anterior superior iliac spine (ASIS) over the iliac wing and extending distally, just lateral to the ASIS for several centimeters. The fascia is then incised lateral and distal to the ASIS, protecting branches of the lateral femoral cutaneous nerve. The musculature of the tensor fascia lata is identified, and blunt dissection is performed medially beneath the fascia to identify the interval between the tensor fascia lata and sartorius muscles. The fascia overlying the rectus femoris is then identified through the interval, and it is incised. Deep dissection initially proceeds lateral to the rectus femoris. The iliocapsularis that overlies the joint capsule is identified and elevated medially off of the capsular tissue. Dissection is then performed medial to the rectus femoris and lateral to the iliocapsularis distally to complete the exposure of the anterior capsule. The interval between the inferomedial capsule (laterally) and the iliopsoas tendon (medially) is identified by dissecting through the iliopsoas bursa. Proximally, the abdominal muscle facial layer overlying the iliac crest and superolateral to the ASIS is incised. A small osteotomy is made at the ASIS using an osteotome in order to mobilize sartorius and the inguinal ligament. Alternatively, a soft tissue sleeve containing the sartorius may be elevated off the ASIS and then repaired with suture to the bone at the conclusion of the procedure. Iliacus is dissected from the inner table of the pelvis toward the sciatic notch. The lateral aspect of the superior pubic ramus is exposed by dissecting medially, leaving intact the origin of the direct head of the rectus femoris. Alternatively, the direct head of the rectus femoris may be incised proximally to improve exposure of the anterior joint capsule if necessary; however, in the author's experience, this is seldom necessary. This tendon is repaired with suture at the conclusion of the procedure if a tenotomy has been performed. The lateral aspect of the superior pubic ramus is exposed by subperiosteal dissection 1.5–2 cm medial to the iliopectineal eminence. A small curved or bent sharp Hohmann retractor may be malleated into the superior ramus at the most medial exposure to maintain access by retracting the iliopsoas. Flexion and adduction of the hip will relax the soft tissues during this exposure, which will also reduce the risk of injury to the femoral nerve that can occur with excessive retraction.

Of the four bony cuts used to complete the periacetabular osteotomy, either the superior ramus or infracotyloid ischial osteotomy are preferably performed first. When osteotomizing the superior ramus, retractors are positioned to protect the obturator neurovascular structures posteriorly. An oscillating saw is used to make the initial cut at the superior ramus. The cut is made in the lateral to medial direction, beginning just medial to the iliopectineal eminence and at an angle of 40°. To minimize the risk of soft tissue injury, an osteotome is used to complete the osteotomy of the ramus.

When performing the first ischial cut at the infracotyloid groove, the hip is flexed to relax soft tissues and improve access. Distally, the interval between the iliopsoas tendon and inferomedial joint capsule that was previously exposed is identified. Long and curved Metzenbaum scissors are placed through the interval and positioned proximal to the obturator externus to palpate the ischium. Avoiding dissection distal to the obturator externus will protect the medial femoral circumflex artery (MFCA), and avoiding medial dissection will minimize the risk to the obturator neurovascular structures. The infracotyloid groove of the ischium, just inferior to the posterior acetabulum, is palpated with the closed scissors. The scissors are removed, and a specialized osteotome with a 30° curvature is placed through the same interval and positioned within the infracotyloid groove, ensuring to avoid any interposed soft tissue. Positioning is confirmed with fluoroscopic imaging. The osteotome is used to make ischial cuts that involve both the medial and lateral cortices within the groove. This is an incomplete osteotomy that must not penetrate through the posterior column. When penetrating the cortex laterally at the infracotyloid groove, the hip is extended and partially abducted to relax and protect the sciatic nerve.

The completion of the periacetabular osteotomy then requires the osteotomy of the iliac wing, which will connect at a corner to the final osteotomy at the quadrilateral surface. At the distal aspect of the ASIS, a small subgluteal window is created posterolaterally, and retractors are placed anteriorly and posteriorly along the iliac crest at the planned osteotomy site to protect the surrounding soft tissues. An oscillating saw is then used to cut the iliac crest, ending medially at the position where the quadrilateral surface osteotomy will begin. A 5-mm Schanz screw is placed proximally into the osteotomized fragment containing the acetabulum, and a T-handle is attached to the screw. This allows for manipulation of the fragment as the final osteotomy is completed. A half-inch osteotome is used to make the osteotomy of the quadrilateral surface, using oblique fluoroscopic imaging to ensure extra-articular positioning. The quadrilateral surface osteotomy should be halfway between the articular surface and the posterior border of the column, which leaves the posterior half of the posterior column intact after completion of the procedure. The distal component of the quadrilateral surface cut is completed with an angled osteotome, with the assistance of fluoroscopy as needed. Manipulating the Schantz screw to provide tension as well as the use of a laminar spreader as this final cut is made will assist to complete this osteotomy, which will meet with the infracotyloid ischial cut performed earlier in the procedure. If the mobility of the fragment is such that there is resistance that limits full alignment correction, the osteotomy is likely incomplete, or there is tethering periosteal tissue, and each osteotomy site should be revisited as needed until the fragment is completely free of attachments that hinder sufficient mobility.

The mobile fragment is positioned under fluoroscopic imaging to normalize femoral head coverage, with particular attention paid to lateral and anterior coverage. The realigned fragment is secured using long fully threaded 3.5 mm screws. Typically, three or four screws will provide sufficient fixation. An open osteochondroplasty of the femoral head-neck junction may be performed as indicated at this time using a burr in order to restore appropriate sphericity if there is concern of impingement. The ASIS osteotomy is reduced and secured with a small fragment screw, or the sartorius is reattached to the ASIS using suture fixation if an ASIS osteotomy had not been performed. Final fluoroscopic imaging and wound closure are performed.

When performing both periacetabular osteotomy and surgical dislocation, patient status is reviewed with the anesthesia team prior to commencing the second approach to ensure it is safe to proceed with additional surgical treatment in the same setting. In these cases, either periacetabular osteotomy or surgical dislocation may be performed first, depending on coexisting pathology. When there is concurrent treatment planned for intra- or extra-articular impingement, it is often beneficial to correct the alignment first with periacetabular osteotomy and then address areas of impingement with surgical dislocation. When there is concurrent treatment planned for chondral or osteochondral injury, performing the surgical dislocation of the hip and chondral/osteochondral repair first can be of benefit so that dynamic examination and radiographic assessment after periacetabular osteotomy can assist with determination of the final hip articulation alignment in such a manner as to limit focal stresses and edge loading at the site of chondral or osteochondral repair. Additionally, there is a role for proximal femoral osteotomy in alignment correction, the specifics of which are not discussed here. Preoperative and postoperative imaging for a case of hip dysplasia in a skeletally mature patient with associated high-grade osteochondral injury are depicted in Figs. 1.2 and 1.3.

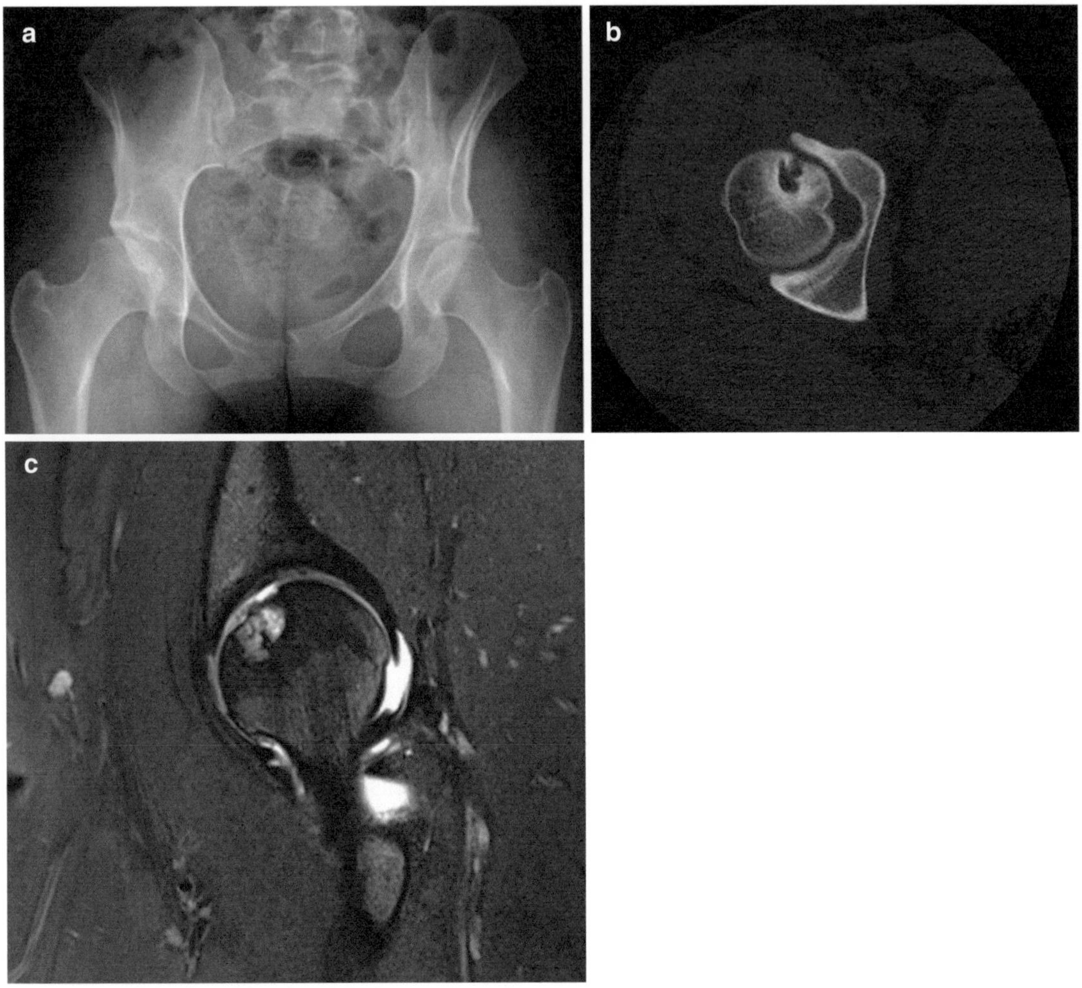

Fig. 1.2 Preoperative AP pelvis radiograph demonstrating hip dysplasia in a skeletally mature patient with right lateral center-edge angle of 11° (**a**); axial CT image demonstrating subchondral bony injury at an associated focal high-grade osteochondral femoral head lesion (**b**); sagittal MRI slice depicting injury to articular cartilage and underlying subchondral bone at the femoral head lesion (**c**)

1.3.2 Surgical Dislocation of the Hip: Surgical Technique

The patient is positioned in the lateral decubitus position, with the operative hip adequately exposed and the ipsilateral extremity incorporated into the sterile field in order to allow manipulation of the lower extremity throughout the procedure.

A straight incision is centered over the greater trochanter. Initial length of incision is made a single handbreadth proximal and distal to the greater trochanter. The incision is extended as necessary during the procedure, with a total length less than 20 cm typically adequate. The fascia lata is split. At the proximal extent of the dissection, the gluteus maximus may be split in a manner consistent with the Kocher-Langenbeck approach, or a Gibson modification may be used to dissect the plane between the gluteus maximus and gluteus medius. The greater trochanter is then identified, and the trochanteric bursa and associated fatty tissue are carefully mobilized at the posterior aspect of the trochanter to expose the short external rotators. Internal rotation of the hip will assist to better visualize soft tissue structures about the posterior greater trochanter.

The posterior aspect of the gluteus medius is then identified. The planned osteotomy site at the

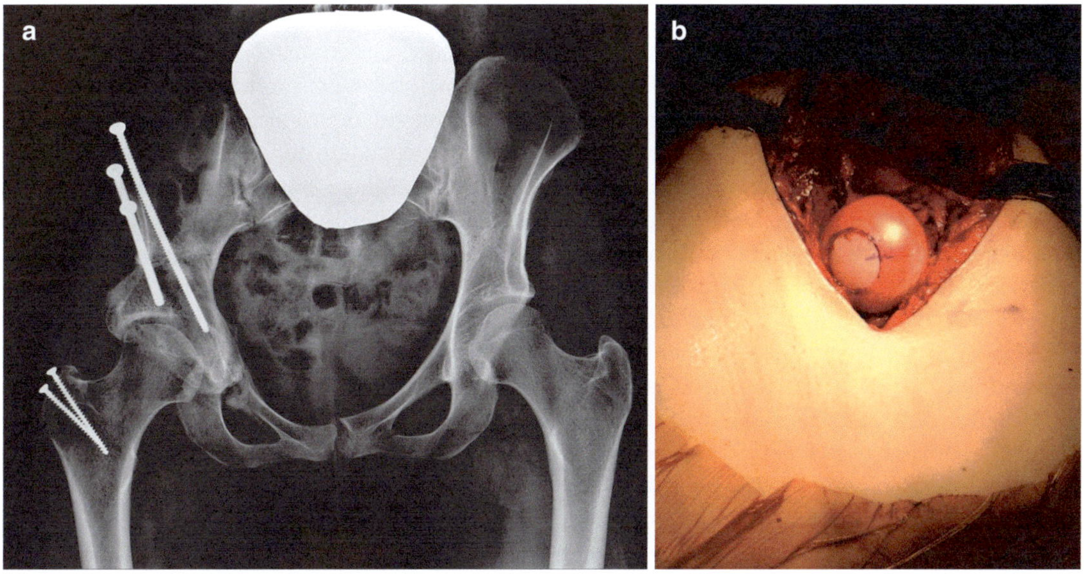

Fig. 1.3 AP pelvis radiograph 3 months postoperatively depicting correction of femoral head coverage in a dysplastic skeletally mature right hip treated with periacetabular osteotomy, surgical dislocation of the hip, and osteochondral allograft transplantation (**a**); intraoperative image depicting exposure after surgical dislocation of the hip and placement of an osteochondral allograft to treat a large focal area of osteochondral injury (**b**)

greater trochanter is marked using electrocautery, beginning at the posterosuperior aspect and proceeding distally, ending at the posterior aspect of the vastus lateralis. The planned thickness of the osteotomized fragment should be least 1 cm, and up to 1.5 cm. A step cut may be made as a component of the osteotomy to improve the stability of the reduced fragment at the conclusion of the procedure. If a relative neck lengthening/trochanteric advancement is planned as a component of the procedure, a straight osteotomy is performed to allow for distalization of the fragment prior to fixation. At the most proximal extent of the osteotomy, the exit point should be slightly anterior to the posterior extent of the gluteus medius tendon. The osteotomy is located anterior to the short external rotators, including the piriformis insertion, as this will protect the deep branch of the MFCA. Once the osteotomy is complete, residual fibers from the anterior extent of the piriformis tendon that remain attached to the fragment are released. Several residual fibers of the posterior gluteus medius tendon may remain attached to the femur, and these should be released. The vastus lateralis and vastus intermedius are elevated from the bone at their proximal aspects, distal to the osteotomy site. The plane between the piriformis tendon and the gluteus minimus is sometimes indistinct at first glance. This plane between the piriformis, which remains attached to the femur, and the gluteus minimus, which is attached to the osteotomized fragment, is carefully delineated.

An osteotome is helpful to complete the osteotomy at the anterior aspect of the greater trochanter and will assist in levering and elevation of the bony fragment. The osteotomized greater trochanteric fragment, with attached gluteus medius, gluteus minimus, and vastus lateralis tendons, is mobilized anteriorly, exposing the joint capsule. Flexing and externally rotating the hip will assist with anterior retraction of the fragment. A “Z” capsulotomy is performed to expose the hip articulation safely, avoiding injury to branches of the MFCA. The initial incision is performed along the femoral neck at the anterolateral aspect. The incision is extended from the distal extent anteroinferiorly, maintaining a position anterior to the lesser trochanter. At the proximal extent, the incision is extended posteriorly and parallel to the acetabular rim. The labrum must be identified and protected when this incision is performed. When completed, the incision should be in the configuration of a "Z" in a right hip and a reverse "Z" in a left hip.

The hip is dislocated anteriorly by flexing and externally rotating the hip. Depending on the location of pathology, the degree of ligamentous laxity, and the available exposure, treatment may proceed without releasing the ligamentum teres. In cases where the femoral head cannot be mobilized sufficiently, the ligamentum teres is incised, allowing for complete dislocation and full exposure of the entire hip articulation. After completing all indicated joint-preserving procedures, the capsule is closed, and the osteotomized greater tuberosity fragment is reduced and fixated using two or three small fragment cortical screws. In the case of an associated relative neck lengthening procedure, the fragment is distalized and fixated in this position after recontouring any bony prominence proximally at the trochanter while ensuring to avoid injury to branches of the MFCA. Final fluoroscopic imaging and wound closure are performed. Surgical dislocation of the hip to perform osteochondral allograft transplantation in association with periacetabular osteotomy to correct alignment is depicted in Fig. 1.3.

1.4 Cartilage Repair in the Setting of Alignment Correction

Articular cartilage allows for joint motion while minimizing friction and distributing joint forces. Chondral tissue must be preserved and repaired whenever possible in order to optimize longevity of the hip joint. Reduced femoral head coverage in the setting of hip dysplasia will lead to altered distribution of these forces across the articular cartilage, which may intensely focus these forces to such an extent that the chondral surface and underlying subchondral bone cannot withstand the stresses. This leads to osteochondral injury in such a pattern that will typically progress, potentially leading to generalized osteochondral injury and joint failure. Normalizing femoral head coverage in cases of hip dysplasia is of primary importance. Unfortunately, by the time alignment is normalized with surgical correction, significant chondral or osteochondral injury may be present. Depending on the pattern and severity of articular cartilage injury, concurrent treatment may be possible using several strategies of repair. Both arthroscopic and open surgical techniques may be employed in conjunction with periacetabular osteotomy to treat labral injury and also osteochondral pathology. Surgical dislocation of the hip is the preferable approach when the size or location of the chondral injury makes complete arthroscopic access suboptimal.

1.4.1 Marrow Stimulation in the Hip

Marrow stimulation techniques such as microfracture have been examined as a treatment option to treat full-thickness focal chondral lesions of the hip. Much clinical research has focused on lesions affecting the acetabular periphery in the setting of femoroacetabular impingement, as these are frequently encountered lesions. While there have been outcome studies demonstrating success in such cases [9], these treatments have typically been evaluated in the setting of associated procedures such osteochondroplasty to correct femoral head-neck asphericity, which makes the determination of specific benefit attributable to microfracture difficult. There are several drilling techniques using small diameter bits/wires that also may be used for marrow stimulation in the hip joint, which may reduce the degree of damage to the subchondral endplate that is associated with microfracture technique using awls. Procedures to treat full-thickness chondral defects in the hip using microfracture in conjunction with scaffolding have been used with success. Successful outcomes using autologous matrix-induced chondrogenesis in the hip was demonstrated by de Girolamo et al., with improvements maintained 8 years postoperatively, in contrast to deteriorating outcomes in a comparison group that underwent microfracture alone [10]. Tahoun et al. reported successful treatment of full-thickness lesions after a minimum 2-year follow-up using microfracture in association with a chitosan solution mixed with whole peripheral blood [11, 12]. In lesions of substantial size, it is preferable to preserve the subchondral endplate when possible in order to promote the restoration of durable articular cartilage. The osteochondral unit is a layered structure with physiologic and metabolic activity involving the interface between subchondral bone and the overlying cartilage, including the tidemark and calcified cartilage layer [13, 14]. Treatment options that best restore this interface between subchondral bone and the articular cartilage are thought to optimize longevity of the repaired cartilage. There are several additional treatments for full-thickness chondral defects in the hip that may be considered. Such techniques have been well studied in the treatment of knee chondral injury and include the use of cell-free scaffolds; autologous minced articular cartilage implanted in a single-stage, two-stage autologous chondrocyte implantation; application of biologic scaffolding embedded with mesenchymal stem cells/signaling cells; and osteochondral grafting.

1.4.2 Autologous Chondrocyte Implantation in the Hip

Cell-based repair of articular cartilage using autologous chondrocyte implantation has been used extensively in the knee, and more recent clinical research has demonstrated the usefulness of this repair technique within the hip joint. Fontana et al. demonstrated successful outcomes of autologous chondrocyte implantation, with improved outcomes being maintained 5 years postoperatively [15]. There has been extensive clinical data supporting the use of autologous chondrocyte implantation in the knee published over recent decades, and it is likely that this technique of cartilage repair can provide full-thickness repair of articular cartilage lesions within the hip consistently. There are, however, socioeconomic considerations and surgical morbidity that must be weighed in the case of autologous chondrocyte implantation, as this is a staged treatment that requires the patient to undergo two surgical procedures.

1.4.3 Mesenchymal Stem Cell/Signaling Cell Treatment of Hip Chondral Defects

Single-stage treatments of full-thickness chondral injury within the hip joint that are capable of restoring durable cartilage repair tissue and that preserve healthy underlying subchondral bone are ideal. Several types of mesenchymal stem cell/signaling cell isolates used with or without biologic scaffolding have been examined most extensively in the treatment of knee chondral injury. Some of these techniques may be modified for minimally invasive use within the hip joint. Mesenchymal stem cells (MSCs) are considered to be a type of signaling cells that exist in a quiescent form, in the vicinity of small blood vessels. These perivascular cells, known as pericytes, become activated in the event of injury and are responsible for modulating inflammatory, trophic, and paracrine activities [16]. These cells are readily isolated from several tissues. Clinically, such isolates that have been used to treat articular cartilage injury include autologous bone marrow aspirate concentrate (BMAC), autologous adipose tissue, and allogeneic cells sourced from umbilical tissue.

Treatment of full-thickness chondral injury using BMAC has been studied fairly extensively in the knee. Activated BMAC embedded onto biologic scaffolding has demonstrated good to excellent clinical outcomes for treatment of large full-thickness chondral injury in the knee using both type I/III collagen matrix and three-dimensional hyaluronic acid-based matrix [17, 18]. Hyaluronic acid-based scaffold embedded with BMAC (HA-BMAC) has demonstrated successful outcomes that are superior compared to microfracture and that are sustained over long-term follow-up [19, 20]. Biologic scaffolding embedded with BMAC can be used to treat full-thickness chondral defects of the acetabulum and femoral head, either through the open approach of surgical dislocation or arthroscopically [21].

Application of biologic scaffolding has been demonstrated to be securely fixated within full-thickness knee chondral defects using fibrin glue [22]. The implantation of these scaffolds within the hip joint at such locations as the anterosuperior acetabulum or femoral head has the additional benefit of continuous compressive loading which may reduce the potential for displacement. Additionally, as these techniques progress in the hip, treatment of lesions with significant injury to both articular cartilage and underlying subchondral bone may be treated with MSC therapies developed to restore the entire osteochondral unit [23, 24].

Lipoaspirate preparations have demonstrated the capability to stimulate outgrowth of cells capable of restoring injured articular cartilage, and this is thought to occur through the cell signaling properties of MSCs [25]. Microfragmented adipose tissue used in a single-stage procedure is available in an injectable form that may be used in conjunction with surgical treatment of hip chondral injury. Jannelli and Fontana reported on the use of autologous microfragmented adipose tissue to treat full-thickness chondral injury within the hip joint [26]. Regarding allograft sources of MSCs, Wharton's jelly preparations have been combined with scaffolding for use in minimally invasive surgery to repair full-thickness chondral defects [27], and this may be used to treat focal high-grade chondral injury of the acetabulum or femoral head.

1.4.4 Osteochondral Transfer and Transplantation in the Hip

Osteochondral injury within the hip joint can present the patient and clinician with a particularly difficult pathology to treat, given the unicompartmental nature of the hip articulation and limited surface area for redistribution of forces elsewhere across the chondral surface. There are a number of different traumatic and atraumatic etiologies associated with hip osteochondral injury. There may be associated femoroacetabular impingement or hip dysplasia contributing to osteochondral injury that requires concurrent treatment, or such injury may be seen in isolation. With regard to high-grade focal osteochondral pathologies that may be identified in isolation, osteonecrosis affecting the hip articulation is frequently encountered, which most commonly affects the femoral head. High-grade focal osteochondral injury of either the acetabulum or femoral head may be treated with osteochondral grafting, although this is a surgical treatment that is preferentially used to treat injuries located to the femoral head. For smaller lesions less than 2–3 cm^2 in size, osteochondral autograft transfer from a non-weight-bearing portion of the anterior femoral head/neck or ipsilateral knee is a treatment option, in addition to the option of osteochondral allograft transfer. In cases of larger lesions, osteochondral allograft transfer is preferentially used, as this avoids donor site morbidity and clinical outcomes have been shown to be generally successful [28].

1.5 Summary

Dysplasia of the adult hip is a major contributing factor for early onset osteoarthritis and rapid progression of degenerative joint changes, often leading to total joint arthroplasty. Correction of this malalignment can be performed surgically using a periacetabular osteotomy and, when accompanied by focal high-grade cartilage injury, may be treated concurrently with surgical dislocation of the hip and a cartilage repair procedure. There have been numerous recent advances in the treatment of high-grade cartilage injury that include cell-based treatments, biologic scaffolds, mesenchymal stem cells/signaling cells, and osteochondral grafting. These techniques may be used in association with complex osteotomy procedures to successfully treat those suffering from hip dysplasia in the setting of high-grade cartilage injury.

References

1. Murphy SB, Ganz R, Müller ME. The prognosis in untreated dysplasia of the hip. A study of radiographic factors that predict the outcome. J Bone Joint Surg Am. 1995;77(7):985–9.
2. Ganz R, Klaue K, Vinh TS, Mast JW. A new periacetabular osteotomy for the treatment of hip dysplasias. Technique and preliminary results. Clin Orthop Relat Res. 1988;232:26–36.
3. Thomas GER, Palmer AJR, Batra RN, Kiran A, Hart D, Spector T, et al. Subclinical deformities of the hip are significant predictors of radiographic osteoarthritis and joint replacement in women. A 20 year longitudinal cohort study. Osteoarthr Cartil. 2014;22(10):1504–10. http://linkinghub.elsevier.com/retrieve/pii/S1063458414011753.
4. Ganz R, Gill TJ, Gautier E, Ganz K, Krügel N, Berlemann U. Surgical dislocation of the adult hip. J Bone Joint Surg (Br). 2001;83-B(8):1119–24. http://online.boneandjoint.org.uk/doi/10.1302/0301-620X.83B8.0831119.
5. Wiberg G. Studies on dysplastic acetabula and congenital subluxation of the hip joint. Acta Chir Scand. 1939;83(Suppl 58):53–68.
6. Lequesne M, de Seze S. False profile of the pelvis. A new radiographic incidence for the study of the hip. Its use in dysplasias and different coxopathies. Rev Rhum Mal Osteoartic. 1961;28:643–52.
7. Tannast M, Fritsch S, Zheng G, Siebenrock KA, Steppacher SD. Which radiographic hip parameters do not have to be corrected for pelvic rotation and tilt? Clin Orthop Relat Res. 2015;473(4):1255–66. http://link.springer.com/10.1007/s11999-014-3936-8.
8. Monazzam S, Bomar JD, Agashe M, Hosalkar HS. Does femoral rotation influence anteroposterior alpha angle, lateral center-edge angle, and medial proximal femoral angle? A pilot study hip. Clin Orthop Relat Res. 2013;471(5):1639–45.
9. MacDonald AE, Bedi A, Horner NS, De Sa D, Simunovic N, Philippon MJ, et al. Indications and outcomes for microfracture as an adjunct to hip arthroscopy for treatment of chondral defects in patients with femoroacetabular impingement: a systematic review. Arthroscopy. 2016;32(1):190–200e2. https://doi.org/10.1016/j.arthro.2015.06.041.
10. de Girolamo L, Jannelli E, Fioruzzi A, Fontana A. Acetabular chondral lesions associated with femoroacetabular impingement treated by autologous matrix-induced chondrogenesis or microfracture: a comparative study at 8-year follow-up. Arthroscopy. 2018;34(11):3012–23. https://doi.org/10.1016/j.arthro.2018.05.035.
11. Tahoun MF, Tey M, Mas J, Abd-Elsattar Eid T, Monllau JC. Arthroscopic repair of acetabular cartilage lesions by chitosan-based scaffold: clinical evaluation at minimum 2 years follow-up. Arthroscopy. 2018;34(10):2821–8. https://linkinghub.elsevier.com/retrieve/pii/S0749806318305255.
12. Whyte GP, Gobbi A. Editorial commentary: acetabular cartilage repair: a critically important frontier in hip preservation. Arthroscopy. 2018;34(10):2829–31. https://doi.org/10.1016/j.arthro.2018.08.001.
13. Blasiak A, Whyte GP, Matlak A, Brzóska R, Sadlik B. Morphologic properties of cartilage lesions in the knee arthroscopically prepared by the standard curette technique are inferior to lesions prepared by specialized chondrectomy instruments. Am J Sports Med. 2018;46(4):908–14. http://www.ncbi.nlm.nih.gov/pubmed/29281796.
14. Sadlik B, Matlak A, Blasiak A, Klon W, Puszkarz M, Whyte GP. Arthroscopic cartilage lesion preparation in the human cadaveric knee using a curette technique demonstrates clinically relevant histologic variation. Arthroscopy. 2018;34(7):2179–88. http://linkinghub.elsevier.com/retrieve/pii/S0749806318301208.
15. Fontana A, Bistolfi A, Crova M, Rosso F, Massazza G. Arthroscopic treatment of hip chondral defects: autologous chondrocyte transplantation versus simple debridement-A pilot study. Arthroscopy. 2012;28(3):322–9.
16. Caplan AI. Mesenchymal stem cells in regenerative medicine. In: Principles of regenerative medicine. Amsterdam: Elsevier Inc.; 2019. p. 219–27. https://doi.org/10.1016/B978-0-12-809880-6.00015-1.
17. Gobbi A, Karnatzikos G, Sankineani SR. One-step surgery with multipotent stem cells for the treatment of large full-thickness chondral defects of the knee. Am J Sports Med. 2014;42(3):648–57. http://ajs.sagepub.com/lookup/doi/10.1177/0363546513518007.
18. Whyte GP, Gobbi A. Biologic knee arthroplasty for cartilage injury and early osteoarthritis. In: Bio-orthopaedics. Berlin: Springer; 2017. p. 517–25. http://link.springer.com/10.1007/978-3-662-54181-4_41.
19. Gobbi A, Whyte GP. One-stage cartilage repair using a hyaluronic acid-based scaffold with activated bone marrow-derived mesenchymal stem cells compared with microfracture: five-year follow-up. Am J Sports Med. 2016;44(11):2846–54. http://www.ncbi.nlm.nih.gov/pubmed/27474386.
20. Gobbi A, Whyte GP. Long-term clinical outcomes of one-stage cartilage repair in the knee with hyaluronic acid–based scaffold embedded with mesenchymal stem cells sourced from bone marrow aspirate concentrate. Am J Sports Med. 2019;47(7):1621–8.
21. Whyte GP, Gobbi A, Sadlik B. Dry arthroscopic single-stage cartilage repair of the knee using a hyaluronic acid-based scaffold with activated bone marrow-derived mesenchymal stem cells. Arthrosc Tech. 2016;5(4):e913–8. http://www.ncbi.nlm.nih.gov/pubmed/27709058.
22. Whyte GP, McGee A, Jazrawi L, Meislin R. Comparison of collagen graft fixation methods in the porcine knee: implications for matrix-assisted chondrocyte implantation and second-generation autologous chondrocyte implantation. Arthroscopy. 2016;32(5):820–7. http://linkinghub.elsevier.com/retrieve/pii/S0749806315008117.

23. Sadlik B, Kolodziej L, Puszkarz M, Laprus H, Mojzesz M, Whyte GP. Surgical repair of osteochondral lesions of the talus using biologic inlay osteochondral reconstruction: clinical outcomes after treatment using a medial malleolar osteotomy approach compared to an arthroscopically-assisted approach. Foot Ankle Surg. 2019;25(4):449–56. http://linkinghub.elsevier.com/retrieve/pii/S1268773118300365.
24. Sadlik B, Gobbi A, Puszkarz M, Klon W, Whyte GP. Biologic inlay osteochondral reconstruction: arthroscopic one-step osteochondral lesion repair in the knee using morselized bone grafting and hyaluronic acid-based scaffold embedded with bone marrow aspirate concentrate. Arthrosc Tech. 2017;6(2):e383–9. http://linkinghub.elsevier.com/retrieve/pii/S2212628716302055.
25. Gobbi A, de Girolamo L, Whyte GP, Sciarretta FV. Clinical applications of adipose tissue-derived stem cells. In: Bio-orthopaedics. Berlin: Springer; 2017. p. 553–9. http://link.springer.com/10.1007/978-3-662-54181-4_44.
26. Jannelli E, Fontana A. Arthroscopic treatment of chondral defects in the hip: AMIC, MACI, microfragmented adipose tissue transplantation (MATT) and other options. SICOT-J. 2017;3:43. http://www.sicot-j.org/10.1051/sicotj/2017029.
27. Sadlik B, Jaroslawski G, Puszkarz M, Blasiak A, Oldak T, Gladysz D, Whyte GP. Cartilage repair in the knee using umbilical cord Wharton's jelly–derived mesenchymal stem cells embedded onto collagen scaffolding and implanted under dry arthroscopy. Arthrosc Tech. 2018;7(1):e57–63. http://linkinghub.elsevier.com/retrieve/pii/S2212628717303237.
28. Meyers MH. Resurfacing of the femoral head with fresh osteochondral allografts long-term results. Clin Orthop Relat Res. 1985;197:111–4. http://journals.lww.com/00003086-198507000-00013.

Anatomy of the Hip Joint Preservation Point of View

2

Łukasz Lipiński

2.1 Introduction

The hip joint is a ball/socket articular connection between the femur and pelvis. It is one of the most exposed joints in our body, and surgical procedures of the hip joint are the most common procedures in orthopedics; thus, surgical anatomy is an important key to success. Morphology of the hip joint is complex and variable depending of anatomic variations.

We can divide anatomical considerations into:

- Bony anatomy
- Soft tissue anatomy

From a surgical point of view, one can palpate different anatomic orientation points and divide each exposure into layers.

There are several anatomic key points in hip surgery:

- Anterosuperior iliac spine
- Anteroinferior iliac spine
- Major trochanter
- Iliac crest
- Posterosuperior iliac spine

Ł. Lipiński (✉)
Orthopedics and Pediatric Orthopedics Clinic, Medical University of Lodz, Lodz, Poland

The acetabulum is created with the connection of three bones: ilium, ischium, and pubis. Spherical orientation of the acetabulum is defined: ±55° of inclination and ± of 20° of anteversion. It covers 70–75% of the femoral head. The femur is the distal part of hip joint created of the femoral head and neck junction covered with joint capsule. Two parameters describe proximal part of the femur: neck/shaft angle with mean value of 130° and anteversion of 15° [1, 2].

The main blood supply comes from internal and external iliac arteries. Deep understanding of vascular supply of the hip is crucial in a safe surgery of the hip.

2.2 Blood Supply

The main blood supply comes from the external iliac artery which is a trunk of common iliac artery. Hip joint procedures are dangerous mainly to the femoral artery which passes directly in front of the hip joint.

Four main branches give blood supply to the hip:

- Medial and lateral circumflex arteries which are the branches of deep femoral artery (Fig. 2.1)
- Superior and inferior gluteal arteries which are both branches of the internal iliac artery

M. Brittberg, K. Slynarski (eds.), *Lower Extremity Joint Preservation*,
https://doi.org/10.1007/978-3-030-57382-9_2

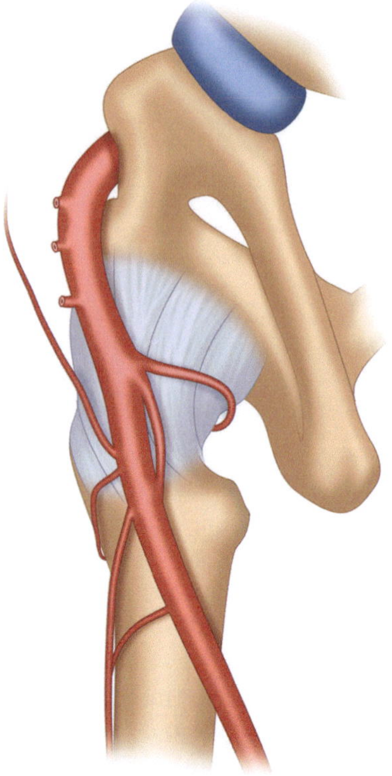

Fig. 2.1 Deep femoral arterty

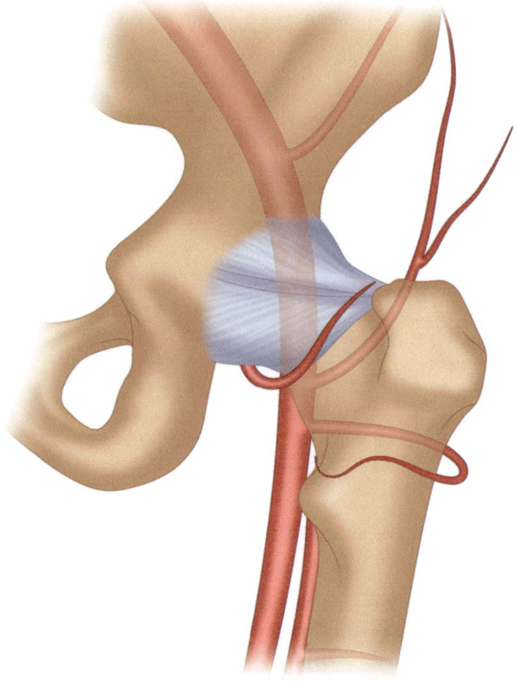

Fig. 2.2 Medial circumflex artery

The common femoral artery is the continuation of the external iliac artery at the level of inguinal ligament. It runs at anteromedial aspect of joint capsule. It is in danger during open and arthroscopic procedures; thus, it is always important to palpate it and respect the anatomy.

The deep femoral artery is the first branch of common femoral artery. It runs deep to the adductor longus muscle and gives perforating arteries to posterior aspect of the femur. The lateral circumflex artery is rather a common branch of the deep femoral artery. The medial circumflex artery is a branch of the deep femoral artery in one-third of cases. Both lateral and medial circumflex arteries supply proximal and distal joint capsule (Fig. 2.2). The superior gluteal artery is a branch of the internal femoral artery; it exits greater sciatic foramen inferior to the gluteus medius and superior to the piriformis muscle. The inferior gluteal artery exits lower part of great sciatic foramen. Both superior and inferior gluteal arteries supply mainly the posterior capsule of the hip. Additional blood supply arises from the obturator artery which branches to the artery of ligamentum teres. It is mostly not important in adults, but we need to remember that one-fifth of patients have the vessel unobstructed during adulthood [3].

In summary, the main blood supply to the hip joint come from medial and lateral femoral arteries entering the hip via synovial folds. Both synovial plicas can be injured after hip-neck fracture and imperfect surgical technique resulting in avascular necrosis of the head.

2.3 Nerves

There are two main nerve crossings to be aware of in relation to the hip joint anatomy: sciatic nerve and femoral nerve. Sciatic nerve arises from L4 to S3 level. Distally it consists of common peroneal and tibial nerves. It gives motor innervation to several muscles:

- Biceps femoris
- Semimembranosus
- Semitendinosus
- Adductor magnus (ischial part)

It enters the hip area through great sciatic foramen under the piriformis muscle. It runs under great gluteal muscle entering medial side of the hip and lower portion of quadratus femoral muscle. The anatomical variants need to be known as the nerve can run also through external rotators of the femur.

The femoral nerve arises from L2 to L4 level. It runs on the iliopsoas muscle and enters the hip region under inguinal ligament and gives motor innervation to muscles:

- Iliac
- Psoas major
- Pectineus
- Quadriceps

It also gives skin sensation innervation to anterior and medial side of the thigh. Sensation innervation around the hip comes also from several nerves: pudendal, genitofemoral, and lateral cutaneous of the thigh (Fig. 2.3). Superior gluteal nerve runs through great sciatic foramen and innervates both abductors of the hip (gluteal medius and minimus muscles) and tensor fasciae latae.

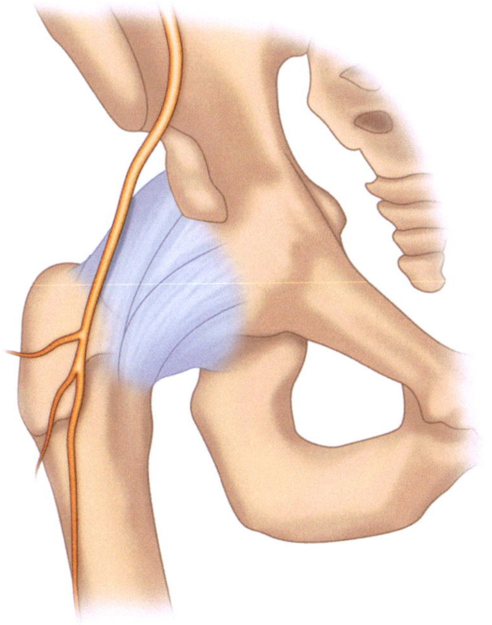

Fig. 2.3 Lateral cutaneous femoral nerve

2.4 Hip Muscles

We can divide hip muscles in different functional groups: flexors, extensors, abductors, adductors, and external and internal rotators.

2.5 Hip Flexors

Main hip flexor muscles are:

- Rectus femoris
- Iliopsoas
- Psoas major
- Psoas minor
- Sartorius

The rectus femoris is muscle located in anterior part of the thigh. It consists of two proximal insertions: upright head and flexed head. The first part originates from anterior inferior iliac spine and the other from acetabular ridge. The muscle belly consists of four separate parts: the rectus femoris, vastus lateralis, vastus medialis, and vastus intermedius with the rectus femoris being the most superficial one. The conjoined distal insertion is located at the proximal part of the patella. The rectus femoris is a hip flexor. Innervation comes from L2 to L4 level.

The Iliopsoas muscle consists of two psoas (major and minor) and iliac muscles. This is the main flexor of the thigh. It acts mostly as a common motor unit. Psoas major originates proximally from transverse processes and lateral surface of the bodies of L1–L4 but can also involve last thoracic vertebra. It reaches iliac fossa and goes deep to inguinal ligament with distal insertion at minor trochanter [4]. Psoas minor originates from last thoracic and first lumbar vertebra bodies. It is not a constant muscle. Distal origin is the same for both psoas muscles. The iliacus muscle originates proximally from two to three of the iliac fossa and from lateral part of the sacrum. It goes under inguinal ligament with distal insertion at minor trochanter. The innervation comes from lumbar plexus L1–L3 (psoas major and minor) and lumbar plexus/femoral nerve L1–L4 (iliacus muscle). Sartorius muscle is the longest muscle in our body crossing both the hip and the knee joints. The proximal insertions come from anterior superior iliac spine and in the muscle tendon crosses the thigh distally and medially. The distal insertion is at superficial pes anserine position. It flexes both the hip and the knee joint and is innervated by the femoral nerve. Other hip muscles can also act as hip flexors, but it is mostly dependent to the degree of starting position of the hip.

2.6 Hip Extensors

Main hip extensors are muscles:

- Gluteus maximus
- Semitendinosus
- Semimembranosus
- Biceps femoris

Gluteus maximus muscle originates proximally from inner part of the ilium, iliac crest, to lower part of the sacrum and coccyx. This is the main muscle responsible for keeping straight position of the body. It also enhances abduction and external rotation. Distal insertions are found at the great trochanter between adductor magnus and vastus lateralis. Innervation comes from L2 to L5 within the inferior gluteal nerve. Hamstring muscles give additional force to extend the hip. Common proximal insertions are at the ischial tuberosity with distal insertion at the pes anserine site. Their common strength of extension is around one-fourth of total extension strength. Innervation comes from sciatic nerve.

2.7 Hip Abductors

There are two main hip abductors:

- Gluteus medius
- Gluteus minimus muscles

The first arises proximally from external iliac surface and crosses the joint capsule laterally with distal insertion at lateral or supero-posterior part of great trochanter. Innervation comes from the superior gluteal nerve. The gluteal minimums muscle runs under the gluteus medius muscle. Distal insertion is more anterior at the great trochanter. Innervation comes from superior gluteal nerve. Additionally tensor fasciae latae and iliotibial band can assist abduction movement, but their role is not crucial [4, 5].

2.8 Hip Adductors

Hip adductors consist of the following muscles:

- Adductor brevis
- Adductor longus
- Adductor magnus (partially)
- Pectineus
- Gracilis

The proximal insertion is located at the inferior part of pubic ramus and ischial tubercle. The common distal insertion is found at medial ridged of the linea aspera and pes anserine (gracilis muscle). All adductor muscles are innervated by the obturator nerve apart from the pectineus muscle (femoral nerve).

2.9 External Rotators

This group consists of muscles:

- Obturator internus
- Obturator externus

- Gemellus superior
- Gemellus inferior
- Quadratus femoris
- Piriformis

The proximal insertion is located at the sacrum and ischial bone. The distal insertion is mainly at great trochanter, intertrochanteric crest, and trochanteric fossa. Innervation comes from L3 to S2 level.

2.10 Internal Rotators

There are *no direct internal rotator muscle groups*. Muscle actions of the tensor fasciae latae, gluteus medius, and gluteus minimus are responsible for this movement.

2.11 Remarks

Surgical treatment of hip pathology within the concept of joint preservation is a difficult decision, and proper anatomy knowledge is crucial. Standard anatomy parameters of X-ray, computed tomography, and magnetic resonance should be evaluated, and their anatomic variances should be well known.

All figures are prepared by the author using commercially available *Atlas of Human Anatomy*.

References

1. Sekiya J, Safran M, Ranawat A, Leunig M. Techniques of hip arthroscopy and joint preservation surgery. Amsterdam: Elsevier; 2011. ISBN 978-1-4160-5642-3.
2. Sylwanowicz W. Bochenek-Reicher--anatomia człowieka [Bochenek-Reicher--the anatomy of man]. Folia Morphol (Warsz). 1972;31(4):585–90.
3. Boraiah S, Dyke JP, Hettrich C, et al. Assessment of vascularity of the femoral head using gadolinium (Gd-DTPA)-enhanced magnetic resonance imaging: a cadaver study. J Bone Joint Surg (Br). 2009;91(1):131–7.
4. Anderson CN. Iliopsoas: pathology, diagnosis, and treatment. Clin Sports Med. 2016;35(3):419–33.
5. Flack NA, Nicholson HD, Woodley SJ. A review of the anatomy of the hip abductor muscles, gluteus medius, gluteus minimus, and tensor fascia lata. Clin Anat. 2012;25(6):697–708.

3 Anatomy, Surgical Management, and Postoperative Outcomes of Acetabular Labral Tears

Lukasz Luboinski, Maciej Pasieczny, Patryk Ulicki, and Tomasz Albrewczyński

3.1 Introduction

The labrum (the cotyloid ligament) is a key anatomical structure in the hip joint. Previous research has suggested that it is crucial to maintaining fluid pressurization and the hip seal, stabilizing the joint to distraction forces, and controlling contact pressure [1]. The hip labrum has been recognized as a common cause of hip pain and dysfunction; it is estimated that the prevalence of labral pathology among clinical populations ranges from 22% to 55% [1].

Because the labrum is commonly involved in patients with FAI, there has been increased interest in the function of the acetabular labrum and its clinical relevance. Over the past 20 years, evidence has emerged suggesting the clinical and mechanical importance of the acetabular labrum. The labrum contributes to overall joint function by limiting the rate of cartilage layer consolidation, thus reducing the solid-on-solid contact stresses between opposing cartilage surfaces [2].

L. Luboinski (✉) · M. Pasieczny · P. Ulicki
T. Albrewczyński
Department of the Orthopedic Surgery and Sports Medicine, Carolina Medical Center, Warsaw, Poland
e-mail: lukasz.luboinski@carolina.pl; maciej.pasieczny@carolina.pl; Patryk.ulicki@carolina.pl; Tomasz.albrewczynski@carolina.pl

3.2 The Anatomy of the Labrum

The acetabular labrum is a triangular fibrocartilaginous structure that forms a horseshoe-shaped attachment to the acetabular rim, which connects the acetabulum to the underlying transverse acetabular ligament. It is approximately 4.7 mm wide at the bony attachment and approximately 5.5 mm tall [3]. The labrum is separated from the capsule by the capsular recess. It merges on the capsular side with the bony acetabulum and on the articular side with the acetabular hyaline cartilage.

Histologically, the fibrocartilaginous labrum is contiguous with the acetabular articular cartilage through a 1–2 mm transition zone. A consistent projection of the bone extends from the bony acetabulum into the substance of the labrum that is attached via a zone of calcified cartilage with a well-defined tidemark [3].

The transverse acetabular ligament is fixed firmly to the two pillars of the acetabular notch. Hip stability results from these two continuous structures encompassing more than half of the femoral head, i.e. extending superiorly or the laterally to the "equator" of the femoral head.

The labrum is primarily composed of two tissue phenotypes: fibrocartilage and dense connective tissue. In the external circumference, there is dense connective tissue. In the inner region, directed towards the articular surface, there is a thin layer of fibrocartilage. The histological results

M. Brittberg, K. Slynarski (eds.), *Lower Extremity Joint Preservation*,
https://doi.org/10.1007/978-3-030-57382-9_3

are consistent with the immunohistochemical analysis of collagen. The dense connective tissue contains type I and III collagen. In the fibrocartilaginous zone, immunostaining for the cartilage-specific type II collagen is also positive [4].

The attachment of the collagen fibres of the labrum to the acetabulum is different anteriorly and posteriorly. The collagen fibres of the labrum in the anterior part of the joint attach to the acetabulum parallel to the edge of the bone. As a result, this attachment can be easily separated by shear forces. By contrast, the posterior attachment is resistant to shear forces as the fibres attach perpendicularly to the edge and merge with the collagen fibres of the bony edge.

In tension, the labrum is much stiffer (by 10–15 times) than the adjoining articular cartilage, and the posterior region of the labrum is significantly stiffer (45%) than the superior region (in a bovine model) [5]. Moreover, 43–60% less force is required to distract the femur by a standardized distance after venting or tearing of the labrum. From the biomechanical data available, it would seem reasonable to conclude that an intact labrum provides a biomechanical advantage to the hip [6].

3.2.1 Innervation

Human acetabular labrum has abundant FNEs and NEOs (Vater-Pacini (pressure), Golgi-Mazzoni (pressure), Ruffini (deep sensation, temperature), and articular (Krause) corpuscles (pressure, pain)). These are more abundant in the antero-superior and postero-superior zones. The labrum, owing to its neural innervation, can potentially mediate pain arising in the hip joint, mediate proprioception of the hip joint, and be involved in neurosecretion that can influence connective tissue repair [7].

3.2.2 The Vascular Supply

Labral blood supply is closely interconnected to that of the hip as a whole as the vascular network surrounding the hip supplies the labrum circumferentially. The structures of the hip labrum are supplied primarily by the superior and inferior gluteal arteries and further supported by connection to the primary circulation to the femoral head, namely, the medial and lateral circumflex arteries and their cervical and epiphyseal branches (from the femoral artery) [8].

The internal circulation of the labrum is divided into the two parts: half closest to the articular surface, Zone II, and the half on the capsular side, Zone I. The part of the capsular side of the labrum closest to the bony acetabular rim, Zone IB, is supplied by the circulation from that bone, which is the main source of labral circulation. The periphery of the capsular side of the labrum, Zone IA, is supplied by the capsular circulation. The same capsular circulation also supplies the periphery of the articular side of the labrum, Zone IIA. The articular part of the labrum, located closest to and merging with the hyaline articular cartilage, Zone IIB, is relatively avascular [9].

3.3 The Aetiology of Hip Labrum Disorders

The labrum can be damaged as a result of a number of pathologies, such as femoroacetabular impingement (FAI), dysplasia, or capsular laxity. Trauma, both acute and chronic, is believed to be the leading cause of labral injury. Another cause is the degeneration and repetitive extreme ranges of motion, as experienced by elite athletes commonly using rotational manoeuvres, in sports like golf, football, and hockey, as well as in ballet, where the hip is repeatedly placed in a position of end movement of rotation [10–13].

In studies of patients with a labral tear, researchers have attributed the injury to a variety of causes. A classification system based on the causes of labral tears was created by Kelly et al. in 2005 and includes the following: (1) trauma, (2) femoroacetabular impingement, (3) capsular laxity and/or hip hypermobility, (4) dysplasia, and (5) degeneration [14].

FAI is known to be the main cause of non-traumatic labral damage and, along with hip instability, a primary precursor to osteoarthritis. There are two subtypes of FAI: cam and pincer. The cam subtype is the deformity of the femoral head-neck junction resulting in the loss of head sphericity, while pincer is a focal or global overcoverage of the acetabulum. The patients can present with elements of both subtypes, resulting in a combined FAI. It is worth noting that the pincer type alone is much less common, with a female predominance [15]. It has been suggested that the migration of the femoral head occurs in the anterolateral chondral region in cam and posterolaterally in pincer impingement. In effect, there is a significant increase in compression forces, especially in cam impingement. The migration may lead to or be a sign of microinstability of the hip joint, which could, in turn, result in a further increase in shear forces [16]. Figure 3.1 shows schematic illustration of a normal hip (a), cam deformity (b), pincer deformity (c), and pathogenesis of mechanical injury of the labrum (d).

A tight iliopsoas tendon is another cause of labral lesions, which may cause impingement on the labrum at a different location than femoroacetabular-induced labral tears. These tears are more common in the anterior region and can be released transecting the iliopsoas tendon using a transcapsular approach [17].

Labral tears occur most frequently in the anterior-superior region of the acetabular labrum [12, 18, 19], with a weak male predominance.

In a study of healthy volunteers with no history of pain, injury, or surgery, labral tears were identified in 69% of hips, chondral defects in 24%, ligamentum teres tears in 2.2%, labral/paralabral cysts in 13%, acetabular bone oedema in 11%, fibrocystic changes of the head-neck junction in 22%, rim fractures in 11%, subchondral cysts in 16%, and osseous bumps in 20%. Participants older than 35 were more likely to have a chondral defect and a subchondral cyst compared with participants at the age of 35 or younger. No other joint lesions were associated with age. Males were 8.5 times more likely to have an osseous bump than females. The alpha angle values were found to be higher in participants with labral tears and also significantly higher in cases of chondral defects, fibrocystic changes of the head-neck junction, osseous bumps, and subchondral cysts [20].

3.3.1 Types of Labral Lesions

There were two main types of labral lesions, lesions at the chondo-labral junction and the intrasubstance tearing of the labrum, leading to a region of separation of the labrum from the articular surface [21, 22]. In the cam subtype, there is a separation between the labrum and the articular hyaline cartilage, often associated with articular cartilage delamination. With pincer subtype, tears occur within the substance of the labrum itself [3]. Labral lesions were observed most commonly in the antero-superior and anterior regions of the acetabulum. Anterior tears are also present in patients after minor trauma [23].

Labral tears can be classified according to their aetiology as degenerative, dysplastic, traumatic, or idiopathic with radial flaps (56.6%), longitudinal peripheral tears (26%), radial fibrillated tears (21.6%), and unstable tears, as described by Lage et al. (5.4%) [24, 25]. Another algorithm was developed by Philippon, whereby labral tears are classified as detached, degenerated, bruised, or torn in small and large labrums, with special emphasis on the importance of preserving the labrum if possible [20].

The Annual Meeting of the American Academy of Orthopaedic Surgeons, San Francisco, 1997, suggested a staged classification of labral injury, consisting of the following stages:

- Stage 0, a contusion of the labrum with adjacent synovitis
- Stage 1, a discreet labral free margin tear with intact articular cartilage
- Stage 2, a labral tear with focal articular damage to the subjacent femoral head but with intact acetabular articular cartilage
- Stage 3, a labral tear with an adjacent focal acetabular articular cartilage lesion with or without femoral head articular cartilage chondromalacia with 3A lesions less than 1 cm of

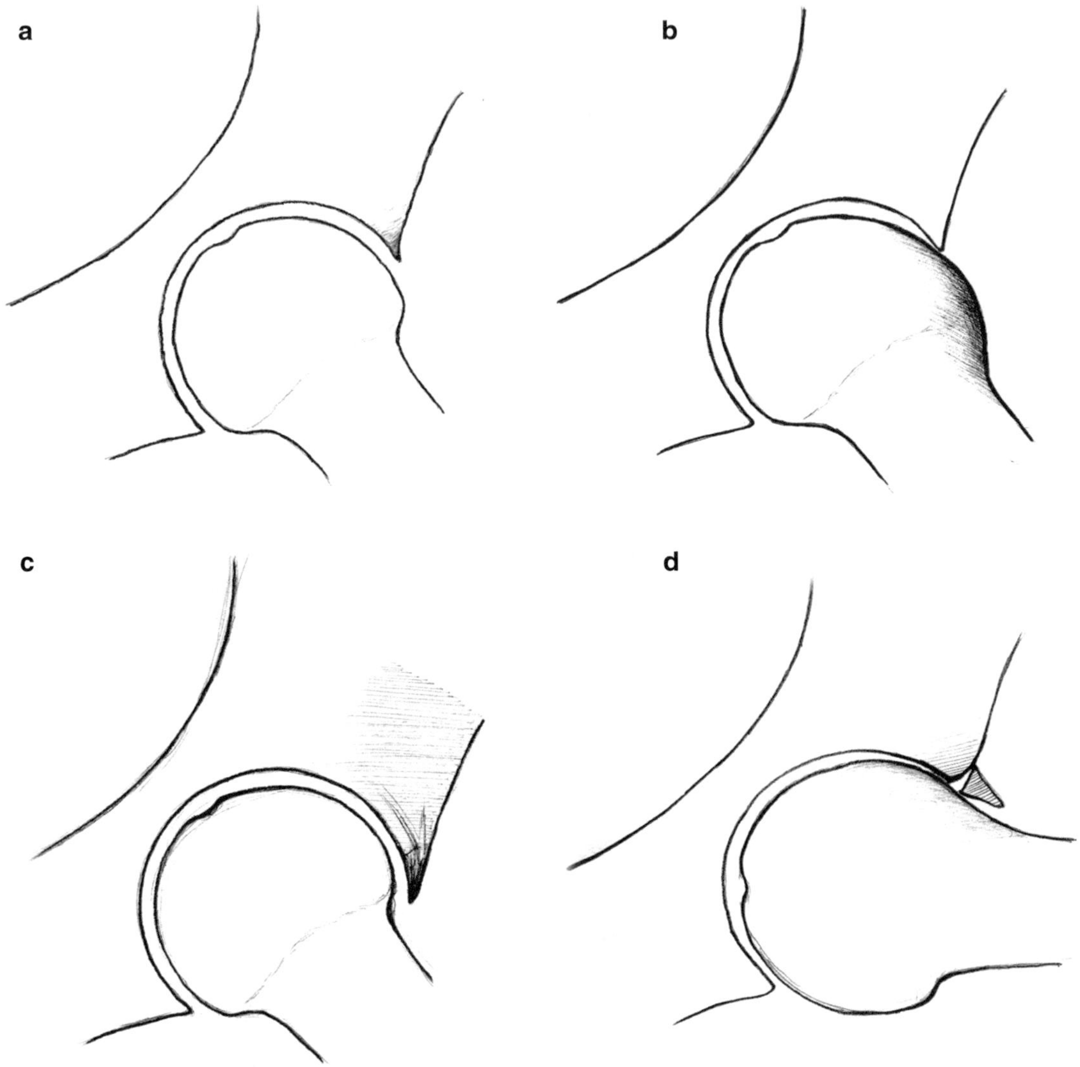

Fig. 3.1 Schematic illustration. (**a**) Normal hip join. (**b**) Cam deformity. (**c**) Pincer deformity. (**d**) Mechanical injury of the labrum

acetabular articular cartilage and 3B greater than 1 cm of acetabular cartilage

- Stage 4, an extensive acetabular labral tear with associated diffuse arthritic articular cartilage changes in the joint

In 95% of cases (59 of 62 hips), labral injury concerned the anterior half of the joint.

Overall, higher-stage tears are associated with more pronounced degenerative changes in the acetabulum and femoral head [20].

Czerny et al. described a classification for the MRA grade consisting of the following, a labrum with no surface tears (I), a labrum with surface tears (II), and a labrum articular cartilage separation (III), distinguishing between an abnormal labrum without intrasubstance cyst-like signals IIIA and with cysts IIIB [26].

However, in the study of Blankenbaker et al., as no correlation was found between Czerny et al.'s classification and Lage et al.'s arthroscopic classification, the authors proposed to describe the morphology of labral tears rather than using a specific classification scheme:

- An irregular labrum, i.e. irregular margins without a tear.
- A flap-type labral tear, may be partial or complete.
- A longitudinal peripheral labral tear, located at the base of the labrum, may be partial or complete.
- A thickened and distorted labrum, in keeping with the instability of the labral lesion.
- A clock-face description to localize tears provides a way to accurately describe a labral tear and define its extent. More than 40% of labral tears extend beyond a quadrant: on a sagittal slice, 12 o'clock is above, 3 o'clock in front, 6 o'clock below, and 9 o'clock behind [25, 27].

3.4 The Role of the Acetabular Labrum in Hip Disorders

3.4.1 The Function of the Labrum

The labrum acts as a secondary stabilizer for external rotation and anterior translation, with the iliofemoral ligament as a primary stabilizing force. What is more important, the labrum seals the hip joint, creating a hydrostatic fluid pressure in the intra-articular space, preventing synovial fluid from leaving the central compartment. This ensures uniform pressurization of the cartilage interstitial fluid and fluid film lubrication and limits the rate of cartilage layer consolidation.

Labral tears lead to a disruption of the labral seal and a reduction in fluid pressurization in the hip joint [28]. Without this fluid film lubrication, loading of the hip would lead to a direct cartilage-to-cartilage contact, increasing the friction of the cartilage surfaces and causing an uneven distribution of the load, thus causing premature articular cartilage degeneration [29].

Biomechanical studies have shown that the removal of the labrum increases the contact stress between the femoral and acetabular cartilage layers up to 92%, which, in turn, increases friction between the joint surfaces [2]. Shear stresses due to cartilage deformation were up to 38% higher throughout the cartilage layers following labrum removal [2]. Moreover, after labrum resection, 43–60% less force is required to distract the femur [6].

In biomechanical studies, the creep consolidation rate of the hip joint cartilage layers was calculated as the rate at which the femur and acetabulum approached each other. This was up to 40% faster in the joint without a labrum, as the labrum adds extra resistance to the flow path for interstitial fluid expression. After 10,000 s the cartilage layers had compressed 35% more in the model without a labrum, and the femur displaced further laterally relative to the model with an intact labrum [2, 29].

From the biomechanical data available, it would seem reasonable to conclude that an intact labrum provides a biomechanical advantage to the hip [6].

3.4.2 Changes in Load Distribution

During activities of daily living, the labrum functions to stabilize the joint, rather than to decrease cartilage contact stresses [30]. The labrum in the normal model supported 1–2% of the applied load, while the labrum in the dysplastic model supported 4–11% of the load, i.e. the labrum in dysplastic hips supported 2.8–4.0 times more of the weight transferred across the joint than in normal hips. The dysplastic hip has been described qualitatively as less congruent than the normal hip based on two-dimensional radiographs. Normal hips had larger cartilage contact stress than dysplastic hips in the few regions that had significant differences [31]. There was qualitatively more lateral loading in dysplastic hips in comparison to normal hips. Contact area on the superior labrum is significantly larger in dysplastic hips than in normal hips. Peak contact stress on the superior labrum is also significantly larger in the dysplastic hips than in the normal hips. There are no significant differences in contact area on the anterior or posterior labrum [31].

3.4.3 The Radiographic Characteristics of Labral Tears

The continuous effect of altered load transfer and shear stress could lead to hypertrophy of the acetabular labrum and secondary damage to the acetabular cartilage connected to the labrum [32, 33]. Most labral tears were found between 1 and 4 o'clock, representing the antero-superior quadrant. Ossifications were observed more often in the hypoplastic labra, while signal alterations and lesions were found to be equally distributed [34].

3.4.4 Labral Tears and OA

Clinical studies show that alterations in labral morphology, such as tears, can contribute to changes in the joint which are consistent with early osteoarthritis [35]. FAI has been recognized as a cause of osteoarthritis; in fact labral tear and subsequent cartilage damage is thought to be the main factor in the pathophysiology of the development of osteoarthritis [36] as the development of osteoarthritis is believed to arise from the repetitive injury to the acetabular rim, involving labrum and cartilage, either at the site of the impingement in cam type or by a subluxing femoral head more posteriorly in pincer type [37, 38]. Since an intact labrum provides a biomechanical advantage to the hip, repair, reattachment, or reconstruction of the labrum may improve the biomechanics of the hip, thereby slowing the progression of arthritis.

3.4.5 Labral Tears and Hip Dysplasia

Dysplasia of the hip is diagnosed radiographically when an anterior and/or lateral centre-edge angle (CEA) is less than 20–25° and an acetabular index is greater than 10°, indicating a shallow acetabulum and an upwardly sloping sourcil, respectively [39].

An estimated 20% of all hip osteoarthritis is secondary to mild to moderate acetabular dysplasia [3], which causes a 4.3-fold increased risk for radiographic hip osteoarthritis [40].

Altered cartilage mechanics is thought to be the link between acetabular dysplasia and hip osteoarthritis; however clinical observation of labral hypertrophy and labral tears in the dysplastic hip suggests that the labrum also experiences altered mechanics [39, 41]. It is suggested that the acetabular labrum undergoes compensatory changes in size in response to variable degrees of acetabular coverage and hip stability [42].

Up to 90% of symptomatic patients with developmental dysplasia of the hip (DDH) have lesions of acetabular labrum, hypertrophy, laceration, and/or cyst formation [43].

The most common finding in acetabular dysplasia is hypertrophy of the anterior labrum with associated infringement on the anterior acetabulum. The hypertrophy and tearing cause impingement of the labrum between the acetabulum and femoral head, accounting for the mechanical symptoms frequently present in this population [23, 34].

3.5 Patient Evaluation

3.5.1 Clinical Examination

Pain is the primary symptom of FAI syndrome, with a wide variation in the location, nature, radiation, severity, and precipitating factors that characterize this pain. Most patients report pain in the groin or hip, but pain may also be felt in the lateral hip, anterior thigh, buttock, knee, lower back, or lateral and posterior thigh. Pain can be both motion-related or position-related [44, 45].

The FADIR (flexion, adduction, internal rotation) test is the most commonly used hip impingement test in the diagnosis of FAI syndrome. The FADIR test has high sensitivity but low specificity. Other typical findings include movement patterns around the hip and pelvis that can result in pain or dysfunction in other regions, such as the spine, pelvis, posterior hip, or abdominal wall. Another common symptom of FAI syndrome is muscle weakness around the hip [45].

The complete FAI examination should be performed, including gait, single-leg control, muscle tenderness around the hip, and hip ROM including internal rotation in flexion as well as external rotation in flexion and abduction—the so-called FABER distance.

Positive impingement testing should reproduce the patient's familiar pain. As the differential diagnosis should include disorders of neighbouring structures, it is essential to examine the groin for other structures that can produce similar pain [45].

3.5.2 Diagnostic Imaging

Standard AP and axial X-ray of the pelvis is the first-line diagnostic imaging test for FAI syndrome. It is generally accepted that alpha angles of 50° or less in the specific plane in which they are measured are considered normal for both genders. (The alpha angle is measured by placing a circle around the femoral head. A line is drawn along the centre of the femoral neck to the centre of the head. The angle is created by drawing a second line from where the first line meets the centre of the femoral head to the point where the bony edge of the femoral head-neck junction meets the anterior margin of the circle. The more the hypertrophic neck changes or the greater the head-neck offset, the smaller the angle.) [46] An increased α angle correlating with articular cartilage injury, labral pathology, and reduced movement is indicative of cam-type FAI [47]. A lateral centre-edge angle over 39° is suggestive of pincer deformity. Other abnormal findings include positive crossover sign, positive posterior wall sign, and positive ischial spine sign [48]. However, with a high prevalence of radiographic findings of FAI in asymptomatic individuals, it is important to correlate the imaging with clinical examination [49, 50]. Figure 3.2 shows different morphology of pincer deformity AP view (a), cam deformity AP view (b), cam deformity axial view (c), and cam deformity after resection axial view (d).

Further imaging assessment includes MRI and MRA. In a study conducted by Czerny et al., 1.5 T MRI was shown to be 30% sensitive and 36% accurate, while MR had a sensitivity of 90% and an accuracy of 91% [26]. Three tesla MRI seems to be equivalent to 1.5 MRA for diagnosis of labral tears and cartilage delimitation and is superior for assessing acetabular cartilage [26].

3.6 Surgical Treatment

3.6.1 Indications for Surgery

The indications for surgical treatment include the presence of symptoms for more than 6 months, radiographic confirmation of FAI abnormalities, and failure of conservative treatment. The main contraindication is arthritis in the form of cartilage damage as well as joint space measurement of less than 2 mm.

Surgical treatment options include labral debridement and refixation, with studies showing better outcomes for repair than for debridement [51].

Labral refixation is achieved with sutures anchored into the acetabular rim [7]. Hip labrum reconstruction is a new technique that showed short-term improvement in patient-reported outcomes and functional scores postoperatively [4]. Among labral reconstruction, several techniques emerge; the iliotibial band, ligamentum teres, and ligamentum gracilis have been successfully utilized as graft sources. Labral reconstruction is a treatment indicated for young, active patients who have undergone previous unsuccessful hip surgery and/or possess an irreparable, degenerative, hypotrophic, or otherwise "non-salvageable" labrum [52]. The patients with signs of instability, in which a labral debridement would worsen the symptoms, may also benefit from the surgery [53]. While long-term results are not yet available, preservation or reconstruction of the labrum is nowadays recommended by most authors in order to preserve the function of the hip joint.

The decision to reconstruct a labrum is made on the basis of MRA/MRI examination, but can be finally confirmed after the arthroscopic examination. Reconstruction should be performed if on arthroscopic examination the labrum is hypotrophic (less than 5 mm of width), with insufficient functional material to perform a repair, or if it has an irreparable/complex tear and/or is unable to

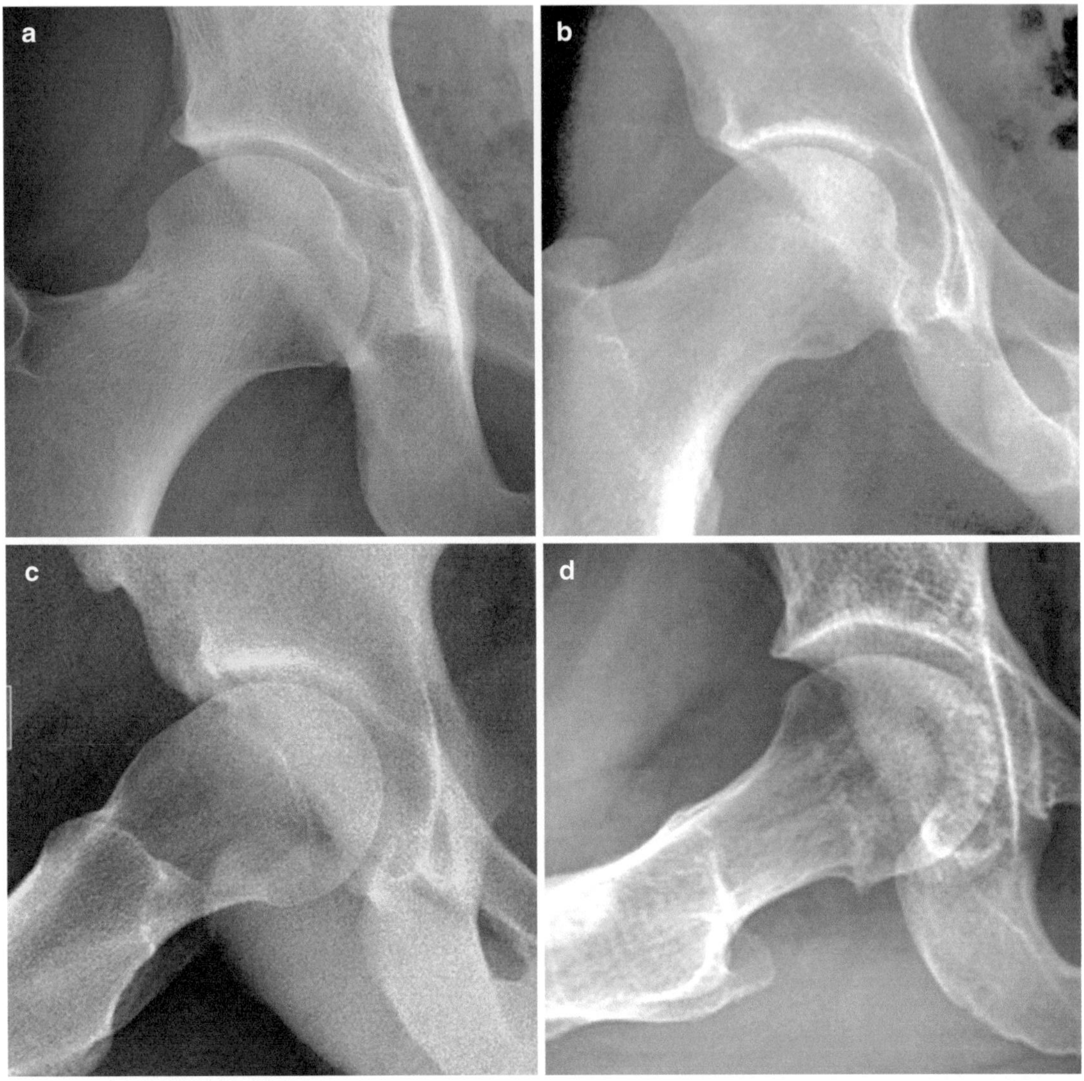

Fig. 3.2 X-ray examination. (**a**) Pincer deformity AP view. (**b**) Cam deformity AP view. (**c**) Cam deformity axial view. (**d**) Cam deformity after resection axial view

form a seal with the femoral head during a dynamic examination [54].

Bone abnormalities present in FAI must be addressed to protect the labrum and cartilage from new injuries. In pincer impingement, it might be necessary to detach the labrum from the acetabular rim. The detached labrum is then treated as a regular labral tear and can be reattached to the trimmed rim using suture anchors. The pincer lesion can also be resected without labral detachment which makes refixation much easier and does not harm chondrolabral junction. cam lesion is addressed in an intra-articular fashion in the lateral compartment at the beginning or end of arthroscopic surgery. In a study conducted by Philippon et al., persistent impingement was shown to be the most common reason for revision hip arthroscopy [55].

3.6.2 Surgical Technique for Labral Reconstruction

Treatment options for labral tears include debridement, repair, and reconstruction. Arthroscopy is performed in a standard fashion using a two- or three-portal approach in a lateral or supine position with the use of traction. The joint is inspected for loose bodies, cartilage wear, synovitis, and labral tears. Any extensive synovitis is debrided and ablated with a shaver and electrocautery. The labrum is assessed with a probe, and tear size is estimated. The ligamentum teres is inspected with a probe, and partial tears are debrided with a curved electrocautery blade [56]. The acetabular rim is trimmed either to correct pincer impingement or to improve the healing response [57]. If a tear is associated with a focal full-thickness chondral defect, the subchondral bone may be drilled or treated with a microfracture technique to enhance fibrocartilage formation [15, 58, 59].

If the remaining labrum is too thin (<3 mm) or extensively damaged, treatment options include resection or reconstruction with grafts. The labrum should be carefully debrided to stabile, healthy tissue. In case of repair, the size and location of the labral tear are further evaluated to plan suture anchor placement. Anchors should be placed 6–8 mm apart, with an average-sized tear requiring 3–4 anchors, drilled 2–3 mm below cartilage surface [60, 61]. Figure 3.3 shows arthroscopic view of injured labrum (a), sutured labrum (b); cam deformity (c); cam deformity after resection (d); pincer deformity, labral bruise (e); and pincer deformity after resection (f).

Simple loop suture should not be used for tear repair as it may cause abrasion of the articular cartilage and lead to a formation of an inverted or everted labrum, resulting in a loss of the optimal seal. Vertical mattress suture should be used instead as it leaves the peripheral edge of the labrum intact to improve the seal of the acetabulum [62, 63].

More challenging situations arise when labral damage is too severe or the tissue is >8–10 mm or <2–3 mm. Revision procedures also present a challenge, as previous labral repairs are often scarred into the hip capsule [64].

At least five different technique variants are reported in literature: Philippon et al. described an arthroscopic technique involving iliotibial band autografts [65], Sierra and Trousdale reported an open approach using the ligamentum teres [66], Matsuda described an arthroscopic technique using gracilis autografts [67], while Park and Ko reported an arthroscopic reconstruction using quadriceps tendon [68]. Domb et al. presented an arthroscopic technique using capsular autografts [69]. Redmond et al. introduced arthroscopic hip labral reconstruction using semitendinosus allograft [70].

In most patients, the length of the labral tear ranges between 20 and 70 mm; hence the length of the graft needed should range between 40 and 140 mm [70].

The graft should resemble the native labrum and should recreate the suction seal of the hip joint [71]. Once obtained, the graft is tubularized to measure roughly 5–6 mm in diameter to ensure adequate tissue is available to form a seal with the femoral head [1].

Preparing the graft on the table and intra-articular arthroscopic insertion of the fully prepared graft provide an advantageous approach to this challenging procedure. The most marginal anchors should be placed in line with the native labrum to allow overlapping of the graft ends in close proximity to the capsular side of the native labral margins, in effect restoring a fluid seal not only at the graft section but also at the graft-native labrum junctions [67]. The graft body is sutured in a standard fashion with anchors and mattress sutures, as in the refixation.

Next, traction is released and the graft is stabilized in the lateral compartment. Sufficient bone is taken from the femoral neck to produce a smooth head-neck offset that prevents elevation of the labrum during flexion [57]. The dynamic examination is then performed to verify that the suction seal has been properly restored [72]. It is crucial to ensure the labrum is stable intraoperatively during the dynamic examination in order to minimize the risk of labral retears during early postoperative rehabilitation [73].

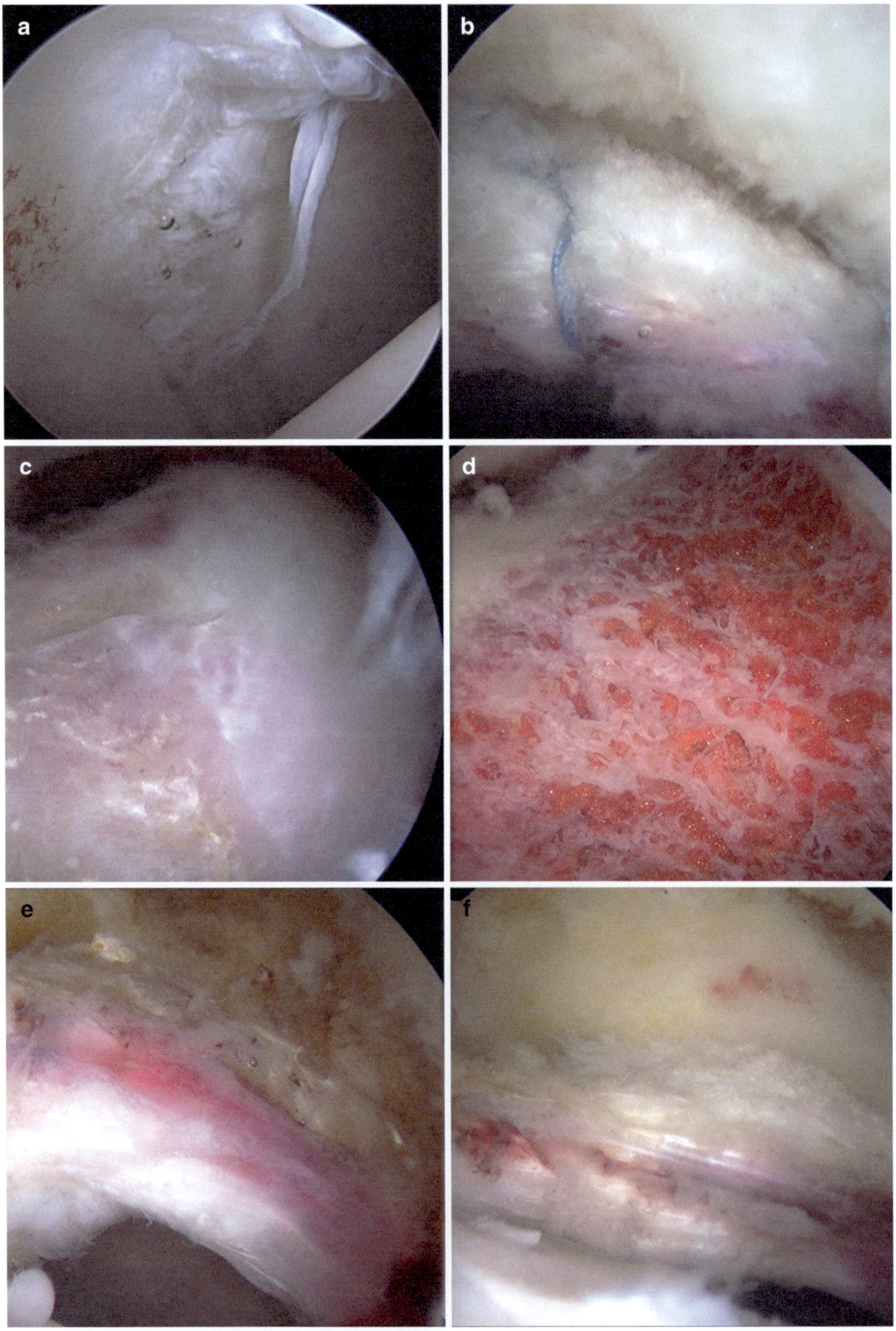

Fig. 3.3 Arthroscopic view. (**a**) Injured labrum. (**b**) Sutured labrum. (**c**) Cam deformity. (**d**) Cam deformity after resection. (**e**) Pincer deformity, labral bruise. (**f**) Pincer deformity after resection, labral bruise

3.6.3 Postoperative Management (Debridement, Repair, Reconstruction)

Postoperative management depends on a performed arthroscopic technique. Usually, the incision care includes a wound check after 2 days and suture removal after 10–14 days. The dressing, provided it is clean and not bloody, is left in place until suture removal. Celecoxib and aspirin are prescribed to prevent heterotopic ossification and venous thromboembolism, respectively.

The extended postoperative weight-bearing limit is not required after arthroscopic labral debridement. A protocol comprising of early low-resistance exercise proves useful in these patients. Cycling is allowed as early as from postoperative day 1; crutch-protected walking is permitted 2 weeks after the procedure, or 6 weeks in cases of microfracture chondroplasty, followed by jogging, freestyle swimming after 4 weeks, and finally running and jumping from 14 weeks onwards.

A standard postoperative protocol used for the patients after labral refixation includes 50% partial weight-bearing. A hinged hip brace might be used for 1 week to prevent hyperextension. The patients are advanced to weight-bearing 4 weeks postoperatively, as tolerated. Initially, flexion is limited to 90°, but after 4 weeks or when the patients can move the hip with minimal or no pain, they can begin extending their range of motion. After approximately 4 months, the patients have typically completed physical therapy, and no further restrictions are recommended.

Postoperative rehabilitation after labral reconstruction includes 10–15 kg of foot-flat weight-bearing with 4 h per day of continuous passive motion. A continuous passive motion machine is also used immediately, and its use is continued for 2–3 weeks postoperatively; the use is increased to 6 h per day for 6–8 weeks if a microfracture was performed. Additionally, a hip brace might be used to restrict extension and external rotation for 14–21 days. Physical therapy is used first, to restore passive motion, then active motion, and finally strength. Passive hip circumduction motions are preferred to prevent adhesions. Full weight-bearing is allowed after 6–8 weeks following a gradual increase of weight-bearing. Endurance training is allowed after maximizing the range of motion and restoring good stability of gait and movement.

3.6.3.1 Outcomes and Prognosis

Over the last decade, hip arthroscopy has gained popularity, for symptoms characteristic for intra-articular pathology; it results in an improvement of function in more than 88% of patients [6]. As a multitude of arthroscopic techniques of treatment FAI-associated pathologies treatment is used, there are many factors that contribute to the expected result [38]. Most promising early and midterm results have been reported with arthroscopic labral reconstruction techniques [74, 75].

Despite the high rate of good to excellent outcomes, hip arthroscopy also has its complications. The rate of complications reported in the literature ranges from 1% to even 20% in some cases, with large reviews of more than 1300 patients reporting the complication rate of 1.21% [76]. The complication rate also includes infrequent complications such as bleeding, occasionally requiring transfusion, infection, deep vein thrombosis, fracture of instruments, and numbness in the scrotum (after traction and post compression).

A growing body of evidence suggests that selective labral debridement, but not segmental labrectomy, may yield durable successful long-term outcomes in selected cases [77, 78]. There is a wide variation in the failure rate of arthroscopic treatment or conversion to total hip arthroplasty, which ranges from 9% to even 20%, perhaps due to the fact that it depends on many factors like surgical technique and patient type, age, sex, comorbidities, severity of arthritic changes, etc.

However, the latest studies show that labral repair and labral reconstruction provide better outcomes and, when possible, should be performed over labral debridement.

Labral repair has proved superior to labral resection and allows for the preservation of more labral tissue. Successful and anatomical labral repair may delay or prevent the development of osteoarthritis of the hip joint in the long term [79]. Usually, at the 10-year follow-up, there is a greater reduction in hip pain with labral reattachment as compared with labral resection. There are many reports in literature that after labral reconstruction using autograft (gracilis, iliotibial band), the modified Harris Hip Score increased by more than 20–25 points, with the median patient satisfaction at about 8–9 out of 10 [65].

3.6.3.2 Return to Sports

Physical activity is an important factor modifying the results of surgical procedures. It is important to note that professional athletes form a large group of arthroscopically treated patients. First of all, the damage of the labrum in athletes is mainly of traumatic aetiology. Moreover, the level of preoperative training is also greater. There have been reported cases of professional athletes returning to sports after arthroscopic treatment for FAI and associated pathologies [80]. More than 93% of the patients returned to professional sport. It is worth noting that around 78% maintain this level of activity at a mean of 1.5 years after follow-up [81].

References

1. White BJ, Herzog MM. Arthroscopic labral reconstruction of the hip using iliotibial band allograft and front-to-back fixation technique. Arthrosc Tech. 2016;5(1):e89–97. https://doi.org/10.1016/j.eats.2015.08.009.
2. Ferguson SJ, Bryant JT, Ganz R, Ito K. The influence of the acetabular labrum on hip joint cartilage consolidation: a poroelastic finite element model. J Biomech. 2000;33(8):953–60.
3. Seldes RM, Tan V, Hunt J, Katz M, Winiarsky R, Fitzgerald RH Jr. Anatomy, histologic features, and vascularity of the adult acetabular labrum. Clin Orthop Relat Res. 2001;(382):232–40.
4. Petersen W, Petersen F, Tillmann B. Structure and vascularization of the acetabular labrum with regard to the pathogenesis and healing of labral lesions. Arch Orthop Trauma Surg. 2003;123:283–8.
5. Ferguson SJ, Bryant JT, Ito K. The material properties of the bovine acetabular labrum. J Orthop Res. 2001;19:887–96.
6. Crawford MJ, Dy CJ, Alexander JW, et al. The 2007 Frank Stinchfield Award. The biomechanics of the hip labrum and the stability of the hip. Clin Orthop Relat Res. 2007;465:16–22.
7. Alzaharani A, Bali K, Gudena R, et al. The innervation of the human acetabular labrum and hip joint: an anatomic study. BMC Musculoskelet Disord. 2014;15:41.
8. Chung SM. The arterial supply of the developing proximal end of the human femur. J Bone Joint Surg Am. 1976;58:961–70.
9. Kelly BT, Shapiro GS, Digiovanni CW, et al. Vascularity of the hip labrum: a cadaveric investigation. Arthroscopy. 2005;21:3–11.
10. Shu B, Safran M. Hip instability: anatomic and clinical considerations of traumatic and atraumatic instability. Clin Sports Med. 2011;30:349–67.
11. Boykin R, Anz A, Bushnell B, et al. Hip instability. J Am Acad Orthop Surg. 2011;19:340–9.
12. McCarthy JC, Noble PC, Schuck MR, et al. The Otto E Aufranc Award the role of labral lesions to development of early degenerative hip disease. Clin Orthop. 2001;393:25–37.
13. Lewis CL, Sahrmann SA. Acetabular labral tears. Phys Ther. 2006;86:110–21.
14. Kelly BT, Weiland DE, Schenker ML, Philippon MJ. Arthroscopic labral repair in the hip: surgical technique and review of the literature. Arthroscopy. 2005;21:1496–504.
15. Beck M, Kalhor M, Leunig M, Ganz R. Hip morphology influences the pattern of damage to the acetabular cartilage: femoroacetabular impingement as a cause of early osteoarthritis of the hip. J Bone Joint Surg (Br). 2005;87(7):1012–8.
16. Kalisvaart MM, Safran MR. Microinstability of the hip-it does exist: etiology, diagnosis and treatment. J Hip Preserv Surg. 2015;2(2):123–35.
17. Philippon M, Peixoto L, Goljan P. Acetabular labral tears: debridement, repair, reconstruction. Operat Tech Sports Med. 2012;20:281–6.
18. Petersilge CA, Haque MA, Petersilge WJ, et al. Acetabular labrum tears: evaluation with MR arthrography. Radiology. 1996;200:225–30.
19. Dorrell JH, Catterall A. The torn acetabular labrum. J Bone Joint Surg. 1986;68B:400–3.
20. Register B, Pennock A, Ho C, Strickland C, Lawand A, Philippon M. Prevalence of abnormal hip findings in asymptomatic participants a prospective, blinded study. Am J Sports Med. 2012;40:2720.
21. McCarthy JC. The diagnosis and treatment of labral and chondral injuries. Instr Course Lect. 2004;53:573–7.
22. Mccarthy J, Noble P, Aluisio F, Schuck M, Wright J, Lee J. Anatomy, pathologic features, and treatment of acetabular labral tears. Clin Orthop Relat Res. 2003;406:38–47.
23. McCarthy JC, Noble P, Schuck M, Alusio FV, Wright J, Lee J. Acetabular and labral pathology. In: Early hip disorders. New York, NY: Springer; 2003.
24. Bharam S. Labral tears, extra-articular injuries, and hip arthroscopy in the athlete. Clin Sports Med. 2006;25(2):279–92.
25. Lage LA, Patel JV, Villar RN. The acetabular labral tear: an arthroscopic classification. Arthroscopy.

1996;12(3):269–72. https://doi.org/10.1016/S0749-8063(96)90057-2.
26. Czerny C, Hofmann S, Neuhold A, Tschauner C, Engel A, Recht MP, Kramer J. Lesions of the acetabular labrum: accuracy of MR imaging and MR arthrography in detection and staging. Radiology. 1996;200:225–30. https://doi.org/10.1148/radiology.200.1.8657916.
27. Blankenbaker DG, Smet AA, Keene JS, Fine JP. Classification and localization of acetabular labral tears. Skelet Radiol. 2007;36(5):391–7.
28. Cadet ER, Chan AK, Vorys GC, et al. Investigation of the preservation of the fluid seal effect in the repaired, partially resected, and reconstructed acetabular labrum in a cadaveric hip model. Am J Sports Med. 2012;40:2218.
29. Ferguson SJ, Bryant JT, Ganz R, Ito K. An in vitro investigation of the acetabular labral seal in hip joint mechanics. J Biomech. 2003;36:171–8.
30. Henak CR, Ellis BJ, Harris MD, et al. Role of the acetabular labrum in load support across the hip joint. J Biomech. 2011;44:2201–6.
31. Henak CR, Abraham CL, Anderson AE, et al. Patient-specific analysis of cartilage and labrum mechanics in human hips with acetabular dysplasia. Osteoarthr Cartil. 2014;22(2):210–7. https://doi.org/10.1016/j.joca.2013.11.003.
32. Hunt D, Clohisy J, Prather H. Acetabular tears of the hip in women. Phys Med Rehabil Clin N Am. 2007;18(3):497–520.
33. Philippon MJ, Stubbs AJ, Schenker ML, Maxwell RB, Ganz R, Leunig M. Arthroscopic management of FAI: osteoplasty technique and literature review. Am J Sports Med. 2007;35(9):1571–80. https://doi.org/10.1177/0363546507300258.
34. Toft F, Anliker E, Beck M. Is labral hypotrophy correlated with increased acetabular depth? J Hip Preserv Surg. 2015;2(2):175–83. https://doi.org/10.1093/jhps/hnv034.
35. McCarthy JC, Busconi B. The role of hip arthroscopy in the diagnosis and treatment of hip disease. Can J Surg. 1995;38(Suppl 1):S13–7.
36. Ganz R, Leunig M, Leunig-Ganz K, Harris WH. The etiology of osteoarthritis of the hip: an integrated mechanical concept. Clin Orthop Relat Res. 2008;466(2):264–72.
37. Beck M, Kalhor M, Leunig M, Ganz R. Hip morphology influences the pattern of damage to the acetabular cartilage. J Bone Joint Surg (Br). 2005;87-B:1012–8.
38. Ganz R, Parvizi J, Beck M, Leunig M, Nötzli H, Siebenrock KA. Femoroacetabular impingement: a cause for osteoarthritis of the hip. Clin Orthop Relat Res. 2004;417:112–20. https://doi.org/10.1097/01.blo.0000096804.78689.c2.
39. Kosuge D, Yamada N, Azegami S, Achan P, Ramachandran M. Management of developmental dysplasia of the hip in young adults: current concepts. Bone Joint J. 2013;95-B:732–7.
40. Solomon L. Patterns of osteoarthritis of the hip. J Bone Joint Surg (Br). 1976;58:176–83.
41. Cooperman D. What is the evidence to support acetabular dysplasia as a cause of osteoarthritis? J Pediatr Orthop. 2013;33(Suppl 1):S2–7.
42. Petersen B, Wolf B, Lambert J, Clayton C, Glueck D, Jesse M, Mei-Dan O. Lateral acetabular labral length is inversely related to acetabular coverage as measured by lateral center edge angle of Wiberg. J Hip Preserv Surg. 2016;3:hnv084. https://doi.org/10.1093/jhps/hnv084.
43. Zhang H-L, Liang J-S, Li L-G, Luo D-Z, Xiao K, Cheng H, Zhang H. Inverted acetabular labrum: an analysis of tissue embedment in hip joint in 15 patients with developmental dysplasia of the hip. Chin Med J. 2017;130:100–3. https://doi.org/10.4103/0366-6999.196582.
44. Burnett RS, Della Rocca GJ, Prather H, Curry M, Maloney WJ, Clohisy JC. Clinical presentation of patients with tears of the acetabular labrum. J Bone Joint Surg Am. 2006;88(7):1448–57.
45. Griffin D, Dickenson E, O'Donnell J, Agricola R, Awan T, Beck M, Clohisy J, Dijkstra P, Falvey E, Gimpel M, Hinman R, Holmich P, Kassarjian A, Martin H, Martin R, Mather R III, Philippon M, Reiman M, Takla A, Bennell K. The Warwick Agreement on femoroacetabular impingement syndrome (FAI syndrome): an international consensus statement. Br J Sports Med. 2016;50:1169–76. https://doi.org/10.1136/bjsports-2016-096743.
46. Grant AD, Sala DA, Davidovitch RI. The labrum: structure, function, and injury with femoro-acetabular impingement. J Child Orthop. 2012;6(5):357–72. https://doi.org/10.1007/s11832-012-0431-1.
47. Johnston TL, Schenker ML, Briggs KK, Philippon MJ. Relationship between offset angle alpha and hip chondral injury in femoracetabular impingement. Arthroscopy. 2008;24:669–75.
48. McCarthy JC, Lee JA. Hip arthroscopy: indications, outcomes, and complications. Instr Course Lect. 2006;55:301–8.
49. Kapron AL, Aoki SK, Peters CL, Anderson AE. In-vivo hip arthrokinematics during supine clinical exams: application to the study of femoroacetabular impingement. J Biomech. 2015;48(11):2879–86. https://doi.org/10.1016/j.jbiomech.2015.04.022.
50. Philippon MJ, Ho CP, Briggs KK, Stull J, LaPrade RF. Prevalence of increased alpha angles as a measure of cam-type femoroacetabular impingement in youth ice hockey players. Am J Sports Med. 2013;41:1357–62.
51. Larson CM, Giveans MR. Arthroscopic debridement versus refixation of the acetabular labrum associated with femoroacetabular impingement. Arthroscopy. 2009;25:369–76.
52. Ayeni O, Alradwan H, de Sa D, Philippon M. The hip labrum reconstruction: indications and outcomes-a systematic review. Knee Surg Sports Traumatol Arthrosc. 2013;22:737. https://doi.org/10.1007/s00167-013-2804-5.
53. Hartigan DE, Perets I, Meghpara MB, et al. Labral debridement, repair and reconstruction: current

concepts. J ISAKOS Jt Disord Orthop Sports Med. 2018;3:155–60.
54. Chahla J, Soares E, Bhatia S, Mitchell JJ, Philippon MJ. Arthroscopic technique for acetabular labral reconstruction using iliotibial band autograft. Arthrosc Tech. 2016;5(3):e671–7. https://doi.org/10.1016/j.eats.2016.02.025.
55. Philippon MJ, Schenker ML, Briggs KK, et al. Revision hip arthroscopy. Am J Sports Med. 2007;35:1918–21.
56. Shenoy K, Dai AZ, Mahure SA, Kaplan DJ, Capogna B, Youm T. Arthroscopic repair of hip labrum with suture anchors. Arthrosc Tech. 2017;6(6):e2143–9. https://doi.org/10.1016/j.eats.2017.08.007.
57. Philippon MJ, Faucet SC, Briggs KK. Arthroscopic hip labral repair. Arthrosc Tech. 2013;2(2):e73–6. https://doi.org/10.1016/j.eats.2012.11.002.
58. Outerbridge RE. The etiology of chondromalacia patellae. J Bone Joint Surg (Br). 1961;43:752–7.
59. Konan S, Rayan F, Meermans G, Witt J, Haddad FS. Validation of the classification system for acetabular chondral lesions identified at arthroscopy in patients with femoroacetabular impingement. J Bone Joint Surg (Br). 2011;93:332–6.
60. Chow RM, Owens CJ, Krych AJ, Levy BA. Arthroscopic labral repair in the treatment of femoroacetabular impingement. Arthrosc Tech. 2013;2(4):e333–6. https://doi.org/10.1016/j.eats.2013.04.009.
61. Fry R, Domb B. Labral base refixation in the hip: rationale and technique for an anatomic approach to labral repair. Arthroscopy. 2010;26(Suppl 1):81–9.
62. Larson CM, Giveans MR. Arthroscopic management of femoroacetabular impingement: early outcomes measures. Arthroscopy. 2008;24:540–6.
63. Ye K, Singh PJ. Arthroscopic labral repair of the hip, using a through-labral double-stranded single-pass suture technique. Arthrosc Tech. 2014;3(5):e615–9. https://doi.org/10.1016/j.eats.2014.07.003.
64. White BJ, Herzog MM. Labral reconstruction: when to perform and how. Front Surg. 2015;2:27. https://doi.org/10.3389/fsurg.2015.00027.
65. Philippon MJ, Briggs KK, Hay CJ, Kuppersmith DA, Dewing CB, Huang MJ. Arthroscopic labral reconstruction in the hip using iliotibial band autograft: technique and early outcomes. Arthroscopy. 2010;26:750–6.
66. Sierra RJ, Trousdale RT. Labral reconstruction using the ligamentum teres capitis: report of a new technique. Clin Orthop Relat Res. 2009;467:753–9.
67. Matsuda DK. Arthroscopic labral reconstruction with gracilis autograft. Arthrosc Tech. 2012;1(1):e15–21. https://doi.org/10.1016/j.eats.2011.12.001.
68. Park SE, Ko Y. Use of the quadriceps tendon in arthroscopic acetabular labral reconstruction: potential and benefits as an autograft option. Arthrosc Tech. 2013;2:e217–9.
69. Domb BG, Gupta A, Stake CE, Hammarstedt JE, Redmond JM. Arthroscopic labral reconstruction of the hip using local capsular autograft. Arthrosc Tech. 2014;3:e355–9.
70. Redmond JM, Cregar WM, Martin TJ, Vemula SP, Gupta A, Domb BG. Arthroscopic labral reconstruction of the hip using semitendinosus allograft. Arthrosc Tech. 2015;4(4):e323–9.
71. Philippon M, Briggs K. Reconstructive techniques in FAI surgery. In: Diagnosis and management of femoroacetabular impingement; 2017. https://doi.org/10.1007/978-3-319-32000-7_13.
72. Frank JM, Chahla J, Mitchell JJ, Soares E, Philippon MJ. Remplissage of the femoral head-neck junction in revision hip arthroscopy: a technique to correct excessive cam resection. Arthrosc Tech. 2016;5(6):e1209–13. https://doi.org/10.1016/j.eats.2016.07.012.
73. Ejnisman L, Philippon M, Lertwanich P. Acetabular labral tears: diagnosis, repair, and a method for labral reconstruction. Clin Sports Med. 2011;30:317–29. https://doi.org/10.1016/j.csm.2010.12.006.
74. Geyer MR, Philippon MJ, Fagrelius TS, Briggs KK. Acetabular labral reconstruction with an iliotibial band autograft: outcome and survivorship analysis at minimum 3-year follow-up. Am J Sports Med. 2013;41:1750–6.
75. Ayeni OR, Alradwan H, de Sa D, Philippon MJ. The hip labrum reconstruction: indications and outcomes—a systematic review. Knee Surg Sports Traumatol Arthrosc. 2014;22:737–43.
76. Kowalczuk M, et al. Complications following hip arthroscopy: a systematic review and meta-analysis. Knee Surg Sports Traumatol Arthrosc. 2013;21(7):1669–75.
77. Byrd JW, Jones KS. Hip arthroscopy for labral pathology: prospective analysis with 10-year follow-up. Arthroscopy. 2009;25:365–8.
78. McCarthy JC, Jarrett BT, Ojeifo O, Lee JA, Bragdon CR. What factors influence long-term survivorship after hip arthroscopy? Clin Orthop Relat Res. 2011;469:362–71.
79. Bowman KF, et al. A clinically relevant review of hip biomechanics. Arthroscopy. 2010;26(8):1118–29.
80. Weiland DE, Philippon MJ. Arthroscopic technique of femoroacetabular impingement. Op Tech Orthop. 2005;15:256–60.
81. Philippon M, Schenker M, Briggs K, Kuppersmith D. Femoroacetabular impingement in 45 professional athletes: associated pathologies and return to sport following arthroscopic decompression. Knee Surg Sports Traumatol Arthrosc. 2007;15(7):908–14. https://doi.org/10.1007/s00167-007-0332-x.

Part II

Knee

4 Bone Marrow Stimulation Techniques for Cartilage Repair

Mats Brittberg

4.1 Introduction

A damaged mesenchymal tissue heals through the bleeding that occurs in the vascularized tissue. A blood clot is formed and acts as a matrix for the growth of repair cells. Eventually a scar tissue is formed which, more or less, is eventually converted to resemble the previously damaged tissue.

As the cartilage lacks blood vessels and also nerves and lymph vessels, the above-described effect is not seen in a pure cartilage injury. On the other hand, a clot formation can occur if the injury is osteochondral and reaches further down into the well-vascularized subchondral bone.

The most common way of attempting to achieve a repair tissue in cartilage lesions is by perforating the underlying bone plate in various ways, thus achieving bleeding, blood clotting, and inducing an ingrowth of progenitor cells from the bone marrow.

In 1959, Pridie [1] described for the first time how to more actively achieve healing in case of widespread cartilage damage. He suggested that through multiple boreholes in damaged area after careful debridement, a connective tissue repair is induced that would at best produce a fibrous cartilage.

Lanny Johnson [2] modified the drilling technique by fraying of the surface layer of the cortical bone in the bone plate with the arthroscopic burr to reach the intracortical vessels. The aim was to achieve a smooth development of the healing tissue. Lanny Johnson developed that technique on the basis of his experience in treating sclerotic arthritis defects. He found that when he treated patients with arthritic cartilage defects with debridement, those with sclerotic bone did not improve, but often required new intervention [2]. He also noted that drilling through a sclerotic surface could not be performed with regard to poor access to the posterior part of the femur condyle. Through his own studies, he found that the intracortical vessels were located at 1–2 mm depth and that they could be reached by scratching hard with a curet. He then proceeded to make multiple pits in the sclerotic bone plate, but the healing was still unsatisfactory. By completing the milling of the entire sclerotic surface, he received a healing that was good. The method now consisted of a discarded surface layer with complementary multiple pits in short exits to reach the intracortical vessels. The procedure was done with motorized cutters, and injuries at the back of the femur condyle as well as on the patella surface could now be transartroscopically treated. The postoperative regimen meant no load bearing for 2 months [2].

M. Brittberg (✉)
Cartilage Research Unit, Region Halland Orthopaedics, Kungsbacka Hospital, University of Gothenburg, Kungsbacka, Sweden
e-mail: mats.brittberg@telia.com

M. Brittberg, K. Slynarski (eds.), *Lower Extremity Joint Preservation*,
https://doi.org/10.1007/978-3-030-57382-9_4

Richard Steadman studied cartilage damage on horses because the horse's cartilage layer resembles the human cartilage layer [3]. When repairing cartilage injuries with bone marrow stimulation, it was found that if calcified cartilage layers were left after treatment, the cartilage damage was impaired. Like Lanny Johnson, Steadman wanted to keep the subchondral bone plate intact in order to reach only the intracortical vessels [3]. With specially angled awls, microfracture defects are made in the cortical bone.

In recent years, microfracture (mfx) technology has become the mode of use for cartilage injuries in different joints. It is often used as the control technique in randomized studies, although the technique is not proven better against other bone marrow stimulation techniques, neither to the debridement nor to the natural course of a cartilage injury.

Steadman has linked a very strict postoperative rehabilitation technique to the technology that has to be followed to achieve the results presented by Steadman's group over the years [3]. However, there are no long-term studies comparing different postoperative rehabilitation methods.

Recent studies indicate that mfx reaches not deep enough to reach large vessels from where chondrogenic cells could migrate easier into the cartilage lesion area [4]. Subsequently today, the techniques are focusing on the depth, and the so-called nano-drillings down to 7–12 mm are becoming more popular when treating defects smaller than 1 cm^2.

4.2 The Different Basic Techniques for Bone Marrow Stimulation

In general, it is best to treat cartilage damage with a surrounding cartilage of good quality. If there is a thin and bad surrounding cartilage, there is a risk that the juvenile repair tissue will be directly affected before it has matured to a good quality.

4.2.1 Subchondral Drilling

Cartilage Damage <1 cm^2

It is good to use when the leg is highly sclerotic as with an osteochondritis or old osteochondral fracture. Multiple drilling with a 2 mm:s drill or alternatively drilling with a 2 mm:s Kirschner pin is recommended. In areas where it is difficult to reach with the drill, special vector guides can be used. Recently, animal experimental studies have shown that in the so-called deep drilling, one will reach larger subchondral blood vessels inducing a better repair performance compared to basic drilling and microfracturing [4]. These studies have induced a renaissance for subchondral drilling as treatment alternative to the popular microfracture technology. With this so-called nano-drilling, a stronger repair tissue may be induced, and it seems that:

- Deep drilling is better than shallow drilling and microfracture.
- Small diameter drill hole is better than large.

Rehabilitation (author's option): If the cartilage damage is greater than 1 cm^2, the patient is given a brace locked in extended mode for 2 weeks. After 2 weeks, the brace is locked up, and the patient is allowed to stay without the use of the brace indoors and at night but must have the open brace on outdoors for an additional 4 weeks to avoid heavy sowing forces and rotational violence. The same mobilization is used for the femur, tibia condyles, and patella.

With load of crutches, weight bearing is allowed to the level of what the pain indicates.

4.2.2 Abrasion Arthroplasty

Cartilage Damage <1 cm^2

This method is rarely used today but may be useful in the treatment of intralesional osteophytes (relatively commonly seen after mfx). With the burr, bone spikes are trimmed away to give a smooth light bleeding surface that can be treated with other repairing techniques afterward.

4.2.3 Microfracture

Cartilage Damage <1 cm^2

Cartilage treatment is still in fashion today because it is easy to perform and cheap. New research findings (see drilling), however, may lead to instead an increased use of drilling.

With different angled awls, you can treat different areas that are difficult to access. The awls are 45°, 60°, and 90° (especially good for the patella and talus). One can use a light hammer unless the handpower is insufficient to fracture the hard superficial subchondral bone plate. Hammers are not recommended when using the 90° awl. The awls are often used by many different doctors in a clinic. It should be borne in mind that the angle of the awls is subjected to excessive stress and fatigue fractures can occur in the angle so that the tip can go off and end up in the joint.

After a thorough revision of the cartilage injury and removal of all the calcified cartilage, multiple microfracture holes are made at 2–4 mm depths (sometimes fat drops can be seen through the holes) and at a distance of 3–4 mm.

4.2.4 Mobilization (According to Steadman [3])

4.2.4.1 Femoral Condyle and Tibia Plateau

Continuous passive motion exercise in CPM (continuous passive motion) machine directly postoperatively. Passive motion is initially set 30–70° and then increased as tolerated at 10–20° increments until full passive motion works. Steadman wants the patient to be treated in CPM 6–8 h every day preferably for 6–8 weeks.

Ten percent of body weight with (touchdown) crushing is allowed for 6–8 weeks.

4.2.4.2 Patella

Recommended orthosis fixed at 0–20° for 8 weeks. CPM is allowed but the orthosis must be on between passive training. It starts with 0–50° in the CPM machine directly postoperatively. These patients are allowed to fully load in their orthosis after 2 weeks.

My own mobilization after microfracture is significantly more aggressive and identical to the treatment described for subchondral drilling.

4.3 Matrix-Associated Bone Marrow Stimulation Techniques (MA-BMS)

Experience has shown that it may be difficult to get a smooth filling of a cartilage injury following the various described bone marrow stimulation methods [1–3]. In recent years, more and more people have been interested in mesenchymal stem cells found in the subchondral bone, and by implanting different porous materials into the debrided cartilage injury, one can induce a stronger and evener growth of cells into the cartilage area. Several matrices for augmented bone marrow repairs are presented below.

4.3.1 Carbon Rods and Pads

Two of the first methods that work in this way are the porous carbon rods and carbon fiber plates that can be used to treat cartilage damage [5–7]. The carbon fiber matrices come from polyester heated to more than 1000° to become carbon filaments woven into porous matrix rods or plates [5–7]. The carbon fiber material gives rise to a highly well-organized connective tissue ingrowth, and the method can be performed transartroscopically.

4.3.2 Trans Arthroscopic Implant

First, you perform a normal debridement of the injury. It is important that the synovitis and vulgar Hoffa's fat body are resected with the shaver instrument for good accessibility.

Drill with 3 mm drill hole to a depth of 12.5 mm (there is a stop on a special drill developed for carbon fiber), and choose the number of holes depending on the size of the cartilage

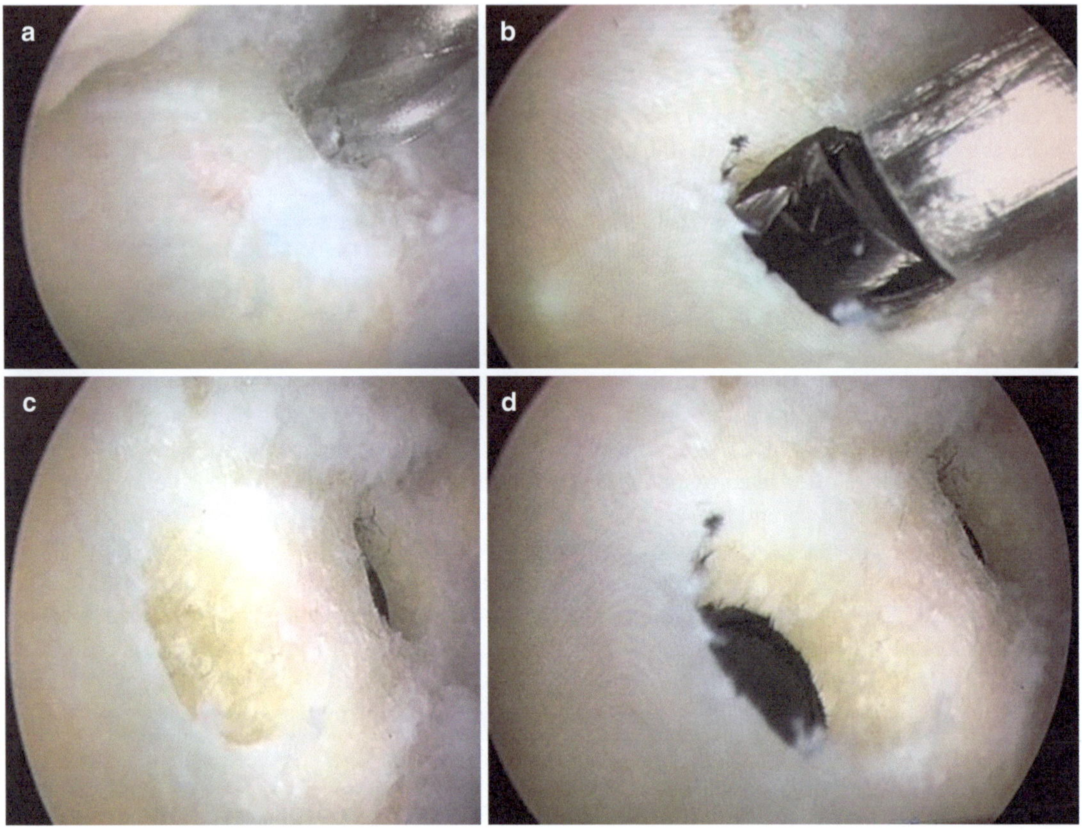

Fig. 4.1 (**a**) A drill hole is made in a trochlear defect. (**b**) A carbon fiber rod has been implanted into the drill hole, slightly below the bony surface. (**c**) A second drill hole has been made. (**d**) A second carbon rod has been implanted

damage. The boreholes should be installed at 8–10 mm intervals. In a defect of the size of 1 cm^2, it is sufficient with a centrally positioned borehole (Fig. 4.1a–d).

In the borehole, a rod is then placed via a special implant cannula so that the rod reaches either the level of the surrounding bone or just below the bone surface. It is important that the implantation guide is kept perpendicular to the bone surface; otherwise, there is a risk that the carbon rod may break when the material is porous and brittle. Before entering the rod in the guide, you can test that the channel is free from debris material with a trocar.

If you need to do a carbon fiber audit, you can easily drill through the carbon pole and then shave with a shaver like a vacuum cleaner to remove carbon particles, then reimplant a new carbon rod, or choose another repair method.

4.3.3 Implant of Carbon Fiber Plate

Carbon fiber plates are more porous than carbon fiber rods. They are used to treat cartilage damage on concave surfaces such as patella's cavity or tibia ceilings.

A bare bone surface is treated by milling the entire subchondral bone plate to a depth of 3 mm, the edges are undermined by a 2 mm edge of the ceiling, and then the plate cut to the right diameter can be implanted into the bone pool underneath the undermined leg edges. No additional fixation required.

Postoperative rehabilitation is as in a microfracture surgery.

4.4 AMIC (Autologous Matrix-Induced Chondrogenesis)

In order to get the blood clot formed in a microfracture procedure to remain as intact as possible, a method has been developed to temporarily cover the blood coagulation during the initial healing. Following a conventional microfracture, the lesion is covered by pasting a collagen-based membrane over the microfracture holes [8]. One can use commercial fibrin glue or own-made so-called partial autologous fibrin (PAF) adhesive.

Postoperatively, it is recommended that the joint is locked in an orthosis in the extended position for 7 days followed by starting with passive movements in CPM for 4–6 weeks. No strain for patients with femur and tibia lesions for 6 weeks, while patella and trochlea injuries are not allowed to load through week 2 and then allow 50% load in weeks 2–4 followed by gradual increase to full load.

The indication is cartilage lesions greater between 1 and 3 cm^2.

4.4.1 Osteochondral Matrix Plugs

Based on the knowledge of how to treat cartilage damage with multiple osteochondral autografts, special matrix materials have been developed to be implanted as one or more cylinders in the cartilage lesion area. Those plugs are synthetic resorbable cylindrical plugs consisting of different materials in different layers. By making the matrices with different layers of different porosity and properties, one tries to mimic the layer of osteochondral region to attract cells to migrate into and to be directed into the osteogenic and chondrogenic direction, depending on the cell's current position in the material. PLA (polylactide) and PLGA (poly-lactide-glycolic acid) in combination with calcium phosphate and hydroxyapatite have been used.

The first used plug of this type was the OBI TruFit [9] where the osseous phase is to be resorbed within 3 months, while the entire polymer is resorbed successively for approximately 9 months, and it is thought that you will gradually get a bone substitution at the bottom of the implantation area. Barber and Dockery [10] have performed a follow-up study, but no such dual repair was performed, but the entire repair area was filled out by a connective tissue mass. As no bony subchondral support material developed, these authors felt that the method was less suitable for a good quality cartilage repair that needs proper subchondral support to develop well. Carmont et al. [11] has reported delayed incorporation of an articular cartilage defect of the lateral femoral condyle treated with three TruFit plugs. The patient reported symptom alleviation and resumption of functional activity after 24 months of continued rehabilitation, meaning that the slow bone healing gives a late improvement.

Another similar synthetic plug is OsseoFit® (OsseoFit Porous Tissue Matrix, Kensey Nash Corp., West Whiteland Township, Pennsylvania, USA) [12] consisting of a layer that resembles the cartilage layer and which consists of bovine collagen, while the bone layer consists of beta-tricalcium phosphate in a network made of PLA. Recently, a third synthetic plug was placed on the market, which consists of a cartilage-like 2-mm thick layer of collagen, glycosaminoglycan, and then a 6-mm bone layer with the same components plus calcium phosphate [13]. In studies, it has been shown that it may be compressed more than the other mentioned plug which may be of importance if some of the plug is slightly prominent. A similar plug with the collagen layer for the cartilage and beta-tricalcium phosphate is BioMatrix® (BioMatrix® Cartilage Repair Device, Arthrex, Karlsfeld, Germany). However, there is still too little documentation for these methods in order to give them a place in the treatment arena.

4.4.2 Coral Exoskeleton

Coral exoskeleton, which consists of $CaCO_3$, has an interconnected pore structure that resembles that of natural human bone. It has been used as scaffold material to fill bone defects in both animal models and humans in almost 50 years [14]. The coral material is biocompatible, osteoconductive, and biodegradable. Calcium carbonate forms as both aragonite and calcite. Recently, an aragonite-hyaluronate (Ar-HA) biphasic scaffold has been described as capable of osteochondral repair [15]. In a small human pilot study, the coral implant was associated with a significant clinical improvement at the 12-month follow-up. Moreover, MRI findings revealed graft integration with good bone and cartilage formation [16].

4.4.3 Blood Clot Augmentation

In addition to focusing on allowing bone marrow cells to migrate into a matrix material, one can focus on improving the clot formation that is the basis of cell growth. One method is based on using the so-called thermo gels. The formed natural blood clots tend to shrink which means that the clot does not fill out the area fully at the edges and the healing can thus become insufficient.

By stabilizing the blood clot so that it retains its volume, it contacts the surrounding cartilage surfaces and allows the cells from the bone marrow to better achieve a more complete healing tissue. One way is to provide coagulation with good volume and strength by supplying a soluble polymer matrix consisting of polysaccharide chitosan with uncoagulated blood. Animal experimental studies and a recent randomized study have shown that this method can provide a satisfactory healing of cartilage damage [17–19].

4.4.4 UV Light Stabilized Gel for Cartilage Repair

A so-called surface erosion scaffold is GelrinC (Regentis, Israel) consisting of a mix of fibrinogen and PEGs (polyethylene glycol diacrylate) forming a gel that when injected to fill up a chondral defects is stabilized by UV light. Via mfx treatment, cells invade the defect area, and enzymes released by the cells degrade the fibrinogen component of GelrinC causing the implant to slowly erode and get smaller. This process allows new surfaces to be exposed, and a new cartilage formation is repeated until the implant is completely resorbed [20]. The method is studied in a clinical trial to be finished in 2019 (Fig. 4.2a–d).

4.4.5 Large Cartilage Bone Damage Treated with Bone Marrow Stimulation

The interest in using "intrinsic" cell-induced repair cells from the bone marrow has been focused on minor injuries <2 cm^2. In case of larger cartilage injuries, surgery with bone marrow stimulation has been difficult. However, a method that is available for such reconstructions is a biomimetic scaffold able to fill large osteochondral injuries with a 2-, 4-, or 6-mm-depth thick layered collagen matrix (MaioRegen© Finceramica, Italy). The collagen matrix is implanted into a subconditional prepared bed where it then swells of the blood that stabilizes the matrix [21]. A multicenter randomized trial with this implant compared with mfx has been performed in 118 patients. Patients affected by deep osteochondral lesions (i.e., Outerbridge grade IV and OCD) showed a superior IKDC subjective outcome ($p = 0.036$) in the scaffold group, and significantly better results were also found for another challenging group, sports-active patients ($p = 0.02$) [22] (Fig. 4.3a–d).

4.5 Conclusion

All methods based on bone marrow cell in growth depend on the number of cells present in the bone marrow and their chondrogenic ability. The number of cells in the bone marrow with the stem cell's character decreases drastically at an increased age. In order to have the greatest chance

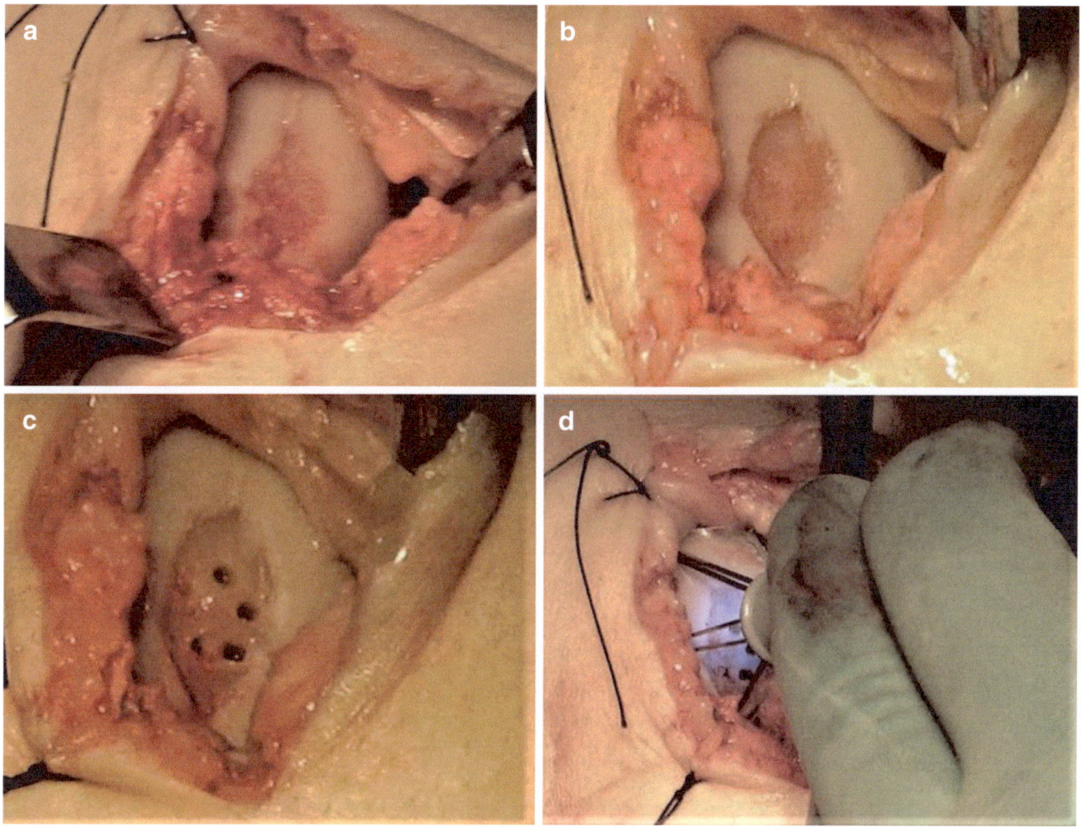

Fig. 4.2 (**a**) A cartilage defect on a femoral condyle will be treated. (**b**) The cartilage defect has been debrided. (**c**) The cartilage defect has been microfractured. (**d**) The cartilage defect has been filled with gel and UV light is used to stabilize the gel

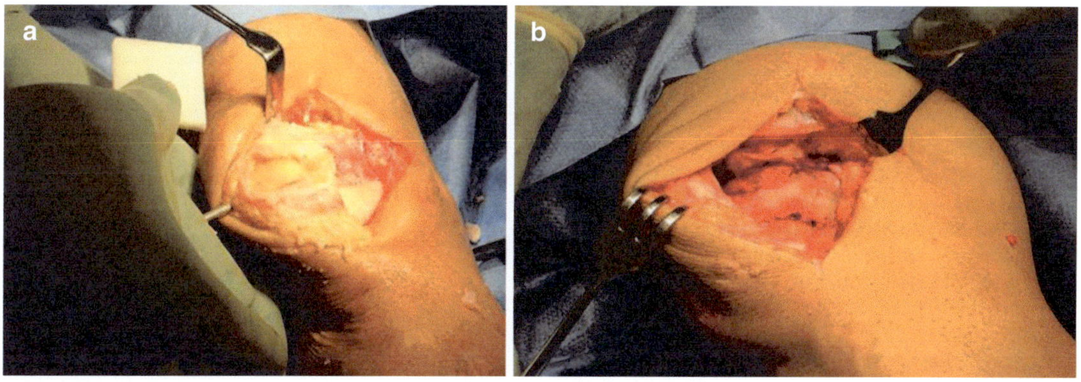

Fig. 4.3 (**a**) A cartilage defect on a patella will be treated by MaioRegen implant. The patella lesion has been debrided. (**b**) A cartilage defect on the trochlea in the same patient has in (**a**) will also be treated by MaioRegen implant. (**c**) The patella defect has been filled with the MaioRegen implant and covered by fibrin glue. (**d**) The trochlea defect has now also be treated by a MaioRegen implant and covered by fibrin glue

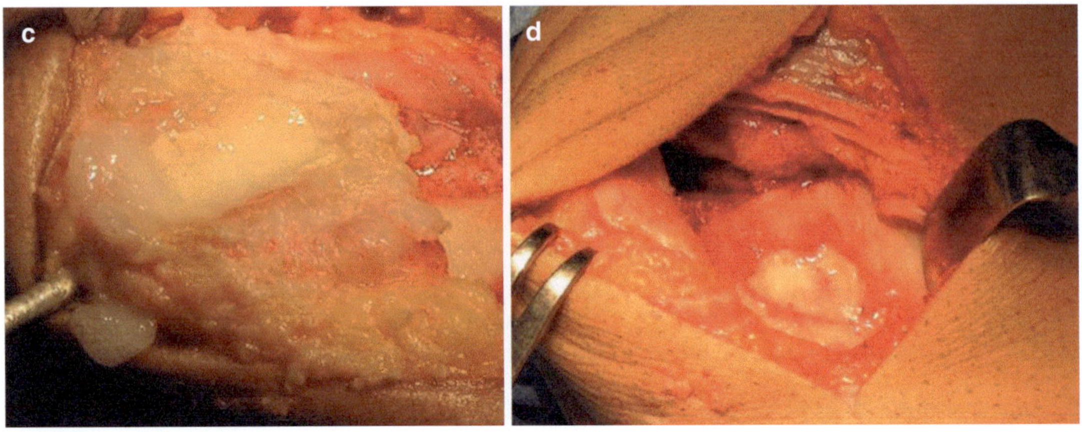

Fig. 4.3 (continued)

of getting a hyaline-like repair tissue, the patient subsequently should be young. The main indications are defects up to 3 cm^2. For defects less than 1 cm, bone marrow stimulation alone as done with thin drilling to a depth of at least 7 mm seems appropriate, while larger lesions need an augmentation to be able to be filled completely with a repair tissue.

References

1. Pridie KH. A method of resurfacing osteoarthritic knee joints. J Bone Joint Surg. 1959;41B:618–9.
2. Johnson LL. Arthroscopic abrasion arthroplasty. Historical and pathological perspective: present status. Arthroscopy. 1986;2:54–9.
3. Steadman JR, Rodkey WG, Rodrigo JJ. Microfracture: surgical technique and rehabilitation to treat chondral defects. Clin Orthop Relat Res. 2001;(391 Suppl):S362–9. Review.
4. Chen H, Chevrier A, Hoemann CD, Sun J, Ouyang W, Buschmann MD. Characterization of subchondral bone repair for marrow-stimulated chondral defects and its relationship to articular cartilage resurfacing. Am J Sports Med. 2011;39(8):1731–40.
5. Brittberg M, Faxén E, Peterson L. Carbon fiber scaffolds in the treatment of early knee osteoarthritis. A prospective 4-year follow-up of 37 patients. Clin Orthop Relat Res. 1994;307:155–64.
6. de Windt TS, Concaro S, Lindahl A, Saris DB, Brittberg M. Strategies for patient profiling in articular cartilage repair of the knee: a prospective cohort of patients treated by one experienced cartilage surgeon. Knee Surg Sports Traumatol Arthrosc. 2012;20:2225.
7. Minns RJ, Brittberg M. The use of carbon fibre rods and pads for the repair of articular cartilage defects. In: Zanasi S, Brittberg M, Marcacchi M, editors. Basic science, clinical repair and reconstruction of articular cartilage defects: current status and prospects, vol. I. Bologna: Timeo; 2006.
8. Benthien JP, Behrens P. The treatment of chondral and osteochondral defects of the knee with autologous matrix-induced chondrogenesis (AMIC): method description and recent developments. Knee Surg Sports Traumatol Arthrosc. 2011;19(8):1316–9.
9. Spalding T. TRUFIT plugs. In: Brittberg M, Gersoff W, editors. Cartilage surgery; an operative manual. Philadelphia, PA: Elsevier Saunders; 2011. p. 51–65.
10. Barber FA, Dockery WD. A computed tomography scan assessment of synthetic multiphase polymer scaffolds used for osteochondral defect repair. Arthroscopy. 2011;27(1):60–4.
11. Carmont MR, Carey-Smith R, Saithna A, Dhillon M, Thompson P, Spalding T. Delayed incorporation of a TruFit plug: perseverance is recommended. Arthroscopy. 2009;25(7):810–4.
12. Elguizaoui S, Flanigan DC, Harris JD, Parsons E, Litsky AS, Siston RA. Proud osteochondral autograft versus synthetic plugs - contact pressures with cyclical loading in a bovine knee model. Knee. 2012;19(6):812–7.
13. TiGenix. A prospective, post-marketing registry on the use of ChondroMimetic for the repair of osteochondral defects. http://clinicaltrials.gov/ct2/show/NCT01209390.
14. Manassero M, Decambron A, Guillemin N, Petite H, Bizios R, Viateau V. Coral scaffolds in bone tissue engineering and bone regeneration. In: Goffredo S, Dubinsky Z, editors. The cnidaria, past, present and future. Cham: Springer; 2016. p. 691–714.
15. Kon E, Filardo G, Shani J, Altschuler N, Levy A, Zaslav K, Eisman JE, Robinson D. Osteochondral regeneration with a novel aragonite-hyaluronate

biphasic scaffold: up to 12-month follow-up study in a goat model. J Orthop Surg Res. 2015;10:81.
16. Kon E, Robinson D, Verdonk P, Drobnic M, Patrascu JM, Dulic O, Gavrilovic G, Filardo G. A novel aragonite-based scaffold for osteochondral regeneration: early experience on human implants and technical developments. Injury. 2016;47(Suppl 6):S27–32.
17. Hoemann CD, Sun J, Légaré A, McKee MD, Buschmann MD. Tissue engineering of cartilage using an injectable and adhesive chitosan-based cell-delivery vehicle. Osteoarthr Cartil. 2005;13(4):318–29.
18. Marchand C, Chen G, Tran-Khanh N, Sun J, Chen H, Buschmann MD, Hoemann CD. Microdrilled cartilage defects treated with thrombin-solidified chitosan/blood implant regenerate a more hyaline, stable, and structurally integrated osteochondral unit compared to drilled controls. Tissue Eng Part A. 2012;18(5-6):508–19.
19. Shive MS, Stanish WD, McCormack R, Forriol F, Mohtadi N, Pelet S, Desnoyers J, Méthot S, Vehik K, Restrepo A. BST-CarGel® treatment maintains cartilage repair superiority over microfracture at 5 years in a multicenter randomized controlled trial. Cartilage. 2015;6(2):62–72.
20. Goldshmid R, Cohen S, Shachaf Y, Kupershmit I, Sarig-Nadir O, Seliktar D, Wechsler R. Steric interference of adhesion supports in-vitro chondrogenesis of mesenchymal stem cells on hydrogels for cartilage repair. Sci Rep. 2015;5:12607.
21. Kon E, Delcogliano M, Filardo G, Busacca M, Di Martino A, Marcacci M. Novel nano-composite multilayered biomaterial for osteochondral regeneration: a pilot clinical trial. Am J Sports Med. 2011;39(6):1180–90.
22. Kon E, Filardo G, Brittberg M, Busacca M, Condello V, Engebretsen L, Marlovits S, Niemeyer P, Platzer P, Posthumus M, Verdonk P, Verdonk R, Victor J, van der Merwe W, Widuchowski W, Zorzi C, Marcacci M. A multilayer biomaterial for osteochondral regeneration shows superiority vs microfractures for the treatment of osteochondral lesions in a multicentre randomized trial at 2 years. Knee Surg Sports Traumatol Arthrosc. 2018;26(9):2704–15.

One-Step Cell-Based Cartilage Repair in the Knee Using Hyaluronic Acid-Based Scaffold Embedded with Mesenchymal Stem Cells Sourced from Bone Marrow Aspirate Concentrate (HA-BMAC)

5

Graeme P. Whyte, Katarzyna Herman, and Alberto Gobbi

5.1 Introduction

Articular cartilage is a highly specialized tissue that minimizes frictional forces when ranging the knee and also distributes load-bearing forces. It is critical that these functions are adequately performed by articular cartilage in order to maintain the health and function of the knee joint, allowing for pain-free physical activity. Due to the avascular anatomic structure of articular cartilage tissue and the physiology of the constituent cells that have low mitotic potential, there is limited capacity for tissue healing. When injured, failure to restore damaged foci of articular cartilage leads to impaired force distribution, and greatly increased loads are sustained by the remaining healthy cartilage tissue, potentially leading to progression of cartilage injury and eventual development of osteoarthritis (OA) [1]. Chondral lesions may arise from acute injury or repetitive microtraumatic insults and may occur in association with other injuries, such as ligament rupture. Apart from discrete injurious events, damage to articular cartilage may be of a progressive nature due to malalignment about the affected joint or chronic joint instability.

When treating injury to articular cartilage, the clinician must recognize the variability of cartilage damage progression. While articular cartilage injury is frequently reported at times of arthroscopic knee surgery, the clinical prognosis can be difficult to specify, and it is difficult to predict progressive disease that would lead to joint failure, particularly in cases of lower-grade injury [1, 2]. It is important, however, to carefully monitor cases of symptomatic articular cartilage injury, as treatment is preferable earlier in the disease course when areas of injury are discrete and there remains healthy cartilage elsewhere about the articulating surfaces.

When faced with large areas of cartilage injury within the knee, and particularly when there are multiple lesions or lesions involving multiple compartments, some surgeons may focus primarily on reconstructive options such as unicompartmental knee arthroplasty (UKA) or total knee arthroplasty (TKA). In younger patients there is

G. P. Whyte (✉)
Orthopaedic Arthroscopic Surgery International (O.A.S.I.), Bioresearch Foundation, Milan, Italy

New York Presbyterian Hospital, Weill Medical College, Cornell University, New York, NY, USA
e-mail: info@whytemd.com

K. Herman · A. Gobbi
Orthopaedic Arthroscopic Surgery International (O.A.S.I.), Bioresearch Foundation, Milan, Italy
e-mail: gobbi@cartilagedoctor.it

M. Brittberg, K. Slynarski (eds.), *Lower Extremity Joint Preservation*,
https://doi.org/10.1007/978-3-030-57382-9_5

concern that TKA will lead to more rapid prosthetic wear, resulting in suboptimal rates of early failure [3, 4]. Moreover, many younger active patients do not want to seriously consider any type of arthroplasty treatment and are highly motivated to undergo treatment that will potentially preserve the native joint over the long-term, or at least delay the need for eventual arthroplasty treatment for a substantial period of time. Cartilage repair procedures are rapidly evolving, and the expected rates of success of such techniques are continually increasing, even in cases of more advanced articular cartilage injury, with or without concomitant injury or malalignment.

5.2 Cartilage Repair: An Ongoing Evolution of Technique

In the event of damaged articular cartilage, restoration of hyaline-like cartilage provides greater durability of the repair tissue which has improved wear characteristics. Prior to the development of more advanced current techniques, surgical treatment to repair cartilage injury initially concentrated on marrow stimulation by methods such as microfracture or subchondral drilling. There may be short-term benefit from marrow stimulation treatment; however, there is concern of a lack of durability of the fibrocartilage repair tissue that develops in response to these techniques [5, 6]. Durability of the repair tissue is of particular concern when using marrow stimulation to treat lesions sized greater than 2–4 cm^2.

Advancements in techniques to repair articular cartilage injury include methods using cell-free scaffolds, scaffolds in association with marrow stimulation, autologous minced cartilage, osteochondral grafting, and cell-based techniques such as autologous chondrocyte implantation (ACI), umbilical cord-derived Wharton's jelly stem cell isolates, and HA-BMAC [7–13].

Of the numerous forms of cartilage repair treatments that have been developed, many have not been shown over long-term clinical follow-up to be well-suited for the treatment of large or multiple chondral lesions within the knee. Regarding methods used to successfully restore high-quality repair tissue within the knee in cases of all sizes and types, cell-based techniques have demonstrated encouraging long-term outcomes.

Cell-based cartilage restoration technologies such as ACI and scaffold-associated bone marrow aspirate concentrate (BMAC) have demonstrated the capability of providing durable cartilage repair tissue [14–21]. Importantly, however, there are several limitations related to use of ACI and matrix-induced autologous chondrocyte implantation (MACI). Due to the harvesting and processing of autologous chondrocytes when performing ACI/MACI, this procedure requires the patient to undergo two surgical procedures, increasing the morbidity of the treatment and also adding substantially to the socioeconomic costs. Preferably, cartilage repair is performed in a single stage and accomplishes the goals of restoring hyaline-like repair tissue that is durable and is of sufficient quality to function long-term.

5.3 Mesenchymal Stem Cells and Associated Bioactive Factors

It is thought that mesenchymal stem cells (MSCs) are a derivative of perivascular cells that reside in close proximity to blood vessels in a quiescent state, which have been called *pericytes* [22, 23]. In the event of blood vessel compromise, which occurs in response to physical injury, pericytes become activated and acquire the phenotype of a MSC. The effects of MSCs on tissue regeneration are thought to be largely related to the trophic and paracrine functions of these cells [22, 24]. These cells are capable of secreting a great array of cytokines and locally active growth factors into the surrounding microenvironment [25, 26], which are capable of influencing articular cartilage regeneration, affecting both reconstitution of cellular elements and also generation of supportive chondral matrix. Activated MSCs release bioactive factors that counteract aggressive immune response, inhibit apoptosis and scar formation, and stimulate angiogenesis and tissue regeneration [25, 27].

MSCs are readily accessible, and this makes them an attractive target for therapeutic use, including for cases of high-grade articular cartilage injury that have traditionally been extraordinarily difficult to treat [28–30]. The regenerative capabilities of MSCs sourced from bone marrow aspirate concentrate are utilized in HA-BMAC cartilage repair.

5.4 HA-BMAC Cartilage Repair

Currently, our preferred technique is a one-stage cartilage repair procedure using a three-dimensional hyaluronic acid-based scaffold (Hyalofast, Anika Therapeutics, Bedford, Massachusetts, USA) that is embedded with activated bone marrow aspirate concentrate (HA-BMAC). Bone marrow aspirate concentrate is an easily assessable source of MSCs, and these cells have been shown to interact with hyaluronic acid-based scaffolding in such a manner that promotes cellular adhesion, proliferation, migration, and the generation of extracellular matrix components [31–33].

Cell-based repair in the setting of a single-stage procedure using MSCs sourced from BMAC has demonstrated comparable outcomes, short- and medium-term, to those expected using methods that are using cultured autologous chondrocytes [10, 19, 21, 34]. Importantly, more recent examination of outcomes at our institution has confirmed that clinical success is maintained long-term. This technique is performed in a single stage, without costly cellular processing and without the socioeconomic costs and increased morbidity to the patient. Analysis of clinical outcomes using the Hyalofast scaffold for MACI compared to HA-BMAC has been examined previously by [10]. After a minimum of 3 years of follow-up, findings demonstrated similar clinical outcomes and histologic quality of repair tissue between these treatment types [10].

A recent prospective analysis of clinical outcomes after HA-BMAC cartilage repair in comparison to microfracture treatment for lesions in the knee at our institution demonstrated superiority of HA-BMAC after medium-term follow-up of 5 years. HA-BMAC led to successful outcomes irrespective of patient age or lesion size. These successful outcomes were maintained from short- to medium-term follow-up in the HA-BMAC group, whereas there was declining success after 2 years of follow-up in the microfracture group [21].

The malleable nature of the HA-BMAC graft and the three-dimensional symmetry allow for this implant to be used arthroscopically in properly indicated lesions and also in cases of osteochondral repair [35, 36]. Sadlik et al. have described a technique of osteochondral repair using HA-BMAC in conjunction with grafting of a morselized bone graft. This technique is referred to as biologic inlay osteochondral reconstruction (BIOR) and has been used to treat large osteochondral lesions in the knee and other joints such as the ankle. BIOR can also be used arthroscopically, given the physical characteristics of the prepared bone graft inlay and the HA-BMAC implant [36, 37].

5.5 HA-BMAC Cartilage Repair: Preoperative Considerations

5.5.1 Diagnostic Imaging

5.5.1.1 Plain Radiography

Plain radiographic imaging of the knee should include anteroposterior, lateral, merchant, and notch views. Full-length lower extremity radiographs are routinely obtained when there is concern of even a small degree of malalignment. In cases of osteochondral injury, plain radiographs can contribute important information related to the size of subchondral injury; however, to best examine the condition of articular cartilage and the status of underlying subchondral bone, more advanced diagnostic imaging is recommended.

5.5.1.2 Magnetic Resonance Imaging

MRI is used to thoroughly examine the status of the articular cartilage at the site of injury and to examine for associated subchondral pathology. Proton density, fast spin echo, and T2-weighted images provide important diagnostic information

[38]. Advances in MRI techniques that use delayed gadolinium-enhanced MRI of cartilage (dGEMRIC) and T2 relaxation time mapping have been developed. These techniques enable examination of glycosaminoglycan and collagen content and map anatomic zones of articular cartilage [39].

5.5.2 Correction of Malalignment: The Role of Osteotomy

Whichever method of cartilage repair is to be used, it is critically important to sufficiently offload the area of repair when there is any degree of malalignment. Redistributing and normalizing the forces that act across the knee compartments will help to optimize the production, maturation, and remodeling of articular cartilage repair tissue. Depending on the correction that is required, realignment treatment options will typically include distal femoral osteotomy (DFO), high tibial osteotomy (HTO), and tibial tubercle osteotomy (TTO). It may be necessary to perform multiple procedures to correct bony malalignment, depending on the degree of deformity. It is important for the treating surgeon to recognize all areas of cartilage injury within the knee joint, as offloading forces to an area affected by injured cartilage may be contraindicated, depending on the extent of injury.

Prior to the expansion in use of cartilage repair techniques, clinical outcomes after osteotomy about the knee have been variable and at times had been shown to be markedly inferior in cases of corrective osteotomy in the setting of associated articular cartilage injury. In treating patellofemoral maltracking abnormalities, there have been poorer outcomes demonstrated when there is associated articular cartilage injury, particularly when located to areas of the articulation that are exposed to increased forces after the osteotomy [40]. Importantly, however, our center and others have shown that good to excellent clinical outcomes may be achieved when bony malalignment involving the patellofemoral articulation is corrected in the setting of significant articular cartilage injury, as long as appropriate articular cartilage repair is performed in conjunction with the realignment procedure [10, 14, 19, 41]. When combined with corrective osteotomy, cell-based articular cartilage repair techniques such as HA-BMAC can be successfully used to treat large and multiple areas of cartilage injury within the knee, even in cases that may have previously been considered only suitable for an arthroplasty procedure.

5.6 HA-BMAC Surgical Technique

The patient is positioned supine as for a standard knee arthroscopy procedure. The ipsilateral iliac crest is exposed and incorporated into the sterile field in anticipation of bone marrow aspiration. General anesthesia is typically used. An examination of the knee is performed under anesthesia to identify or confirm associated injury that will be treated concurrently. A diagnostic arthroscopy is performed to carefully examine all areas of articular cartilage injury. The appropriate surgical approach is determined. Arthroscopic treatment may be considered if the entirety of all cartilage lesions are visualized and are positioned such that the defects can be completely prepared about the periphery, as would be performed in the case of exposure by arthrotomy. The cartilage lesion(s) is prepared by removing unstable chondral tissue about the site of injury and creating vertical walls of healthy cartilage about the defect. The base of the lesion is debrided evenly by removing the calcified cartilage layer while avoiding penetration of the subchondral end plate. The technique of cartilage lesion preparation is a crucial component to the cartilage repair procedure that will impact the quality of the regenerated repair tissue, and this should be performed in meticulous fashion [42]. Specialized instruments may be used to assist with lesion preparation if an arthroscopic approach is used [43], and the security of graft fixation within the prepared defect must also be carefully considered when using an arthroscopic approach [44]. Bone marrow aspirate is obtained from the ipsilateral iliac crest and is processed in a commercially available system (BMAC Harvest Smart PreP2

System®—Harvest Technologies, Plymouth, MA) to produce an isolate of BMAC. Typically, 60 cm^3 of bone marrow aspirate is used to create the final isolate. The dimensions of the defect(s) are measured, and the lesion(s) is templated. Sterile aluminum foil or a sterile dental dam can assist to template the lesion. The hyaluronic acid-based scaffold (Hyalofast, Anika Therapeutics, Bedford, Massachusetts, USA) is size-matched to the defect(s). BMAC is clot-activated with batroxobin enzyme (Plateltex Act, Plateltex SRO, Bratislava, Slovakia) and is combined with the size-matched scaffold to create the HA-BMAC graft. In the absence of batroxobin enzyme, autologous thrombin may be used. The HA-BMAC graft is then implanted into the defect(s). In cases of arthroscopic implantation, a valveless cannula will assist to equalize pressure within the joint and to improve visualization, as the graft is implanted under dry arthroscopy. Whether an open or arthroscopic approach is used, the repair site must be examined under direct visualization while ranging the knee through flexion and extension to ensure that the implant is secured. Fibrin glue and/or 6-0 absorbable suture may be used at the surgeon's discretion to improve the stability of implant fixation if required. HA-BMAC cartilage repair is depicted in Fig. 5.1.

5.6.1 Rehabilitation Protocol

The initial postoperative period up to 6 weeks will focus on restoring full range of motion and strength/conditioning while also minimizing joint effusion. Continuous passive motion (CPM) begins on the second postoperative day and is prescribed for 6 h per day until 90° of knee flexion is regained. When HA-BMAC cartilage repair is performed in the patellofemoral compartment, partial weight-bearing begins on postoperative day 1 with the knee immobilized in full extension. When repair is performed in the medial or lateral compartment, weight bearing is restricted for the first 4 weeks postoperatively and then is progressed to full weight bearing by 6 weeks. There is focus on isometric and isotonic exercises during the early postoperative period.

Active functional training will begin 9 weeks postoperatively. There is progression of strength and endurance training from 3 to 8 months postoperatively, and straight-line running at a moderate pace is expected to be pain-free by 8 months. The patient will then progress to agility and sport-specific training exercises, with return to sport expected at 10 months, after appropriate restoration of strength, endurance, and proprioception.

5.7 Summary

Cartilage repair procedures are performed to restore articular cartilage to areas of high-grade injury in order to prevent, or slow the progression of, degenerative cartilage injury that will eventually lead to significant functional limitation in many of those affected. Marrow stimulations techniques are simple to perform; however, the repair tissue is of predominantly fibrocartilage and is not of sufficient quality to reliably provide long-term benefit, particularly in larger lesions. Cell-based techniques, such as those that use autologous chondrocyte culture and implantation, have demonstrated encouraging long-term results and can be used in the case of large lesions and in cases of associated bony malalignment that is corrected at the time of cartilage repair. There are numerous disadvantages of two-stage procedures such as ACI, given the costs associated with cell processing and multiple surgeries, as well as the socioeconomic impact and increased surgical risk to the patient. There is ongoing investigation into the development of single-stage cartilage repair procedures that dependably restore durable articular cartilage tissue. Cartilage repair using a hyaluronic acid-based scaffold embedded with bone marrow aspirate concentrate (HA-BMAC) has been used at our institution to treat a wide range of cartilage lesions types, including multiple lesions that affect multiple knee compartments, and in cases of bony malalignment that require operative

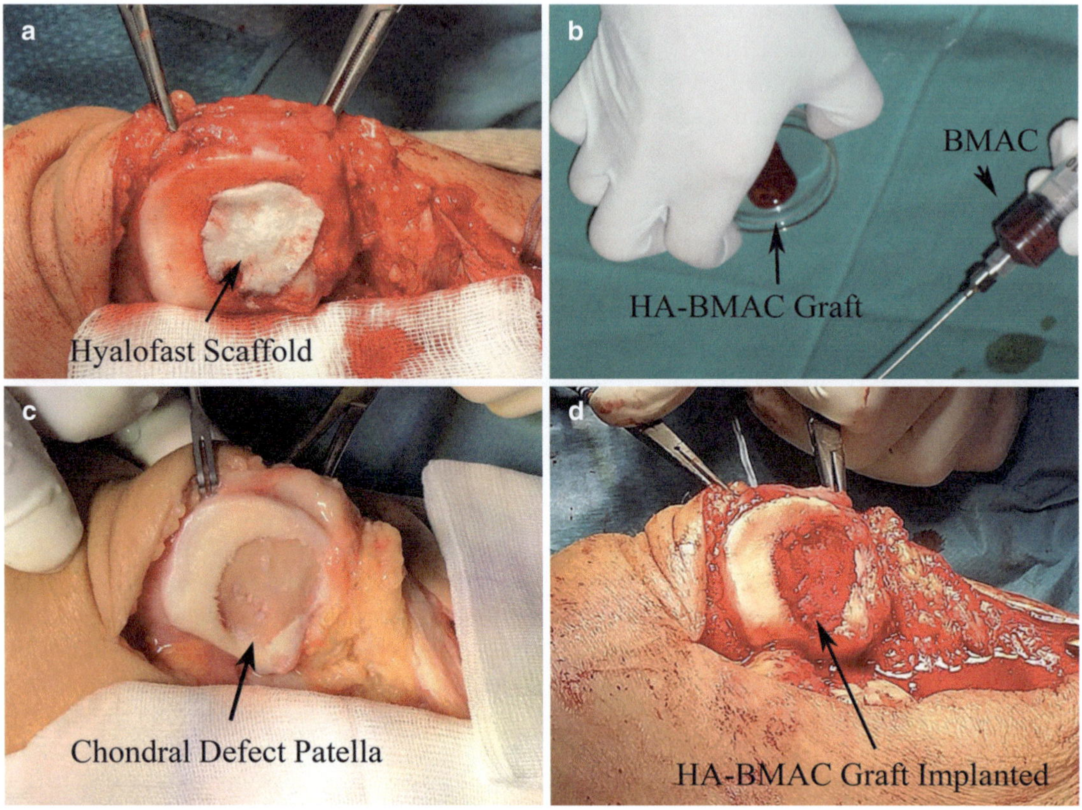

Fig. 5.1 (**a**) Hyaluronic acid-based scaffold (Hyalofast) size-matched to chondral defect of patella. (**b**) Bone marrow aspirate concentrate (BMAC) combined with hyaluronic acid-based scaffold to create HA-BMAC graft. (**c**) Prepared chondral defect of patella. (**d**) HA-BMAC graft secured within patellar chondral defect

correction. Moreover, success of this procedure has been demonstrated across a wide range of patient ages. Further investigation into these single-stage methods of cell-based cartilage repair is necessary to better develop currently available techniques and to clearly delineate the limitations that need to be improved upon.

References

1. Mankin HJ. The response of articular cartilage to mechanical injury. J Bone Joint Surg Am. 1982;64(3):460–6. http://www.ncbi.nlm.nih.gov/pubmed/6174527.
2. Widuchowski W, Widuchowski J, Trzaska T. Articular cartilage defects: study of 25,124 knee arthroscopies. Knee. 2007;14(3):177–82. http://linkinghub.elsevier.com/retrieve/pii/S0968016007000270.
3. Julin J, Jämsen E, Puolakka T, Konttinen YT, Moilanen T. Younger age increases the risk of early prosthesis failure following primary total knee replacement for osteoarthritis. A follow-up study of 32,019 total knee replacements in the Finnish Arthroplasty Register. Acta Orthop. 2010;81(4):413–9. http://www.pubmedcentral.nih.gov/articlerender.fcgi?artid=2917562&tool=pmcentrez&rendertype=abstract.
4. Odland AN, Callaghan JJ, Liu SS, Wells CW. Wear and lysis is the problem in modular TKA in the young OA patient at 10 years. Clin Orthop Relat Res. 2011;469(1):41–7. http://www.pubmedcentral.nih.gov/articlerender.fcgi?artid=3008910&tool=pmcentrez&rendertype=abstract.
5. Gobbi A, Karnatzikos G, Kumar A. Long-term results after microfracture treatment for full-thickness knee chondral lesions in athletes. Knee Surg Sport Traumatol Arthrosc. 2014;22(9):1986–96. http://link.springer.com/10.1007/s00167-013-2676-8.
6. Gobbi A, Nunag P, Malinowski K. Treatment of full thickness chondral lesions of the knee with microfracture in a group of athletes. Knee Surg Sport Traumatol Arthrosc. 2005;13(3):213–21. http://link.springer.com/10.1007/s00167-004-0499-3.
7. Efe T, Theisen C, Fuchs-Winkelmann S, Stein T, Getgood A, Rominger MB, et al. Cell-free collagen type I matrix for repair of cartilage defects—clinical and magnetic resonance imaging results. Knee Surg

Sport Traumatol Arthrosc. 2012;20(10):1915–22. http://link.springer.com/10.1007/s00167-011-1777-5.
8. Sadlik B, Wiewiorski M. Implantation of a collagen matrix for an AMIC repair during dry arthroscopy. Knee Surg Sport Traumatol Arthrosc. 2015;23(8):2349–52. http://link.springer.com/10.1007/s00167-014-3062-x.
9. Cole BJ, Farr J, Winalski CS, Hosea T, Richmond J, Mandelbaum B, et al. Outcomes after a single-stage procedure for cell-based cartilage repair: a prospective clinical safety trial with 2-year follow-up. Am J Sports Med. 2011;39(6):1170–9. http://ajs.sagepub.com/lookup/doi/10.1177/0363546511399382.
10. Gobbi A, Chaurasia S, Karnatzikos G, Nakamura N. Matrix-induced autologous chondrocyte implantation versus multipotent stem cells for the treatment of large patellofemoral chondral lesions: a nonrandomized prospective trial. Cartilage. 2015;6(2):82–97. http://car.sagepub.com/cgi/doi/10.1177/1947603514563597.
11. Gobbi A, Scotti C, Lane JG, Peretti GM. Fresh osteochondral allografts in the knee: only a salvage procedure? Ann Transl Med. 2015;3(12):164.
12. Murphy RT, Pennock AT, Bugbee WD. Osteochondral allograft transplantation of the Knee in the pediatric and adolescent population. Am J Sports Med. 2014;42(3):635–40. http://ajs.sagepub.com/lookup/doi/10.1177/0363546513516747.
13. Sadlik B, Jaroslawski G, Puszkarz M, Blasiak A, Oldak T, Gladysz D, Whyte GP. Cartilage repair in the knee using umbilical cord Wharton's jelly–derived mesenchymal stem cells embedded onto collagen scaffolding and implanted under dry arthroscopy. Arthrosc Tech. 2018;7(1):e57–63. http://linkinghub.elsevier.com/retrieve/pii/S2212628717303237.
14. Gomoll AH, Gillogly SD, Cole BJ, Farr J, Arnold R, Hussey K, et al. Autologous chondrocyte implantation in the patella: a multicenter experience. Am J Sports Med. 2014;42(5):1074–81. http://ajs.sagepub.com/lookup/doi/10.1177/0363546514523927.
15. Gobbi A, Bathan L. Biological approaches for cartilage repair. J Knee Surg. 2009;22(01):36–44. http://www.thieme-connect.de/DOI/DOI?10.1055/s-0030-1247726.
16. Kon E, Gobbi A, Filardo G, Delcogliano M, Zaffagnini S, Marcacci M. Arthroscopic second-generation autologous chondrocyte implantation compared with microfracture for chondral lesions of the knee: prospective nonrandomized study at 5 Years. Am J Sports Med. 2009;37(1):33–41. http://ajs.sagepub.com/lookup/doi/10.1177/0363546508323256.
17. Filardo G, Vannini F, Marcacci M, Andriolo L, Ferruzzi A, Giannini S, et al. Matrix-assisted autologous chondrocyte transplantation for cartilage regeneration in osteoarthritic knees: results and failures at midterm follow-up. Am J Sports Med. 2013;41(1):95–100. http://ajs.sagepub.com/lookup/doi/10.1177/0363546512463675.
18. Marcacci M, Berruto M, Brocchetta D, Delcogliano A, Ghinelli D, Gobbi A, et al. Articular cartilage engineering with Hyalograft(R) C: 3-year clinical results. Clin Orthop Relat Res. 2005;(435):96–105. http://ovidsp.dc2.ovid.com/ovid-b/ovidweb.cgi?QS2=434f4e1a73d37e8c51165efa93679dd0a5c34306f560e888dcd4c289708cbd8f2a374e69ece52cfa9d56ff5038571ef84d7091dfca3b9e0d9def3ecd7e6b25b727a2b3a4b-9b9a6c58a5ee253612a945f32c5a652e4c53c4347a3c0019da7d012e0817871f8526.
19. Gobbi A, Karnatzikos G, Sankineani SR. One-step surgery with multipotent stem cells for the treatment of large full-thickness chondral defects of the knee. Am J Sports Med. 2014;42(3):648–57. http://ajs.sagepub.com/lookup/doi/10.1177/0363546513518007.
20. Gobbi A, Karnatzikos G, Scotti C, Mahajan V, Mazzucco L, Grigolo B. One-step cartilage repair with bone marrow aspirate concentrated cells and collagen matrix in full-thickness knee cartilage lesions: results at 2-year follow-up. Cartilage. 2011;2(3):286–99. http://www.pubmedcentral.nih.gov/articlerender.fcgi?artid=4300809&tool=pmcentrez&rendertype=abstract.
21. Gobbi A, Whyte GP. One-stage cartilage repair using a hyaluronic acid-based scaffold with activated bone marrow-derived mesenchymal stem cells compared with microfracture: five-year follow-up. Am J Sports Med. 2016;44(11):2846–54. http://www.ncbi.nlm.nih.gov/pubmed/27474386.
22. Caplan AI. MSCs: the sentinel and safe-guards of injury. J Cell Physiol. 2016;231(7):1413–6. http://www.ncbi.nlm.nih.gov/pubmed/26565391.
23. Chen WCW, Péault B, Huard J. Regenerative translation of human blood-vessel-derived MSC precursors. Stem Cells Int. 2015;2015:375187. http://www.ncbi.nlm.nih.gov/pubmed/26273304.
24. Caplan AI. Adult mesenchymal stem cells: when, where, and how. Stem Cells Int. 2015;2015:628767. http://www.ncbi.nlm.nih.gov/pubmed/26273305.
25. Caplan AI, Correa D. The MSC: an injury drugstore. Cell Stem Cell. 2011;9(1):11–5. http://www.ncbi.nlm.nih.gov/pubmed/21726829.
26. de Girolamo L, Lucarelli E, Alessandri G, Avanzini MA, Bernardo ME, Biagi E, et al. Mesenchymal stem/stromal cells: a new "'cells as drugs'" paradigm. Efficacy and critical aspects in cell therapy. Curr Pharm Des. 2013;19(13):2459–73. http://www.ncbi.nlm.nih.gov/pubmed/23278600.
27. Kean TJ, Lin P, Caplan AI, Dennis JE. MSCs: delivery routes and engraftment, cell-targeting strategies, and immune modulation. Stem Cells Int. 2013;2013:732742. http://www.ncbi.nlm.nih.gov/pubmed/24000286.
28. Whyte GP, Gobbi A. Biologic knee arthroplasty for cartilage injury and early osteoarthritis. In: Bio-orthopaedics. Berlin: Springer; 2017. p. 517–25. http://link.springer.com/10.1007/978-3-662-54181-4_41.
29. Gobbi A, Whyte GP. Osteochondritis dissecans: pathoanatomy, classification, and advances in biologic surgical treatment. In: Bio-orthopaedics. Berlin: Springer; 2017. p. 489–501. http://link.springer.com/10.1007/978-3-662-54181-4_39.
30. Gobbi A, Espregueira-Mendes J, Karahan M, Cohen M, Whyte GP. Osteochondritis dissecans of the knee

in football players. In: Injuries and health problems in football. Berlin: Springer; 2017. p. 189–200. http://link.springer.com/10.1007/978-3-662-53924-8_17.
31. Pasquinelli G, Orrico C, Foroni L, Bonafè F, Carboni M, Guarnieri C, et al. Mesenchymal stem cell interaction with a non-woven hyaluronan-based scaffold suitable for tissue repair. J Anat. 2008;213(5):520–30. http://www.ncbi.nlm.nih.gov/pubmed/19014359.
32. Lisignoli G, Cristino S, Piacentini A, Zini N, Noël D, Jorgensen C, et al. Chondrogenic differentiation of murine and human mesenchymal stromal cells in a hyaluronic acid scaffold: differences in gene expression and cell morphology. J Biomed Mater Res A. 2006;77(3):497–506. http://www.ncbi.nlm.nih.gov/pubmed/16482549.
33. Facchini A, Lisignoli G, Cristino S, Roseti L, De Franceschi L, Marconi E, et al. Human chondrocytes and mesenchymal stem cells grown onto engineered scaffold. Biorheology. 2006;43(3–4):471–80.
34. Gobbi A, Scotti C, Karnatzikos G, Mudhigere A, Castro M, Peretti GM. One-step surgery with multipotent stem cells and Hyaluronan-based scaffold for the treatment of full-thickness chondral defects of the knee in patients older than 45 years. Knee Surg Sports Traumatol Arthrosc. 2017;25(8):2494–501. http://www.ncbi.nlm.nih.gov/pubmed/26768608.
35. Whyte GP, Gobbi A, Sadlik B. Dry arthroscopic single-stage cartilage repair of the knee using a hyaluronic acid-based scaffold with activated bone marrow-derived mesenchymal stem cells. Arthrosc Tech. 2016;5(4):e913–8. http://www.ncbi.nlm.nih.gov/pubmed/27709058.
36. Sadlik B, Gobbi A, Puszkarz M, Klon W, Whyte GP. Biologic inlay osteochondral reconstruction: arthroscopic one-step osteochondral lesion repair in the knee using morselized bone grafting and hyaluronic acid-based scaffold embedded with bone marrow aspirate concentrate. Arthrosc Tech. 2017;6(2):e383–9. http://linkinghub.elsevier.com/retrieve/pii/S2212628716302055.
37. Sadlik B, Kolodziej L, Puszkarz M, Laprus H, Mojzesz M, Whyte GP. Surgical repair of osteochondral lesions of the talus using biologic inlay osteochondral reconstruction: clinical outcomes after treatment using a medial malleolar osteotomy approach compared to an arthroscopically-assisted approach. Foot Ankle Surg. 2019;25:449. http://linkinghub.elsevier.com/retrieve/pii/S1268773118300365.
38. Schwarz C, Blazina ME, Sisto DJ, Hirsh LC. The results of operative treatment of osteochondritis dissecans of the patella. Am J Sports Med. 1988;16(5):522–9. http://www.ncbi.nlm.nih.gov/pubmed/3189687.
39. Aglietti P, Buzzi R, Bassi PB, Fioriti M. Arthroscopic drilling in juvenile osteochondritis dissecans of the medial femoral condyle. Arthrosc. 1994;10(3):286–91. http://www.ncbi.nlm.nih.gov/pubmed/8086022.
40. Pidoriano AJ, Weinstein RN, Buuck DA, Fulkerson JP. Correlation of patellar articular lesions with results from anteromedial tibial tubercle transfer. Am J Sports Med. 1997;25(4):533–7.
41. Gobbi A, Kon E, Berruto M, Francisco R, Filardo G, Marcacci M. Patellofemoral full-thickness chondral defects treated with Hyalograft-C: a clinical, arthroscopic, and histologic review. Am J Sports Med. 2006;34(11):1763–73. http://ajs.sagepub.com/lookup/doi/10.1177/0363546506288853.
42. Sadlik B, Matlak A, Blasiak A, Klon W, Puszkarz M, Whyte GP. Arthroscopic cartilage lesion preparation in the human cadaveric knee using a curette technique demonstrates clinically relevant histologic variation. Arthroscopy. 2018;34:2179. http://linkinghub.elsevier.com/retrieve/pii/S0749806318301208.
43. Blasiak A, Whyte GP, Matlak A, Brzóska R, Sadlik B. Morphologic properties of cartilage lesions in the knee arthroscopically prepared by the standard curette technique are inferior to lesions prepared by specialized chondrectomy instruments. Am J Sports Med. 2017;1:363546517745489. http://www.ncbi.nlm.nih.gov/pubmed/29281796.
44. Whyte GP, McGee A, Jazrawi L, Meislin R. Comparison of collagen graft fixation methods in the porcine knee: implications for matrix-assisted chondrocyte implantation and second-generation autologous chondrocyte implantation. Arthroscopy. 2016;32(5):820–7. http://linkinghub.elsevier.com/retrieve/pii/S0749806315008117.

6 Chondrocyte Implantation

Mats Brittberg

6.1 Indication and Basic Science

The repair capacity of injured cartilage is poor [1, 2], and damaged cartilage could by time give substantial joint disability and pain. Basic in all tissue repairs is the involvement of cells. When a vascularized tissue is damaged, cells are migrating into the hematomas formed. Cartilage, a tissue being without blood vessels, is subsequently lacking such forming hematomas important for attracting cells when injured [3].

Most often chondral and osteochondral injuries have been treated by introducing chondrogenic cells from the bone marrow [4]. The results are unpredictable as the amount of cells migrating from the bone marrow is depending on many variables such as number of existing cells, age of patients, and quality of scaffolds used for repair augmentation.

As the chondrocytes are few and their migratory capacity in the matrix is low, use of single chondrocytes for repair for long was not attractive. However with the knowledge of how to isolate chondrocytes from their matrix [5] and expand the cells in vitro [6–11], the possibility to use the true cartilage repair cells increased. Through increased experience of the chondrocytes behaviors in in vitro and an in vivo animal experiments [6–11], the first autologous chondrocyte implantation in humans was performed in October, 1987 [12]. Since that first operation, the technique has been developed, and there are now four generations of ACI to know about with generation 3 being the most used. The fourth-generation ACI is mainly one-stage procedures with direct isolation of cells and implantation. Included into that group of ACI also belongs Cartilage Autograft Implantation system (CAIS).

In vitro cell expansion and scaffold seeding are expensive procedures, and, subsequently, ACI has been mainly used for failed other cartilage procedures, so-called secondhand surgeries. However, the main indications today are:

1. Large chondral defects >3 cm
2. Large osteochondral defects >3 + bone grafting if defect depth >8 mm
3. All types of chondral and osteochondral defects with failed other types of cartilage repair

There is no special age limit besides that the surrounding cartilage should be of good quality.

It might then be important to differ between:

- Healthy cartilage
- Degenerative cartilage (e.g., this type of cartilage could be seen after ACL and meniscal injuries and after repeated patella dislocation

M. Brittberg (✉)
Cartilage Research Unit, Region Halland Orthopaedics, Kungsbacka Hospital, University of Gothenburg, Kungsbacka, Sweden
e-mail: mats.brittberg@telia.com

M. Brittberg, K. Slynarski (eds.), *Lower Extremity Joint Preservation*,
https://doi.org/10.1007/978-3-030-57382-9_6

with local derangement of cartilage structure but not a generalized joint disease)
- OA cartilage (pre-OA, early OA, late OA)

ACI treatments can be used with surrounding healthy and also with surrounding degenerative cartilage sometimes on its way to pre-OA/early localized OA. A generalized early OA and further on to established full OA are not indications for an ACI.

As with other cartilage repairs, concomitant malalignment should be treated by unloading osteotomies in combination with the ACI procedure.

Very large cartilage defects may also benefit for an ACI in conjunction with an unloading osteotomy.

The gold standard for determining if a patient is a suitable candidate for ACI has to finally to be done by an arthroscopic evaluation as MRI is still not having enough sensitivity or specificity for a complete cartilage injury evaluation.

Important to evaluate with an arthroscopic procedure are:

- Location
- Depth
- Size of the lesion
- The quality of the surrounding cartilage
- The degree of undermining cartilage
- Status of opposing chondral surface

6.2 General Techniques

Common for all cartilage repairs is a meticulous debridement of the cartilage lesion area. The first generation of ACI was a combination therapy with into the debrided lesion, injection of in vitro expanded chondrocytes in a suspension under a sutured membrane of thin periosteum [11, 12]. The cambium layer containing chondrogenic cells was facing the defect [11, 12] (Fig. 6.1a, b).

The operative techniques for both open procedure with periosteum or collagen membrane and new-generation techniques with trans-arthroscopic scaffolds are briefly presented.

6.2.1 Cartilage Harvest

The steps include an initial arthroscopically harvested cartilage biopsy from which chondrocytes can be isolated by enzymatic digestion and in in vitro culture expanded several times the initial number of cells. In a clinical setting today, the aim is to transplant in a density of 30×10^6 cells/mL or at least 2×10^6 cells/cm^2 (suspension ACI, first generation).

6.2.2 Harvest Sites

The most common sites for cartilage biopsy are the superomedial edge of the femoral condyle and the lateral intercondylar notch in the same location where a notchplasty is performed during anterior cruciate ligament (ACL) reconstruction. Another recommended area is the super lateral edge of the femoral condyle that is non-articulating with the tibia or patella. An arthroscopic gouge or ring curette is used to obtain two or three small pieces of partial to full-thickness cartilage with the size of a fingernail clipping (200–300 mg). At the same time, 16×6 mL of autologous venous blood is collected for preparation of serum to be used together with the culture medium. Osteochondral loose bodies might also be used as a possible cell source [13].

6.2.3 In Vitro Cell Expansion

The goal of in vitro chondrocyte manipulation is to increase the cell number. The culture technique has been developed first for implantation of cells in suspensions, first generation of ACI with periosteal or collagen membrane covering. However, today both second- and third-generation ACI exist with cells cultured on a carrier membrane (MACI) [14] or with cells in a 3D scaffold like Hyaff-11 [15].

In common for all generations is that the chondrocytes are isolated by collagenase digestion overnight and cultured in DMEM/F12 with

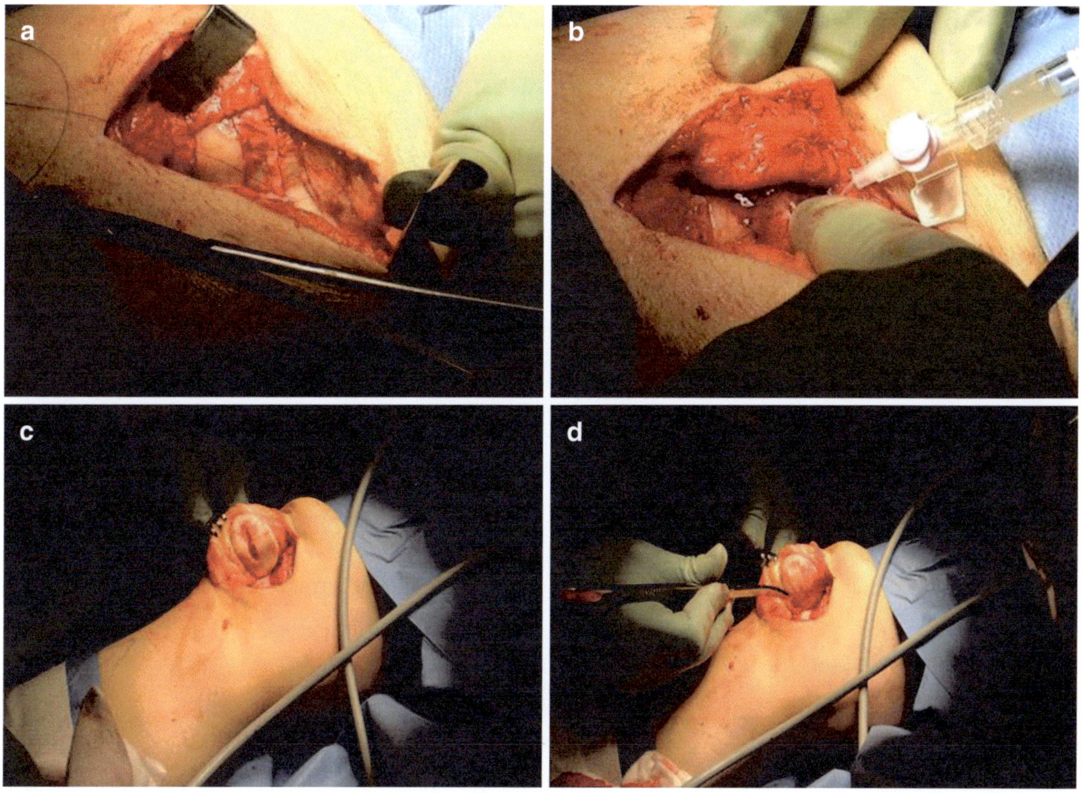

Fig. 6.1 (**a**) Cartilage lesion on a femoral condyle treated by first-generation ACI with periosteum sutured over the defect. (**b**) The lesion on (**a**) is now treated by injection of a suspension of chondrocytes into the defect area covered by a suture periosteum. (**c**) A cartilage lesion on a patella has been debrided. (**d**) The patella cartilage lesion has been filled with a chondrocyte-seeded Hyaff-11 graft and smoothed to fit exact the defect area

10% autologous serum supplement. Primary cultures are performed in 25 cm^2 culture flasks, and after 1 week cell expansion, the cells are trypsinized and passaged to 75 cm^2 culture flasks at a cell density of 8000 cells/cm^2.

For the suspension culture, after another 2 weeks of cell culture, the cells are trypsinized, washed, and resuspended to a treatment density of 30 million cells/mL. The cells are under sterile conditions put into a syringe to be used as a suspension injection of cells into a defect covered by a periosteal or collagen membrane.

For cells on a carrier membrane like MACI, the cells are cultured for about 3–5 weeks before being seeded on an I–III collagen membrane [14]. Regarding a 3D scaffold as an example, Hyaff-11 can be used. Here the biopsy material is taken to the laboratory for in vitro isolation and expansion of autologous chondrocytes for a duration of 1 week. Finally, the cells are seeded into the Hyaff-11 scaffold (HYAFF, Anika Therapeutics, Bedford, MA, USA) for 3–4-week culture, where they adhere, continue to proliferate, and redifferentiate into mature chondrocytes capable of producing their own extracellular matrix. This nonwoven 3D structure consists of a network of 20-μm-thick fibers with interstices of variable sizes, which constitute an optimal physical support to allow cell-to-cell contact, cluster formation, and extracellular matrix deposition [16].

There are other scaffolds used for chondrocytes in a similar manner [17, 18].

6.2.4 The Chondrocyte Implantation

For ACI generation 1 [12], implantation consists of an arthrotomy, defect preparation, periosteal flap harvest, fixation of periosteal flap to defect, securing a watertight seal with fibrin glue, implanting the chondrocytes, and wound closure (Fig. 6.1a, b). However, the periosteum was after a while replaced by a resorbable membrane such as collagen I/III membrane Chondro-Gide (Geistlich, Wolhausen, Switzerland) or Restore (DePuy, Warzaw, Indiana). Those implants are called second-generation ACI.

The cells are distributed in the defect area in the fibrin glue to establish an even distribution.

Third-generation ACIs are cell-seeded membranes such as matrix-induced ACI (MACI© Vericel, Boston, MA, USA) and chondrocytes cultured in 3D matrices such as in a hyaluronic acid ester (Hyalograft©, Anika Therapeutics, Bedford, MA, USA). Such techniques have facilitated the procedure as those methods can be used transarthroscopically and there is no need for fixation with sutures (Figs. 6.1c, d, 6.2a, b, 6.3a–d).

The MACI implant is a cell carrier where the cells are growing on the surface of the implant [14]. The implant is placed in the defect with the cell side facing the defect. The defect has prior to implantation been filled with fibrin glue. Quite fast after implantation, the cells leave the scaffold in migrate into the glue to start chondrogenesis. Other scaffolds, like Hyaff-11, have allowed the cells during the in vitro culture to migrate into the scaffold. A scaffold like Hyaff-11 can subsequently be implanted with any surface fac-

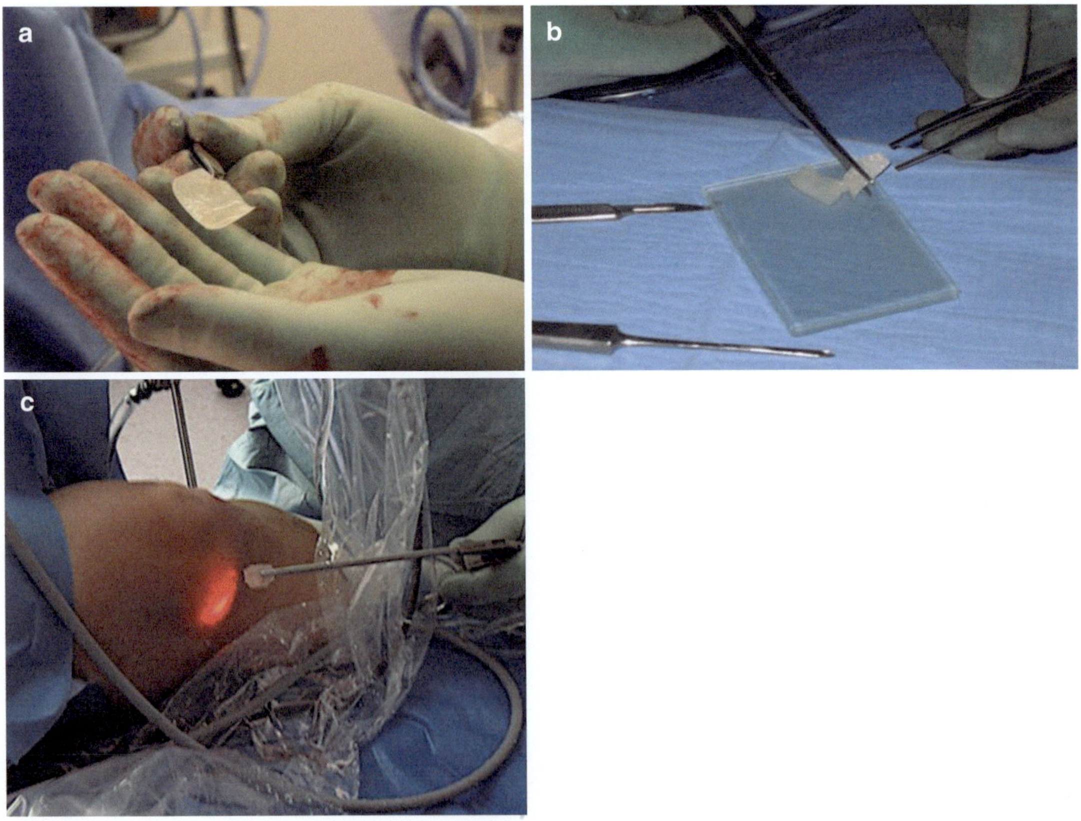

Fig. 6.2 (**a**) A chondrocyte-seeded Hyaff-11 scaffold is gripped and should be cut into the size of a trochlea cartilage defect. (**b**) The cell-seeded graft is now cut into an approximate size of the debrided lesion. (**c**) The cell-seeded graft has been caught by a grasper with plain surfaces and should now be implanted via the arthroscopic portal

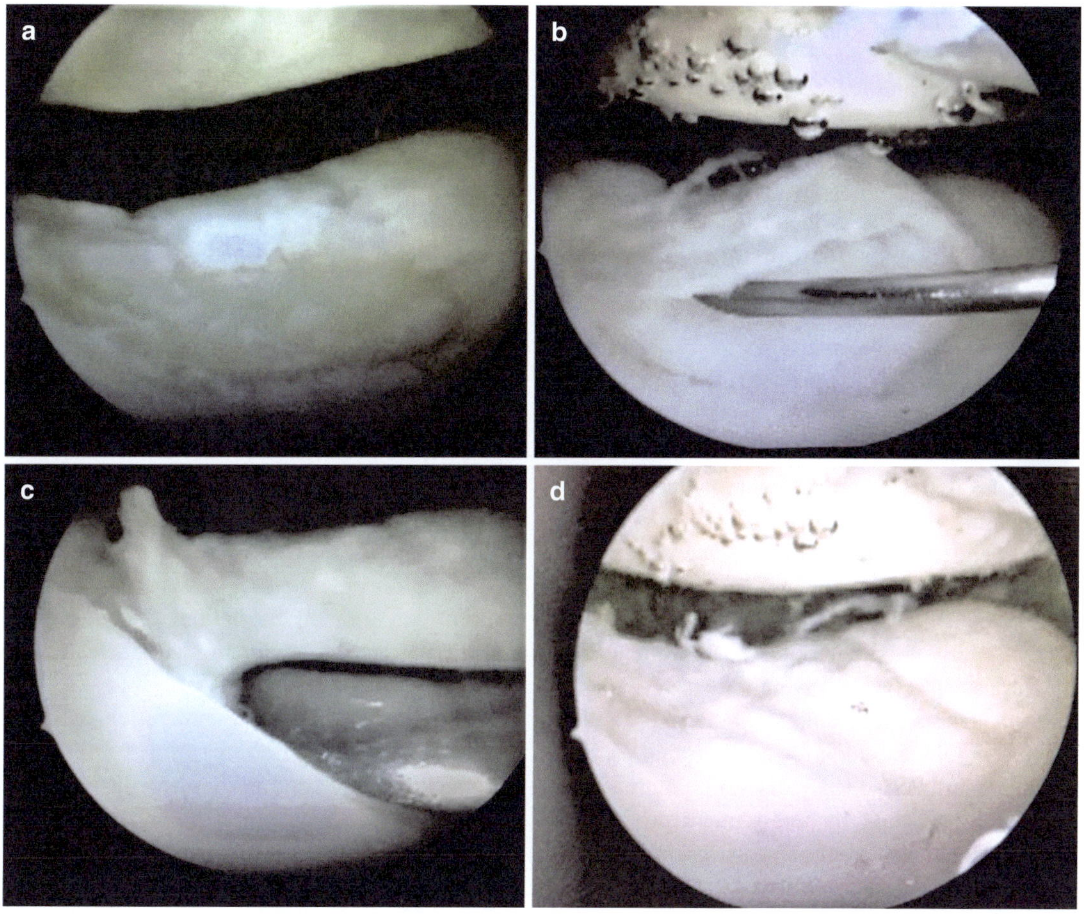

Fig. 6.3 (**a**) The trochlea cartilage lesion area has been debrided into a clean defect. (**b**) The cell-seeded graft is now in the knee joint and pushed into the defect area with the arthroscopic smooth probe. (**c**) The cell-seeded graft is smoothed slightly with a curved tonsil elevator. (**d**) The cell-seeded graft is now securely in place, and its stability has been tested by flexion and extension movements

ing the lesion bottom. Such a scaffold also allows to be folded and with an easier handling trans-arthroscopically [19, 20].

The fourth-generation ACIs are one-stage procedures and allow no cell expansion meaning that there are fewer chondrocytes used, but the combination with additional autologous or allogeneic MSCs should increase the chondrogenic activity. Also those techniques utilize fibrin glue and scaffolds which may be intruded trans-arthroscopically [21, 22].

The fragment ACI (CAIS) is also a fourth-generation ACI where autologous cartilage fragments are implanted into the defect area filled with fibrin glue and covered with a biological resorbable membrane [23, 24].

6.2.5 Coexisting Knee Pathology

Cartilage lesions are often seen combined with other injuries such as menisci, cruciate ligaments, and patellar instabilities, and as with any cartilage repair method, good results should not be expected if coexisting knee pathology is not carefully taken care of. Taking care of such coexisting pathologies is part of the joint restoration philosophy.

Biomechanical malalignment and ligamentous insufficiency can lead to excessive forces and abnormal compressive loads that can destroy the induced repair tissue.

Subsequently, it is crucial that any associated knee pathology responsible for or contributing to the cartilage defect is identified and corrected prior to or in conjunction with the cells and scaffolds are being implanted.

6.2.6 Biomechanical Malalignment

If the mechanical axis on long-standing X-rays passes through the compartment in which the cartilage injury is located, an unloading osteotomy is recommended to shift abnormal forces away from that compartment. Unloading osteotomies should also be considered when the lesions on the condyles are large even without a malalignment or as an alternate use, protect weight bearing with the use of a custom-made unloader brace.

One should also look for an abnormal patellar tracking and if needed consider to unload the patellofemoral joint by realignment procedures shifting the distal patella tendon insertion medially/laterally and or anteriorly.

6.2.7 Joint Stability

Ligamentous instabilities produce excessive shear forces in the knee, which may negatively influence the process of repair tissue maturation. If performed concomitantly, it is best that cruciate ligament reconstruction precede ACI and the ligament reconstruction should be performed in a standard fashion with the desired technique of the surgeon and patient.

6.2.8 Meniscal Damage and Loss

Damaged meniscus should if possible be preserved or repaired. When a total meniscectomy is required, meniscus transplantation may be considered. The meniscal allograft will help reduce the concentrated forces in the involved compartment and help protect the cartilage repair tissue area.

6.2.9 Osteochondral Defects

Bone grafting can be done at the time of arthroscopic evaluation and chondral biopsy. However, the most common is to do the procedure as a one-stage procedure with ACI in combination with bone grafting via the so-called "sandwich" technique [25] in which the bony defect is filled with bone grafts, periosteum is on top of the bone grafts in level with the subchondral bone plate, and periosteum is also on top of the cartilage defect with the cells in between the both cell layers.

The author places the periosteum with the cambium layer facing the bone in the bottom and the second layer of periosteum with the cambium layer facing the defect area.

For the third- and fourth-generation ACI, one should first perform bone grafting followed by placing the cell-seeded graft with cells/cartilage fragments over the bone grafts.

6.3 More Exact Technical Descriptions

6.3.1 First- and Second-Generation ACI

The damaged joint is opened through a mini-arthrotomy, and the cartilage injury is debrided to a slightly oval defect with vertical walls and a clean bony bottom. The debrided lesion size needs to be measured. In order to obtain the right size for a periosteal or a collagen patch, a template made from either sterile paper or aluminum can be placed over the defect and outlined with a sterile marking pen, oversizing by 1–2 mm. The template is cut out to be used during the periosteal patch harvest to help insure an accurate size and shape. Similar technique is used for the sizing of a collagen membrane to cover the defect prior to implantation of the cell suspension; a flap of periosteum or a collagen membrane is to be sutured over the defect.

6.3.2 Harvest of Periosteum

The periosteal patch is obtained through a separate incision from the proximal medial tibia, two fingers distal to the pes anserinus location. All fat and fascia layers are removed from the periosteum. A sharp periosteal elevator is then used to slowly dissect the periosteum from the bone using the template.

6.3.3 Periosteal or Collagen Patch Suturing (Fig. 6.1a–d)

The periosteum should be attached to the defect using 5-0 or 6-0 Vicryl sutures (Ethicon Vicryl polyglactin 910 P-1 cutting needle, Johnson-Johnson Intl) using interrupted sutures with the chondrogenic cell layer facing into the lesion area.

The suture needle should be passed through the periosteum from outside to inside about 2 mm from the edge of the periosteum and then passed through the cartilage from inside to outside with the needle entering the cartilage approximately 2 mm in the defect and perpendicular to the defect wall. An approximately 2–3 mm bites from the defect edge is recommended. The sutures are then placed alternately around the defect and spaced approximately 3–4 mm from each other.

An 18 gauge catheter attached to a saline-filled 1 mL syringe is placed under the periosteum or collagen membrane, and the defect area is slowly filled with saline to test water tightness. Any leakage is blocked with additional sutures. The space may then be filled with fibrin glue. Finally the sutured area is sealed with fibrin glue acting for water tightness.

The surgeon introduces the cell-filled syringe through the small opening of the cartilage defect and advanced to the distal end of the defect, and the cells may then be injected under the periosteal or collagen patch as the catheter is slowly withdrawn to the opening of the defect. The small opening is then closed with one or two additional sutures and then sealed with fibrin glue.

6.3.4 ACI Third-Generation ACI

6.3.4.1 Chondrocytes Grown Inside a Scaffold

One such type of scaffold is the Hyaff-11 scaffold [15, 16]. Such a scaffold is allowing the chondrocytes to grow inside the porous Matricel and could be implanted by press fitting directly into the lesion as described by Marcacci et al. [26]. Fibrin glue is needed for a secure positioning. The author's technique, the "folded blanket" technique, for the knee is here described below.

Cartilage biopsies are harvested from a minor weight-bearing area and sent to the cell laboratories. After 4–5 weeks, the scaffold is sent to the surgeon as 2 × 2 cm large patches. Anteromedial or anterolateral portals are created, and an arthroscopy is performed in supine position. The chondrocyte-seeded matrix is prepared with a scissor or scalpel to an appropriate size of the defect (Fig. 6.2a–c).

The lesion is filled with fibrin glue at the bottom with a syringe. The scaffold is caught with an arthroscopic grasper with plain surfaces and introduced into the joint through a clear portal, released and pushed with the smooth trocar into the fibrin glue-covered debrided lesion area. Some extra fibrin glue is injected over the implanted graft, and the graft is compressed toward the defect bottom with a curved tonsil elevator (Fig. 6.3a–d). When there is a graft being oversized, the edges may be folded like a blanket into the defect to fill it up entirely, the folded blanket technique [26].

If the defect is very large, several cut pieces of the scaffold are implanted to fill the defect like a patchwork quilt. Several layers of the cell graft may be used to fill the defect up to surrounding cartilage, the mille-feuille technique [26].

Graft position stability is controlled by flexion and extension movements, and the scaffold should either be in level with surrounding cartilage or slightly below.

6.3.4.2 Chondrocyte Implantation as a Cell Carrier

Such a scaffold is the MACI implant [14]. Many surgeons use mini-open technique to implant the graft. With arthroscopic implantation, a more precise measurement of the lesion is needed as the scaffold cannot be folded. The size of the defect is measured with a ruler, and the measurements are used to shape the membrane to get exact the size of the measured defect. The defect bottom is filled with fibrin glue.

With MACI, the cells are grown only on the surface of one side of the scaffold material. Colored dots need to be placed onto the cell side to guide the orientation once the graft is inside the knee. The cell-seeded graft may then be introduced into the knee via an arthroscopic cannula like a half-pipe instrument.

The graft is positioned into the defect using a probe with care to get the cell side of the membrane the right way up. Fibrin glue is finally injected over the exact fitted implant.

For the cell seeding on matrices direct at time of surgery, similar operative techniques as described above may be used depending on type of scaffold, similar with one-stage fourth-generation ACI.

6.4 Postoperative Rehabilitation

The extremity is immobilized in a brace locked in extension for 2 weeks. Full weight bearing is allowed in the brace as to a level what pain allows. After 2 weeks, the brace is used outdoors and unlocked for another 4 weeks to avoid shearing forces on the grafted area.

A very large defect may be protected by an unloader brace for a longer period, or one may even consider to perform a concomitant permanent unloading with osteotomy.

In general, knowledge of the need of slow gradual time course of maturation of the repair is critical to understand how to rehabilitate patients following autologous chondrocyte implantation. A well-protected graft area will allow the maturation of the induced tissue, an ongoing process of remodeling of the tissue to continue safely.

If the graft is overloaded, a thinning of the repair may occur with a final failure, progressive matrix thinning (PMT). There is always a degree of individual variation to be considered meaning that the rehabilitation program needs to be designed according to the patient's status and needs, weight and age as well as such factors as the size and location of the lesion, and any possible concomitant operations performed.

Protection of the repair tissue from excessive intra-articular forces is critical during the early postoperative period, avoiding twisting rotational shearing forces.

A gradually increased weight-bearing status should be the initial steps of the rehabilitation process. Isometric quadriceps training, straight leg raises, and hamstring strengthening should be introduced early and progressively advanced to resisted exercises and return to greater degrees of functional activities. From 3 weeks post-surgery start progressive closed chain exercises with light resistance. Open chain exercises can be initiated around the 8th week. Running is not advised until the 8th or 9th month post ACI with high-level activities being initiated at the 12th month.

6.5 Expected Outcomes

Autologous chondrocyte implantation (ACI) has since the report from Brittberg et al. with the first 23 patients in 1994 [12] been performed in more than 30,000 patients throughout the world. The clinical results have been reported from numerous centers worldwide.

In a clinical evaluation of 244 patients with 2–10-years follow-up [27], subjective and objective improvements were seen in high numbers of patients with femoral condyle lesions and osteochondritis dissecans. There was a high percentage of good to excellent results (84–90%) in patients with different types of single femoral condyle lesions, while other types of lesions had a lower degree of success (mean 74%).

To study the long-term durability of ACI-treated patients, 61 patients that had passed 2 years post-surgery were followed for at least 5 years up to 11 years post-surgery (mean 7.4 years) [27]. After 2 years, 50 out of 61 patients were graded good–excellent. At the 5- to 11-year follow-up, 51 of the 61 were graded good–excellent. The total failure rate was 16% (10/61) at mean 7.4 years. All ACI failures occurred in the first 2 years, and patients showing good to excellent improvement at 2 years had a high percentage of good results at long-term follow-up [27].

Since, the first performed ACI, more than 30 years ago, ACI has been studied in up to date 18 randomized studies [23, 24, 27–42]. In eight of those studies, different generations of ACI were compared against microfracture (MFX) [23, 24, 31, 36–40]. In 6/8 of those studies, ACI was significantly better clinically than MFX in different parameters evaluated [23, 24, 36, 37, 39, 40].

The most recent study is the SUMMIT trial where a third-generation ACI, a cell carrier (MACI), is compared with MFX [43]. At 2, 3, and 5 years post-surgery, the ACI had significantly better outcomes in co-primary endpoints KOOS and function compared with MFX [40, 43].

Included in the presented RCTs is one of the four generations of ACI. It is the CAIS (Cartilage Autograft Implantation System) where cartilage is harvested and crushed into small fragments, placed on a resorbable membrane, and implanted into the defect area covered by fibrin glue. Two randomized studies have shown statistical superiority with the cartilage fragments versus MFX treatments [23, 24]. Same technology has recently been developed with juvenile allogeneic fragments.

6.5.1 Imaging Evaluation of the Cartilage Repair

High morphologic integrity and quality of the ACI at medium-term follow-ups have been shown by using the Mocart Score and T2 mapping [17, 44]. Graft maturation after ACI in the knee joint needs at least 1 year [17, 44].

In a long-term follow-up with MRI, 9–18 years posttreatment, the quality of the repair tissue was found to be similar to the surrounding normal cartilage, but intralesional osteophytes, subchondral cysts, and bone marrow edema were common. The defect areas were restored in most patients. However, there was no correlation between the dGEMRIC values and the clinical outcome scores [45].

Roberts et al. [46] studied patients operated on with ACI using a comparison between MRI and histology biopsies. They found that the repair tissue was on average 2.5 mm thick. It was of varying morphology ranging from predominantly hyaline in 22% of biopsy specimens, mixed in 48%, through to predominantly fibrocartilage, in 30%. The repair tissue showed maturation improving with increasing time post-grafting. Repair tissue was also well integrated with the host tissue in all aspects viewed [46].

6.6 Conclusion

Autologous chondrocyte implantation (ACI) has been in use for cartilage repair in more than 30 years. The different generations of ACI seem to be useful techniques for chondral and osteochondral lesions of the knee with satisfactory results at long-term follow-ups. Furthermore, the different generations have also shown superiority versus microfracture treatment in several randomized studies. The evidence base for ACI has improved, and recently the National Institute for Health and Care Excellence made a new evaluation. Their survival analysis suggests that long-term results are better with ACI than with microfracture operations. Economic modeling suggested that ACI was also cost-effective compared with MF across a range of scenarios [47]. However, in another study, next-generation ACI had a statistically greater improvement in functional outcome scores as compared with the other three procedures, while microfracture technique was found to be the most cost-effective treatment option and first-generation ACI the least cost-effective [48]. A similar more cost-effectiveness for microfracture has also been reported by Aae et al. [49].

However, finally one could use the conclusions from the working group "Clinical Tissue Regeneration" of the German Society for Orthopaedics and Trauma (DGOU) who summarized the indication for ACI to be used for symptomatic cartilage defects starting from defect sizes of more than 3 cm^2, in the case of young and active sports patients at 2.5 cm^2, while advanced degenerative joint disease needs to be considered as the most important contraindication [50].

References

1. Mankin HJ. The reaction of articular cartilage to injury and osteoarthritis (first of two parts). N Engl J Med. 1974;291(24):1285–92. Review.
2. Mankin HJ. The reaction of articular cartilage to injury and osteoarthritis (second of two parts). N Engl J Med. 1974;291(25):1335–40. Review.
3. Mankin HJ. The structure, chemistry and metabolism of articular cartilage. Bull Rheum Dis. 1967;17(7):447–52. Review.
4. Pridie KH. A method of resurfacing osteoarthritic knee joints. J Bone Joint Surg. 1959;41B:618–9.
5. Smith AU. Survival of frozen chondrocytes isolated from cartilage of adult mammals. Nature. 1965;205:782–4.
6. Chesterman PJ, Smith AU. Homotransplantation of articular cartilage and isolated chondrocytes. An experimental study in rabbits. J Bone Joint Surg (Br). 1968;50(1):184–9.
7. Bentley G, Greer RB III. Homotransplantation of isolated epiphyseal and articular cartilage chondrocytes into joint surfaces of rabbits. Nature. 1971;230(5293):385–8.
8. Green WT. Articular cartilage repair, behaviour of rabbit chondrocytes during tissue culture and subsequent allografting. Clin Orthop. 1977;124:237–50.
9. Peterson L, Menche D, Grande D, Pitman M. Chondrocyte transplantation; an experimental model in the rabbit. In: Transactionfrom the 30th Annual Meeting Orthopaedic Research Society, Atlanta, Feb 7–9; 1984. p. 218.
10. Grande DA, Pitman MI, Peterson L, Menche D, Klein M. The repair of experimentally produced defects in rabbit articular cartilage by autologous chondrocyte transplantation. J Orthop Res. 1989;7(2):208–18.
11. Brittberg M, Nilsson A, Lindahl A, Ohlsson C, Peterson L. Rabbit articular cartilage defects treated with autologous cultured chondrocytes. Clin Orthop Relat Res. 1996;326:270–83.
12. Brittberg M, Lindahl A, Nilsson A, Ohlsson C, Isaksson O, Peterson L. Treatment of deep cartilage defects in the knee with autologous chondrocyte transplantation. N Engl J Med. 1994;331(14):889–95.
13. Melrose J. The knee joint loose body as a source of viable autologous human chondrocytes. Eur J Histochem. 2016;60(2):2645.
14. Brittberg M. Cell carriers as the next generation of cell therapy for cartilage repair: a review of the matrix-induced autologous chondrocyte implantation procedure. Am J Sports Med. 2010;38(6):1259–71.
15. Grigolo B, Roseti L, Fiorini M, Fini M, Giavaresi G, Aldini NN, Giardino R, Facchini A. Transplantation of chondrocytes seeded on a hyaluronan derivative (hyaff-11) into cartilage defects in rabbits. Biomaterials. 2001;22(17):2417–24.
16. Grigolo B, Lisignoli G, Piacentini A, Fiorini M, Gobbi P, Mazzotti G, Duca M, Pavesio A, Facchini A. Evidence for redifferentiation of human chondrocytes grown on a hyaluronan-based biomaterial (HYAff 11): molecular, immunohistochemical and ultrastructural analysis. Biomaterials. 2002;23(4):1187–95.
17. Siebold R, Suezer F, Schmitt B, Trattnig S, Essig M. Good clinical and MRI outcome after arthroscopic autologous chondrocyte implantation for cartilage repair in the knee. Knee Surg Sports Traumatol Arthrosc. 2018;26(3):831–9.
18. Zak L, Albrecht C, Wondrasch B, Widhalm H, Vekszler G, Trattnig S, Marlovits S, Aldrian S. Results 2 years after matrix-associated autologous chondrocyte transplantation using the novocart 3D scaffold: an analysis of clinical and radiological data. Am J Sports Med. 2014;42(7):1618–27.
19. Brittberg M, Peterson L, Sjögren-Jansson E, Tallheden T, Lindahl A. Articular cartilage engineering with autologous chondrocyte transplantation. A review of recent developments. J Bone Joint Surg Am. 2003;85-A(Suppl 3):109–15. Review.
20. Brittberg M, Concaro S. Transarthroscopic implantation of Hyalograft (Hyaff 11) with autologous chondrocytes. In: Brittberg M, Gersoff W, editors. Cartilage surgery. An operative manual. Philadelphia, PA: Elsevier Saunders; 2011. p. 147–60.
21. Hendriks J, Verdonk P, Widuchowski W, et al. First clinical experience with INSTRUCT - a single surgery, autologous cell based technology for cartilage repair. In: ICRS Abstract Proceedings. Electronic Poster P187. 2013. https://cposter.ctimeetingtech.com/get/pdf/icrs/5931/.
22. de Windt TS, Vonk LA, Slaper-Cortenbach ICM, et al. Allogeneic MSCs and recycled autologous chondrons mixed in a one-stage cartilage cell transplantation: a first-in-man trial in 35 patients. Stem Cells. 2017;35(8):1984–93.
23. Cole BJ, Farr J, Winalski CS, et al. Outcomes after a single-stage procedure for cell-based cartilage repair: a prospective clinical safety trial with 2-year follow-up. Am J Sports Med. 2011;39(6):1170–9.
24. Spalding T, Almqvist F, Brittberg M, et al. The CAIS project: European multicenter randomized controlled pilot study of a one stage procedure for cell-based cartilage repair. Orthop Proc. 2011;93-B(Suppl III):292.
25. Bartlett W, Gooding CR, Carrington RW, Skinner JA, Briggs TW, Bentley G. Autologous chondrocyte implantation at the knee using a bilayer collagen membrane with bone graft. A preliminary report. J Bone Joint Surg (Br). 2005;87(3):330–2.
26. Marcacci M, Kon E, Zaffagnini S, Filardo G, Delcogliano M, Neri MP, Iacono F, Hollander AP. Arthroscopic second generation autologous chondrocyte implantation. Knee Surg Sports Traumatol Arthrosc. 2007;15(5):610–9.
27. Horas U, Pelinkovic D, Herr G, et al. Autologous chondrocyte implantation and osteochondral cylinder transplantation in cartilage repair of the knee joint. A prospective, comparative trial. J Bone Joint Surg Am. 2003;85-A(2):185–92.
28. Schneider U, Andereya S. [First results of a prospective randomized clinical trial on traditional chondro-

cyte transplantation vs CaReS-Technology]. Z Orthop Ihre Grenzgeb. 2003;141(5):496–7.
29. Bentley G, Biant LC, Carrington RW, et al. A prospective, randomised comparison of autologous chondrocyte implantation versus mosaicplasty for osteochondral defects in the knee. J Bone Joint Surg (Br). 2003;85(2):223–30.
30. Visna P, Pasa L, Cizmár I, et al. Treatment of deep cartilage defects of the knee using autologous chondrograft transplantation and by abrasive techniques--a randomized controlled study. Acta Chir Belg. 2004;104(6):709–14.
31. Knutsen G, Engebretsen L, Ludvigsen TC, et al. Autologous chondrocyte implantation compared with microfracture in the knee. A randomized trial. J Bone Joint Surg Am. 2004;86-A(3):455–64.
32. Bartlett W, Skinner JA, Gooding CR, Carrington RW, et al. Autologous chondrocyte implantation versus matrix-induced autologous chondrocyte implantation for osteochondral defects of the knee: a prospective, randomised study. J Bone Joint Surg (Br). 2005;87(5):640–5.
33. Dozin B, Malpeli M, Cancedda R, et al. Comparative evaluation of autologous chondrocyte implantation and mosaicplasty: a multicentered randomized clinical trial. Clin J Sport Med. 2005;15(4):220–6.
34. Gooding CR, Bartlett W, Bentley G. A prospective, randomised study comparing two techniques of autologous chondrocyte implantation for osteochondral defects in the knee: periosteum covered versus type I/III collagen covered. Knee. 2006;13(3):203–10.
35. Zeifang F, Oberle D, Nierhoff C, et al. Autologous chondrocyte implantation using the original periosteum-cover technique versus matrix-associated autologous chondrocyte implantation: a randomized clinical trial. Am J Sports Med. 2010;38(5):924–33.
36. Basad E, Ishaque B, Bachmann G, et al. Matrix-induced autologous chondrocyte implantation versus microfracture in the treatment of cartilage defects of the knee: a 2-year randomised study. Knee Surg Sports Traumatol Arthrosc. 2010;18(4):519–27.
37. Vanlauwe J, Saris DB, Victor J, et al. Five-year outcome of characterized chondrocyte implantation versus microfracture for symptomatic cartilage defects of the knee: early treatment matters. Am J Sports Med. 2011;39(12):2566–74.
38. Lim HC, Bae JH, Song SH, et al. Current treatments of isolated articular cartilage lesions of the knee achieve similar outcomes. Clin Orthop Relat Res. 2012;470(8):2261–7.
39. Crawford DC, DeBerardino TM, Williams RJ III. NeoCart, an autologous cartilage tissue implant, compared with microfracture for treatment of distal femoral cartilage lesions: an FDA phase-II prospective, randomized clinical trial after two years. J Bone Joint Surg Am. 2012;94(11):979–89.
40. Saris D, Price A, Widuchowski W, et al. Matrix-applied characterized autologous cultured chondrocytes versus microfracture: two-year follow-up of a prospective randomized trial. Am J Sports Med. 2014;42(6):1384–94.
41. Akgun I, Unlu MC, Erdal OA, et al. Matrix-induced autologous mesenchymal stem cell implantation versus matrix-induced autologous chondrocyte implantation in the treatment of chondral defects of the knee: a 2-year randomized study. Arch Orthop Trauma Surg. 2015;135(2):251–63.
42. Clavé A, Potel JF, Servien E, et al. Third-generation autologous chondrocyte implantation versus mosaicplasty for knee cartilage injury: 2-year randomized trial. J Orthop Res. 2016;34(4):658–65.
43. Brittberg M, Recker D, Ilgenfritz J, et al. Matrix-applied characterized autologous cultured chondrocytes versus microfracture: five-year follow-up of a prospective randomized trial. Am J Sports Med. 2018;46(6):1343–51.
44. Niethammer TR, Safi E, Ficklscherer A, Horng A, Feist M, Feist-Pagenstert I, Jansson V, Pietschmann MF, Müller PE. Graft maturation of autologous chondrocyte implantation: magnetic resonance investigation with T2 mapping. Am J Sports Med. 2014;42(9):2199–204.
45. Vasiliadis HS, Danielson B, Ljungberg M, McKeon B, Lindahl A, Peterson L. Autologous chondrocyte implantation in cartilage lesions of the knee: long-term evaluation with magnetic resonance imaging and delayed gadolinium-enhanced magnetic resonance imaging technique. Am J Sports Med. 2010;38(5):943–9.
46. Roberts S, McCall IW, Darby AJ, Menage J, Evans H, Harrison PE, Richardson JB. Autologous chondrocyte implantation for cartilage repair: monitoring its success by magnetic resonance imaging and histology. Arthritis Res Ther. 2003;5(1):R60–73.
47. Mistry H, Connock M, Pink J, Shyangdan D, Clar C, Royle P, Court R, Biant LC, Metcalfe A, Waugh N. Autologous chondrocyte implantation in the knee: systematic review and economic evaluation. Health Technol Assess. 2017;21(6):1–294.
48. Kraeutler MJ, Belk JW, Purcell JM, McCarty EC. Microfracture versus autologous chondrocyte implantation for articular cartilage lesions in the knee: a systematic review of 5-year outcomes. Am J Sports Med. 2018;46(4):995–9.
49. Aae TF, Randsborg PH, Lurås H, Årøen A, Lian ØB. Microfracture is more cost-effective than autologous chondrocyte implantation: a review of level 1 and level 2 studies with 5 year follow-up. Knee Surg Sports Traumatol Arthrosc. 2018;26(4):1044–52.
50. Niemeyer P, Albrecht D, Andereya S, Angele P, Ateschrang A, Aurich M, Baumann M, Bosch U, Erggelet C, Fickert S, Gebhard H, Gelse K, Günther D, Hoburg A, Kasten P, Kolombe T, Madry H, Marlovits S, Meenen NM, Müller PE, Nöth U, Petersen JP, Pietschmann M, Richter W, Rolauffs B, Rhunau K, Schewe B, Steinert A, Steinwachs MR, Welsch GH, Zinser W, Fritz J. Autologous chondrocyte implantation (ACI) for cartilage defects of the knee: a guideline by the working group "Clinical Tissue Regeneration" of the German Society of Orthopaedics and Trauma (DGOU). Knee. 2016;23(3):426–35.

Joint Preservation with Stem Cells

7

Konrad Slynarski and Willem Cornelis de Jong

7.1 Introduction

Spontaneous repair of an articular cartilage lesion that does not penetrate below the calcified zone into the subchondral bone appears to be non-existent. If the lesion does cross the calcified zone and penetrates into the subchondral bone, the circulatory system comes into play, and a complete necrosis-inflammation-repair response is initiated, usually resulting in repair tissue that is roughly a combination of fibrocartilage and hyaline cartilage [1]. Sparse evidence exists that during developmental stages, a spontaneous repair process resulting in new hyaline articular cartilage may still occur: artificially created partial-thickness lesions of femoral articular cartilage in foetal lambs mostly healed in utero [2]. To some extent, spontaneous repair may also occur in adult rabbits: artificially created osteochondral lesions filled up with new hyaline cartilage, containing chondroblasts, chondrocytes, and glycosaminoglycans [3]. For man, however, no such reports exist.

Since long, the ultimate desire of joint medicine has been to find a treatment for articular cartilage lesions that would result in new cartilage remodelled to precisely have the anatomical and biochemical properties of the native hyaline cartilage whilst being perfectly integrated to the original surrounding cartilage. To accomplish this, many strategies may be considered, but cells must be our main actors.

Chondroblasts and chondrocytes are the cells that make cartilage tissue. Isolation of these cells from a cartilage biopsy yields cell numbers deemed insufficient to treat an articular cartilage lesion. In addition, using a biopsy from healthy cartilage would only create a new lesion. Expansion in vitro would remedy the need for more cells, but dedifferentiation of the cells into a fibroblastic phenotype is challenging to prevent or reverse [4, 5]. To circumvent these problems, cells that can become chondroblasts or chondrocytes may be used: stem cells.

7.2 The Stem Cells

Stem cells are undifferentiated cells that can divide indefinitely and, when they divide, produce either two new stem cells or a new stem cell and a more specialised cell. The range of specialised cells a stem cell can produce defines its level of potency, of which several are defined. A totipotent stem cell gives rise to all the tissues of an embryo and the extraembryonic tissues; a pluripotent stem cell gives rise to all the tissues of an embryo except for the extraembryonic tissues; a

K. Slynarski (✉)
Słynarski Knee Clinic, Warsaw, Poland
e-mail: konrad@slynarski.pl

W. C. de Jong
CellCoTec BV, Bilthoven, The Netherlands

M. Brittberg, K. Slynarski (eds.), *Lower Extremity Joint Preservation*,
https://doi.org/10.1007/978-3-030-57382-9_7

multipotent stem cell gives rise to a limited set of cell types; a unipotent stem cell gives rise to just one specific cell type. Because of the natural role of stem cells in cell replenishment and tissue renewal, their application in regenerative medicine, including that of cartilage, appears obvious.

Stem cells can be sourced from quite a few tissues, e.g. bone marrow aspirate (historically most widely used), adipose tissue (easily accessible, also from the infrapatellar fat pad), synovial membrane [6], but also dental pulp [7] and umbilical cord blood. After harvest, the stem cells can be kept in culture and expanded relatively easily to build up a stem cell bank with ready-for-use cell populations. To induce stem cells to become chondroblasts or chondrocytes, however, is not straightforward.

For many years existed a hypothesis according to which mature organisms have a population of cells possessing the properties of stem cells, destined for self-repair and self-renewal processes, referred to as mesenchymal stem cells (MSCs) [8]. According to this hypothesis, MSCs can differentiate into individual end-stage cell types, such as those that fabricate specific mesenchymal tissues including bone, cartilage, muscle, bone marrow stroma, tendon/ligament, fat, dermis, and other connective tissues [8–10]. Those cells also secrete a broad spectrum of bioactive macromolecules that are both immunoregulatory and serve to erect regenerative microenvironments in case of tissue injury [11]. According to the current research on mesenchymal stem cell physiology, these cells are actually pericytes (perivascular cells) which are activated in response to trauma or local inflammation and act to repair the damage using various types of chemotactic factors [12]. These secreted bioactive factors suppress the local immune system, inhibit fibrosis (inhibit scar formation) and apoptosis, enhance angiogenesis, and stimulate mitosis and differentiation of tissue-intrinsic reparative or stem cells [13]. It has been proposed that the pericyte is released from its position on a vascular tube in the case of a focal injury and, as such, it functions as an immunomodulatory and trophic MSC [14]. MSC-induced immune modulation turns off T-cell supervision of the injured area and blocks autoimmunological reactions. Its trophic activity limits the field of damage so that scarring does not occur and that tissue-intrinsic progenitors replace the expired cells.

7.3 Stem Cell Sources and Delivery

Historically, the most often used source of MSCs has been the bone marrow. According to the new concept, whereby MSCs are pericytes found on capillaries, they can be harvested from practically any tissue. However, taking into account the ease of harvesting, minimal invasiveness, as well as high cell concentration, adipose tissue seems to be the optimal source of MSCs. Studies have shown that 1 g of adipose tissue can yield approximately 5000 stem cells, which is 500 times more cells than can be obtained from an equivalent amount of bone marrow [15]. In keeping with this understanding of the role of pericytes, it seems to follow logically that the therapeutic process could be based on such a natural, easily available source for body regeneration. To this end, cells could be harvested, condensed, and administered in large quantities to the injured area, stimulating the surrounding tissue to heal. With regard to the impact of intraarticular administration of stem cells on the healing of articular cartilage damage, research studies have concentrated mainly on the knee joint [16–19]. In literature, we encounter two general methods of stem cell administration. Stem cells can be delivered directly into the joint without prior preparation of the damaged area (typically used for systemic degenerative disease), or such delivery may be preceded by the debridement of the focal chondral defect (arthroscopy), potentially with the additional application of tissue adhesive as sealant or carrier [20]. Yong-Gon Koh et al. [21] treated a group of patients aged over 65 by administering a single application of stem cells extracted from adipose tissue following arthroscopic debridement. Improvement was reported in all clinical outcomes (KOOS, VAS), the progression of lesions was found to be delayed in radiographic assessment according to the Kellgren-Lawrence scale, and the quality of cartilage was found to improve on second-look arthroscopy.

7.4 The Mode of Action of Stem Cells

The MSCs respond to inflammation and fibrotic environment, but also control nociceptive pathways. Kouroupis et al. studied human infrapatellar fat pad (IFP)-derived MSC (IFP-MSC) reaction to inflammatory and pro-fibrotic environments (cell priming by TNF-α/IFNγ and TNF-α/IFNγ/CTGF exposure, respectively) [22]. Primed cells experienced dramatic phenotypic changes, including a sharp increase in CD10 (surface neutral endopeptidase expressed in multiple cell types including the immune system and MSC, with enzymatic activity neutralising various signalling substrates including SP), upregulation of key immunomodulatory transcripts, and secreted factors affecting key pathways (IL10, TNF-α, MAPK, Ras, and PI3K-Akt). Naïve and more so primed MSC (both) induced Substance P (SP) degradation in vitro. These findings were reproduced in vivo in a rat model of acute synovitis, where transiently engrafted human IFP-MSC induced local SP reduction. Substance P is secreted by sensory nerve fibres in the synovium and IFP and associated with nociceptive pathways and is also a key modulator of local inflammatory/immune and fibrotic responses. The possibilities of simultaneous inhibition of pain pathways, modulation of immune response, and inflammation make these cells interesting, non-invasive, treatment option for osteoarthritis and other inflammatory joint diseases.

In natural chondrogenesis, mesenchymal cells from mesodermal or neural crest origin crowd together, enlarge, and then produce the initial hyaline extracellular matrix. This is followed up by further interstitial growth and appositional growth if a perichondrium is present. This embryological process is a three-dimensional process during which generous amounts of cell-cell contact, mechanical stimuli, inducer molecules, differential membrane affinities for such inducers, morphogen concentration gradients, etc., together orchestrate the morphogenesis of a cartilage tissue. A vast amount of research has been performed to study the biological, chemical, and physical factors that contribute to chondrogenic differentiation of stem cells in vitro. Much attention has gone out to signalling molecules such as Sonic hedgehog (Shh), bone morphogenetic proteins (BMPs), and transforming growth factor (TGF)-β, as well as to culturing under hypoxic conditions and culturing in a 3D fashion instead of on a flat surface.

7.5 Stem Cells, Chondrocytes, or Chondrons in Cocultures

One way to simulate a chondrogenic microenvironment for stem cells is to coculture them with chondrocytes. Coculturing provides the stem cells with multiple biochemical and biophysical signals at physiological levels, as well as live feedback by the cocultured cells. This approach has the potential to at least partly mimic the sequential cellular interactions that form the basis of natural cartilage growth.

Over the past 15 years, many different stem cell species, as well as stem cell-containing cell fractions, have been cocultured with chondrocytes in various experimental setups. The following are some of the results that were obtained with coculture setups in which no TGF-β or dexamethasone was used. Rat bone marrow stromal cells cocultured for 8 weeks with rat rib cartilage chondrocytes (at a ratio of 80% + 20%, respectively) on a scaffold in vitro produced a tissue abundant with type II collagen, mature cartilage lacunae, and glycosaminoglycan (GAG) at levels of 70–80% of chondrocyte-only cultures [23]. Immortalised human mesenchymal stem cells cocultured with immortalised human chondrocytes upregulate the expression of genes involved in chondrogenesis, SOX9, and COL2A1, but not of RUNX2, a gene involved in osteogenesis. In the stem cell monoculture, such a shift in gene expression was absent [24]. Human mesenchymal stem cells cocultured with human osteoarthritic chondrocytes increase expression of aggrecan and type II collagen, decrease expression of type I collagen, and produce GAGs, all indicators of a chondrogenic differentiation [25]. In a nude mouse model, pig bone marrow stromal cells (BMSCs) co-implanted subcutaneously with pig articular chondrocytes (70% BMSCs and 30% chondrocytes) had, after 8 weeks, produced just as much GAGs as articular chondrocytes implanted alone [26]. In vitro 4-week micromass coculture of mouse embryonic stem cells (80%) mixed with primary bovine articular chondrocytes (20%) resulted in a GAG production that was at a level of 76% of that of the chondrocytes alone. This meant that the GAG production per initial chondrocyte seeding percentage had been five times greater in the coculture group [27].

Although the coculture approach was initially meant to induce stem cells to differentiate into chondrocytes, cocultures reveal that over time, the number of stem cells decreases—sometimes dramatically—whereas the number of chondrocytes increases [28, 29]. Combined with the finding that cocultures outperform chondrocyte monocultures in terms of glycosaminoglycan production per initial chondrocyte seeding percentage, a trophic effect of the stem cells on the chondrocytes has been assumed. One such trophic mediator possibly is fibroblast growth factor 1 [30]. Direct cell-cell contact between the two cell species appears a requirement for coculture-induced enhanced chondrogenesis as well [31]. The function of stem cells in coculture appears to be more auxiliary (helping out) than primary (forming the target tissue) and corresponds well with the reported trophic and immunomodulatory behaviour of mesenchymal stem cells (MSCs) in situations of heart injury, brain injury, and meniscus injury [13]. Moreover, despite the well-known ability of mesenchymal stem cells to differentiate in vitro into various lineages under the "right" culture conditions, differentiation in vivo does not appear to be part of their behaviour [32]. MSCs actually being perivascular cells, which build up a substantial part of the walls of blood capillaries [33], migrate off in case of an injury to provide their trophic and immunomodulatory powers. Because of this, the term "medicinal signalling cell" has been proposed to be used instead of "mesenchymal stem cell" as the full name of "MSCs" [34].

7.6 One-Stage Procedures

The coculture strategy has been applied clinically in several co-implantation cohort studies. These co-implantation studies report on single-stage treatments, made possible by a fast-isolation protocol of chondrocytes and chondrons. Autologous mononucleated bone marrow cells mixed with autologous articular chondrocytes were combined with a load-bearing porous scaffold to treat symptomatic focal cartilage lesions of the knee in the 40-patient INSTRUCT trial [35]. The scaffold was three-dimensionally printed, porous, biocompatible, and biodegradable; composed of a copolymer of polyethylene glycol terephthalate and polybutylene terephthalate (PolyActive; PolyVation BV); and designed to have mechanical properties similar to native articular cartilage. A cartilage biopsy specimen of approximately 0.3 g was collected from a low load-bearing region of the femoral condyle in a similar fashion to ACI. The cartilage lesion was then prepared with specifically designed instrumentation to punch out a circular defect, and debrided cartilage was collected and added to the low load-bearing cartilage biopsy specimen. From the ipsilateral iliac crest, 14 mL of bone marrow was aspirated. A technician intraoperatively processed the cartilage pieces and bone marrow aspirate to isolate primary chondrocytes (PCs) and mononucleated cells (MNCs), respectively, within approximately 60 min (CartiONE Cell Service; Cartilage Repair Systems, LLC). The cells were washed and counted to determine if sufficient numbers had been retrieved to satisfy (1) the predetermined total cell-seeding density of 30×10^6 cells/cm^3 in the defect and (2) the minimum PC:MNC ratio requirements based on preclinical research. All isolated PCs were used; the number of MNCs added was controlled so that the PC:MNC ratio did not fall below the minimum. The cell mixture was seeded into a scaffold, which was placed into the defect with a press-fit technique and secured to the surrounding cartilage with two to five sutures and fibrin glue. The subchondral part of the scaffold was filled and sealed with fibrin glue before the cells were seeded into its chondral part. A standard ACI rehabilitation protocol was applied. Magnetic resonance images were made when the patient was discharged from hospital at 3, 6, 12, and 24 months. Patient-reported measures of pain, general and knee-specific quality of life, and functional activity levels were collected at baseline and 3, 6, 12, 18, and 24 months after surgery with the visual analog scale for pain, the Knee Injury and Osteoarthritis Outcome Score (KOOS), and the International Knee Documentation Committee (IKDC) score. Second-look arthroscopies were performed on subsets of patients at 6, 12, or 24 months, during which gross appearance of the repair tissue was assessed according to macroscopic ICRS scoring criteria. The patient reported symptom, function, and quality-of-life scores from the self-administered KOOS, IKDC, and visual analog scale pain scales improved clinically and statistically significantly over the 24 months after the surgery. The nature, frequency, and severity of reported adverse events were comparable with those reported for ACI and microfracture. Arthralgia was reported for 12 patients (30%), joint effusion for 7 (17.5%), and joint swelling for 5 (12.5%). Postoperative pain caused by the surgical procedure but not related to the joint (e.g. wound pain) was reported for five patients as well. Two patients (5%) reported a decreased ROM of the operated knee. Arthrofibrosis was also reported for two patients. Delamination of the scaffold in one patient and postoperative adhesions in another led to removal of the scaffold at 4 months and 20 months, respectively. Magnetic resonance imaging revealed sustained lesion filling in nearly all patients at all time points from discharge to the final follow-up at 24 months. MRI scans were assessed by two readers independently, using the MOCART variables and grades. Integration of the repair tissue with the surrounding native tissue at the border zone was scored mostly as either "complete" or "demarcating" by reader 1 and primarily as "complete" by reader 2. Surface of the repair tissue was scored mostly as either "intact" or "damaged/50% of depth" by reader 1; reader 2 scored this variable predominantly as "intact". Structure of the repair tissue shifted from "homogeneous" to "inhomogeneous" by reader 1; the ratio between the grades was fairly constant in reader 2's assessment. Both readers assessed the repair tissue's signal intensity as improving over the 24 months, on dual T2 fast spin echo and three-dimensional gradient echo fat suppression images.

Hyaline neocartilage was found in 22 of the 31 biopsy specimens available. Structural evaluation of the repair tissue by MOCART, macroscopic scoring at second-look arthroscopies, and histological evaluation of biopsy specimens supported these findings. The sustained lesion filling indicated that the generation of repair tissue was in concert with the degradation of the scaffold material, a process that takes place mostly within the first year after implantation.

Allogeneic bone marrow MSCs mixed with autologous articular chondrons were combined with fibrin glue to treat symptomatic focal cartilage lesions of the knee in the 35-patient IMPACT trial [36, 37]. De Windt et al. used primary autologous chondrons instead of chondrocytes and cultured allogeneic mesenchymal stromal cells instead of primary autologous bone marrow MNCs. Furthermore, their cell-carrying material was a fibrin glue. The approximate areal density of the deployed chondrons in the De Windt et al. study varied between 0.14 and 0.36 million chondrons/cm^2. The presence of the pericellular matrix around chondrocytes possibly increases their chondrogenicity after treatment, but more clinical research and results are needed.

These treatments are safe and have provided early efficacy in terms of patient-reported outcome measures, repair tissue histology, and MRI results. The chondrocyte fast isolation protocol enables implantation of primary autologous chondrocytes, circumventing the need for chondrogenic in vitro cultured expansion or redifferentiation. The fast isolation protocol of autologous chondrocytes, as well as the chondrocytes' combination with autologous mononucleated bone marrow cells, is now commercially available for use in the clinic. Currently, the tissue processing, cell isolation, counting, and mixing handlings take up to 75–85 min after collection of the cartilage pieces. Despite the OR time, the procedure costs less than two-stage ACI and may have health-economic advantages over it. Further investigation of comparative health economics is needed. Many factors will influence the success rate of co-implantation treatments for articular cartilage lesions: a.o., areal cell-seeding densities, MSC source, chondrocyte/chondron quality, chondrocyte/chondron percentage, characteristics of the cell carrier, lesion location and size, as well as patient demographics and the physical rehabilitation schedule.

Supplementing the chondrocytes with bone marrow MNCs ensures a minimum cell density in the lesion and benefits from coculture-induced increased chondrogenic potential. The adult stem cells from the MNC fraction of the aspirate likely do not differentiate into new chondrocytes but have immunosuppressive and trophic effects on the chondrocytes that allow for increased regenerative potential before the MNC fraction disappears [36, 37]. Similar conclusions from other studies seem to confirm that stem cells support cartilage transplants rather than differentiate into chondrocytes after their transplantation in place of cartilage damage. Zhao et al. investigated the viability of bone marrow MSCs and chondrocytes after co-implantation into a rat osteochondral defect model. Results of sulphated glycosaminoglycans (GAGs) and collagen quantification demonstrated that coculture pellets of BMSCs and chondrocytes have more GAG deposition than that of BMSCs or chondrocytes alone [38]. Implantation of MSCs with allogeneic cartilage is superior to implantation of MSCs alone in cartilage regeneration accompanied with better clinical outcomes [39]. In this study 80 patients treated with cartilage repair procedures and concomitant HTO were prospectively randomised into two groups: MSC implantation (MSC group) and MSC implantation with allogeneic cartilage (MSC-AC group). Clinical outcomes at the second-look arthroscopy at mean 12 months improved significantly in both groups; however outcomes from the second-look arthroscopy to the final follow-up at mean 27 months improved further only in the MSC-AC group.

7.7 Summary

Although most of research on use of MSCs for cartilage regeneration in last 30 years was focusing almost exclusively on tissue engineering approach, where MSCs were considered as cells that directly contributed to formation of a new tissue by differentiation to specific phenotypes, we are now appreciating their true, much wider potential for clinical use. It now seems that their trophic activities are much more important and will be used in the clinics on much larger scale in the near future.

References

1. Mankin HJ. The response of articular cartilage to mechanical injury. J Bone Joint Surg Am. 1982;64(3):460–6.
2. Namba RS, Meuli M, Sullivan KM, Le AX, Adzick NS. Spontaneous repair of superficial defects in articular cartilage in a fetal lamb model. J Bone Joint Surg Am. 1998;80(1):4–10.
3. Shapiro F, Koide S, Glimcher MJ. Cell origin and differentiation in the repair of full-thickness defects of articular cartilage. J Bone Joint Surg Am. 1993;75(4):532–53.
4. Schulze-Tanzil G. Activation and dedifferentiation of chondrocytes: implications in cartilage injury and repair. Ann Anat. 2009;191:325–38.
5. Duan L, Ma B, Liang Y, Chen J, Zhu W, Li M, Wang D. Cytokine networking of chondrocyte dedifferentiation in vitro and its implications for cell-based cartilage therapy. Am J Transl Res. 2015;7(2):194–208.
6. De Bari C, Dell'Accio F, Tylzanowski P, Luyten FP. Multipotent mesenchymal stem cells from adult human synovial membrane. Arthritis Rheum. 2001;44(8):1928–42.
7. Kerkis I, Kerkis A, Dozortsev D, Stukart-Parsons GC, Massironi SMG, Pereira LV, Caplan AI, Cerruti HF. Isolation and characterization of a population of immature dental pulp stem cells expressing OCT-4 and other embryonic stem cell markers. Cells Tissues Organs. 2006;184(3-4):105–16.
8. Caplan A. Mesenchymal stem cells. J Orthop Res. 1991;9:641–50.

9. Caplan AI. Cell delivery and tissue regeneration. J Control Release. 1989;11:157–65.
10. Caplan AI. Review: mesenchymal stem cells: cell-based reconstructive therapy in orthopedics. Tissue Eng. 2005;11:1198–211.
11. Haynesworth SE, Baber MA, Caplan AI. Cytokine expression by human marrow-derived mesenchymal progenitor cells in vitro: effects of dexamethasone and IL-1 alpha. J Cell Physiol. 1996;166:585–92.
12. Caplan AI, Correa D. The MSC: an injury drugstore. Cell Stem Cell Perspect. 2011;9(1):11–5. https://doi.org/10.1016/j.stem.2011.06.008.
13. Caplan AI, Dennis JE. Mesenchymal stem cells as trophic mediators. J Cell Biochem. 2006;98(5):1076–84.
14. Caplan AI. All MSCs are pericytes? Cell Stem Cell. 2008;3(3):229–30.
15. Salem HK, Thiemermann C. Mesenchymal stromal cells: current understanding and clinical status. Stem Cells. 2010;28:585–6.
16. Filardo G, Madry H, Jelic M, Roffi A, Cucchiarini M, Kon E. Mesenchymal stem cells for the treatment of cartilage lesions: from preclinical findings to clinical application in orthopaedics. Knee Surg Sports Traumatol Arthrosc. 2013;21(8):1717–29. https://doi.org/10.1007/s00167-012-2329-3.
17. de Girolamo L, Kon E, Filardo G, Marmotti AG, Soler F, Peretti GM, Vannini F, Madry H, Chubinskaya S. Regenerative approaches for the treatment of early OA. Knee Surg Sports Traumatol Arthrosc. 2016;24(6):1826–35. https://doi.org/10.1007/s00167-016-4125-y.
18. Nakamura N, Miyama T, Engebretsen L, Yoshikawa H, Shino K. Evidence-based medicine series systematic review cell-based therapy in articular cartilage lesions of the knee. Arthroscopy. 2009;25(5):531–52. https://doi.org/10.1016/j.arthro.2009.02.007.
19. Koga H, Engebretsen L, Brinchmann JE, Muneta T, Sekiya I. Mesenchymal stem cell-based therapy for cartilage repair: a review. Knee Surg Sports Traumatol Arthrosc. 2009;17(11):1289–97. https://doi.org/10.1007/s00167-009-0782-4.
20. Kim YS, Kwon OR, Choi YJ, Suh DS, Heo DB, Koh YG. Comparative matched-pair analysis of the injection versus implantation of mesenchymal stem cells for knee osteoarthritis. Am J Sports Med. 2015;43:2738.
21. Koh YG, Choi YJ, Kwon SK, Kim YS, Yeo JE. Clinical results and second-look arthroscopic findings after treatment with adipose-derived stem cells for knee osteoarthritis. Knee Surg Sports Traumatol Arthrosc. 2015;23(5):1308–16. https://doi.org/10.1007/s00167-013-2807-2.
22. Kouroupis D, Bowles A, Willman M, Orfei C, Colombini A, Best T, Kaplan L, Correa D. Infrapatellar fat pad-derived MSC response to inflammation and fibrosis induces an immunomodulatory phenotype involving CD10-mediated Substance P degradation. Sci Rep. 2019;9(1):10864. https://doi.org/10.1038/s41598-019-47391-2.
23. Miao C, Mu S, Duan P, Liang X, Yang B, Zhou G, Tang S. Effects of chondrogenic microenvironment on construction of cartilage tissues using marrow stromal cells in vitro. Artif Cells Blood Substit Immobil Biotechnol. 2009;37(5):214–21.
24. Chen WH, Lai MT, Wu ATH, Wu CC, Gelovani JG, Lin CT, Hung SC, Chiu WT, Deng WP. In vitro stage-specific chondrogenesis of mesenchymal stem cells committed to chondrocytes. Arthritis Rheum. 2009;60(2):450–9.
25. Aung A, Gupta G, Majid G, Varghese S. Osteoarthritic chondrocyte-secreted morphogens induce chondrogenic differentiation of human mesenchymal stem cells. Arthritis Rheum. 2011;63(1):148–58.
26. Liu X, Sun H, Yan D, Zhang L, Lv X, Liu T, Zhang W, Liu W, Cao Y, Zhou G. In vivo ectopic chondrogenesis of BMSCs directed by mature chondrocytes. Biomaterials. 2010;31(36):9406–14.
27. Hendriks JAA, Miclea RL, Schotel R, de Bruijn E, Moroni L, Karperien M, Riesle J, van Blitterswijk CA. Primary chondrocytes enhance cartilage tissue formation upon co-culture with a range of cell types. Soft Matter. 2010;6:5080–8.
28. Wu L, Leijten JCH, Georgi N, Post JN, van Blitterswijk CA, Karperien M. Trophic effects of mesenchymal stem cells increase chondrocyte proliferation and matrix formation. Tissue Eng Part A. 2011;17(9–10):1425–36.
29. Wu L, Prins HJ, Helder MN, van Blitterswijk CA, Karperien M. Trophic effects of mesenchymal stem cells in chondrocyte co-cultures are independent of culture conditions and cell sources. Tissue Eng Part A. 2012;18(15–16):1542–51.
30. Wu L, Leijten J, van Blitterswijk CA, Karperien M. Fibroblast growth factor-1 is a mesenchymal stromal cell-secreted factor stimulating proliferation of osteoarthritic chondrocytes in co-culture. Stem Cells Dev. 2013;22(17):2356–67.
31. De Windt TS, Saris DBF, Slaper-Cortenbach ICM, van Rijen MHP, Gawlitta D, Creemers LB, de Weger RA, Dhert WJA, Vonk LA. Direct cell-cell contact with chondrocytes is a key mechanism in multipotent mesenchymal stromal cell-mediated chondrogenesis. Tissue Eng Part A. 2015;21(19–20):2536–47.
32. Guimarães-Camboa N, Cattaneo P, Sun Y, Moore-Morris T, Gu Y, Dalton ND, Rockenstein E, Masliah E, Peterson KL, Stallcup WB, Chen J, Evans SM. Pericytes of multiple organs do not behave as mesenchymal stem cells in vivo. Cell Stem Cell. 2017;20(3):345–59.
33. Crisan M, Yap S, Casteilla L, Chen CW, Corselli M, Park TS, Andriolo G, Sun B, Zheng B, Zhang L, Norotte C, Teng PN, Traas J, Schugar R, Deasy BM, Badylak S, Bühring HJ, Giacobino JP, Lazzari L, Huard J, Péault B. A perivascular origin for mesenchymal stem cells in multiple human organs. Cell Stem Cell. 2008;3(3):301–13.
34. Caplan AI. Mesenchymal stem cells: time to change the name! Stem Cells Transl Med. 2017;6(6):1445–51.

35. Słynarski K, de Jong WC, Snow M, Hendriks JAA, Wilson CE, Verdonk P. Single-stage autologous chondrocyte-based treatment for the repair of knee cartilage lesions: two-year follow-up of a prospective single-arm multicenter study. Am J Sports Med. 2020;48(6):1327–37. https://doi.org/10.1177/0363546520912444.
36. De Windt TS, Vonk LA, Slaper-Cortenbach ICM, van den Broek MPH, Nizak R, van Rijen MHP, de Weger RA, Dhert WJA, Saris DBF. Allogeneic mesenchymal stem cells stimulate cartilage regeneration and are safe for single-stage cartilage repair in humans upon mixture with recycled autologous chondrons. Stem Cells. 2017a;35(1):256–64.
37. De Windt TS, Vonk LA, Slaper-Cortenbach ICM, Nizak R, van Rijen MHP, Saris DBF. Allogeneic MSCs and recycled autologous chondrons mixed in a one-stage cartilage cell transplantation: a first-in-man trial in 35 patients. Stem Cells. 2017b;35(8):1984–93.
38. Zhao Z, Zhou X, Guan J, Wu M, Zhou J. Co-implantation of bone marrow mesenchymal stem cells and chondrocytes increase the viability of chondrocytes in rat osteo-chondral defects. Oncol Lett. 2018;15(5):7021–7. https://doi.org/10.3892/ol.2018.8195.
39. Kim YS, Chung PK, Suh DS, Heo DB, Tak DH, Koh YG. Implantation of mesenchymal stem cells in combination with allogenic cartilage improves cartilage regeneration and clinical outcomes in patients with concomitant high tibial osteotomy. Knee Surg Sports Traumatol Arthrosc. 2020;28(2):544–54. https://doi.org/10.1007/s00167-019-05729-3.

Cartilage Pathology and Repair: Fresh Allografts

8

Florian Gaul, Luís Eduardo Tírico, and William Bugbee

8.1 Introduction

Chondral and osteochondral defects of the knee joint are common problems for orthopaedic surgeons worldwide. They often occur in young and active patients after traumatic events or are diagnosed as part of the clinical spectrum of osteochondritis dissecans (OCD). If left untreated, these lesions can heavily impair quality of life and can promote the development of early stage osteoarthritis (OA) [1].

Besides the classic palliative treatment options for these lesions, there is a growing interest in biologic restoration techniques. One such technique is the transplantation of fresh osteochondral allograft (OCA) tissue, which has been successfully used in a wide variety of clinical situations involving diseased, damaged, or missing articular cartilage. Hyaline cartilage represents an attractive candidate for transplantation because it is an avascular and aneural tissue without the need for blood supply or innervation for normal function. Furthermore, it is relatively immunoprivileged because chondrocytes are imbedded within a matrix which protects them from host immune surveillance.

F. Gaul
Department for Orthopaedics, Trauma and Plastic Surgery, University Hospital Leipzig, Leipzig, Germany

L. E. Tírico
Orthopedic and Traumatology Institute, University of Sao Paulo Medical School, Sao Paulo, Brazil
e-mail: Luis.tirico@hc.fm.usp.br

W. Bugbee (✉)
Joint Reconstruction, Joint Preservation and Cartilage Repair Service, Orthopaedic Research, Department of Orthopaedic Surgery, Scripps Clinic, La Jolla, CA, USA
e-mail: bugbee.william@scrippshealth.org

► Osteochondral allografting is the transplantation of an intact structural and functional unit consisting of architecturally mature hyaline cartilage with living chondrocytes and a non-living subchondral bone portion which generally functions as a scaffold to allow attachment and fixation of the graft to the host by creeping substitution (similar to other types of bone graft).

It has been shown that chondrocytes remain viable for many weeks during hypothermal storage in nutritive culture medium containing human serum, providing the surgeon an acceptable therapeutic window [2–8]. Furthermore, current clinical evidence suggests no difference in outcome between the transplantation of OCA tissue with prolonged storage up to 28 days in comparison to the transplantation of early (less than 7 days) release grafts [9].

► The advantage of an OCA is that large deep lesions can be treated in a one-stage procedure without having the issue of donor site morbidity. For the patient, it provides predictable symptomatic pain relief and lasting functional improvements with the possibility of delaying or eliminating the need for arthroplasty [10, 11].

M. Brittberg, K. Slynarski (eds.), *Lower Extremity Joint Preservation*,
https://doi.org/10.1007/978-3-030-57382-9_8

8.2 Indications (Table 8.1)

▶ Major indications for an OCA transplantation as a primary treatment are symptomatic full-thickness chondral and subchondral defects greater than 2–3 cm^2 in diameter or focal lesions of ICRS grade III–IV with subchondral damage greater than 6–10 mm (i.e. OCD, focal avascular osteonecrosis, posttraumatic defects) (Figs. 8.1 and 8.2). Furthermore, OCA is indicated as a salvage procedure after failure of other cartilage restoration techniques, such as microfracture, osteochondral autograft transplantation (OAT), autologous chondrocyte implantation (ACI) or primary failed OCA transplantation.

Table 8.1 Indications for OCA transplantation in the knee joint

Primary treatment
Full-thickness chondral/subchondral defects > 2–3 cm^2
Focal lesion ICRS grade III–IV with subchondral damage greater than 6–10 mm
OCD
Avascular necrosis
Posttraumatic defects
Salvage procedure after primary failed cartilage restoration technique
Microfracture
OAT
ACI
OCA transplantation

ACI autologous chondrocyte implantation, *OAT* osteochondral autograft transplantation, *OCA* osteochondral allograft transplantation, *OCD* osteochondritis dissecans

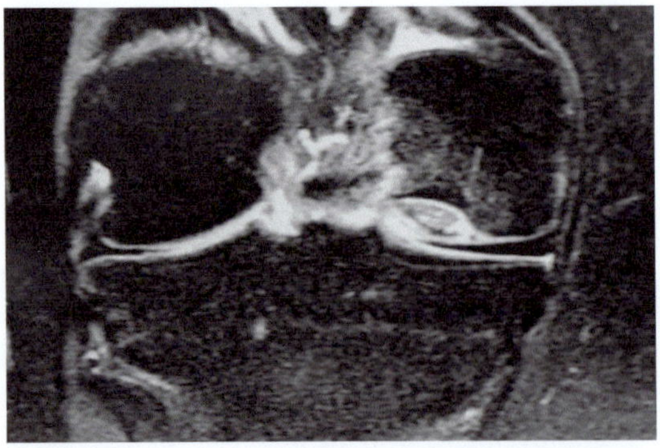

Fig. 8.1 MR image of typical osteochondritis lesion of the medial femoral condyle amenable to osteochondral allografting

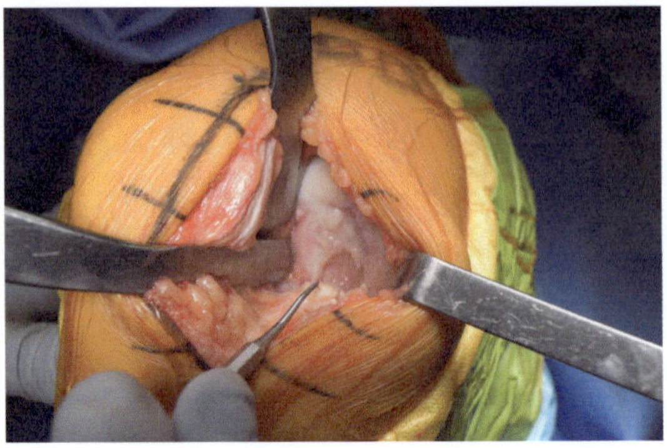

Fig. 8.2 Intraoperative image demonstrating large lesion size and bone involvement

Most commonly, OCA transplantation is used to treat femoral defects, but in selected cases it is also possible to address tibial chondral defects (entire tibial and meniscal surface may be transplanted) or bipolar ("kissing") lesions of the femur and tibia (less successful than the treatment of unipolar defects [12, 13]). Osteochondral allografts are versatile when addressing even very large, complex, or multiple lesions in topographically challenging environments, especially if they involve an osseous component.

8.3 Contraindications

▶ Such as for all osteochondral grafting and cartilage restoration techniques, some absolute contraindications are advanced multicompartmental OA and inflammatory arthropathies [14]. Relative contraindications include smoking, alcohol abuse, uncorrected ligamentous instability, uncorrected joint malalignment and obesity (BMI > 30 kg/m^2). Typically, there are no absolute age limitations but inferior outcomes have been reported in patients >40 years [14–16].

8.4 Preoperative Planning

Besides a detailed case history and an accurate clinical examination, one of the main steps in planning an OCA procedure is matching the donor with the recipient. This is done by size alone. In the current practice, small-fragment fresh osteochondral allografts are not human leukocyte antigen-(HLA-) or blood type-matched between donor and recipient, and no immunosuppression is used. For exact perioperative planning, antero-posterior radiographs of the knee joint in full extension (weight bearing) with a magnification marker are routinely used. The medio-lateral dimension of the tibia, just below the joint surface is measured, correcting for magnification. The donor graft is measured at the tissue bank performing a direct measurement on the donor tibial plateau using a caliper. Matching donor and recipient is usually considered acceptable if the difference is between ±2 mm. In order to assess additional pathologies, a series of standard radiographs needs to be done (including weight bearing AP view with 45° knee flexion, lateral view, patellar view and standing bilateral long-leg alignment view). Additionally, CT and MRI scans can be helpful to assess the cartilage integrity, the extent of bone involvement, as well as concomitant ligamentous and/or meniscal pathologies.

► We want to emphasize that the true size of the articular lesion is often underestimated (up to 60%) within the imaging diagnostics [17, 18]. Therefore, if applicable it is always helpful to examine images recorded during previous surgical procedures (i.e. arthroscopy). However, it should be noted that there is a significant variability in anatomy, which is not reflected in any preoperative imaging. In particular, this is applicable to OCD patients in which the affected condyle is typically larger, flatter and wider. In these cases, a larger donor generally should be used. It is the responsibility of the surgeon to inspect the graft and to confirm the adequacy of the size match and quality of the allograft tissue prior to surgery.

8.5 Operative Procedures

Currently, the two widely used techniques for preparation and implantation of fresh OCA are the press fit dowel technique (plug technique) and the shell graft technique. Both procedures have advantages and disadvantages. The dowel or plug technique which is similar in principle to osteochondral autograft transfer systems is typically used for contained lesions between 15 and 35 mm in diameter and generally does not require fixation due to the press fit primary stability. Many commercially available systems are available to harvest and prepare the cylindrical graft with the use of coring reamers. This technique has its limitations because posterior femoral condyle and tibial plateau lesions are not conducive to the use of a circular coring system and may be more amenable to shell allografts. Additionally, the more ovoid or elongated a lesion is in shape, the more normal cartilage needs to be sacrificed at the recipient site in order to accommodate the circular donor plug. In a case of an elliptical-shaped lesion on the femoral condyle, two allografts plugs can be shaped to cover the defect, usually requiring an overlap of the grafts at the interface between them.

The shell graft technique is a free-hand technique which is typically used for large uncontained, asymmetric lesions or lesions in locations on the femur that are difficult to access and therefore more difficult to perform. Additional fixation of the graft with bioabsorbable pins or compression screws is generally needed. However, depending on the technique employed, with this procedure, less normal cartilage may need to be sacrificed.

► Although the dowel or plug allograft method is generally preferred for most lesions, the surgeon should always be prepared to perform a shell graft if the lesion size or location do not allow for proper placement of the dowel graft instruments.

8.6 Surgical Techniques

For both techniques, the patient is placed in supine position and a proximal thigh tourniquet is affixed. A leg or foot holder is extremely helpful to keep the knee in a position between 70° and 120° of flexion. For most lesions of the femoral condyle, eversion of the patella is not necessary.

The standard approach is done by a midline incision followed by a lateral or medial parapatellar arthrotomy, depending on the location of the lesion. If the lesion is far posterior or very large, it might be necessary to detach and reflect the meniscus which can be done safely by leaving a small tissue portion adjacent to the anterior attachment of the meniscus to allow later refixation. After incising the joint capsule, retractors are carefully placed and the knee is brought into a position that allows exposure of the condyle and a direct access to the lesion.

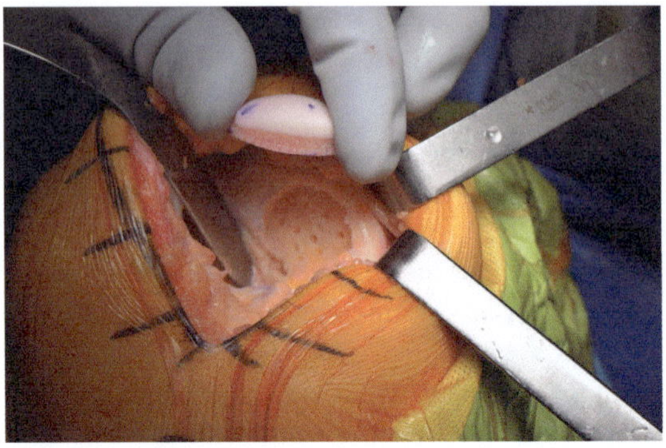

Fig. 8.4 Side view of allograft. Note the relatively thin bone portion of the allograft

8.6.1 Dowel Technique (Plug Technique) (Figs. 8.3, 8.4, and 8.5)

For preparation and implantation of press fit dowel allografts, many different commercial instrumentation systems are available for lesion

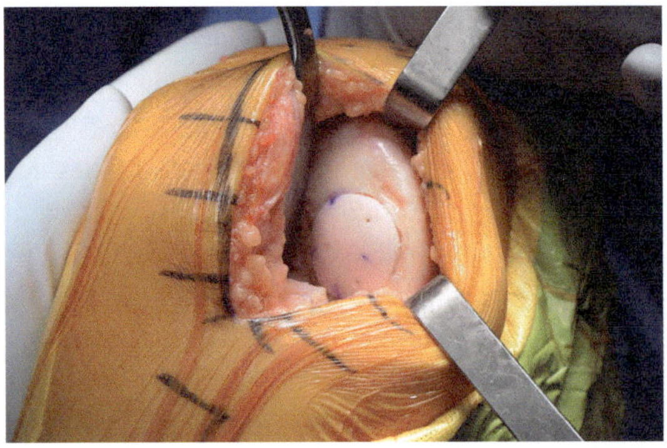

Fig. 8.5 After insertion of the allograft. Interference fit precludes the need for additional fixation

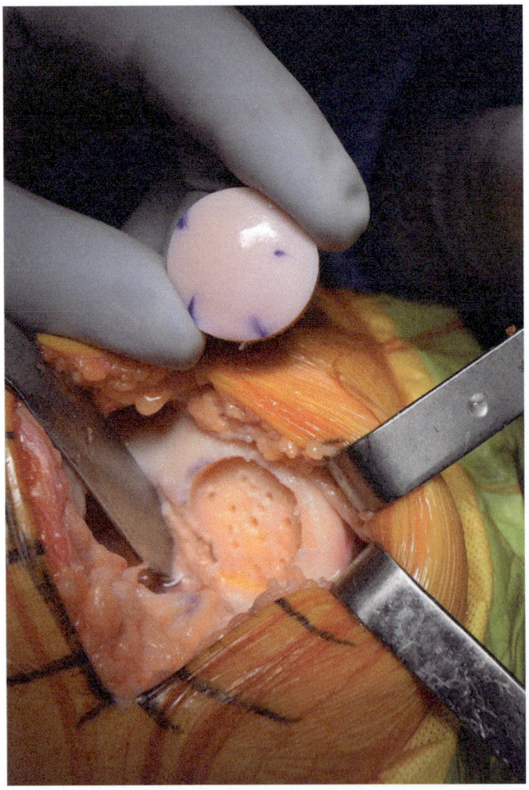

Fig. 8.3 Intraoperative view of lesion seen in Figs. 8.1 and 8.2 after preparation of both recipient site and allograft plug

sizes up to 35 mm in diameter and surgical techniques are similar. It is important to examine the lesion with a probe and determine the actual size by identifying healthy and stable cartilage walls which are necessary for good graft integration. Then a guidewire is driven into the centre of the lesion, perpendicular to the curvature of the articular surface, and the size of the proposed graft is determined, utilizing different sizing dowels. If the lesion falls between two sizes, it is generally preferred to start with the smaller size. The dowel and the socket are drilled with a reamer to an ideal depth of 5–6 mm without exceeding 10 mm.

► **It is critical for the surgeon to take care not to inadvertently ream too deep as the bone becomes much softer once the subchondral plate is removed and cancellous bone is encountered.**

If the lesion is deeper than 10 mm, pathologic bone is removed with a curette until there is healthy, bleeding bone. Cancellous bone from reaming can be collected for bone grafting to fill deeper defects or to modify the fit of the graft. Bone graft from the proximal tibia or iliac crest can be used in cases of large cystic lesions. At this point, the guide pin can be removed and depth of the prepared recipient site is measured and recorded in the four quadrants (12, 3, 6, and 9 o'clock positions).

Next, the corresponding anatomic location of the recipient site has to be identified on the graft. After the graft is placed into a graft holder (or alternately, held with bone-holding forceps), a circular saw guide is placed perpendicular to the articular surface, and an appropriate-sized tube saw is used to core out the graft. Before removing the plug from the condyle, identifying marks are made to ensure proper orientation. Next, the allograft plug thickness has to be adjusted manually by trimming excess bone with a saw according to the depth measurements from the recipient site. The graft should be irrigated copiously with a high-pressure lavage to remove all marrow elements [19]. In order to ease the insertion of the graft, the recipient site is dilated using a slightly oversized tamp. This may also prevent excessive impact loading of the articular surface when the graft is inserted while compacting the subchondral bone to prevent subsidence of the graft. The graft is then inserted by hand in the appropriate rotation and is gently tamped into place until it is flush. Some careful cycling of the knee through a range of motion allows the opposing articular surface to further seat the graft. Usually, no further fixation is required, but if the graft is large or has an exposed edge within the notch, additional fixation with absorbable pins may be added. In cases in which a single plug is not enough to cover the whole lesion, the procedure can be repeated ("snowman technique"). In that situation, the first graft should be temporarily secured with small k-wires to prevent dislocation during preparation of the second overlapping site. Finally, the knee is cycled through a full range of motion in order to verify graft stability and potential impingements, and a standard closure is performed.

8.6.2 Shell Graft Technique

For the shell graft technique, the same surgical approach is used (as described above), the lesion is identified and its dimensions are marked with a surgical pen. In order to minimize the sacrifice of healthy cartilage, a geometric shape (i.e., rectangular or trapezoid) should be created in order to simplify hand grafting the shell allograft. A #15 scalpel is then used to demarcate the lesion, and sharp ring curettes are used to remove all tissue inside this mark. The subchondral bone is removed to a depth of 4–5 mm by using sharp curettes, electric burrs and osteotomies. Stable side walls should be present. The final size of the created defect is measured by length, width and depth, or a foil template is used. Based on that, the basic graft shape is free-hand cut with an oscillating saw, initially slightly over sized by a few millimetres. Excess bone and cartilage are removed as necessary through multiple trial fittings, and the graft is finally placed flush to the articular surface after extensive irrigation of the osseous bed. The graft should also be irrigated copiously with a high-pressure lavage to remove all marrow elements [19]. Depending on the local situation and degree of inherent stability, the graft is additionally fixated using absorbable pins or compression screws. After cycling the knee through a full range of motion to ensure graft stability, a standard closure is performed.

8.7 Postoperative Care

Depending on the size and location of the graft as well as the stability of fixation, patients are typically restricted to touch-down weight bearing for 4–6 weeks with free range of motion (ROM) to promote the healing process and graft vascularization. After 2–4 weeks, closed chain exercise such as cycling is introduced. For patients with patellofemoral grafts, weight bearing in extension (as tolerated) is allowed with limitation of 45° knee flexion for the first 4 weeks after the surgery, utilizing an immobilizer or ROM brace. Weight bearing is progressed slowly between the second and fourth month until full weight bearing (with the use of crutches) which generally is allowed 6–8 weeks after the surgery. Patients with large or complex grafts are restricted to partial weight bearing for 8–12 weeks. Full weight bearing without medical aids and normal gait pattern are generally tolerated between the third and fourth month. In case of concomitant surgical procedures, the postoperative care has to be individually modified accordingly.

8.8 Outcomes

Recent literature shows significant improvement in clinical scores with good to excellent outcomes and graft survival rates in the mid- and long-term after OCA transplantations in the knee joint [10, 20]. In one of the largest studies to date, Sadr et al. reported our experience in the treatment of OCD of the medial and lateral femoral condyle [21]. One hundred and forty-nine knees in 135 patients with a mean follow-up of 6.3 years after the surgery were evaluated. The majority of patients were male (75.8%), the median age at the time of surgery was 21 years, and 82% of the patients had undergone previous surgical interventions with a median of one surgery before the OCA transplantation (arthroscopic debridement, marrow stimulation, loose body removal, among others). The mean size of the lesion was 7.3 cm^2 (range, 2.2–25 cm^2). Regarding the location of the lesion, the majority involved the femoral condyle (62% medial, 29% lateral) followed by the trochlea (6%) and the patella (1%). Of all operated knees, 34 (23%) required reoperations, and 12 (8%) were considered as failures with a mean time to failure of 6.1 ± 1.3 years (seven revision OCA transplantations, three unicompartmental arthroplasties, and two total knee arthroplasties). The overall OCA survivorship was 95% at 5 years and 93% at 10 years. Ninety-five percent of the patients reported satisfaction with their treatment and improved subjective knee function.

In another large study, Levy et al. assessed the outcomes of 129 patients who underwent osteochondral allografting of the femoral condyle [22]. Indications for the procedure included OCD (45%), traumatic chondral injuries (22.5%), degenerative chondral injuries (15.5%), avascular necrosis (14.7%) and osteochondral fractures (2.3%). The majority of patients underwent prior surgical procedures. The mean age of the cohort was 33 years and 53% of the patients were male. After a mean follow-up of 13.5 years, the authors reported a significant improvement of the modified Merle d'Aubigné-Postel score from 12.1 ± 2.1 points preoperatively to 16.0 ± 2.2 points postoperatively as well as a graft survivorship of 82% at 10 years (74% at 15 years). Sixty-one knees (47%) underwent reoperations, and 31 (24%) were considered clinical failures at a mean of 7.2 years.

In the study with the longest follow-up period to date, Raz et al. reported on the Toronto experience with fresh osteochondral allografts of the femoral condyle [11]. A total of 58 knees were reviewed with a mean follow-up of 21.8 years (range 15–22 years). The etiology of the osteochondral lesion was posttraumatic disease (76%) and osteochondritis dissecans (24%). Realignment osteotomy was performed in 36 patients (62%). In 23 (64%) of these cases, a high tibial closing-wedge osteotomy was performed, and in the other 13 cases (36%), a distal femoral varus closing-wedge osteotomy was performed. Thirteen of the 58 grafts failed at a mean of 11 years; three patients underwent graft removal, nine cases were converted to total knee arthroplasty, and one patient underwent multiple debridements followed by above-the-knee amputation. The authors reported 91% graft survivorship at 10 years.

Furthermore, in a series of 156 knees in 143 patients with a mean age of 29.6 years, a mean follow-up of 6 years and a mean lesion size of 6.2 cm^2 (range, 2.3–11.5 cm^2), we found that the size of the lesion does not influence the outcomes after OCA transplantation for isolated femoral condyle lesions of the knee [23]. Regarding the outcomes of OCA transplantations for patellofemoral lesions, which are typically rare, a recent study reported decreased clinical improvement and more frequent reoperations in comparison to OCA transplantations for symptomatic femoral or tibial lesions [10].

The majority of publications are focused on isolated osteochondral lesions, while patients often have significant comorbidities in the knee joint which might need a treatment as well.

In a large recent study, Frank et al. report on outcomes of OCA transplantation with and without concomitant meniscus allograft transplantation (MAT) [24]. The authors found no significant difference between the two groups in terms of failure rates (14% OCA with MAT; 14% for OCA without MAT), reoperation rate (34% OCA with MAT, 36% OCA without MAT), time to reoperation (2.2 ± 2.4 years for OCA with MAT; 3.4 ± 2.7 years for OCA without MAT) and patient-reported clinical outcome scores at final follow-up.

Furthermore, in our two latest studies, we found that a history of anterior cruciate ligament reconstruction does not affect the outcomes of an OCA transplantation and that an OCA and a simultaneous high tibial osteotomy is safe and effective in properly selected patients [25, 26].

8.9 Return to Sports

Due to technical advancements and better donor graft availability over the last decades, OCA transplantations have become a more common treatment especially for osteochondral defects in young and highly active patients. Usually, patients are allowed to return to sports in 4–6 months after the surgery if complete graft healing and incorporation has been demonstrated radiographically and full ROM and optimal quadriceps strength, complete stability and no effusion are achieved. In a recent large literature review on return to sport after the treatment of cartilage lesions in the knee joint, Krych et al. found that OCA transplantations had the second highest return to sport rate (88%) in comparison to OAT (93%), ACI (82%) and microfracture (58%) [27]. In the analysis of 2549 patients with an average age of 35 years and a follow-up period of 47 months, patients receiving an OCA transplantation returned to sport after an average of 9.6 ± 3.0 months (5.2 ± 1.8 months for OAT, 9.1 ± 2.2 months for microfracture and 11.8 ± 3.8 months for ACI).

In another recent systematic literature review of 1117 patients, Campbell et al. also reported a return to sport rate of 88% after OCA transplantation (89% for OAT, 84% for ACI and 75% for microfracture) [28]. Furthermore, the authors reported that athletes who were younger, had a shorter preoperative duration of symptoms, underwent no previous surgical interventions, participated in a more rigorous rehabilitation protocol, and had a smaller cartilage defect had a significantly better prognosis after surgery.

In our OCA database, we identified 142 patients (149 knees) who were highly competitive athletes (45%) or well trained and frequently exercising (55%) who received an OCA transplantation without any concomitant procedure for a symptomatic osteochondral lesion of the knee joint [29]. The mean age of the cohort was 31.2 years, 58.4% of the patients were male, and indications for the surgery included osteochondritis dissecans (65%), degenerative chondral lesions (38%), traumatic chondral injuries (29%), avascular necrosis (6%), fracture (6%) and osteoarthritis (5%). At a mean follow-up of 6 years, 75.2% of the knees had returned to sport or recreational activity following the OCA. Among those who did not return to sport, knee-related issues and lifestyle changes were cited as reasons why. Patients who did not return to sport were more likely to be female, have injured their knee in an activity other than sport, and have a larger graft size. However, among the entire cohort, regardless of return to sport status, 71% achieved "very good" to "excellent" knee function following the OCA, and 79% were able to participate in a high level of activity (moderate, strenuous, or very strenuous activities) as assessed on the IKDC subjective evaluation form.

8.10 Complications

Overall, complications after OCA transplantation are rare. The risk of disease transmission from graft tissue is low. Zou et al. estimated a risk of viral transmission of 1/63,000 for hepatitis B, 1/103,000 for hepatitis C and 1/493,000 for human immunodeficiency virus (HIV) in the United States [30]. In our experience of transplanting over 1000 grafts during the last 35 years, we have not had a single case of disease transmission from the transplanted allograft.

Postoperative infections are also rare but, as with most procedures, can cause serious problems. Infections can occur anytime from days to weeks after surgery, and it is important to distinguish between a deep joint infection requiring further surgery and a superficial wound infection. It is not clear whether a deep infection requires removal of the graft tissue unless it is obviously the source of infection. Fortunately, because of the relative health of the younger patients and short surgery times, surgical site infections have been rare in our experience.

Another complication is graft failure, which we define as the need for an additional operative procedure following the primary OCA transplantation that requires the removal of the graft. In most cases this is due to a subchondral collapse or a non-union at the bone-to-bone interface which is diagnosed by a visible graft-host interface on serial radiographic evaluation.

> However, we note many clinical cases in which radiographic or advanced imaging suggests graft failure, but clinically the patient has few symptoms. In these cases we recommend a cautious approach with closer follow up to determine if clinical failure occurs and surgical intervention is necessary.

If a delayed union is suspicious, patience is essential because complete healing or recovery may take an extended period of time. Decreasing activities, the reintroduction of weight bearing or the use of braces may be helpful in the early management. Furthermore, close radiographic follow-up examinations are important to track the healing process. MRI scans are often not helpful, especially within the first 6 months after the primary allografting procedure due to extensive signal abnormalities. These are difficult to interpret, because even normal, well-functioning grafts often show signal abnormalities.

Treatment options for failed allografts include observation, if the patient is minimally symptomatic and the joint is thought to be at low risk for further progression of the disease. Further options for salvage procedures are (arthroscopic) debridement, removal of fragmented areas of the graft, revision OCA transplantation or conversion to arthroplasty. We found, that outcomes of revision OCA were not inferior when compared to primary transplantation [31, 32].

8.11 Conclusion

Osteochondral allograft transplantation is a useful and important technique for the treatment of a wide variety of knee joint pathologies. Fresh allografts can be fashioned to fit most anatomic knee sites and are versatile in that they can restore both chondral and osseous pathology. Surgical techniques are generally straightforward. Clinical outcome data is very favourable with excellent survivorship, patient satisfaction and important clinical improvement in the majority of patients.

References

1. Heir S, Nerhus TK, Rotterud JH, et al. Focal cartilage defects in the knee impair quality of life as much as severe osteoarthritis: a comparison of knee injury and osteoarthritis outcome score in 4 patient categories scheduled for knee surgery. Am J Sports Med. 2010;38:231–7. https://doi.org/10.1177/0363546509352157.
2. Ball ST, Amiel D, Williams SK, et al. The effects of storage on fresh human osteochondral allografts. Clin Orthop Relat Res. 2004:246–52.
3. Czitrom AA, Keating S, Gross AE. The viability of articular cartilage in fresh osteochondral allografts after clinical transplantation. J Bone Joint Surg Am. 1990;72:574–81.
4. Pennock AT, Wagner F, Robertson CM, et al. Prolonged storage of osteochondral allografts: does the addition of fetal bovine serum improve chondrocyte viability? J Knee Surg. 2006;19:265–72.
5. Robertson CM, Allen RT, Pennock AT, Bugbee WD, Amiel D. Upregulation of apoptotic and matrix-related gene expression during fresh osteochondral allograft storage. Clin Orthop Relat Res. 2006;442:260–6.

6. Williams RJ III, Dreese JC, Chen CT. Chondrocyte survival and material properties of hypothermically stored cartilage: an evaluation of tissue used for osteochondral allograft transplantation. Am J Sports Med. 2004;32:132–9. https://doi.org/10.1177/0095399703258733.
7. Williams RJ III, Ranawat AS, Potter HG, Carter T, Warren RF. Fresh stored allografts for the treatment of osteochondral defects of the knee. J Bone Joint Surg Am. 2007;89:718–26. https://doi.org/10.2106/jbjs.f.00625.
8. Williams SK, Amiel D, Ball ST, et al. Prolonged storage effects on the articular cartilage of fresh human osteochondral allografts. J Bone Joint Surg Am. 2003;85-a:2111–20.
9. Schmidt KJ, Tirico LE, McCauley JC, Bugbee WD. Fresh osteochondral allograft transplantation: is graft storage time associated with clinical outcomes and graft survivorship? Am J Sports Med. 2017;45:2260–6. https://doi.org/10.1177/0363546517704846.
10. Assenmacher AT, Pareek A, Reardon PJ, et al. Long-term outcomes after osteochondral allograft: a systematic review at long-term follow-up of 12.3 years. Arthroscopy. 2016;32:2160–8. https://doi.org/10.1016/j.arthro.2016.04.020.
11. Raz G, Safir OA, Backstein DJ, Lee PT, Gross AE. Distal femoral fresh osteochondral allografts: follow-up at a mean of twenty-two years. J Bone Joint Surg Am. 2014;96:1101–7. https://doi.org/10.2106/jbjs.m.00769.
12. Bakay A, Csonge L, Papp G, Fekete L. Osteochondral resurfacing of the knee joint with allograft. Clinical analysis of 33 cases. Int Orthop. 1998;22:277–81.
13. Beaver RJ, Mahomed M, Backstein D, et al. Fresh osteochondral allografts for post-traumatic defects in the knee. A survivorship analysis. J Bone Joint Surg Br. 1992;74:105–10.
14. Chui K, Jeys L, Snow M. Knee salvage procedures: the indications, techniques and outcomes of large osteochondral allografts. World journal of orthopedics. 2015;6:340–50. https://doi.org/10.5312/wjo.v6.i3.340.
15. Behery O, Siston RA, Harris JD, Flanigan DC. Treatment of cartilage defects of the knee: expanding on the existing algorithm. Clin J Sport Med. 2014;24:21–30. https://doi.org/10.1097/jsm.0000000000000004.
16. Capeci CM, Turchiano M, Strauss EJ, Youm T. Osteochondral allografts: applications in treating articular cartilage defects in the knee. Bulletin of the Hospital for Joint Disease. 2013;71:60–7.
17. Campbell AB, Knopp MV, Kolovich GP, et al. Preoperative MRI underestimates articular cartilage defect size compared with findings at arthroscopic knee surgery. Am J Sports Med. 2013;41:590–5. https://doi.org/10.1177/0363546512472044.
18. Gomoll AH, Yoshioka H, Watanabe A, Dunn JC, Minas T. Preoperative measurement of cartilage defects by MRI underestimates lesion size. Cartilage. 2011;2:389–93. https://doi.org/10.1177/1947603510397534.
19. Sun Y, Jiang W, Cory E, et al. Pulsed lavage cleansing of osteochondral grafts depends on lavage duration, flow intensity, and graft storage condition. PLoS One. 2017;12:e0176934. https://doi.org/10.1371/journal.pone.0176934.
20. Pisanu G, Cottino U, Rosso F, et al. Large osteochondral allografts of the knee: surgical technique and indications. Joints. 2018;6:42–53. https://doi.org/10.1055/s-0038-1636925.
21. Sadr KN, Pulido PA, McCauley JC, Bugbee WD. Osteochondral allograft transplantation in patients with osteochondritis dissecans of the knee. Am J Sports Med. 2016;44:2870–5. https://doi.org/10.1177/0363546516657526.
22. Levy YD, Gortz S, Pulido PA, McCauley JC, Bugbee WD. Do fresh osteochondral allografts successfully treat femoral condyle lesions? Clin Orthop Relat Res. 2013;471:231–7. https://doi.org/10.1007/s11999-012-2556-4.
23. Tirico LEP, McCauley JC, Pulido PA, Bugbee WD. Lesion size does not predict outcomes in fresh osteochondral allograft transplantation. Am J Sports Med. 2018;46:900–7. https://doi.org/10.1177/0363546517746106.
24. Frank RM, Lee S, Cotter EJ, et al. Outcomes of osteochondral allograft transplantation with and without concomitant meniscus allograft transplantation: a comparative matched group analysis. Am J Sports Med. 2018;46:573–80. https://doi.org/10.1177/0363546517744202.
25. Hsu AC, Tirico LEP, Lin AG, Pulido PA, Bugbee WD. Osteochondral allograft transplantation and opening wedge tibial osteotomy: clinical results of a combined single procedure. Cartilage. 2018;9:248–54. https://doi.org/10.1177/1947603517710307.
26. Tirico LEP, McCauley JC, Pulido PA, Bugbee WD. Does anterior cruciate ligament reconstruction affect the outcome of osteochondral allograft transplantation? A matched cohort study with a mean follow-up of 6 years. Am J Sports Med. 2018;46:1836–43. https://doi.org/10.1177/0363546518767636.
27. Krych AJ, Pareek A, King AH, et al. Return to sport after the surgical management of articular cartilage lesions in the knee: a meta-analysis. Knee Surg Sports Traumatol Arthrosc. 2017;25:3186–96. https://doi.org/10.1007/s00167-016-4262-3.
28. Campbell AB, Pineda M, Harris JD, Flanigan DC. Return to sport after articular cartilage repair in athletes' knees: a systematic review. Arthroscopy. 2016;32:651–668.e651. https://doi.org/10.1016/j.arthro.2015.08.028.
29. Nielsen ES, McCauley JC, Pulido PA, Bugbee WD. Return to sport and recreational activity after osteochondral allograft transplantation in the knee. Am J Sports Med. 2017;45:1608–14. https://doi.org/10.1177/0363546517694857.

30. Zou S, Dodd RY, Stramer SL, Strong DM. Probability of viremia with HBV, HCV, HIV, and HTLV among tissue donors in the United States. N Engl J Med. 2004;351:751–9. https://doi.org/10.1056/NEJMoa032510.
31. Gaul F, Tirico LEP, McCauley JC, Bugbee WD. Long-term follow-up of revision osteochondral allograft transplantation of the ankle. Foot Ankle Int. 2018;39:522. https://doi.org/10.1177/1071100717750578.
32. Horton MT, Pulido PA, McCauley JC, Bugbee WD. Revision osteochondral allograft transplantations: do they work? Am J Sports Med. 2013;41:2507–11. https://doi.org/10.1177/0363546513500628.

9 Synthetic and Mini-metal Implants in the Knee

Tim Spalding, Iswadi Damasena, and Leif Ryd

9.1 Introduction

The treatment of isolated chondral and osteochondral lesions remains a clinical challenge, with multiple proposed algorithms [1]. Chondral regenerative procedures do best in younger patients, while older patients with progressive osteoarthritis are treated with arthroplasty. A "gap" has been identified, where some patients with focal knee lesions are considered too old for biological treatment or already have failed biological treatment, but too young for unicompartmental or total arthroplasty (UKA/TKA) [2]. Mini-metal implants have been proposed as a solution to fill this gap.

Around for more than 15 years, there are three current products on the market in this area: HemiCAP/UniCAP (Arthrosurface Inc., Franklin, Massachusetts, USA), Episealer (Episurf, Sweden), and the BioPoly RS Knee system (Schwartz Biomedical, Fort Wayne, USA). The HemiCAP implant was introduced in 2003, and in 2006 the UniCAP was approved for larger cartilage lesions, with the ability to address both the medial and lateral compartments of the knee [3]. The BioPoly and the Episealer systems have subsequently followed and have been in clinical use since 2013. This chapter reviews these three products describing the implants and the surgical technique for implantation, rehabilitation, and available results.

T. Spalding (✉) · I. Damasena
Department of Trauma & Orthopaedic Surgery, University Hospital Coventry and Warwickshire NHS Trust, Coventry, Warwickshire, UK
e-mail: tim.spalding@uhcw.nhs.uk; iswadi.damasena@uhcw.nhs.uk

L. Ryd
Karolinska Institute, Stockholm, Sweden

Episurf Medical AB, Stockholm, Sweden
e-mail: Leif.Ryd@episurf.com

9.2 Indications

Mini-metal and synthetic implants are indicated for the treatment of focal chondral defects on the medial and lateral femoral condyle and the trochlea. The intention is for the implant to share load through the joint by filling a chondral defect matching the surrounding articular surface. Patient profiling is important, and the ideal candidate is a patient with specific compartmental knee pain, usually aged between 40 and 65 years of age, and who has failed previous conservative treatment for a primary chondral or osteochondral lesion or failed previous biologic resurfacing procedures. There should be no or minimal degenerative change on the opposing joint surface (max should be ICRS grade 2 partial thickness loss), and weight-bearing X-rays should show normal joint space as measured by joint height. Range of motion should show within 5° full extension and only 10° loss of flexion.

M. Brittberg, K. Slynarski (eds.), *Lower Extremity Joint Preservation*,
https://doi.org/10.1007/978-3-030-57382-9_9

Malalignment up to 5° is allowed, but over that alignment should be corrected by osteotomy.

For the status of the meniscus, it is generally accepted that there should be 50% or more remaining without significant extrusion. There should not be any evidence of bony deformities, erosions, or cystic formations. Diagnosis and suitability for the potential of using partial resurfacing are made on MRI preoperatively where measurement of the damaged area and state of the corresponding surface can be evaluated. Standard anteroposterior, lateral radiographs and the Rosenberg standing posteroanterior 45-degree view should show no loss of joint space.

Patient expectations are important to consider as it is generally advised that impact activities and sport are not appropriate following surgery. High BMI (body mass index) and smoking are also risk factors to be considered, and there should be no significant ligament laxity and no metabolic disorders affecting bone quality.

9.3 Episealer Implant (Episurf, Sweden)

The Episealer (Episurf Medical, Stockholm, Sweden) is an innovative, patient-specific metal implant designed from MRI that is sized and shaped to fill the surface defect (Fig. 9.1a, b). The family of resurfacing implants include the Episealer Condyle Solo (CE-marked, Class IIb, year 2013), the Episealer Trochlea Solo (CE-marked, Class IIb, year 2014) and the Episealer Femoral Twin (CE-marked, Class IIb, year 2015).

Customization of the Episealer with respect to implant size (shape, diameter, and thickness) and articular surface curvature is achieved by the creation of a Damage Marking Report (Fig. 9.2a, b). This report is generated from the MRI resulting in creation of a virtual 3D model which is a replica of the patient's knee. This allows preoperative planning and individual customization of implant and surgical tools. The toolkit includes reaming and insertion instrumentation and an individualized 3D printed cutting guide to enable exact perpendicular insertion and correct depth of implantation. MRI sequences required are specific for the system and need to include a 3D volume sequence. Production of the patient specific implant and instruments takes approximately 5 weeks.

The mini-prosthesis is manufactured from cobalt-chrome alloy. The articulating surface is individualized to the curvature of the affected condyle (Fig. 9.1a, b) utilizing a CAD/CAM process based on the MRI. The surface is polished down to Ra = 0.05 μm (5 times better than industry standard). The under surface has an undercut peripheral edge and a flat underside designed to rest on the subchondral bone. The surface is double coated with a layer of hydroxyapatite on top of a layer of titanium, both 60 μm thick. For location and fixation there is a 3-mm-wide, 15-mm-long peg which inserts into an undersized drill

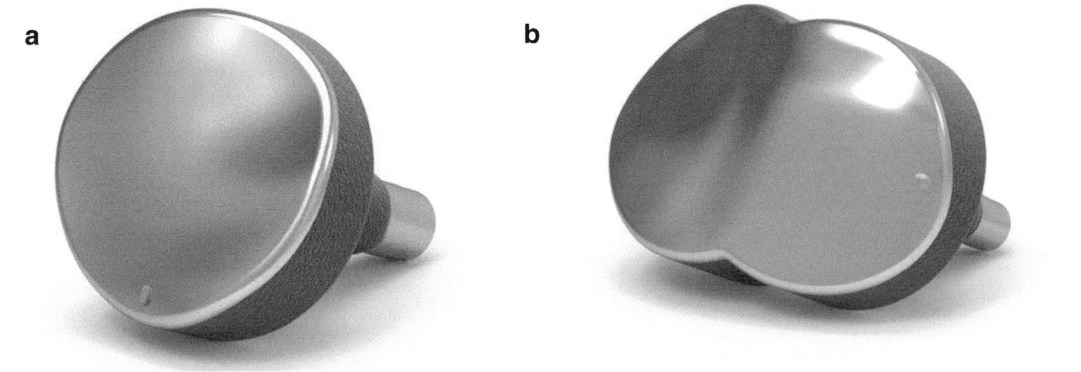

Fig. 9.1 (**a**) Episealer Solo implant (reproduced with permission from Episurf). (**b**) Episealer Twin implant (reproduced with permission from Episurf)

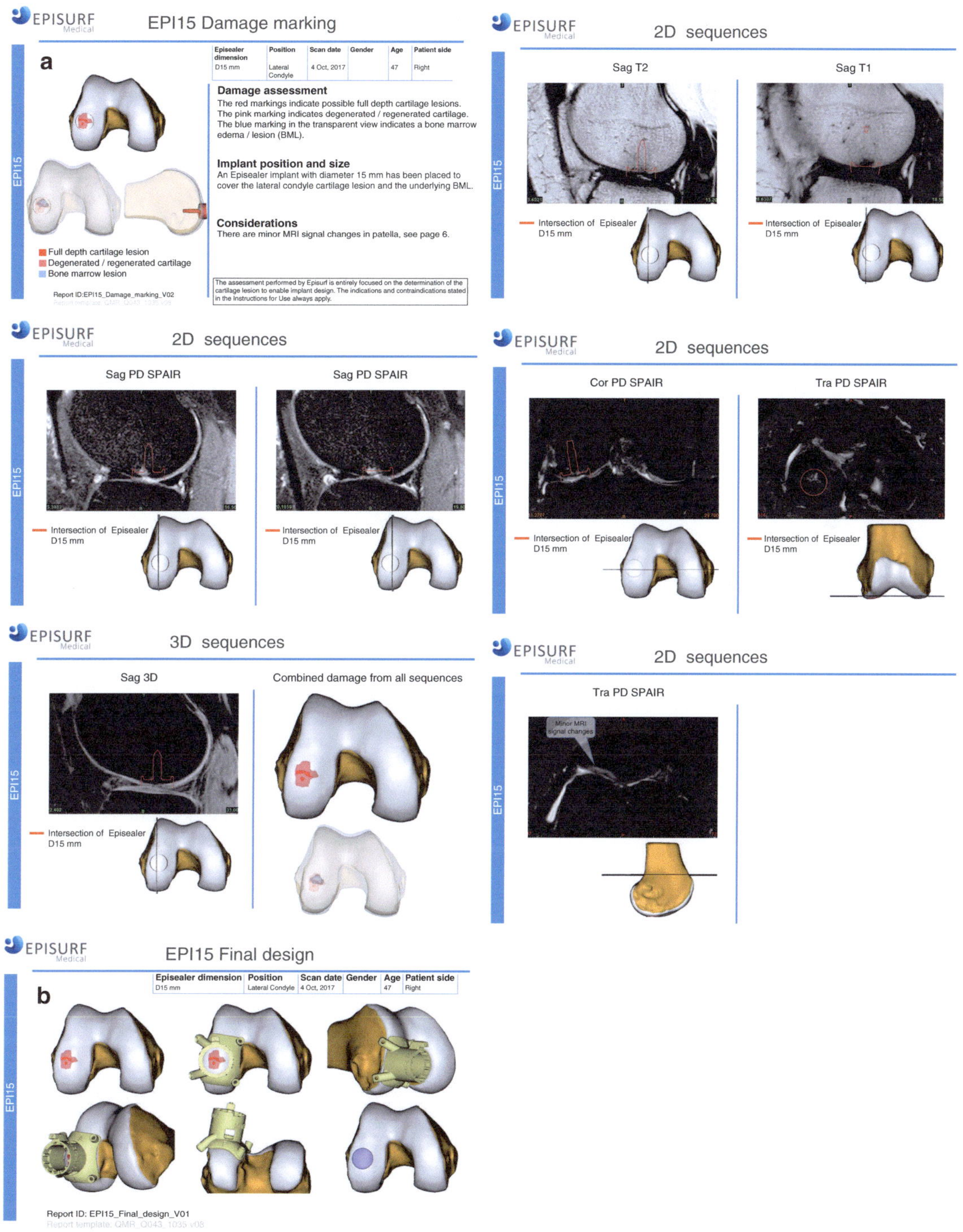

Fig. 9.2 (**a**) Episealer damage marking report illustration showing area of articular cartilage damage (reproduced with permission from Episurf). (**b**) Episealer design report with drill guide in place prepared for surgeon to approve before manufacture (reproduced with permission from Episurf)

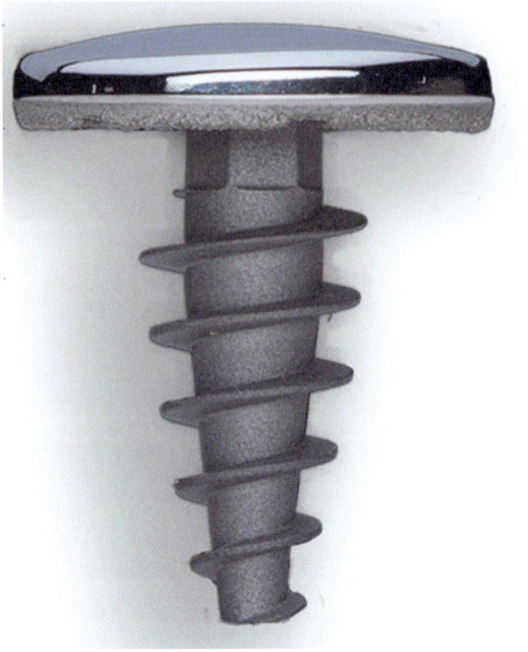

Fig. 9.3 HemiCap Implant with permission from Arthrosurface

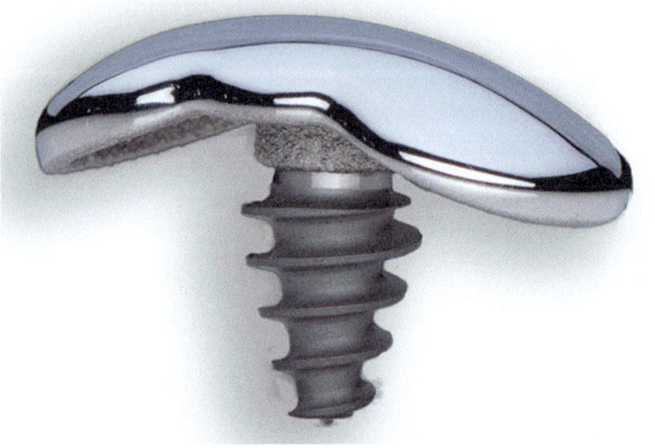

Fig. 9.4 UniCap implants with permission from Arthrosurface

hole to provide immediate interference fixation (Fig. 9.1a, b).

Correct positioning of the implant is aided by means of a corresponding, patient-specific toolkit, to assist the surgeon during surgery. A guiding tool (Epiguide) is made patient-specific from the MR images. This guide is delivered together with the implant and six more tools in a complete kit of surgical instruments. The tools are referred to as Epiguide, Epidummy, Drilling socket, Adjustment socket, Epimandrel, Epidrill, and Epicut. Recently, the Epidrill has been updated with a new cutting edge, and the Epicut has been excluded from the kit.

9.4 HemiCAP/UniCAP System (Arthrosurface, USA)

The system, introduced in 2004, uses novel knee resurfacing technology and has more than six different implant shapes and 70 different convexities. It is an inlay prosthetic system that preserves healthy surrounding tissues. The system is modular such that an off-the-shelf implant can be implanted, based on convexity measurements taken at surgery subsequently matched as close as possible to the inventory of sizes.

The femoral articulating component is made of cobalt chrome (CoCrMo) with a titanium plasma spray undercoating. The circular HemiCAP component has two diameters: 15 and 20 mm (Fig. 9.3). There is a range of over 16 surface convexities and symmetrical and asymmetrical curvatures, which match the intraoperative surface measurements of the defect determined at the time of surgery. A tapered screw post made from titanium alloy (Ti-6Al-4V) and bead blasted is placed in the bone, and the implant is then "press fit" onto the screw by means of a morse taper, in order to interlock the components and provide implant stability within a shallow bone bed.

The UniCAP component is available in two lengths (27 or 40 mm) and essentially is a larger length implant combining two circular implants on one fixation screw (Fig. 9.4). In addition, the system allows for damage on the tibial surface to be covered by a 20 mm tibial polyethylene component (UHMWPE) cemented into place, after retro-drilling the tibia. Many surgeons, however, have chosen not to implant the tibial component, and this is in part due to the technical difficulty of socket preparation and implant insertion.

As with most new technologies, proper indications and technique have as much to do with outcomes as the implant itself. Placing the implants recessed to the surface goes counterintuitive to a surgeons' desire for perfect placement as the immediate intraoperative visual fit looks "imperfect" or incongruent. However, cartilage compresses with load and metal does not. Congruency under load is the objective. In a way, it is contrary to OC grafting where the principle is to leave it slightly proud as a certain amount of biological subsidence is assumed postoperatively.

As a key part of the design, careful intraoperative measuring of the defect shape is required to match the implant curvature to the curvature of the articular surface. There needs to be an intact bony rim to ensure bony stability. The locating screw in this system is aligned strictly perpendicular via an effective cannulated system of guides and reamers. Similar to the other implant systems, it is important to place the implant slightly recessed below the articular surface (0.5 mm) to avoid damage to the opposing articular surfaces.

9.5 BioPoly (Schwartz Biomedical, USA)

The BioPoly RS Partial Resurfacing Knee Implant was also developed for the management of symptomatic chondral lesions. BioPoly is a biosynthetic implant and is a microcomposite manufactured from ultrahigh molecular weight polyethylene in combination with hyaluronic acid—a hydrophilic lubricating molecule (Fig. 9.5). The product is overmolded onto a grit-blasted titanium-alloy base plate and stem. Three sizes (15 mm diameter, 20 mm diameter, and a 15 × 24 mm racetrack-shaped implant) are available, and the implant articulates on the tibial and meniscal surfaces. Like the metal implants, rehabilitation is faster than biologic components, and less resection is required in comparison with partial or total arthroplasty.

9.6 Mini-metal Implants Basic Science

From a basic scientific perspective, there are three challenges that need to be met for a metal implant to be successful. The implant must bond to the bone, the opposing cartilage must be able to withstand a hard surface and thirdly the surrounding cartilage must react favourably to the implant. Bonding to the bone can be achieved in a few ways. Cementation, using polymethylmethacrylate (PMA), is a time-honoured mode of fixation. Screw fixation is currently used in the HemiCAP and UniCAP implant systems [1]. Titanium has been shown to function long term in tooth implants resulting in so-called osseointegration [4]. Finally, hydroxyapatite (HA) has been shown to result in bony ongrowth in a very consistent way [5].

The Episealer implant features a double coating, with HA on top of titanium. This combination has been studied in sheep and shown to result in excellent bone-to-implant contact of 90%+ after 12 months [6]. The same double coating has also resulted in zero migration, using RSA-measurements, in a clinical trial after 24 months indicating that consistent bonding to bone can be achieved [7].

For cartilage to articulate against a hard metal surface may appear counter-intuitive at first sight.

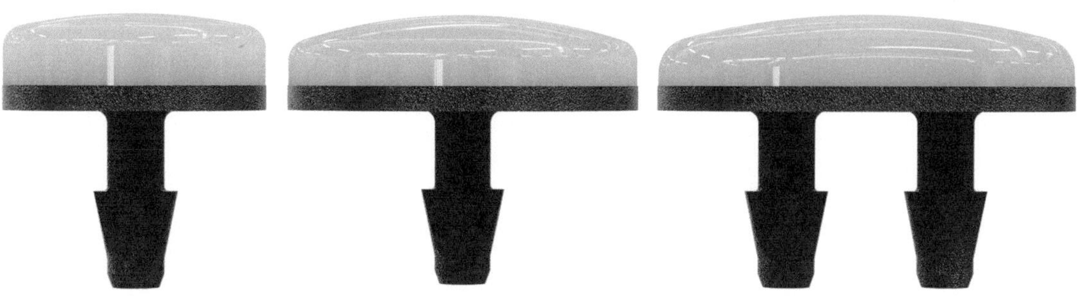

Fig. 9.5 BioPoly implants with permission from Schwartz Biomedical

This wear couple is, however, often existing in TKA, where hyaline cartilage is articulating against prosthetic metal (chrome-cobalt) when the arthroplasty is performed without a patellar button. The Swedish Knee Registry reports this to be a valid alternative with long-term data [8]. In the field of small implants, the opposing cartilage has been shown to be sensitive to implant placement, and the implant must be counter sunk by 0.5–1.0 mm—it should not protrude [9].

The reaction of the surrounding cartilage is arguably the most crucial aspect of small implant surgery, and the preparation of this junction is of the utmost importance. Contrary to any other modes of treatment, a hard implant will support the cartilaginous edges and, hence, counteract the "pot hole effect" of progressive cartilage loss. The reaction of cartilage to the double coating in the Episealer implant (HA—on-top-of-titanium) has been studied in a sheep model and close adherence of cartilage to the implant was reported [6]. These authors suggested the "chondro-integration" occurred between cartilage and HA, which was further confirmed in a controlled study [10].

9.7 Surgical Technique

9.7.1 Episealer Technique

A specific MR examination including diagnostic and 3D sequences (total scan time usually less than 20 min) is uploaded on a dedicated web platform and analysed by a software engineer at the company headquarters. Using these images, a 3D graphic and "damage report" is produced specifying the cartilage damage and bone marrow lesions (Fig. 9.2a, b). A proposed implant is overlaid on the damage report and returned to the surgeon over the web platform. Once this is approved by the surgeon, individualized implants and guide instruments are manufactured and supplied.

At surgery a limited arthrotomy is created determined by the location of the defect. Enough exposure is required to allow safe seating of the guide sleeve. Retractors can be used to manipulate the capsule around the base of the Epiguide system. Supports on the operating table must be positioned to hold the knee in the exact position required. Medially, a sub-vastus approach provides excellent exposure and reduces morbidity associated with a longer mid rectus incision. The incision is made adjacent to the patella and then extended under the vastus medialis opening up the capsule. Appropriate retractors are then inserted to sublux the patella laterally and a second retractor to hold the capsule medially. For a lateral approach, the incision may need to be longer due to the patella covering the condyle. Trochlea lesions are ideally exposed through a medial approach, either sub-vastus or mid-vastus.

The procedure can be broken down into key stages:

1. The abnormal area on the articular surface is identified and outlined.
2. The Epiguide is then inserted and exactly positioned according to the pre-op plan (Fig. 9.6a). It is held in place using three sharp pins that are supplied in the instrumentation. Looking down the Epiguide sleeve, the abnormal area is then identified and correlated once more with the pre-op plan. It is useful to have this plan clearly visible in the operating room.
3. The drill socket is then inserted at the zero point, and the Epidrill is inserted and drilled down until the metal touches the edge of the rim (Fig. 9.6b). The guide is then removed.
4. The adjustable socket is inserted at the zero marking (Fig. 9.6c), and the Epidrill is used once more bottoming out on to the guide (Fig. 9.6d). The Epiguide is then removed and the prepared area inspected. Debris from the reaming is removed by use of suction and irrigation, and the Epidummy, which matches the final implant, is inserted to assess the coverage depth (Fig. 9.6e).
5. The superior margin of the socket is marked with a sterile pen to enable accurate positioning of the implant.
6. A blunt end of the pin is used to probe the edge at this stage. It is usually slightly proud, and so the adjustable socket guide is then

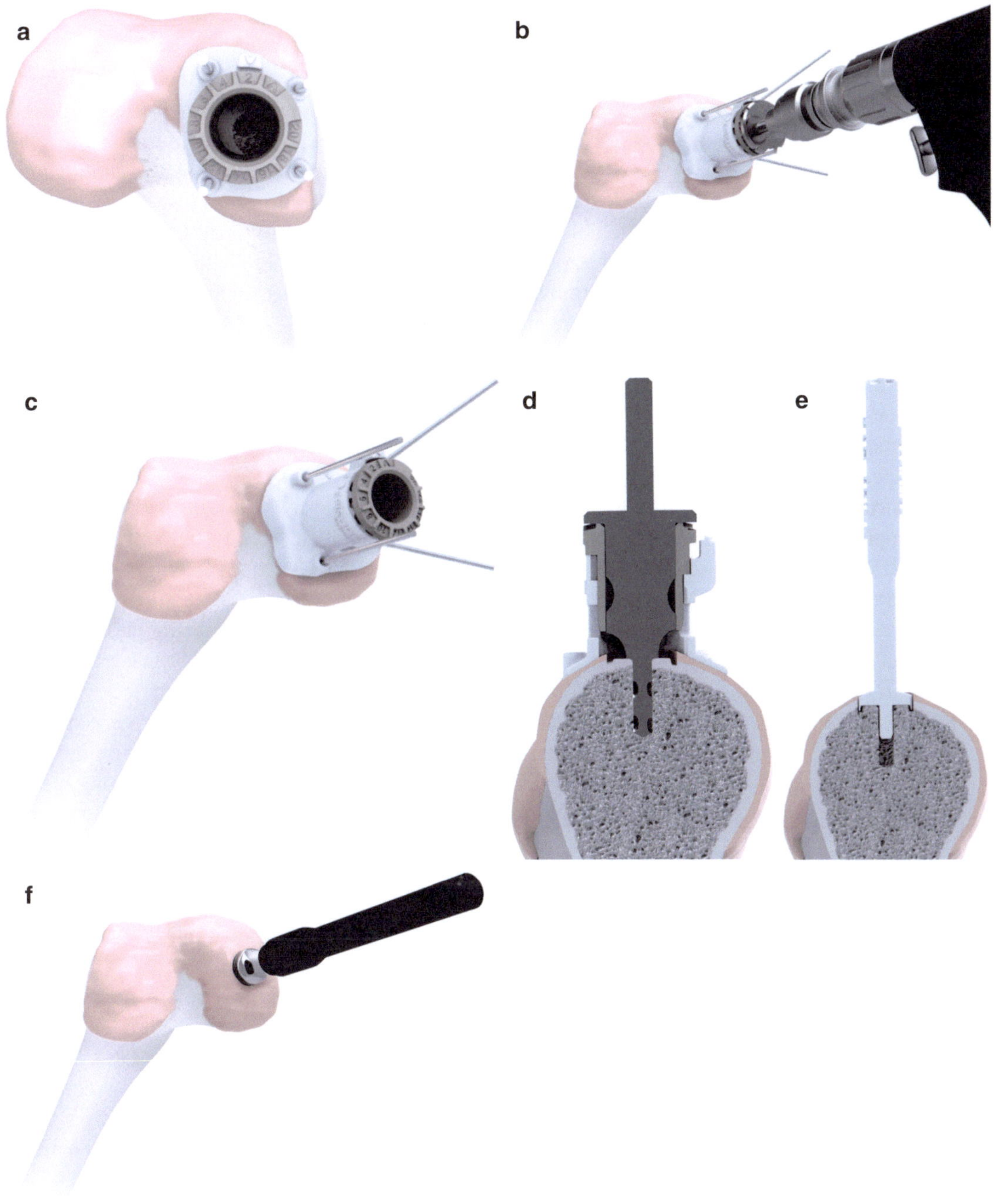

Fig. 9.6 Episealer technique for Solo implant (all image reproduced with permission from Episurf). (**a**) Epiguide attached according to preoperative plan. (**b**) Epidrill inserted and drilled to the guide rim. (**c**) Adjustable socket in place for drilling. (**d**) Epidrill creating socket. (**e**) Trial implant for depth—insertion of Epidummy. (**f**) Insertion and impaction of implant

rotated to a new point. Each 2 mm marking represents a further depth cut of 0.2 mm and the socket is redrilled and reamed prior to checking with the Epidummy once more. This step can be repeated to achieve the correct depth of resection.

7. The arthroscope can be used to inspect the guide, and the aim is to achieve the guide sitting about 0.5–1 mm below the level of the articular surface. The guide is then removed, and the Epidummy is checked once more and any prominent edge of the articular surface can be tidied up. The defect is now ready for insertion of the Episealer implant which is positioned according to the premarked superior aspect of the articular margin. This mark is important.
8. The implant is positioned manually and then tapped in to place using the Epimandrel inserter (Fig. 9.6f). It is inserted until it is just recessed under the edge of the articular surface, as set by the reaming. The edge is carefully probed to see it is beneath the margin.
9. For closure, the sub-vastus approach or lateral arthrotomy is brought together. Extensive local anaesthetic infiltration is performed with closure according to the surgeon's preference.

9.7.1.1 Technique for Insertion of Twin Episealer

When the twin Episealer is to be implanted, there are additional few steps to ensure optimal positioning, and slightly more exposure is required than when using a single Episealer (Fig. 9.7a–d).

1. The Epiguide is oval in shape (Fig. 9.7a) with a central cutting element, and the guide needs to be rotated with the drill 180° to create the oval socket. The depth preparation is performed in a similar manner to the solo.
2. A key point is to rotate both the guide and adjustable drill socket tubes to drill the inferior area. Care is taken to ensure the same depth is reamed in both areas (Fig. 9.7b).
3. Viewing the Episealer twin is easier as there is more space around the Epidummy trial. The blunt ended guide pin is used to probe the interface in order to achieve the optimal depth 0.5 mm below the surrounding articular cartilage is achieved.
4. There is no need to mark the area for orientation as the superior aspect is clear from the implant shape. The twin implant is inserted tapping it into place (Fig. 9.7c), and it should sit at the desired height just below the joint surface (Fig. 9.7d). Any edge of prominent articular surface or fibrillation can be removed prior to local anaesthetic infiltrated and closure of the joint.

9.7.2 HemiCAP and UniCAP Surgical Technique

A small arthrotomy is established exposing the affected medial or lateral compartment and the chondral lesion. The knee is positioned in a stable hold by means of good table supports to allow perpendicular access. The technique consists of the detailed stages below. In overview, a femoral drill guide is placed over the defect with four points of contact to establish a perpendicular working axis for a guide pin. Specific measurements are made, which determine the specific implant to be inserted. A specific fixation screw is inserted using the guide system and the HemiCAP implant impacted onto the morse taper of the screw.

The key stages as shown in Fig. 9.8 are:

1. The appropriate drill guide is used to locate the axis perpendicular to the articular surface and covering the defect (Fig. 9.8a). This is a key step as it determines both coverage and exact alignment of the implant.
2. The Guide Pin is inserted to the etch marking on the Guide Pin, aligned on the guide.
3. A cannulated drill is placed over the Guide Pin and inserted until the proximal shoulder of drill is flush to the articular surface (Fig. 9.8b). It is important to use lavage for this stage.
4. The hole is then tapped to the etched depth mark on the Tap (Fig. 9.8c).
5. The screw fixation component is inserted until the line on the Driver is flushed with the

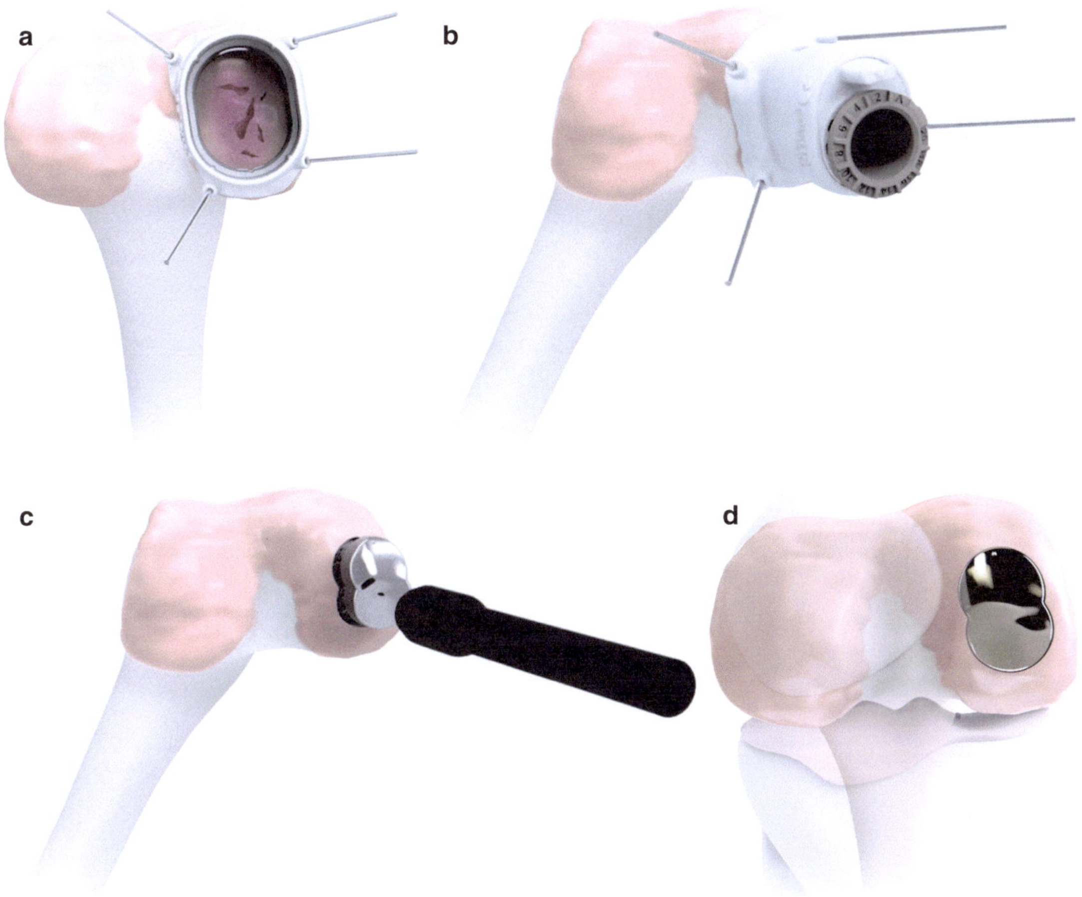

Fig. 9.7 Episealer technique for Twin implant (all images reproduced with permission from Episurf). (**a**) Positioning of guide. (**b**) Oval-shaped guide and drill system. (**c**) Insertion of Episealer implant. (**d**) Final view of implant

contour of the adjacent cartilage surface (Fig. 9.8d).

6. The Guide Pin is removed, and the Trial Cap attached to the screw to confirm correct depth of the Fixation Component—slightly below the adjacent articular cartilage surface (Fig. 9.8e). The screw can be inserted further if necessary. The Trial Cap is then removed.
7. Next the femoral surface is prepared. The Centring Shaft is reinserted into the screw Fixation Component and the Contact Probe inserted over the Centring Shaft. This is rotated around to measure offsets at four indexing points (Fig. 9.8f), noting the numbers on the appropriate Sizing Card (15 or 20 mm diameter guide).
8. From the card the appropriate Articular Component is selected.
9. The Guide Pin replaces the Centring Shaft and the Circle Cutter applied to score the articular cartilage.
10. The correct Surface Reamer is chosen dependant on the measured offsets (matching colour codes) and drilled until it contacts the top surface on the Fixation Component (Fig. 9.8g). A useful tip is to begin reaming before contact with bone to prevent chipping of articular rim.
11. The Sizing Trial is inserted (Fig. 9.8h), and the fit is checked to be slightly recessed. It can be adjusted using the next reamer. The Sizing Trials must match the Surface Reamer's offset size.

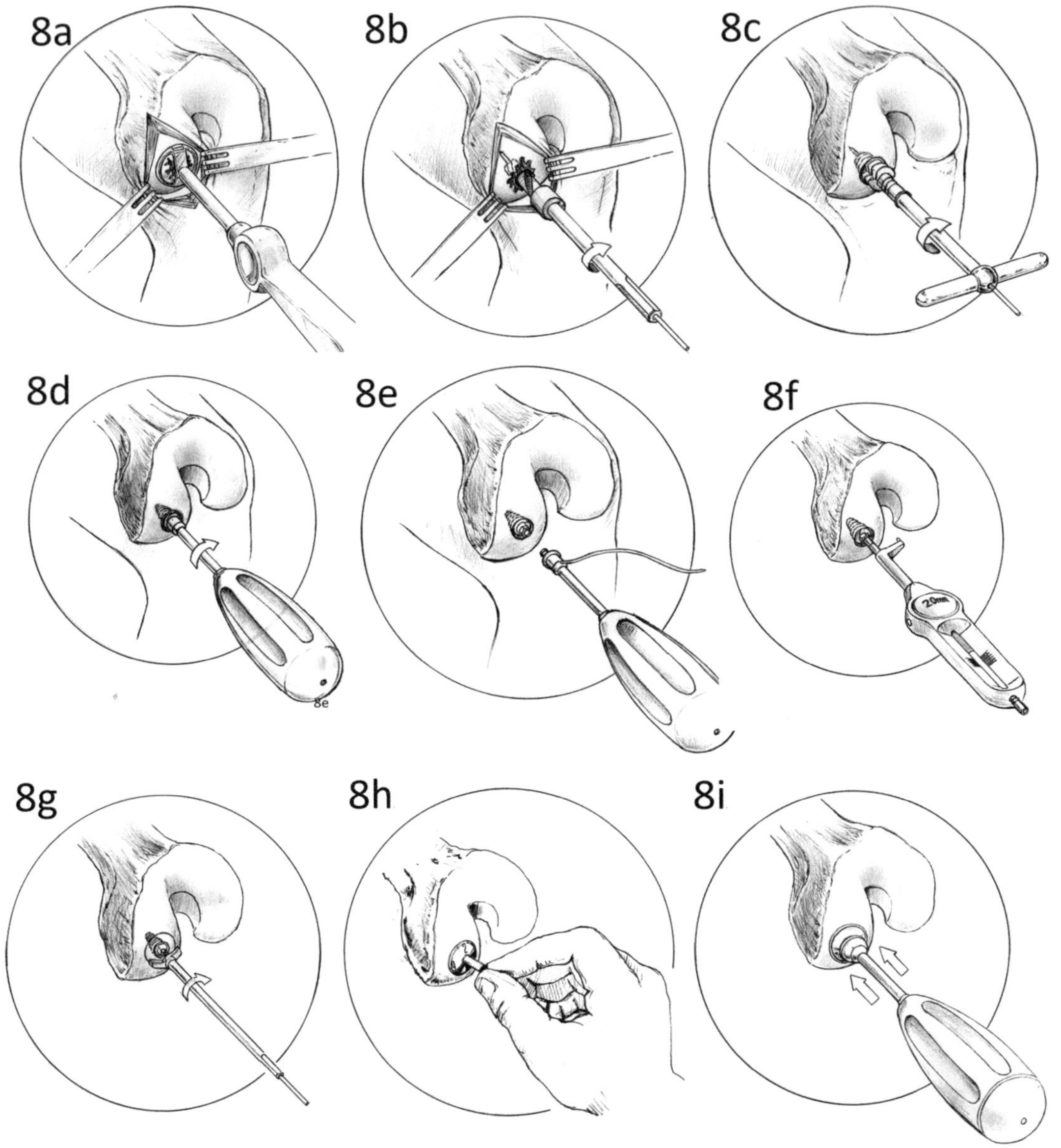

Fig. 9.8 (**a**–**i**) HemiCap implant technique, see text for description of stages (all images reproduced with permission from Arthrosurface)

12. Finally, the Articular Component is firmly impacted into place, seated on the bone (Fig. 9.8i).
13. Cement is applied to the underside of the component, and the Articular Component is aligned on the handle of the Implant Holder prior to insertion onto the taper of the Fixation Component. The component is then firmly impacted onto the morse taper connection on the screw.
14. After irrigation of the knee joint, routine closure is performed according to the surgeon's choice

For the UniCAP procedure, a different guide block is used, determined by the sizing guide.

This guide allows insertion of guide wires for over-reaming to allow accurate depth position of the larger implant.

9.7.3 BioPoly Surgical Technique

The surgical technique for the BioPoly RS Partial Resurfacing Knee Implant involves preparation of a specific socket, similar to the techniques for the mini-metal implants. A simple, bone-sparing technique is used to establish the correct implant orientation and depth relative to surrounding anatomy, and the BioPoly implant is press fit into place.

The key stages are illustrated in Fig. 9.9:

1. Implant sizing is determined by placing the appropriately sized trial over the defect to ensure adequate cover (Fig. 9.9a).
2. The drill guide is applied to the articular cartilage (Fig. 9.9b), centred on the defect, and a drill pin is inserted to the etched line. It is vital that this step achieves perpendicular alignment, and this can be adjusted by checking the guide for movement as the wire is inserted.
3. The drill guide is removed, and an appropriately sized guide tube is placed over the pilot nail (Fig. 9.9b). A cutting cannula is then

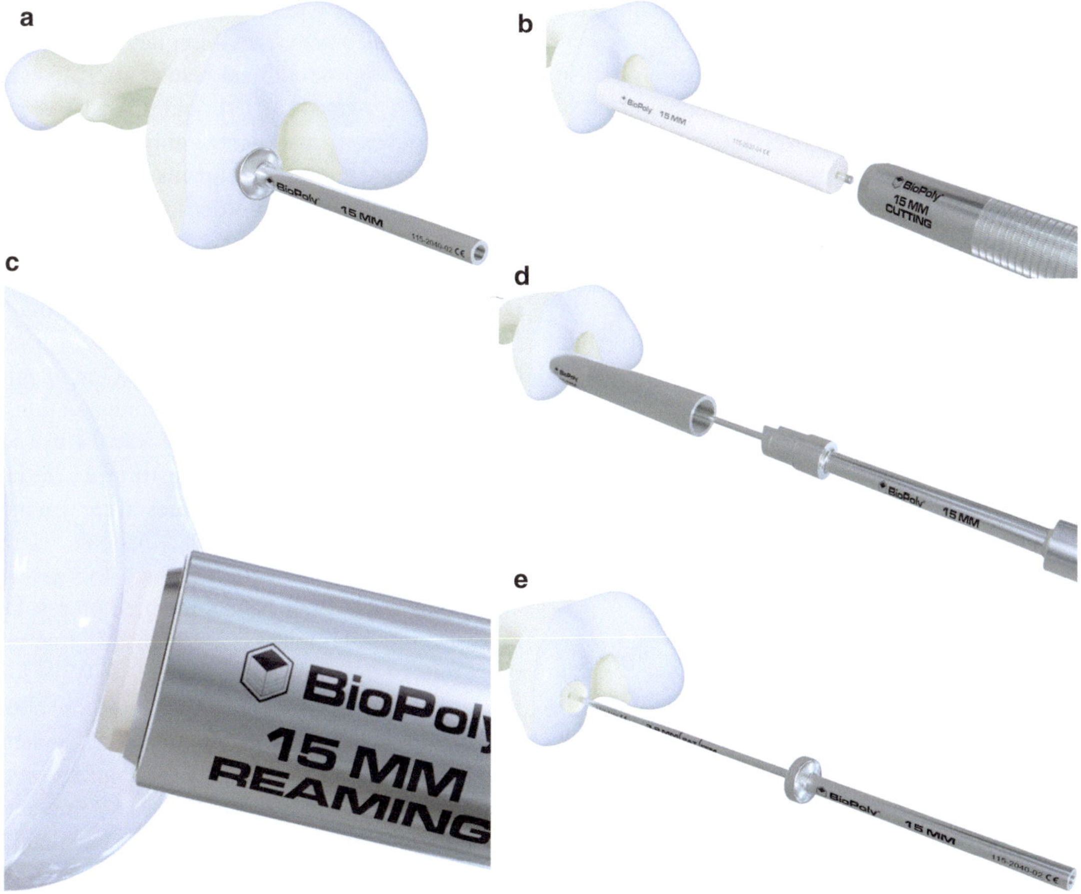

Fig. 9.9 BioPoly implant technique (all images reproduced with permission from Schwartz Biomedical). (**a**) Sizing guide applied to defect determining cover. (**b**) Insertion cutting guide to score the articular cartilage. (**c**) Reaming cannula applied. (**d**) Insertion of reamer through reaming cannula. (**e**) Trial inserted over guide wire

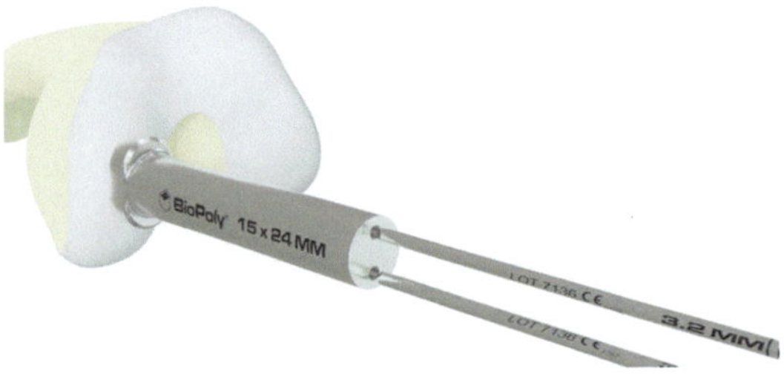

Fig. 9.10 Guide for preparation of Biopoly 15 × 24 implant

positioned over the guide tube and manually twisted to cut the cartilage (Fig. 9.9c).

4. The reaming cannula is then placed over the guide tube, and the inner guide tube is removed, to be replaced by a cannulated reamer on the pilot nail (Fig. 9.9d).
5. The reamer is drilled under irrigation until it contacts the top of the reaming cannula.
6. The trial is inserted over the pilot nail and checked to be 0.5 mm recessed below the articulating cartilage (Fig. 9.9e).
7. Finally, the trial and guide wire are removed, and the implant is inserted by pressing the distal end of the matching inserter over the implant and pushing into the site and gently impacting.

When using the 15 mm × 24 mm implant, two pilot nails are inserted using the 15 mm × 24 mm drill guide that has two holes (Fig. 9.10), and a second reaming is required for the shape of the implant. Intervening cartilage is removed using a blade.

9.8 Postoperative Care and Rehabilitation

For all implants on the distal femoral condyle, the rehabilitation is essentially the same as the implants are stable under load. A gradual return to activities is allowed. Partial weight bearing as tolerated is encouraged for 6 weeks before weaning off crutches, in order to help bony ingrowth. If a patient cannot comply with rehabilitation, then the femoral implant should be cemented in place to prevent micromotion.

Cycling can commence as soon as range of flexion allows, and swelling is used as a guide allowing introduction of strength work with physiotherapy. Return to sport activities, avoiding impact running, starts when full flexion is achieved and there is no pain or swelling. The total recovery time is variable, and because the approach is minimally invasive, return to activity can be very quick at 10–12 weeks though in some patients it can take up to 6–9 months for full resolution to be obtained.

9.9 Published Clinical Results

With exact placement, metal implants have been shown to give good clinical results after 2 years [11], after 5 years [12, 13], and after 12 years [14]. However, there is inevitably a failure or conversion rate with such implants and the results need to be understood in order to better quantify and optimise the indications.

HemiCAP and UniCAP Implants Around 50,000 HemiCAP® and UniCAP® devices have been inserted worldwide according to the manufacturing company (personal communication). Malahias et al. [15] conducted a systematic and comprehensive review analysing 10 of 21 initial studies. No Level I or II studies were found. Three hundred and thirty-four patients were included in the review with mean age 43.5 years, 48% being male. Four papers reported on results of the HemiCAP implant [12, 13, 16, 17], four on the results of the resurfacing HemiCAP-Wave for trochlea defects [18–21], one reported on both [19], and one reported on the UniCAP implant [20]. Overall use of the UniCAP implants showed inferior clinical results to the HemiCAP implant, and three out of four studies which statistically assessed the radiographic osteoarthritic changes reported significant worsening of the OA grade at the follow-up end point. The mean VAS pain score improved from 7.3 preoperative to 2.4. The total mean preoperative KSS was 50.5 which improved to 89 (used in two studies), and the total mean WOMAC improved from 42 to 86.

Failure rates were not analysed in this review to give a clear figure for expected survival.

The review noted that there was a lack of mid- to long-term, well-designed clinical studies, and any published studies were small [14]. In addition, the progression of osteoarthritis seemed to be a major drawback of the procedure. The authors concluded that partial resurfacing for femoral or patellofemoral compartments resulted in good short-term outcomes for middle-aged patients, and the procedure lies between biological treatments and arthroplasty. Patients should be aware of the failure rates, or conversion rate, buying time before joint replacement surgery.

For the femoral condyle lesions, Bollars et al. [13] reported excellent results in 18 middle aged patients after a mean follow up of 34 months. Becher et al. [12] reported on 5-year results in 21 patients also noting excellent results. Dhollander et al. [17] reported good clinical results but looked at radiological changes and found that the HemiCAP resulted in osteoarthritic changes after a mean follow up period of 26.1 months in 14 patients. Pascual-Garrido et al. [16] compared the HemiCAP in 32 patients to alternative biological treatment in 30 patients showing similar clinical improvement.

Laursen has comprehensively studied a prospective cohort of patients with outcome at 3 months, 1 year, and 2 years [20]. Radiologic status (Kellgren–Lawrence system), American Knee Society Scores (AKSS) with objective and function subscales, and the visual analogue scale (VAS) pain scores were evaluated. Sixty-one patients with trochlear and condylar cartilage lesions were treated with the HemiCAP® implant [22], and 64 patients were treated with the femoral component of the UniCAP® implant for either full-thickness cartilage lesions or early OA [20]. The cohorts were subsequently reported with up to 10 years clinical and radiographic results (126 patients aged 35–65 who were operated on with either the HemiCAP® or UniCAP® resurfacing mini-prosthesis). These studies demonstrated that the implants had a conversion rates of 40% and 60%, respectively, after 10 years of follow-up [23, 24]. The author noted that although seemingly high failure rates, or perhaps better termed conversion rates, the patients were younger than the normal age for arthroplasty and had a high level of symptoms. The author concluded from the analysis that the femoral surface replacing implants can be a temporary or even a long-term treatment for symptomatic patients, as they show improvement in disability and function even over lengthy periods.

It is important to note, however, that in the UniCAP series from Laursen et al., the tibial polyethylene button was not used, and the state of the opposing tibial surface was not recorded. While a good proportion of patients stayed happy with good function, this observation may explain the high conversion rate to arthroplasty, and it serves to help optimise indications for the procedure.

Most recently, Nahas et al. [25] reported on 14 patients with mean 10 year follow-up after HemiCAP implantation. Mean age at implantation was 40 (28–49), with ten implanted on the medial femoral condyle, two on lateral condyle, and two bicondylar. Of ten reviewed, two were revised (one to TKR and one to UKR) giving survival rate of 80% at 9.4 years.

BioPoly Implant Nathwani et al. [26] reported on the prospective results of 33 patients with focal cartilage lesions affecting the femoral condyle treated with the BioPoly implant. Outcomes were collected at 6 months, 1 year, and 2 years postoperatively and were compared with historical outcomes following microfracture treatment. More than 50% had a previous failure of cartilage-repair procedures. Significant and clinically meaningful improvements in the KOOS scores, VAS pain score, and SF-36 physical component score ($p < 0.025$) were reported for each time points compared with the preoperative scores. The Tegner activity score was significantly improved at 2 years compared with the preoperative score ($p < 0.025$). No significant differences were detected between younger patients (≤40 years) and older patients (>40 years). When compared with historical microfracture data, the BioPoly RS Implant demonstrated significantly superior KOOS scores for quality of life and sports. The authors concluded that improvement was sustained for 2 years regardless of patient age and allowed better function than after microfracture. Clearly longer-term results are required.

Episealer Implant For the Episealer, data is currently being collected as part of a controlled product launch with comprehensive analysis for factors determining outcome at 2-year follow-up. Recently published data on 80 patients with focal cartilage lesions ICRS grade 3 or 4 who were prospectively analysed at 3 months, 1 year, and 2 years postoperatively shows a low failure rate and excellent clinical scores [27]. Seventy-five patients were evaluated at a minimum 24 months following implantation. Two patients had undergone revision (2.5%), 1 declined participation, and 2 had not completed the full data requirements, leaving 75 of the 80 with complete data for analysis. The mean age was 48 years (range 27–69) and 41% were male. In 48 patients (64%), Episealer® implants were performed following failed prior articular cartilage repair procedures. Forty patients were treated with the Episealer condyle Solo implant, 25 with the Episealer condyle Twin implant and 10 were treated for defects on the trochlea (either Episealer Femoral Twin or Episealer Trochlea Solo implants). Sixty were implanted on the medial femoral condyle and 5 on the lateral condyle. Assessing the results in this comprehensive series showed that all 5 KOOS domain mean scores were significantly improved at 1 and 2 years ($p < 0.001$–0.002). Mean preoperative aggregated KOOS4 of 35 improved to 57 and 59 at 12 and 24 months respectively ($p < 0.05$). Mean VAS score improved from 63 preoperatively to 32 at 24 months. The improvement exceeded the minimal clinically important difference (MCID) and this improvement was maintained over time. Location of defect and history of previous cartilage repair did not significantly affect the outcome ($p > 0.05$), however it was accepted that this was a small study not powered to detect such differences with the factors. In discussion the authors noted the good results could be attributed to the individualised design and the specific customised and appropriate accurate guides for implantation. A low failure rate of 2.5% at 24 months was considered to indicate that mini-metal implants appear to have a definitive place in the management of focal femoral chondral and osteochondral defects in the knee [27].

9.10 Discussion

Mini-metal implants are a well-tested treatment for specific chondral defects. From a basic scientific perspective, the use of a hard metal implant may be warranted and implants have shown good tolerance in the joint. Precise surgical techniques are required to ensure optimal positioning with recession below the articular cartilage height. The key factor in long-term success is patient indications that are narrowly defined based on joint alignment, focal or localised disease rather than progressive OA, meniscal integrity, BMI, and grade ICRS 2 or less damage to the tibia. It is important to emphasize and remind that these partial implants were designed as a bridge for patients that are beyond the treatment scope of biologics and too early for a complete joint replacement. Results should not necessarily be compared to unicompartmental or total joint arthroplasty as the indications are very different. The likely ideal patient is an individual between 40 and 60 years of age, active, unwilling or unable to comply with a long postoperative biological rehabilitation protocol and the where the articular cartilage damage is localised rather than diffuse.

Clinical results from the HemiCAP and UniCAP implants, which have the longest follow-up, are concerning, but the longer-term papers report on implantation with poor description of the tibial surface. Results from the BioPOLY implant and the Episealer implant show that at short-term follow-up clinical improvement is encouraging, and failure rates are low.

9.11 Conclusion

Adherence to strict indications is important and for the right patient, especially those with failed previous cartilage repair and facing revision of articular cartilage repair; this surgery may be an excellent option, buying time and quality of active life and bridging the gap before arthroplasty. It is clear, however, that more work on outcome analysis for specific cohorts of patients with all the implants discussed is required.

References

1. Biant LC, McNicholas MJ, Sprowson AP, Spalding T. The surgical management of symptomatic articular cartilage defects of the knee: consensus statements from United Kingdom knee surgeons. Knee. 2015;22(5):446–9.
2. Li CS, Karlsson J, Winemaker M, Sancheti P, Bhandari M. Orthopedic surgeons feel that there is a treatment gap in management of early OA: international survey. Knee Surg Sports Traumatol Arthrosc. 2014;22:363–78.
3. Miniaci A. UniCAP as an alternative for unicompartmental arthritis. Clin Sports Med. 2014;33(1):57–65.
4. Adell R, Lekholm U, Rockler B, Branemark PI. A 15-year study of osseointegrated implants in the treatment of the edentulous jaw. Int J Oral Surg. 1981;10(6):387–416.
5. Soballe K. Hydroxyapatite ceramic coating for bone implant fixation. Mechanical and histological studies in dogs. Acta Orthop Scand. 1993;64(Suppl. 255):1–58.
6. Martinez-Carranza N, Berg HA, Lagerstedt AS, Nurmi-Sandh H, Schupbach P, Ryd L. Fixation of a double-coated titanium-hydroxiapatite focal knee resurfacing implant A 12-month study in sheep. Osteoarthr Cart. 2014;22(6):836–44.
7. Stålman A, Martinez-Carranza N, Roberts D, Högström M. A customized femoral resurfacing metal implant for focal chondral lesions. Short term results of the first 10 patients. Proc ICRS. 2016;2017:23–30.
8. Robertsson O, Ranstam J, Sundberg M, W-Dhal A, Lidgren L. The Swedish Knee Arthroplasty Register: a review. Bone Joint Res. 2014;3(7):217–22.
9. Martinez-Carranza N, Berg HE, Hultenby K, Nurmi-Sandh H, Ryd L, Lagerstedt AS. Focal knee resurfacing and effects of surgical precision on opposing cartilage. A pilot study on 12 sheep. Osteoarthr Cartil. 2013;21(5):739–45.
10. Schell H, Jung T, Ryd L, Duda G. On the attachment of cartilage to HA: signs of "chondrointegration". Studies on the Episealer mini-prosthesis in the sheep knee. In: Proceedings of the 17th congress of European Society of SportsTraumatology, Knee Surgery and Arthroscopy; 2016.
11. Stålman A, Sköldenberg O, Martinez-Carranza N, Roberts D, Högström M, Ryd L. No implant migration and good subjective outcome of a novel customized femoral resurfacing metal implant for focal chondral lesions. Knee Surg Sports Traumatol Arthrosc. 2018;26(7):2196–204.
12. Becher C, Kalbe C, Thermann H, Paessler HH, Laprell H, Kaiser T, et al. Minimum 5-year results of focal articular prosthetic resurfacing for the treatment of full-thickness articular cartilage defects in the knee. Arch Orthop Trauma Surg. 2011;131(8):1135–43.
13. Bollars P, Bosquet M, Vandekerckhove B, Hardeman F, Bellemans J. Prosthetic inlay resurfacing for the treatment of focal, full thickness cartilage defects of the femoral condyle: a bridge between biologics and conventional arthroplasty. Knee Surg Sports Traumatol Arthrosc. 2012;20(09):1753–9.
14. Becher C, Cantiller EB. Focal articular prosthetic resurfacing for the treatment of full-thickness articular cartilage defects in the knee: 12-year follow-up of two cases and review of the literature. Arch Orthop Trauma Surg. 2017;137(09):1307–17.
15. Malahias MA, Chytas D, Thorey F. The clinical outcome of the different HemiCAP and UniCAP knee implants: a systematic and comprehensive review. Orthop Rev. 2018;10(2):7531.
16. Pascual-Garrido C, Daley E, Verma NN, Cole BJ. A comparison of the outcomes for cartilage defects of the knee treated with biologic resurfacing versus focal metallic implants. Arthroscopy. 2017;33:364–73.
17. Dhollander AA, Almqvist KF, Moens K, et al. The use of a prosthetic inlay resurfacing as a salvage procedure for a failed cartilage repair. Knee Surg Sports Traumatol Arthrosc. 2015;23:2208–12.
18. Patel A, Haider Z, Anand A, Spicer D. Early results of patellofemoral inlay resurfacing arthroplasty using the HemiCap Wave prosthesis. J Orthop Surg. 2017;25(1):1–5.
19. Imhoff AB, Feucht MJ, Meidinger G, et al. Prospective evaluation of anatomic patellofemoral inlay resurfacing: clinical, radiographic, and sports-related results after 24 months. Knee Surg Sports Traumatol Arthrosc. 2015;23:1299–307.
20. Laursen JO. Treatment of full-thickness cartilage lesions and early OA using large condyle resurfacing prosthesis: UniCAP. Knee Surg Sports Traumatol Arthrosc. 2016;24(5):1695–701.
21. Feucht MJ, Cotic M, Beitzel K, et al. A matched-pair comparison of inlay and onlay trochlear designs for patellofemoral arthroplasty: no differences in clinical outcome but less progression of osteoarthritis with inlay designs. Knee Surg Sports Traumatol Arthrosc. 2017;25(09):2784–91.
22. Laursen JO, Lind M. Treatment of full-thickness femoral cartilage lesions using condyle resurfacing prosthesis. Knee Surg Sports Traumatol Arthrosc. 2017;25:746–51.
23. Laursen JO, Skjøt-Arkil H, Mogensen CB. Ten-year cohort study of 62 HemiCAP® patients showing initial high revision rates but good clinical outcomes and long-term survival after five years in "Treatment of full-thickness cartilage lesions and early OA in the knee using condylar resurfacing prosthesis in the middle-aged patient". PhD Thesis. University of Southern Denmark. 2019.

24. Laursen JO, Skjøt-Arkil H, Mogensen CB. UniCAP offers a long term treatment for middle-aged patients, who are not revised within the first nine years. Knee Surg Sports Traumatol Arthrosc. 2019;27(5):1693–7.
25. Nahas S, Monem M, Li L, Patel A, Parmar H. Ten-year average full follow-up and evaluation of a contoured focal resurface prosthesis (HemiCAP) in patients in the United Kingdom. J Knee Surg. 2019; https://doi.org/10.1055/s-0039-168892.
26. Nathwani D, McNicholas M, Hart A, Miles J, Bobic V, et al. Partial resurfacing of the knee with the biopoly implant: interim report at 2 years. JBJS Open Access. 2017;2(2) https://doi.org/10.2106/JBJS.OA.16.00011.
27. Holz J, Spalding T, Boutefnouchet T, et al. Patient-specific metal implants for focal chondral and osteochondral lesions in the knee; excellent clinical results at 2 years. Knee Surg Sports Traumatol Arthrosc. 2020. https://doi.org/10.1007/s00167-020-06289-7.

10 Knee Joint Preservation Rehabilitation

Karen Hambly, Jay Ebert, Barbara Wondrasch, and Holly Silvers-Granelli

10.1 Introduction and Background

10.1.1 Principles of Knee Joint Preservation Rehabilitation

Mechanical stimulation is essential for local adaptation and nutrition of the knee joint [1]. Knee injury or surgery alters the physiological load-bearing abilities of tissue and disrupts the homeostasis of the joint. The aim of knee joint preservation rehabilitation is to provide a mechanical environment for healing responses that will facilitate the restoration of joint homeostasis and the return to optimal function [2]. The frequency and intensity of load that can be applied across the knee joint without supra-physiologic overload or failure of the tissue structure in a given time period will change as rehabilitation progresses. Rehabilitation is thus a stepwise process with load progressions that reflect the biologic healing phases of the affected tissues and individual patient characteristics [1].

10.1.1.1 Overview of the Rehabilitation Process

An increasing range of knee joint preservation surgical interventions are available for osteochondral repair, all of which consider the rehabilitation process as critical for a successful outcome.

The **rehabilitation components** and when they are introduced should be **individualised** based on:

- The nature and extent of tissue damage (location, size, and quality of surrounding tissue)
- The surgical procedure (number of surgeries, type, and concomitant pathologies)
- The individual characteristics of the patient (demands of activities of daily living/sport, age, sex, symptom duration, body mass index (BMI), and general health)

Rehabilitation programmes vary considerably between patients in terms of their content and timings of progressions, but they all adhere to common principles. The **rehabilitation process** needs to reflect **the healing timescales of the**

K. Hambly (✉)
School of Sport and Exercise Sciences, University of Kent, Kent, UK
e-mail: K.Hambly@kent.ac.uk

J. Ebert
School of Human Sciences (Exercise and Sport Science), University of Western Australia, Perth, WA, Australia
e-mail: Jay@hfrc.com.au

B. Wondrasch
Department of Health Sciences, St. Poelten University of Applied Sciences, St. Poelten, Austria
e-mail: Barbara.Wondrasch@fhstp.ac.at

H. Silvers-Granelli
Research, Velocity Physical Therapy, Los Angeles, CA, USA

M. Brittberg, K. Slynarski (eds.), *Lower Extremity Joint Preservation*, https://doi.org/10.1007/978-3-030-57382-9_10

tissue which can be considered as **four overlapping phases**:

1. Inflammation
2. Proliferation
3. Remodelling
4. Maturation

The load-bearing abilities of the tissues change during these healing phases make controlling and monitoring the response to loading a core principle in the rehabilitation. The loading on an injured knee can be controlled through the application of thorough knowledge of the functional anatomy and the principles of biomechanics and exercise prescription to the selection of exercises [3]. The content of the rehabilitation programme should address restoration of full range of motion (ROM); full weight bearing (FWB); strength; neuromuscular control; and return to activity.

10.1.2 Pre-operative Rehabilitation Management (Prehabilitation)

Whereas there is strong agreement on the importance of post-operative rehabilitation after cartilage repair [2, 4], pre-operative rehabilitation is still underestimated.

Pre-operative rehabilitation should include patient education and conditioning with preparing patients mentally and physically for the surgical procedure and the post-operative period [4, 5]. Several studies including patients awaiting various surgical procedures of the lower extremity have shown that good pre-operative function can positively affect post-operative results, the duration of hospital stay and general health while reducing the risks of peri-operative complications [6, 7]. Further, a study evaluating the effects of an active rehabilitation programme for patients with cartilage defects demonstrated such an improvement of knee function that 63% of the patients postponed surgery [5].

10.1.2.1 Education

Knowledge on the nature of the chondral (or osteochondral) defect (size, geometry and location) and on knee biomechanics is essential to better understand how contraindicated knee movements and loads may affect the healing cartilage tissue in the early post-operative period [2, 4].

Teaching of proficient ambulation with crutches under different weight-bearing (WB) modalities (in percentage of body weight) should be exercised in the pre-operative period, enabling a smoother post-operative transition for the patient. Further, the stepwise rehabilitation process and load progression including progression criteria should be explained including the importance of joint homeostasis (control of pain and effusion) and the risk of permanent overloading.

10.1.2.2 Conditioning

Rehabilitation in this pre-operative phase should focus on improving muscle strength and neuromuscular control of the knee joint muscles, mobility in the tibiofemoral (TFJ) and patellofemoral (PFJ) joint and, if present, reduction of pain and effusion to enable proper knee joint function [5].

Weakness of the quadriceps, the hamstrings and the hip musculature may be significant for proceeding degenerative changes and play a role in the pathogenesis of knee osteoarthritis (KOA) [8, 9] and should therefore be addressed in all stages of the rehabilitation process. Muscle strength exercises should be performed and adjusted according to pain and other symptoms. Both open (OKC) and closed (CKC) kinetic chain exercises should be implemented and with focus on movement quality to avoid unfavourable loading patterns in the knee joint. Neuromuscular exercises should start with static and non-complex exercises with progression from double to single leg, eyes open to eyes closed and the use of unstable WB surfaces. To avoid a decrease in the proprioceptive ability of the non-affected leg, the exercises should be performed on both legs. Further, muscle strength of the core and the upper limbs should be a further focus to assist early post-operative tasks such as bed and chair transfers and crutch ambulation.

To enhance mobility in the TFJ and PFJ both **active** and **passive** modalities are recommended.

- **Passive techniques** include manual therapy with gliding techniques and soft tissue treatment to provide joint arthrokinematics, which is essential for physiological loading of the articular cartilage tissue [10].
- **Active mobility** exercises in non-weight-bearing (NWB) positions and emphasises mechanical stimulation of the cells and synovial fluid and nutrition of the cartilage tissue [11]. To prevent excessive shear forces, which might generate effusion and pain due to a symptomatic chondral lesion, active mobility exercises are recommended to be performed in a CKC system.

10.1.3 Post-operative Rehabilitation Management

10.1.3.1 Progressive Motion

Sufficient ROM of a joint is an essential prerequisite for everyday life including activities of daily living (ADLs) and sports activity. Early restoration of ROM after cartilage repair techniques is indicated to prevent adhesions, to aid in pain relief and to normalise joint arthrokinematics which is important to provide physiological loading of articular cartilage tissue [12].

Studies have shown that controlled early resumption of ROM by joint circulation exercises is beneficial in regard to knee function, whereas immobilisation will delay recovery and adversely affects cartilage tissues' physiology [13]. As chondrocytes derive their nutrition mainly from synovial fluid, quantity and quality of synovial fluid play an important role in cartilage metabolism. Joint circulation exercises are exercises with the focus of improving joint homeostasis and with the ability to stimulate synovial production. However, as the healing cartilage tissue is vulnerable in the first 4–6 weeks post-operatively, the tissue should be protected from excessive load, in particular avoidance of shear forces combined with compressive forces. Therefore, an understanding of the knee biomechanics is essential to appreciate the forces that will be exerted on the healing cartilage tissue in designing rehabilitation exercises after cartilage repair.

The flexion and extension movement within the TFJ involves a combination of rolling and gliding of the surfaces of the femur and the tibia, linked up with a spin movement at the end of flexion and extension. The TFJ is exposed to high mechanical load during vertical WB activities (e.g. during walking, standing and stair climbing) [14], which should therefore be avoided in the early post-operative phase. However, ROM exercises in unloaded or partial loaded positions produce low to moderate load and are therefore recommended. The PFJ is a sellar joint composed of the patella and the underlying femoral trochlea. In higher knee flexion angles, particularly in WB positions, the load within the PFJ increases implying increased loading of the healing cartilage tissue. ROM exercises between 0° and 90° of knee flexion in unloaded or partial loaded position are considered safe with respect to the healing tissue [15, 16].

In general, both active and passive ROM exercises are recommended and should be performed in a CKC system without substantial load to minimise shear forces over the repair site [4, 17]. Further, these exercises are safe and easy for the patient to undertake and should be performed daily and for a longer period of time. Several modalities are possible such as continuous passive motion (CPM), heel slides, cycling and rowing.

10.1.3.2 Progressing Weight Bearing

While there are several important components of the post-operative rehabilitation algorithm, the gradual progression of the patient back to full weight-bearing (FWB) gait is critical, with particular relevance to cartilage procedures in the TFJ. Clinically, an overly aggressive approach may increase pain and inflammation while risking early graft failure or tissue degradation as may be the case with autologous chondrocyte implantation (ACI) and microfracture. An approach that is too conservative may not provide the best mechanical stimulus for early tissue proliferation, subsequent maturation and longer-term durability.

With the evolving nature of cartilage repair procedures, together with clinical experience and a growing appreciation of the phases of repair tissue maturation, proposed WB protocols have become more accelerated without apparent detriment to patient outcome. While a period of tissue protection is warranted after cartilage repair, it is generally accepted that the early primitive repair tissue following procedures such as marrow stimulation (microfracture and autologous matrix-induced chondrogenesis—AMIC) and ACI needs progressive stimulation. For example, repair tissue quality after ACI may be affected by the mechanical loading stimulus in the initial post-operative period [18, 19].

In basic science research, **cyclic compressive loading** has been shown to **enhance**:

- Chondrogenesis
- Matrix synthesis
- Gene expression

Static compression and immobilisation have been demonstrating a catabolic cellular response [20–24].

Therefore, lengthy periods of knee joint immobilisation and NWB after cartilage repair are no longer advocated, with an early progressive WB programme recommended. While a conservative 6-week period of toe-touch ambulation and increase towards FWB at 11–12 weeks post-operatively was proposed initially after traditional periosteal-covered ACI [25], second-generation collagen-covered ACI techniques looked to introduce earlier WB [26], while third-generation matrix-induced ACI techniques have proven safe with accelerated WB protocols resulting in a 6–8-week return to FWB [27–29].

An initial period of tissue protection has been advocated for microfracture, with many studies recommending a return to FWB around 4–8 weeks [30], though some studies still outline a period of non-weight bearing (NWB) for up to 4 weeks post-surgery [30]. However, it has been suggested that much like the acceleration in WB demonstrated in ACI studies, scaffold-augmented microfracture techniques may also permit faster rehabilitation pathways [31]. Osteochondral autografts and allografts permit the immediate filling of the chondral defects [32]. However, despite the lack of a primitive early tissue repair and the theoretical ability to accelerate WB, studies after these procedures often still recommend an early period of NWB, with an additional period of 2–3 weeks of partial WB (PWB) [33].

Individualised WB and rehabilitation protocols remain imperative given the array of factors that will influence progression (i.e. patient demographics and physical conditioning, specific lesion size and location, concomitant surgeries, etc.). WB timelines remain varied across different surgical procedures as well as studies (i.e. randomised studies or published protocols as part of a prospective evaluation of a particular procedure). However, an element of early tissue protection throughout the proliferation phase remains, followed by a gradual increase in load as the tissue develops and matures, with a transition towards high loading (i.e. jogging, jumping, etc.) once the tissue is considered able to better absorb these loads and protect the underlying bone.

10.1.3.3 Muscle Strengthening

The **progressive muscular loading programme** aims to serve multiple functions in cartilage repair surgery, dependent on the pre- and/or post-operative timeline. This includes:

1. Addressing ROM, neuromuscular, gait and other biomechanical deficits in preparation for surgery (pre-surgery).
2. Early cellular and tissue loading to enhance tissue development, combined with minimising muscle atrophy and general limb de-conditioning in the earlier post-operative stages (0–6 weeks).

3. Graduated tissue and knee loading, combined with restoration of strength during the mid-post-operative stages (6 weeks to 3–6 months) to improve the ability to undertake daily activities and better prepare for later stage rehabilitation and return to sport.
4. Higher level loading and sport-specific strengthening exercises (5–6 months onwards) to restore optimal lower limb and trunk mechanics, thereby improving movement and reducing the risk of further injury. While the most optimal introduction of varied strengthening exercises is unknown, largely due to the lack of specific studies comparing protocols, as well as the wide array of variables that will demand a more individualised strength and conditioning programme, existing work has demonstrated good patient outcomes when following the aforementioned principles [4, 27, 34–36].

The quality of the repair tissue after cartilage repair procedures such as marrow stimulation and ACI may be, at least in part, dependent on the mechanical loading stimulus throughout the post-operative period [18, 19]. The effect of exercise on articular cartilage and the physiological responses to loading provide strong rationale for post-operative exercise rehabilitation after cartilage repair [4]. However, the most appropriate selection of exercises may be critical to accommodate the aforementioned factors, without jeopardising the integrity of the primitive tissue repair in the early stages or risking further knee injury as a result of advancing too quickly on a knee (and musculoskeletal system) poorly conditioned for higher level strengthening activities.

When considering the progression of strengthening exercises and mode of exercise to prescribe (isometric or isotonic, OKC or CKC, etc.), one must understand TFJ and PFJ arthrokinematics. This must be combined with a range of other factors including the stage of tissue healing, size, containment and specific location of the repair site, patient body weight, physical conditioning, movement coordination, activity history and compliance, as well as the close monitoring of classic signs of overload (i.e. pain, effusion) [4]. Of particular further importance to cartilage defects, these patients often endure a lengthy pre-operative duration of symptoms, unlike those who may undergo anterior cruciate ligament (ACL) reconstruction almost immediately after an acute ACL injury. Therefore, these patients often present pre-operatively with excessive muscular weakness, poor neuromuscular control and knee function [5, 37], making post-surgical strengthening even more important in order to address post-operative (and already existing pre-operative) muscular deficits. In considering these factors, the therapist can manipulate the exercise(s) selected to deliver an individualised programme that improves physical function while minimising detrimental forces across the tissue repair.

In summary, progressive strengthening should accommodate the phases of tissue development and plays an important role in repair tissue stimulation and the restoration of strength and functional deficits that must be addressed to ensure a full and unrestricted return to work and/or sporting activities.

10.1.3.4 Neuromuscular Re-education

Neuromuscular re-education addresses many critical factors following a cartilage repair surgery. Generalised exercise and strength training have served as the gold standard for the conservative management of diagnosed cartilage lesions and for both pre- and post-operative interventions. These interventions have been shown to impart positive effects demonstrated by a reduction in pain, effusion and overall improved patient function [38, 39]. However, strength training in isolation does not adequately address the functional instability or the deficiencies in neuromuscular stabilisation of the affected joint [40]. Historically, neuromuscular training exercises have been successfully integrated into injury prevention programmes, in order to mitigate risk to ligamentous and cartilage structures in the knee joint [41–44].

The **primary goal of neuromuscular training** is to improve:

- Sensorimotor cortical control
- Improve overall biomechanical movement
- Achieve sufficient functional stability of the joint [45, 46]

Alterations in joint kinetics and kinematics, joint laxity and instability, inefficient kinaesthesia and proprioception and antalgic gait may be found in patients presenting with deficient neuromuscular control [47, 48]. The addition of functional exercises that replicate the demands of daily living and sport should be included during the rehabilitation period. These exercises should be performed at a variety of joint angles and on varying surfaces to further challenge the proprioceptive capacity of the kinematic chain. It is critical that these exercises are performed and assessed qualitatively, as optimal technique of performance should supersede the quantity of repetitions in order to restore optimal function. Progressions to neuromuscular training exercises should be qualitatively based, and functional milestones should be reached without adverse reaction to the joint before the patient is allowed to proceed.

It is critical to continually address any diagnosed underlying pathokinematics, measurable strength imbalances and proprioceptive deficiencies during the rehabilitation process [49, 50]. Restoring optimal gluteal, posterior hip and lateral hip strength and neuromuscular control is essential if any dynamic valgus, hip internal rotation or adduction or excessive lateral compartment loading at the knee was recognised during the evaluation or rehabilitation process [51]. Deficiencies in kinaesthesia and proprioception can be addressed simultaneously to inadequacies in muscular strength and power [2, 5]. It is paramount that the neuromuscular training exercises prescribed must be highly individualised, taking into account the patient's specific goals and generalised condition, consideration of the size and location of the cartilage lesion, any concomitant injury and relevant past medical history. Self-reported pain and outcome scores and adverse events should be closely monitored during this phase.

Dependent upon the needs and goals of the patient, appropriate biomechanical clinical tests, such as the six-minute walk, dynamic balance, single leg squat and single-legged hop tests that may elucidate a patient's functional deficiencies, both quantitative and qualitative, in relationship to their pain, function and disability should be included to adequately assess improvements in neuromuscular control [37]. In addition, these tests allow the clinician to determine a patient's physical and psychological readiness to return to specific activities while monitoring the functional improvements throughout the course of the rehabilitation phase [37, 52].

10.1.3.5 Therapeutic Exercises and Return to Activity

Following a cartilage repair procedure, patients typically progress through the rehabilitation **process at varying rates**, depending upon a **multitude of factors** that include:

- The patient's age
- Sex
- Ethnicity
- Prior level of function
- Presence of systemic illness
- Traumatic onset
- BMI
- The lesion site location and severity
- Any concomitant pathology(ies) [53–55]

These variables are directly correlated to the patient outcome after articular cartilage repair. When prescribing exercise to patients after cartilage repair, it is critical to be mindful of patient age, prior level of activity and BMI [39, 56, 57]. Declines in metabolic activity and matrix synthesis are notable with increasing age, as differentiated chondrocytes have difficulty during cell multiplication and are largely unable to migrate to the site of the lesion in the extracellular matrix [58]. Patients that present with a BMI greater than 30 kg/m^2 typically need modifications to the intensity of their therapeutic protocol, since increased BMI has been correlated to increased risk for knee and hip osteoarthritis and cartilage loading and deleterious changes to cartilage volume [59, 60]. History of participating in contact sports and history of injury may increase the incidence of cartilage degeneration secondary to the exposure of high biomechanical loading from exposure to repetitive joint loading associated with cutting, deceleration and pivoting [61]. The history of prior ACL or meniscal injury statistically increases a patient's likelihood of an articular cartilage lesion [62, 63].

The prescription of therapeutic exercise will depend upon the site and severity of the lesion. If the patient presents with an elevated BMI, the intervention must be inclusive of a BMI reduction plan [59, 64]. Specific exercise selection must be defined by the clinician in order to avoid excessive loading of the articular cartilage repair site. In addition, a functional progression must be in place that takes into consideration the patient's prior level of function and conditioning, their functional goals and their specific loading response to exercise. When deemed appropriate, the inclusion of a walking protocol is an easy, cost-effective way to assess lower extremity functional progression, as healthy and healing knee cartilage is thought to adapt to progressive biomechanical loading [65]. Speed, distance covered and biomechanical performance can easily be assessed and monitored by a clinician, and it allows for patient autonomy and empowerment. Utilisation of an elliptical machine and stationary bicycle are two additional options to increase patient endurance and aerobic capacity during the post-operative phase(s).

Progressive strengthening exercises have been shown to mitigate pain, decrease joint loading, increase ROM and restore function and to support cartilage health, when loaded appropriately [66]. Inclusion of a stretching protocol is important to decrease any excessive loads that may be applied to the joint due to adaptive shortening of the musculature. Suggested strengthening exercises should occur in the frontal, sagittal and transverse plane: squats (varying angles depending on lesion site) with no anterior shear or genu valgum, knee extension, hip abduction, hip extension, hip external rotation and calf raises. Stretches may include, but are not limited to, hamstrings, quadriceps, hip flexor, hip external rotators and gastrocnemius/soleus. Stretches should be performed at least once a day and should be held for a duration of 30–60 s.

Psychosocial factors directly impact the rate of return to sport after injury and similarly can be projected to influence rehabilitation and athletic activity after articular cartilage repair. These **psychological factors** include:

- Fear of re-injury
- Kinesiophobia
- Decreased confidence
- Anxiety
- Commitment
- Patient's inability to control the outcome [67]

After an injury is sustained, a patient is often subject to a range of psychological responses in addition to the functional impairment, including stress, hesitancy, alterations in self-esteem, depression, fear of re-injury and anxiety [68–70]. The aforementioned responses are often at their height in the time immediately following the injury and/or surgery and generally subside over time during the rehabilitation process [71]. However, these elements may persist, or even increase, in the later stages of the rehabilitation process as the topic of return to prior level of activity is discussed [72, 73]. If these fears are left unresolved, there can be a significant delay incurred during the rehabilitation process which might ultimately jeopardise the successful return to activity.

10.2 Rehabilitation Outcome Measures

Clinical practice guidelines recommend the use of a validated-patient reported outcome measure, a general health questionnaire and a validated activity scale [37]. The standard of rehabilitation reporting after knee cartilage repair procedures remains lower than the standard of the reporting for surgery [74], and there is a need to standardise the documentation of outcome measures in rehabilitation. Rehabilitation outcome measures should be documented as a minimum at baseline and return to activity with further midpoints desirable.

Recommended **measures of physical impairment** include:

- Assessment of modified stroke test for effusion
- Knee active ROM
- Maximum voluntary isometric or isokinetic quadriceps strength testing
- Joint-line tenderness [37]

Currently, there are no **cartilage-specific performance-based tests** of physical function, but it is recommended for use:

- 30-s sit to stand.
- Stair-climb.
- Timed-up-and-go.
- 6-min walk tests in the early rehabilitation phase [37].
- Single-leg hop tests are recommended in the later return to activity rehabilitation phase [37].

Patient-reported outcome measures (PROMs) are routinely used to measure a person's health status and as primary end points in clinical trials and can be categorised as being site-specific, generic, disease-specific, population-specific or generic.

The **knee site-specific PROMs** that have been recommended **for use in cartilage repair** [75] are:

- ***The International Knee Documentation Committee Subjective Knee Form (IKDC)*** *[76]*
- ***The Knee injury and Osteoarthritis and Outcome Score (KOOS)*** *[77]*

Currently, there is no disease-specific PROM for articular cartilage defects. Generic PROMs are not able to directly evaluate the rehabilitation, but they do allow for the analysis of health-related quality of life and health economics.

The 36-item (SF-36) and 12-item (SF-12) Short Form Health Surveys, as well as the EuroQol (e.g. EQ-5D) surveys, are commonly used generic PROMs in cartilage repair studies.

Pre-operative PROMs have been shown to be able to provide accurate expectations for post-operative global levels of function following ACI surgery [78]. However, the standard of rehabilitation reporting after knee cartilage repair procedures remains lower than the standard of the reporting for the surgery [74], and validated minimal clinically important difference (MCID) thresholds for cartilage repair populations are limited. Activity rating scales such as the Marx or Tegner are frequently used in cartilage repair studies, but often without adjustment for age or gender, and normative data from people who have undergone cartilage repair procedures is not available [79].

The rehabilitation process after cartilage repair surgery is a lengthy and emotional experience for many patients [80]. The psychological response to rehabilitation after surgery has the potential to influence functional outcomes. It is important to consider **specific outcome measures for psychosocial aspects**, especially those that are temporal and open to change during the course of the rehabilitation. Self-efficacy beliefs have been found to influence rehabilitation outcome following joint surgery:

- *The Self-Efficacy for Rehabilitation Scale* was designed specifically for people undergoing lower limb orthopaedic surgery [81]
- *The Knee Self-Efficacy Scale* measures perceived knee function self-efficacy both in the present and for the future [82].
- *The Tampa Scale of Kinesiophobia* [83] can be used to quantify fear of movement and re-injury and their association with poorer knee-related quality of life after rehabilitation [84].

10.3 Summary

Knee joint preservation rehabilitation aims to provide a mechanical environment for healing responses that will facilitate the restoration of joint homeostasis and a return to optimal function. It is a stepwise process with load progressions reflecting the biologic healing phases of the affected tissues and individual patient characteristics. The principles of applied biomechanics and exercise prescription are core to the individualisation of the rehabilitation programme.

References

1. Mithoefer K, Hambly K, Logerstedt D, Ricci M, Silvers H, Della VS. Current concepts for rehabilitation and return to sport after knee articular cartilage repair in the athlete. J Orthop Sports Phys Ther. 2012;42(3):254–73.
2. Hambly K, Bobic V, Wondrasch B, Van Assche D, Marlovits S. Autologous chondrocyte implantation postoperative care and rehabilitation: science and practice. Am J Sports Med. 2006;34(6):1020–38.
3. van Rossom S, Smith CR, Thelen DG, Vanwanseele B, Van Assche D, Jonkers I. Knee joint loading in healthy adults during functional exercises: implications for rehabilitation guidelines. J Orthop Sports Phys Ther. 2018;48(3):162–73.
4. Edwards PK, Ackland T, Ebert JR. Clinical rehabilitation guidelines for matrix-induced autologous chondrocyte implantation on the tibiofemoral joint. J Orthop Sports Phys Ther. 2014;44(2):102–19.
5. Wondrasch B, Aroen A, Rotterud JH, Hoysveen T, Bolstad K, Risberg MA. The feasibility of a 3 month active rehabilitation program for patients with knee full-thickness articular cartilage lesions: the Oslo CARE study. J Orthop Sports Phys Ther. 2013;43(5):310–24.
6. Topp R, Swank AM, Quesada PM, Nyland J, Malkani A. The effect of prehabilitation exercise on strength and functioning after total knee arthroplasty. PM R. 2009;1(8):729–35.
7. Santa Mina D, Scheede-Bergdahl C, Gillis C, Carli F. Optimization of surgical outcomes with prehabilitation. Appl Physiol Nutr Metab. 2015;40(9):966–9.
8. Costa RA, Oliveira LM, Watanabe SH, Jones A, Natour J. Isokinetic assessment of the hip muscles in patients with osteoarthritis of the knee. Clinics. 2010;65(12):1253–9.
9. Hinman RS, Hunt MA, Creaby MW, Wrigley TV, McManus FJ, Bennell KL. Hip muscle weakness in individuals with medial knee osteoarthritis. Arthritis Care Res. 2010;62(8):1190–3.
10. Beumer L, Wong J, Warden SJ, Kemp JL, Foster P, Crossley KM. Effects of exercise and manual therapy on pain associated with hip osteoarthritis: a systematic review and meta-analysis. Br J Sports Med. 2016;50(8):458–63.
11. Alford JW, Cole BJ. Cartilage restoration, Part 1: Basic science, historical perspective, patient evaluation, and treatment options. Am J Sports Med. 2005;33(2):295–306.
12. Williams JM, Moran M, Thonar EJ, Salter RB. Continuous passive motion stimulates repair of rabbit knee articular cartilage after matrix proteoglycan loss. Clin Orthop. 1994;304:252–62.
13. Buckwalter JA. Effects of early motion on healing of musculoskeletal tissues. Hand Clin. 1996;12(1):13–24.
14. McGinty G, Irrgang JJ, Pezzullo D. Biomechanical considerations for rehabilitation of the knee. Clin Biomech. 2000;15(3):160–6.
15. Grelsamer RP, Weinstein C. Applied biomechanics of the patella. Clin Orthop. 2001;389:9–14.
16. Wallace DA, Salem GJ, Salinas R, Powers CM. Patellofemoral joint kinetics while squatting with and without an external load. J Orthop Sports Phys Ther. 2002;32(4):141–8.
17. Fitzgerald GK, Axe MJ, Snyder-Mackler L. Proposed practice guidelines for nonoperative anterior cruciate ligament rehabilitation of physically active individuals. J Orthop Sports Phys Ther. 2000;30(4):194–203.
18. Khan KM, Scott A. Mechanotherapy: how physical therapists' prescription of exercise promotes tissue repair. Br J Sports Med. 2009;43(4):247–52.
19. Carter DR, Beaupre GS, Wong M, Smith RL, Andriacchi TP, Schurman DJ. The mechanobiology of articular cartilage development and degeneration. Clin Orthop. 2004;(427 Suppl):S69–77.
20. Elder SH, Goldstein SA, Kimura JH, Soslowsky LJ, Spengler DM. Chondrocyte differentiation is modulated by frequency and duration of cyclic compressive loading. Ann Biomed Eng. 2001;29(6):476–82.
21. Quinn TM, Grodzinsky AJ, Buschmann MD, Kim YJ, Hunziker EB. Mechanical compression alters proteoglycan deposition and matrix deformation around individual cells in cartilage explants. J Cell Sci. 1998;111(Pt 5):573–83.
22. Sah RL, Kim YJ, Doong JY, Grodzinsky AJ, Plaas AH, Sandy JD. Biosynthetic response of cartilage explants to dynamic compression. J Orthop Res. 1989;7(5):619–36.
23. Ragan PM, Chin VI, Hung HH, Masuda K, Thonar EJ, Arner EC, et al. Chondrocyte extracellular matrix synthesis and turnover are influenced by static compression in a new alginate disk culture system. Arch Biochem Biophys. 2000;383(2):256–64.
24. Grumbles RM, Howell DS, Howard GA, Roos BA, Setton LA, Mow VC, et al. Cartilage metalloproteases in disuse atrophy. J Rheumatol Suppl. 1995;43:146–8.
25. Minas T, Peterson L. Advanced techniques in autologous chondrocyte transplantation. Clin Sports Med. 1999;18(1):13–44, v–vi.
26. Robertson WB, Fick D, Wood DJ, Linklater JM, Zheng MH, Ackland TR. MRI and clinical evaluation of collagen-covered autologous chondrocyte implantation (CACI) at two years. Knee. 2007;14(2):117–27.
27. Ebert JR, Fallon M, Zheng MH, Wood DJ, Ackland TR. A randomized trial comparing accelerated and traditional approaches to postoperative weightbearing

rehabilitation after matrix-induced autologous chondrocyte implantation: findings at 5 years. Am J Sports Med. 2012;40(7):1527–37.
28. Edwards PK, Ackland TR, Ebert JR. Accelerated weightbearing rehabilitation after matrix-induced autologous chondrocyte implantation in the tibiofemoral joint: early clinical and radiological outcomes. Am J Sports Med. 2013;41:2314. https://doi.org/10.1177/0363546513495637.
29. Wondrasch B, Zak L, Welsch GH, Marlovits S. Effect of accelerated weightbearing after matrix-associated autologous chondrocyte implantation on the femoral condyle on radiographic and clinical outcome after 2 years: a prospective, randomized controlled pilot study. Am J Sports Med. 2009;37(Suppl 1):88S–96S.
30. Negrin L, Kutscha-Lissberg F, Gartlehner G, Vecsei V. Clinical outcome after microfracture of the knee: a meta-analysis of before/after-data of controlled studies. Int Orthop. 2012;36(1):43–50.
31. Erggelet C, Vavken P. Microfracture for the treatment of cartilage defects in the knee joint - a golden standard? J Clin Orthop Trauma. 2016;7(3):145–52.
32. Camp CL, Stuart MJ, Krych AJ. Current concepts of articular cartilage restoration techniques in the knee. Sports Health. 2014;6(3):265–73.
33. Hangody L, Fules P. Autologous osteochondral mosaicplasty for the treatment of full-thickness defects of weight-bearing joints: ten years of experimental and clinical experience. J Bone Joint Surg Am. 2003;85(90002):25–32.
34. Van Assche D, Caspel DV, Staes F, Saris DB, Bellemans J, Vanlauwe J, et al. Implementing one standardized rehabilitation protocol following autologous chondrocyte implantation or microfracture in the knee results in comparable physical therapy management. Physiother Theory Pract. 2011;27(2):125–36.
35. Della Villa S, Kon E, Filardo G, Ricci M, Vincentelli F, Delcogliano M, et al. Does intensive rehabilitation permit early return to sport without compromising the clinical outcome after arthroscopic autologous chondrocyte implantation in highly competitive athletes? Am J Sports Med. 2010;38(1):68–77.
36. Tyler TF, Lung JY. Rehabilitation following osteochondral injury to the knee. Curr Rev Musculoskelet Med. 2012;5:72.
37. Logerstedt DS, Scalzitti DA, Bennell KL, Hinman RS, Silvers-Granelli H, Ebert J, et al. Knee pain and mobility impairments: meniscal and articular cartilage lesions revision 2018. J Orthop Sports Phys Ther. 2018;48(2):A1–A50.
38. Beaufils P, Hulet C, Dhenain M, Nizard R, Nourissat G, Pujol N. Clinical practice guidelines for the management of meniscal lesions and isolated lesions of the anterior cruciate ligament of the knee in adults. Orthop Traumatol Surg Res. 2009;95(6):437–42.
39. Zhang W, Moskowitz RW, Nuki G, Abramson S, Altman RD, Arden N, et al. OARSI recommendations for the management of hip and knee osteoarthritis, part I: critical appraisal of existing treatment guidelines and systematic review of current research evidence. Osteoarthr Cartil. 2007;15(9):981–1000.
40. Fitzgerald GK, Piva SR, Irrgang JJ. Reports of joint instability in knee osteoarthritis: its prevalence and relationship to physical function. Arthritis Rheum. 2004;51(6):941–6.
41. Mandelbaum BR, Silvers HJ, Watanabe DS, Knarr JF, Thomas SD, Griffin LY, et al. Effectiveness of a neuromuscular and proprioceptive training program in preventing anterior cruciate ligament injuries in female athletes. Am J Sports Med. 2005;33:1003.
42. Myer GD, Ford KR, Palumbo JP, Hewett TE. Neuromuscular training improves performance and lower-extremity biomechanics in female athletes. J Strength Cond Res. 2005;19(1):51–60.
43. Noyes FR, Barber-Westin SD, Smith ST, Campbell T, Garrison TT. A training program to improve neuromuscular and performance indices in female high school basketball players. J Strength Cond Res. 2012;26(3):709–19.
44. Silvers-Granelli HJ, Bizzini M, Arundale A, Mandelbaum BR, Snyder-Mackler L. Higher compliance to a neuromuscular injury prevention program improves overall injury rate in male football players. Knee Surg Sports Traumatol Arthrosc. 2018;26:1975–83.
45. Hewett TE, Myer GD, Ford KR, Heidt RS Jr, Colosimo AJ, McLean SG, et al. Biomechanical measures of neuromuscular control and valgus loading of the knee predict anterior cruciate ligament injury risk in female athletes: a prospective study. Am J Sports Med. 2005;33(4):492–501.
46. Lindblom H, Walden M, Carlfjord S, Hagglund M. Implementation of a neuromuscular training programme in female adolescent football: 3-year follow-up study after a randomised controlled trial. Br J Sports Med. 2014;48(19):1425–30.
47. Madhavan S, Shields RK. Neuromuscular responses in individuals with anterior cruciate ligament repair. Clin Neurophysiol. 2011;122(5):997–1004.
48. Olson TJ, Chebny C, Willson JD, Kernozek TW, Straker JS. Comparison of 2D and 3D kinematic changes during a single leg step down following neuromuscular training. Phys Ther Sport. 2011;12(2):93–9.
49. Thorlund JB, Aagaard P, Roos EM. Thigh muscle strength, functional capacity, and self-reported function in patients at high risk of knee osteoarthritis compared with controls. Arthritis Care Res. 2010;62(9):1244–51.
50. Thorlund JB, Aagaard P, Roos EM. Muscle strength and functional performance in patients at high risk of knee osteoarthritis: a follow-up study. Knee Surg Sports Traumatol Arthrosc. 2012;20(6):1110–7.
51. Myer GD, Ford KR, Di Stasi SL, Foss KD, Micheli LJ, Hewett TE. High knee abduction moments are common risk factors for patellofemoral pain (PFP) and anterior cruciate ligament (ACL) injury in girls: is PFP itself a predictor for subsequent ACL injury? Br J Sports Med. 2015;49(2):118–22.

52. Cacolice PA, Carcia CR, Scibek JS, Phelps AL. The use of functional tests to predict sagittal plane knee kinematics in NCAA-D1 female athletes. Int J Sports Phys Ther. 2015;10(4):493–504.
53. Chan CX, Wong KL, Toh SJ, Krishna L. Chinese ethnicity is associated with concomitant cartilage injuries in anterior cruciate ligament tears. Orthop J Sports Med. 2018;6(1):2325967117750083.
54. Jimenez G, Cobo-Molinos J, Antich C, Lopez-Ruiz E. Osteoarthritis: trauma vs disease. Adv Exp Med Biol. 2018;1059:63–83.
55. Neumann J, Hofmann FC, Heilmeier U, Ashmeik W, Tang K, Gersing AS, et al. Type 2 diabetes patients have accelerated cartilage matrix degeneration compared to diabetes free controls: data from the Osteoarthritis Initiative. Osteoarthr Cartil. 2018;26(6):751–61.
56. Janakiramanan N, Teichtahl AJ, Wluka AE, Ding C, Jones G, Davis SR, et al. Static knee alignment is associated with the risk of unicompartmental knee cartilage defects. J Orthop Res. 2008;26(2):225–30.
57. Rosenberger P, Dhabhar F, Epel E, Jokl P, Ickovics J. Sex differences in factors influencing recovery from arthroscopic knee surgery. Clin Orthop Relat Res. 2010;468(12):3399–405.
58. Hambly K, Silvers-Granelli H, Steinwachs M. Rehabilitation after articular cartilage repair of the knee in the football (soccer) player. Cartilage. 2012;3(S):50S–6S.
59. Hangaard S, Gudbergsen H, Skougaard M, Bliddal H, Nybing JD, Tiderius CJ, et al. Point of no return for improvement of cartilage quality indicated by dGEMRIC before and after weight loss in patients with knee osteoarthritis: a cohort study. Acta Radiol. 2018;59(3):336–40.
60. Gersing AS, Schwaiger BJ, Nevitt MC, Joseph GB, Chanchek N, Guimaraes JB, et al. Is weight loss associated with less progression of changes in knee articular cartilage among obese and overweight patients as assessed with MR imaging over 48 months? Data from the Osteoarthritis Initiative. Radiology. 2017;284(2):508–20.
61. Fernandes GS, Parekh SM, Moses J, Fuller C, Scammell B, Batt ME, et al. Prevalence of knee pain, radiographic osteoarthritis and arthroplasty in retired professional footballers compared with men in the general population: a cross-sectional study. Br J Sports Med. 2018;52:678.
62. Frobell RB, Le Graverand MP, Buck R, Roos EM, Roos HP, Tamez-Pena J, et al. The acutely ACL injured knee assessed by MRI: changes in joint fluid, bone marrow lesions, and cartilage during the first year. Osteoarthr Cartil. 2009;17(2):161–7.
63. Reinke EK, Spindler KP, Lorring D, Jones MH, Schmitz L, Flanigan DC, et al. Hop tests correlate with IKDC and KOOS at minimum of 2 years after primary ACL reconstruction. Knee Surg Sports Traumatol Arthrosc. 2011;19(11):1806–16.
64. Hussain SM, Tan MC, Stathakopoulos K, Cicuttini FM, Wang Y, Chou L, et al. How are obesity and body composition related to patellar cartilage? A systematic review. J Rheumatol. 2017;44(7):1071–82.
65. Harkey MS, Blackburn JT, Davis H, Sierra-Arevalo L, Nissman D, Pietrosimone B. The association between habitual walking speed and medial femoral cartilage deformation following 30minutes of walking. Gait Posture. 2018;59:128–33.
66. Hernandez-Molina G, Reichenbach S, Zhang B, Lavalley M, Felson DT. Effect of therapeutic exercise for hip osteoarthritis pain: results of a meta-analysis. Arthritis Rheum. 2008;59(9):1221–8.
67. Ardern CL, Taylor NF, Feller JA, Webster KE. Fear of re-injury in people who have returned to sport following anterior cruciate ligament reconstruction surgery. J Sci Med Sport. 2012;15(6):488–95.
68. Ardern CL, Taylor NF, Feller JA, Whitehead TS, Webster KE. Psychological responses matter in returning to preinjury level of sport after anterior cruciate ligament reconstruction surgery. Am J Sports Med. 2013;41(7):1549–58.
69. Hsu CJ, George SZ, Chmielewski TL. Association of quadriceps strength and psychosocial factors with single-leg hop performance in patients with meniscectomy. Orthop J Sports Med. 2016;4(12):2325967116676078.
70. Hsu CJ, Meierbachtol A, George SZ, Chmielewski TL. Fear of reinjury in athletes. Sports Health. 2017;9(2):162–7.
71. Rosenthal BD, Boody BS, Hsu WK. Return to play for athletes. Neurosurg Clin N Am. 2017;28(1):163–71.
72. Chmielewski TLZG, Lentz TA, et al. Longitudinal changes in psychosocial factors and their association with knee pain and function after anterior cruciate ligament reconstruction. Phys Ther. 2011;91:1355–66.
73. Christino MA, Fantry AJ, Vopat BG. Psychological aspects of recovery following anterior cruciate ligament reconstruction. J Am Acad Orthop Surg. 2015;23(8):501–9.
74. Bright P, Hambly K. A systematic review of reporting of rehabilitation in articular-cartilage-repair studies of third-generation autologous chondrocyte implantation in the knee. J Sport Rehabil. 2014;23(3):182–91.
75. Roos EM, Engelhart L, Ranstam J, Anderson AF, Irrgang JJ, Marx RG, et al. ICRS recommendation document: patient-reported outcome instruments for use in patients with articular cartilage defects. Cartilage. 2011;2(2):122–36.
76. Irrgang JJ, Anderson AF, Boland AL, Harner CD, Kurosaka M, Neyret P, et al. Development and validation of the International Knee Documentation Committee subjective knee form. Am J Sports Med. 2001;29(5):600–13.
77. Roos EM, Roos HP, Lohmander LS, Ekdahl C, Beynnon BD. Knee Injury and Osteoarthritis Outcome Score (KOOS)--development of a self-administered outcome measure. J Orthop Sports Phys Ther. 1998;28(2):88–96.
78. Howard JS, Lattermann C. Use of preoperative patient reported outcome scores to predict outcome following

autologous chondrocyte implantation. Orthop J Sports Med. 2014;2(2 Suppl):2325967114S00050.
79. Hambly K. The use of the Tegner Activity Scale for articular cartilage repair of the knee: a systematic review. Knee Surg Sports Traumatol Arthrosc. 2011;19(4):604–14.
80. Toonstra JL, Howell D, English RA, Lattermann C, Mattacola CG. Patient experiences of recovery after autologous chondrocyte implantation: a qualitative study. J Athl Train. 2016;51:1028.
81. Waldrop D, Lightsey O, Ethington C, Woemmel C, Coke A. Self-efficacy, optimism, health competence and recovery from orthopaedic surgery. J Couns Psychol. 2001;48:233–8.
82. Thomee P, Wahrborg P, Borjesson M, Thomee R, Eriksson BI, Karlsson J. A new instrument for measuring self-efficacy in patients with an anterior cruciate ligament injury. Scand J Med Sci Sports. 2006;16(3):181–7.
83. Miller R, Kori S, Todd D. The Tampa Scale. In: Book M, editor. Serial; 1991. Unpublished Report.
84. Kvist J, Ek A, Sporrstedt K, Good L. Fear of re-injury: a hindrance for returning to sports after anterior cruciate ligament reconstruction. Knee Surg Sports Traumatol Arthrosc. 2005;13(5):393–7.

11 Meniscus Anatomy

Urszula Zdanowicz

11.1 Medial Meniscus

In his study Śmigielski et al. [1] proposed dividing the medial meniscus into five anatomical zones: the anterior root (zone 1), the anteromedial zone (zones 2a and 2b), the medial zone (zone 3), the posterior zone (zone 4), and the posterior root (zone 5) (Fig. 11.1). This division is based on different anatomical appearances within each zone.

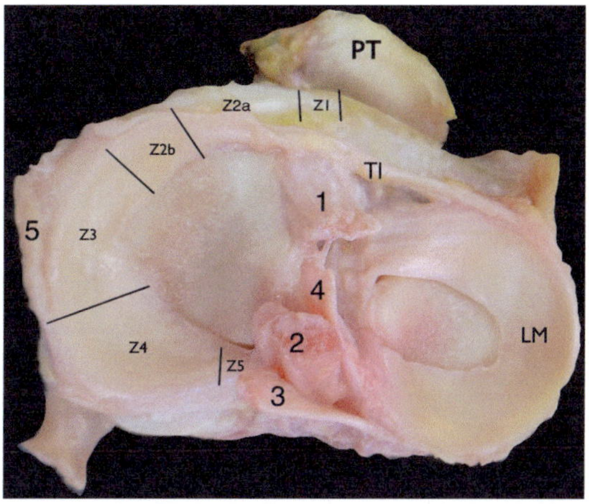

Fig. 11.1 Anatomic dissection of the right knee. Division of medial meniscus into five zones is presented (Z1; Z2a,b; Z3; Z4; Z5). (1) Anterior cruciate ligament. (2) Posterior cruciate ligament. (3) Posterior menisco-femoral ligament (Wrisberg lig.). (4) Anterior menisco-femoral ligament (Humphrey ligament). (5) Medial collateral ligament. *LM* lateral meniscus, *TL* transverse ligament, *PT* patellar tendon

11.1.1 Zone 1 Anterior Root

The center of anterior root of the medial meniscus is anterior to the apex of the medial tibial spine (average distance 27.5 mm), anterolateral to the cartilage surface of the medial tibial condyle (average 7.6 mm), and anterior to the nearest edge of the ACL (average of 9.2 mm) [2].

Berlet et al. [3] distinguished four types of anterior root locations of the medial meniscus. In the most frequent type I, the anterior root is situated in the flat intercondylar region of the tibial plateau. In the remaining types, the location of the anterior root descends down the tibial plateau, up to type IV, where no firm bony attachment may be observed [4].

11.1.2 Zone 2 Anteromedial Zone

The anteromedial zone may be further divided [1] by the transverse ligament into two subzones: 2a and 2b. Within zone 2 the medial meniscus is attached to the tibia via the coronary ligament

U. Zdanowicz (✉)
Carolina Medical Center, Warsaw, Poland

McGowan Institute for Regenerative Medicine, University of Pittsburgh, Pittsburgh, PA, USA
e-mail: u.zdanowicz@icloud.com

M. Brittberg, K. Slynarski (eds.), *Lower Extremity Joint Preservation*,
https://doi.org/10.1007/978-3-030-57382-9_11

(also called the menisco-tibial ligament). The superior edge of the medial meniscus has loose attachment to synovial tissue.

11.1.3 Zone 3 Medial Zone

The medial zone is situated at the level of the medial collateral ligament (MCL). At this level both meniscal edges (superior and inferior), as well as the outer part, are attached to deep layer of MCL (which is also often considered as the reinforcement of joint capsule) [1, 5] (Figs. 11.2 and 11.3).

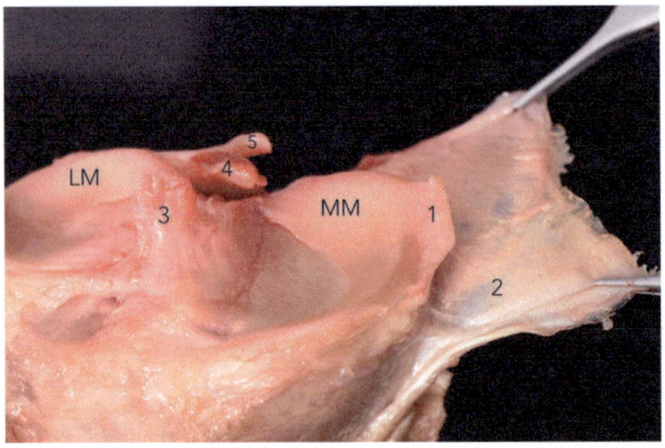

Fig. 11.2 Anatomic dissection of the right knee joint. *MM* medial meniscus, *LM* lateral meniscus. (1) Deep layer of the medial collateral ligament (MCL); notice how firmly it is attached to zone 3 of the medial meniscus. (2) Superficial layer of the MCL. (3) ACL. (4) PCL. (5) posterior menisco-femoral ligament

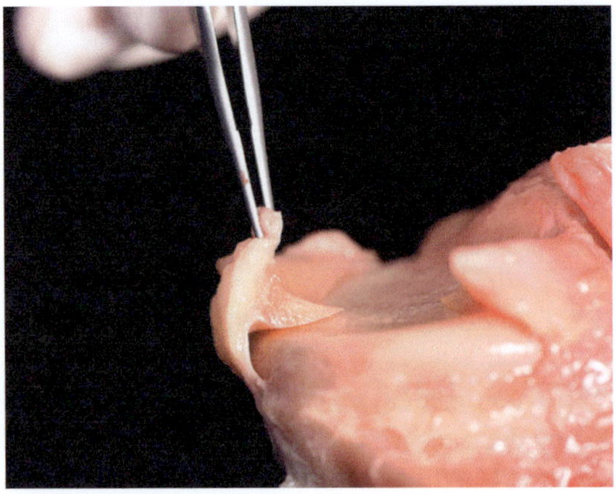

Fig. 11.3 Anatomical dissection. Cross-section of the medial meniscus in zone 3, at the level of MCL. Notice how meniscus is attached to the deep layer of MCL

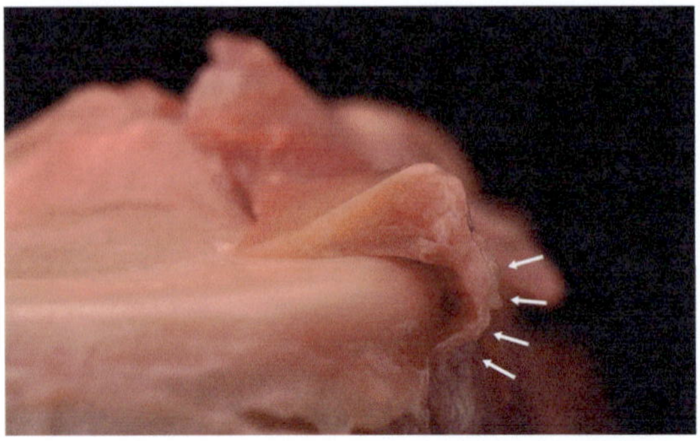

Fig. 11.4 Anatomical dissection. Cross-section of the posterior horn (zone 4) of the medial meniscus is showed. The coronary ligament (menisco-tibial ligament) is marked with white arrows. Notice that the superior edge of meniscus in this area is not attached to anything

11.1.4 Zone 4 Posterior Zone

Within the posterior zone, the medial meniscus is stabilized by the coronary ligament (menisco-tibial ligament) to the tibia. Contrary, its superior edge is free and does not attach to anything [1, 6] (Fig. 11.4), which may be important in cases of meniscal suturing.

11.1.5 Zone 5 Posterior Root

Posterior root attachment of the medial meniscus is situated anteromedial to tibial insertion of the posterior cruciate ligament and posterior to posterior root attachment of the lateral meniscus as well as posterior from the medial tibial eminence apex [7] (Fig. 11.5). Taking into consideration the most reproductible distances from arthroscopic landmarks, the most significant and practical were [7]:

1. The distance from the medial tibial eminence, which was 9.6 mm posterior and 0.7 mm lateral
2. The medial tibial plateau articular cartilage inflection point, where the medial meniscus posterior root attachment center was 3.5 mm lateral
3. The most proximal PCL tibial attachment, which was directly 8.2 mm from the medial posterior root attachment center

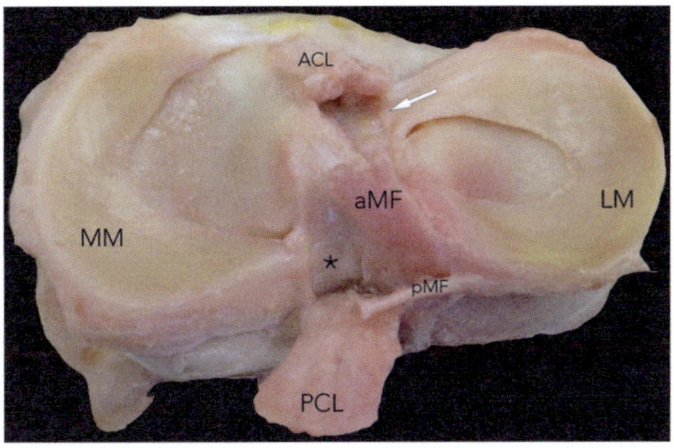

Fig. 11.5 Anatomical dissection of the right knee joint. Notice: Posterior root attachment of the medial meniscus (*) is situated anteromedial to tibial insertion of the posterior cruciate ligament (PCL). Also see how the anterior root of the lateral meniscus inserts beneath tibial attachment of the anterior cruciate ligament (ACL) (marked with white arrow). *MM* medial meniscus, *LM* lateral meniscus, *aMFL* anterior menisco-femoral ligament (Humphrey ligament), *pMFL* posterior menisco-femoral ligament (Wrisberg ligament)

11.1.6 Differences Between Male and Female

Vrancken et al. [8] performed a 3D analysis of the medial meniscus. He describes two different meniscal shapes, which differ mainly in height. He also stated that the main difference between the male and female meniscus is the size of it. However further research is needed to determine whether the meniscal shape variations might influence its function.

11.2 Lateral Meniscus

11.2.1 Anterior Root

The anterior root of the lateral meniscus inserts beneath the tibial attachment of the ACL, anteromedial from the apex of the lateral tibial eminence [2, 9]. The outer fibers of anterior and posterior horn of the lateral meniscus blend with a "C"-shaped ACL tibial insertion. The center of the "C" is the place of the wide bony insertion of the anterior root of the lateral meniscus [9] (Fig. 11.4).

11.2.2 Anterior Horn

In the area of anterior horn, the lateral meniscus is loosely attached to the tibia with very thin coronary ligament (menisco-tibial ligament), which allows for this great mobility the lateral meniscus had.

11.2.3 Popliteus Hiatus Area

Area at the level of popliteus hiatus is one of the most complex and fascinating areas within the knee.

Evolutionary and developmental anatomy is the key to understand the complicated morphology of the posterior-lateral corner structures and its relationship to the lateral meniscus. Three hundred and sixty million years ago in vertebrates as well as during human embryonic development, the fibula articulated with the femur. However, as the vertebrate knee evolved, the fibula and the attached lateral portion of the joint capsule moved distally, resulting in the popliteal hiatus and an intra-articular popliteus tendon. In early evolution—in the moment where the fibula still articulated with the femur—the popliteus tendon had its proximal attachment on the fibular head. In the course of the distal migration of the fibula, the popliteus tendon acquired a new femoral attachment, while retaining its original fibular one [10, 11].

The menisco-fibular ligament is a thick fibrous band connecting the inferior edge of the posterior part of the lateral meniscus with the head of the fibula (Fig. 11.6). It is to certain part a reinforcement of the coronary ligament (menisco-tibial ligament). However the coronary ligament attaches just below articular margin of proximal lateral tibial condyle, while distal attachment of the menisco-fibular ligament is on fibular head [12, 13]. This relatively large, often underestimated ligament is believed to position the lateral meniscus and thus having a great impact on its biomechanics, as well as likely relation to lateral meniscal tears.

According to Kimura et al. [14] at the level of popliteus hiatus there might be two types of

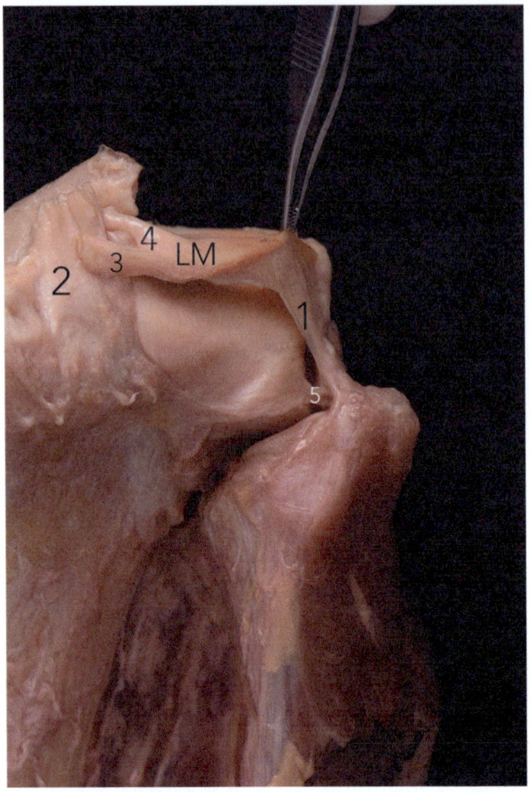

Fig. 11.6 Anatomical dissection of the right knee joint, posterior view. *LM* lateral meniscus. (1) Menisco-fibular ligament. (2) Posterior cruciate ligament. (3) Posterior menisco-femoral ligament. (4) Anterior menisco-femoral ligament. (5) Superior capsule of the proximal tibiofibular joint

menisco-tibial (coronary) ligament: type I (21%), in which coronary ligament is covering the entire popliteal tendon beneath meniscus, and more frequent (79%) type II, in which the coronary ligament has a defect through which popliteal tendon is visible. Kimura also recognised menisco-femoral coronary ligament, what we call today superior menisco-popliteal fasicles. He did not recognised at the time menisco-fibular ligament.

11.2.4 Menisco-femoral Ligaments

There are two ligaments that connect the posterior horn of the lateral meniscus to the intercondylar area: **anterior menisco-femoral ligament** (also called **Humphrey** ligament) (aMFL) and **posterior menisco-femoral** ligament (**Wrisberg** ligament) (pMFL). Proximal attachment Humphrey ligament lies between the distal margin of the femoral attachment of the PCL and the edge of the condylar articular cartilage. The posterior menisco-femoral ligament inserts more posteriorly than the aMFL, at the proximal margin of the attachment of the PCL [15].

In his study Kato et al. [16] measured the mean width of these ligaments, and Humphrey ligament had a mean width of 8.7 mm and Wrisberg ligament of 6.8 mm, whereas PCL in the same study had a mean width of 13.3 mm, which clearly shows how big and thick these ligaments are.

The incidence of presence of menisco-femoral ligaments varies between studies. The average incidence of both ligaments' presence is 31.8%; at least one is present in 92% of cases, aMFL alone in 21.7% whereas pMFL alone in 38.4% [15]. According to Parsons [17] presence and function of menisco-femoral ligaments is closely related to knee rotational movements. Parsons did a comperative study of the knee joint anatomy betweem human and other mammals. In lower monkeys (e.g., rhesus), in which much more rotation in the knee is present than in humans—the posterior part of the lateral meniscus is not connected to the tibia, but (with the oblique ligament, running posterior to the posterior cruciate ligament) is connected to the femur. On the other hand in mammals with no rotation in the knee (e.g., fruit bat), all menisco-femoral ligaments, menisci, and even popliteus muscle are absent. According to the theory of Heller and Langman with internal rotation of the knee in flex position, menisco-femoral ligaments pull the posterior horn medially and anteriorly, whereas the popliteus, through **menisco-popliteal fascicles**, works as antagonist to that movement [15, 18].

11.2.5 Posterior Root

The posterior root attachment is situated posteromedial to the lateral tibial eminence apex. Taking into consideration the most reproductible distances from arthroscopic landmarks were [7]:

1. 1.5 mm posterior and 4.2 mm medial to the lateral tibial eminence apex
2. 4.3 mm medial to the lateral tibial plateau articular cartilage edge
3. Directly 12.7 mm to the most proximal edge of the PCL tibial attachment

Acknowledgments I would like to thank Dr Marek Tramś for his help with anatomical dissection and Maciej Śmiarowski for wonderful pictures. I would also like to thank the Center for Medical Education (www.cem-med.pl) for support.

References

1. Śmigielski R, Becker R, Zdanowicz U, Ciszek B. Medial meniscus anatomy-from basic science to treatment. Knee Surg Sports Traumatol Arthrosc. 2015;23:8–14.
2. LaPrade CM, Ellman MB, Rasmussen MT, James EW, Wijdicks CA, Engebretsen L, LaPrade RF. Anatomy of the anterior root attachments of the medial and lateral menisci: a quantitative analysis. Am J Sports Med. 2014;42:2386–92.
3. Berlet GC, Fowler PJ. The anterior horn of the medical meniscus. An anatomic study of its insertion. Am J Sports Med. 1998;26:540–3.
4. Hatayama K, Higuchi H, Kimura M, Takeda M, Ono H, Watanabe H, Takagishi K. Histologic changes after meniscal repair using radiofrequency energy in rabbits. Arthroscopy. 2007;23:299–304.
5. Wymenga AB, Kats JJ, Kooloos J, Hillen B. Surgical anatomy of the medial collateral ligament and the posteromedial capsule of the knee. Knee Surg Sports Traumatol Arthrosc. 2006;14:229–34.
6. Fenn S, Datir A, Saifuddin A. Synovial recesses of the knee: MR imaging review of anatomical and pathological features. Skeletal Radiol. 2009;38:317–28.
7. Johannsen AM, Civitarese DM, Padalecki JR, Goldsmith MT, Wijdicks CA, LaPrade RF. Qualitative and quantitative anatomic analysis of the posterior root attachments of the medial and lateral menisci. Am J Sports Med. 2012;40:2342–7.
8. Vrancken ACT, Crijns SPM, Ploegmakers MJM, O'Kane C, van Tienen TG, Janssen D, Buma P, Verdonschot N. 3D geometry analysis of the medial meniscus - a statistical shape modeling approach. J Anat. 2014;225:395–402.
9. Siebold R, Schuhmacher P, Fernandez F, Śmigielski R, Fink C, Brehmer A, Kirsch J. Flat midsubstance of the anterior cruciate ligament with tibial "C"-shaped insertion site. Knee Surg Sports Traumatol Arthrosc. 2015;23:3136–42.
10. Covey DC. Injuries of the posterolateral corner of the knee: the journal of bone and joint surgery-american volume. 2001;83(1):106–18. https://doi.org/10.2106/00004623-200101000-00015.
11. Haines RW. The tetrapod knee joint. J Anat. 1942;76:270–301.
12. Natsis K, Paraskevas G, Anastasopoulos N, Papamitsou T, Sioga A. Meniscofibular ligament: morphology and functional significance of a relatively unknown anatomical structure. Anat Res Int. 2012;2012:214784.
13. Zdanowicz UE, Ciszkowska-Łysoń B, Krajewski P, Ciszek B, Badylak SF. Menisco-fibular ligament — an overview: cadaveric dissection, clinical and MRI diagnosis, arthroscopic visualization and treatment. Folia morphologica. Ahead of print. 2020. https://doi.org/10.5603/FM.a2020.0127.
14. Kimura M, Shirakura K, Hasegawa A, Kobayashi Y, Udagawa E. Anatomy and pathophysiology of the popliteal tendon area in the lateral meniscus: 1. Arthroscopic and anatomical investigation. Arthroscopy. 1992;8:419–23.
15. Gupte CM, Bull AM, Thomas RD, Amis AA. A review of the function and biomechanics of the meniscofemoral ligaments. Arthroscopy. 2003;19:161–71.
16. Kato T, Śmigielski R, Ge Y, Zdanowicz U, Ciszek B, Ochi M. Posterior cruciate ligament is twisted and flat structure: new prospective on anatomical morphology. Knee Surg Sports Traumatol Arthrosc. 2018;26:31–9.
17. Parsons FG. The joints of mammals compared with those of man: a course of lectures delivered at the Royal College of Surgeons of England. J Anat Physiol. 1899;34:41–68.
18. Heller L, Langman J. The menisco-femoral ligaments of the human knee. J Bone Joint Surg (Br). 1964;46:307–13.

12 Current Concepts in Meniscus Pathology and Repair

R. Kyle Martin, Devin Leland, and Aaron J. Krych

12.1 Introduction

The medial and lateral menisci are important structures in the knee that were once thought to be functionless and expendable. Partial and subtotal resection of the injured meniscus was used liberally in the past for the management of tears. This was performed because of concern regarding the healing potential of these injuries due to the poor vascularity of the meniscus. The menisci are now known to contribute to load distribution, stability, and arthritis prevention of the healthy knee. The ramifications of the excision of significant portions of these structures have since been established, and the focus has shifted to meniscus preservation. Advancements in meniscal repair techniques and the introduction of adjunctive biologic treatments has resulted in improved healing potential and clinical outcomes. In this chapter, we will outline the various meniscal tear patterns seen in clinical practice and discuss the indications, techniques, and outcomes for meniscal repair.

R. K. Martin (✉)
Department of Orthopaedic Surgery, University of Minnesota, Minneapolis, MN, USA

Department of Orthopaedic Surgery, CentraCare, Saint Cloud, MN, USA

D. Leland · A. J. Krych
Department of Orthopaedic Surgery and Sports Medicine, Mayo Clinic, Rochester, MN, USA
e-mail: Leland.Devin@mayo.edu; Krych.Aaron@mayo.edu

12.2 Meniscus Pathology

12.2.1 Typical Meniscus Injuries and Healing Potential

Several classification systems for meniscal injury have been developed with varying degrees of success. In general, meniscal tears can be described based on the mechanism of injury (traumatic versus degenerative), vascularity, the presence of concomitant injuries, or the morphology of the tear. All of these systems take into consideration factors that influence the healing potential of the meniscus.

Traumatic meniscus tears typically involve acute injuries that the patient can recall and may be associated with concomitant injuries. In contrast, degenerative meniscus tears occur secondary to repetitive movements in a knee with osteoarthritic changes. Whereas traumatic meniscus injuries are considered for surgical intervention, the standard approach to degenerative meniscus tears is non-operative in nature, depending on symptoms and presentation.

The central two-thirds of the meniscus is avascular and acellular, limiting the healing potential of the meniscus most significantly in this region [1]. In contrast, blood supply to the peripheral third occurs via the perimeniscal capillary plexus and is believed

M. Brittberg, K. Slynarski (eds.), *Lower Extremity Joint Preservation*,
https://doi.org/10.1007/978-3-030-57382-9_12

to foster healing [2]. Several studies have supported this [3, 4], and the proximity of the tear to the peripheral meniscal rim has been identified as the greatest predictor of meniscal healing [5]. Despite the poor vascularity in the central portion of the meniscus, repair of tears in the avascular zone can still provide relief of symptoms as has been demonstrated by Noyes and Barber-Westin [6–8].

The presence of concomitant injuries to the knee has been found to influence the rate of healing following meniscal repair. Cannon and Vittori reported healing rates of 91% if meniscus repair was performed concurrently with anterior cruciate ligament (ACL) reconstruction compared to only 50% among those undergoing isolated meniscus repair in the setting of a stable knee [9]. The improved knee stability imparts an optimal environment for meniscus healing, and the release of growth factors and pluripotent cells during tunnel drilling is thought to provide biologic augmentation at the repair site. Conversely, if knee instability is missed or neglected at the time of meniscal repair, the ongoing knee instability has an adverse effect on meniscus healing [10–12].

The typical morphology of meniscus tears can be described as:

- Vertical/longitudinal
- Radial, oblique/flap
- Horizontal cleavage

Of these patterns, the vertical longitudinal tears have the highest healing potential [13, 14]. The exception to this occurs when the longitudinal tear extends from anterior to posterior allowing the meniscal fragment to flip on itself, also known as a bucket-handle meniscus tear. This bucket-handle configuration reduces the healing rate of the meniscal repair [9].

The radial, oblique/flap, and horizontal tears all involve the central avascular portion of the meniscus to some degree, limiting the healing potential of these tear patterns. Additionally, the horizontal cleavage tear is most commonly a degenerative meniscus lesion found in older patients.

Recently, the International Society of Arthroscopy, Knee Surgery, and Orthopaedic Sports Medicine (ISAKOS) proposed a comprehensive classification system of meniscal tears in an attempt to standardize the reporting of meniscal injuries and improve consistency across studies. The classification is divided into:

- Tear depth
- Rim width
- Location, tear pattern
- Tissue quality

The classification has been demonstrated to have sufficient interrater reliability [15].

12.2.2 Meniscus Root Injuries

A meniscal root injury is defined as a meniscal detachment from the insertion point on the tibia or a radial meniscal tear within 1 cm of this attachment point [16]. The meniscal root attachments play an essential role in the function of the menisci, and injury to these structures has been reported to be comparable to a meniscal deficient state [17–20]. If left untreated, these meniscal injuries can lead to the rapid development of osteoarthritis due to meniscal extrusion and the loss of resistance to hoop stress [21]. LaPrade et al. developed a classification system for meniscal root tears and reported that most injuries involved the posterior root attachments, specifically of the type 2 morphology. Posterior lateral meniscal root injuries are most commonly associated with anterior cruciate ligament (ACL) tears, while patients with posterior medial meniscal root injuries are more likely to have concomitant articular cartilage defects [22]. Careful probing of the posterior meniscal roots coupled with a high index of suspicion for a tear is recommended during arthroscopy as a high percentage of these tears are missed on pre-operative MRI [23].

12.2.3 Ramp Lesions

A "ramp" lesion is an injury involving the peripheral attachment of the posterior horn of the medial meniscus at the meniscocapsular junction.

These injuries most commonly occur in the setting of an ACL rupture with reported rates of 9–17% [24–26]. Magnetic resonance imaging (MRI) has a low sensitivity for identifying ramp lesions, which is possibly related to reduction of the lesion with the knee in the extended position during imaging [24, 26]. An associated bone bruise in the posteromedial tibial plateau on MRI may suggest the presence of a ramp lesion and was seen in 72% of patients with this injury in one study [26].

These lesions can also be difficult to identify during arthroscopy, and some authors recommend routine evaluation with the use of an accessory posteromedial portal [27]. Others report sufficient visualization obtained with the scope passed from the anterolateral portal through the intercondylar notch with the knee in 30° of flexion [26]. Biomechanically, ramp lesions have been demonstrated to increase anterior tibial translation and external rotation in an ACL deficient knee and have been postulated to increase ACL graft strain if not repaired at the time of ACL reconstruction [28–30].

12.2.4 Discoid Meniscus

The discoid meniscus is a congenital variant resulting in abnormal meniscal morphology and is present in 0.4–16.6% of the population [31, 32]. The abnormality is most common in the Asian population and is bilateral in 15–25% of cases [33–35]. Discoid morphology most often involves the lateral meniscus, whereas a discoid medial meniscus is rarely seen [36, 37]. The abnormal morphology leads to an increased risk of meniscal injury and instability [38], which can manifest as knee pain or mechanical symptoms. In younger children, the primary presentation is one of spontaneous knee snapping or popping, while older children and adults are more likely to present with a torn discoid meniscus [39, 40]. The classification system described by Watanabe remains the most commonly used [41].

12.3 Meniscus Repair

12.3.1 Typical Meniscus Injuries

12.3.1.1 Indications

Laboratory biomechanical testing suggests that meniscal repair should always be performed; however, this fails to consider the aforementioned challenges regarding healing potential. Failed meniscal repair can lead to persistent pain and lower outcome scores, while reoperation exposes the patient to additional surgical risks and morbidity. Surgical indications therefore revolve around the factors associated with meniscal healing. These include tear morphology, location, acuity, and the presence of concomitant injuries. Adding to the complexity of the decision making process is the fact that meniscal healing is not well defined, with clinical, radiographic, and second-look-arthroscopy healing demonstrating variable correlation [5].

Patient-related factors may also largely influence the decision of whether or not to repair a meniscal tear. Since post-operative rehabilitation protocols often limit weight bearing and range of motion for several weeks or months following a meniscal repair, patients must be committed to the lengthy recovery period following surgery. This may be undesirable for those who wish to return to jobs of a physical nature immediately after surgery, such as manual laborers or professional athletes. However, the short-term rehabilitation must be balanced with the long-term function of the knee. Recently, accelerated rehabilitation protocols have been developed with promising results and in some patients may allow earlier range of motion and weight bearing [42, 43]. Overall, however, patients unwilling to comply with the prescribed post-operative restrictions should be counselled on the long-term risks associated with partial meniscectomy and may be considered for partial resection rather than repair [44–46]. Tobacco use has also been shown to decrease healing rates of meniscal repairs, and patients should be encouraged to quit smoking if a meniscal repair is to be performed [47].

12.3.1.2 Techniques

Meniscal repair is most often performed using arthroscopic:

- Inside-out
- Outside-in
- All-inside techniques

The choice of technique is depending on tear pattern and location. Some tears may require a combination of any or all of these techniques.

The outside-in approach is most often utilized for tears of the anterior horn or midportion of the meniscus but has limited applicability for tears of the posterior third due to suboptimal needle trajectory [48]. Posterior meniscal tears require inside-out or all-inside meniscal repair techniques (Fig. 12.1).

Inside-out sutures are less expensive and are most useful for large tears where multiple sutures may be needed. All-inside suture devices typically utilize either anchor-based fixation with pre-tied slip knots or self-retrieving suture-passing devices combined with subsequent intra-articular knot tying. All-inside sutures do not require an additional skin incision, and device evolution has improved the ease of use. Both techniques share similar indications and outcomes [49].

In general, vertical mattress configurations are biomechanically superior to horizontal meniscal repair sutures. Vertical longitudinal tears are best repaired using stacked vertical mattress sutures placed 3–5 mm apart [50]. Circumferential compression through the placement of vertical sutures can be used to preserve both leaflets during repair of horizontal cleavage meniscus tears (Fig. 12.2). To achieve compression across a radial meniscus tear, all-inside sutures can be placed in a vertical configuration with a self-retrieving suture-passing device. An anatomic transtibial meniscal repair technique utilizing crossed traction sutures through tibial tunnels has also been described for radial meniscus tears [51]. Figure 12.3 demonstrates meniscal repair technique options for radial meniscus tears.

12.3.1.3 Outcomes

Outcomes of meniscal repair vary based on a number of factors including tear morphology, size, and repair technique. Vertical longitudinal tears have an excellent capacity for healing,

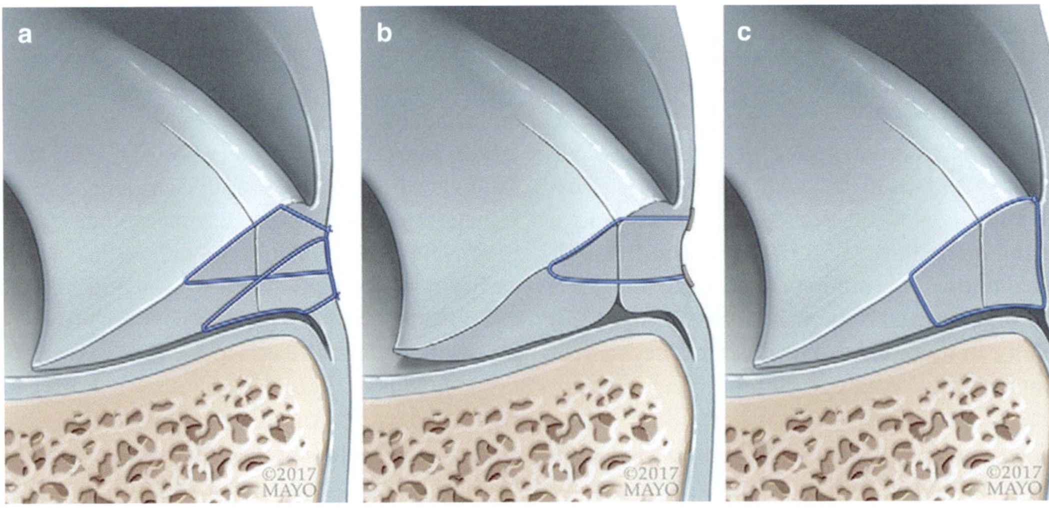

Fig. 12.1 Schematic diagrams demonstrating the suture configuration that results following surgical repair of a vertical longitudinal meniscal tears using an inside-out repair with knots tied over the capsule (**a**), all-inside anchor-based construct (**b**), and all-inside knot-tying technique (**c**). ©2017 MAYO. (With permissions from Mayo Foundation for Medical Education and Research. All rights reserved)

especially in the setting of an acute peripheral tear. A recent study evaluating 80 patients with vertical longitudinal meniscal tears reported a healing rate of 85% at a mean of 51.2 months post-repair [47].

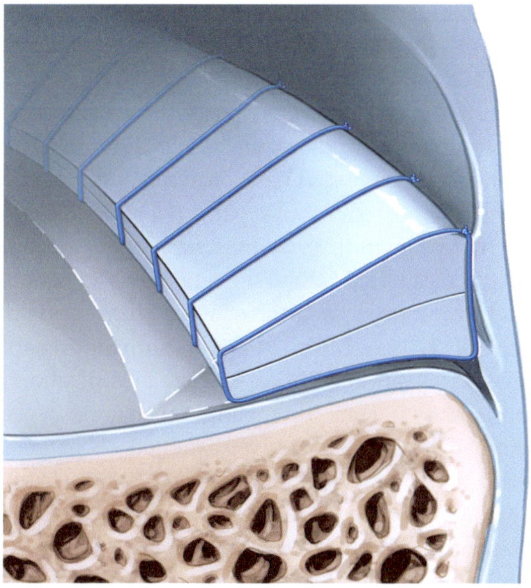

Fig. 12.2 Schematic image demonstrating repair of a horizontal cleavage meniscal tear using multiple all-inside circumferential compression sutures placed with a self-retrieving suture-passing device followed by arthroscopic knot tying ©2017 MAYO. (With permissions from Mayo Foundation for Medical Education and Research. All rights reserved)

Horizontal meniscal tears are often considered for non-operative treatment or partial meniscectomy due to the relatively limited healing potential versus the vertical longitudinal configurations. In younger patients in whom the horizontal meniscus tear should be differentiated from the degenerative tear patterns seen in those over the age of 50 with associated arthritis, repair can provide excellent outcomes and acceptable healing rates. A systematic review of these tears reported an overall healing rate of 78.6%, and the authors advocated for consideration of surgical repair in these patients [52].

The described all-inside repair technique for radial meniscus tears has demonstrated lower displacement, higher load to failure, and greater stiffness than an all-inside repair which relies on fixation to the periphery of the meniscus or capsule and creates a horizontal suture configuration [53]. The transtibial technique for radial tears has also been shown to produce less tear gapping and higher load to failure than an inside-out repair technique [51]. Additionally, clinical outcomes were similar to those for vertical longitudinal tears repaired using inside-out sutures [54].

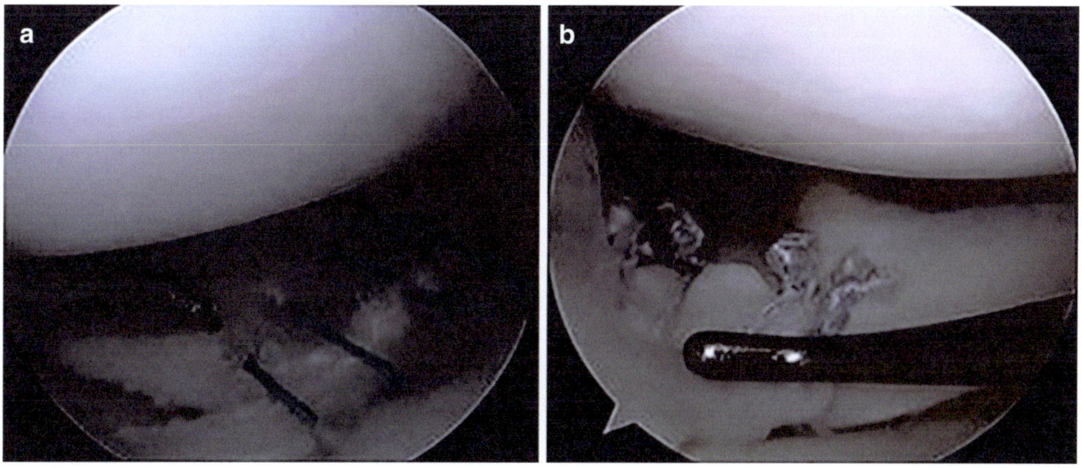

Fig. 12.3 Radial meniscal tear repair techniques. Arthroscopic image following inside-out repair of a right radial medial meniscal tear with horizontal mattress sutures (**a**). Arthroscopic image following all-inside repair with knot tying of a right radial medial meniscal tear (**b**)

12.3.2 Meniscus Root Injuries

12.3.2.1 Indications

Meniscus root repair is advocated in young (<50 years old) patients with a reasonable level of activity and a relatively acute injury with intact articular cartilage. Chronic symptomatic meniscal root injuries can be considered for surgical repair; however, the integrity of the meniscal tissue may not be suitable. Patients who are scheduled to undergo knee ligament reconstruction with signs of an extruded meniscus are also good candidates. Contraindications include Outerbridge grade ≥3 osteoarthritic changes, joint space narrowing, malalignment, and patient comorbidities precluding elective surgical intervention [55–57].

12.3.2.2 Techniques

Arthroscopic posterior meniscal root repairs are divided into two techniques:

- Transosseous suture repairs
- Suture anchor repairs

Several different transosseous methods have been described in the literature including both one and two-tunnel options or with a socket created with a retrograde reaming device [55, 58–62]. Numerous meniscal root aiming guides are now available to aid in tunnel creation, or a standard ACL tibial aiming guide can be used.

Sutures are typically passed through the meniscal root with a suture passing device and retrieved through the tibial tunnel(s). Various suture configurations in the meniscal root have also been described and compared in the literature. Simple cinch (luggage strap) [63], locking loop [64], double locking-loop [65], and modified Kessler [66] suture patterns have performed the best in comparison studies to date. Fixation can be achieved by tying the sutures over a bone bridge, button, or washer and screw construct or secured with an anchor in the tibia.

The suture anchor repair technique involves the insertion of one or more suture anchors near the meniscal root footprint through a posteromedial accessory portal. Sutures are then passed through the meniscal root and sliding knots are tied from the anteromedial portal. This technique avoids the risk of tunnel collision in the setting of concomitant ligament reconstruction and suture failure due to abrasion in the tibial tunnel [55].

12.3.2.3 Outcomes

Overall, outcomes following posterior meniscal root repair have been favorable [19, 67–71]. Chung et al. reported on 91 patients with medial meniscus posterior root repairs at a mean follow-up of 7 years [68]. Lysholm scores improved significantly at final follow-up, and only one patient had conversion to arthroplasty. They reported overall Kaplan-Meier survival probabilities of 99% at 5 years and 92% at 8 years. Not all studies have shown such promising results, however. Kaplan et al. retrospectively studied 18 patients who underwent posterior medial meniscus root repair, and while they observed improved clinical outcomes, they also noted increased extrusion and progression of degenerative changes on MRI at a mean follow-up of 2 years. This variability in outcome is likely multifactorial but depends upon patient selection in a well-aligned, stable knee without cartilage wear.

12.3.3 Ramp Lesions

12.3.3.1 Indications

The surgical indication for repair of an identified ramp lesion remains controversial. Some authors suggest that the favorable vascularity and stability of these lesions precludes the need for surgical repair, especially if identified during ACL reconstruction [25]. Several studies have supported this notion, demonstrating good outcomes when ACL reconstruction was performed without repair of ramp lesions [72–74]. Persistent rotational laxity and increased tibiofemoral contact pressures remain a concern, however, and some authors suggest ramp repair in order to restore the normal kinematics [28, 30, 75, 76]. Less controversy exists for ramp lesions in the setting of a chronic ACL deficient knee, when meniscal repair is advocated in conjunction with ACL reconstruction [27].

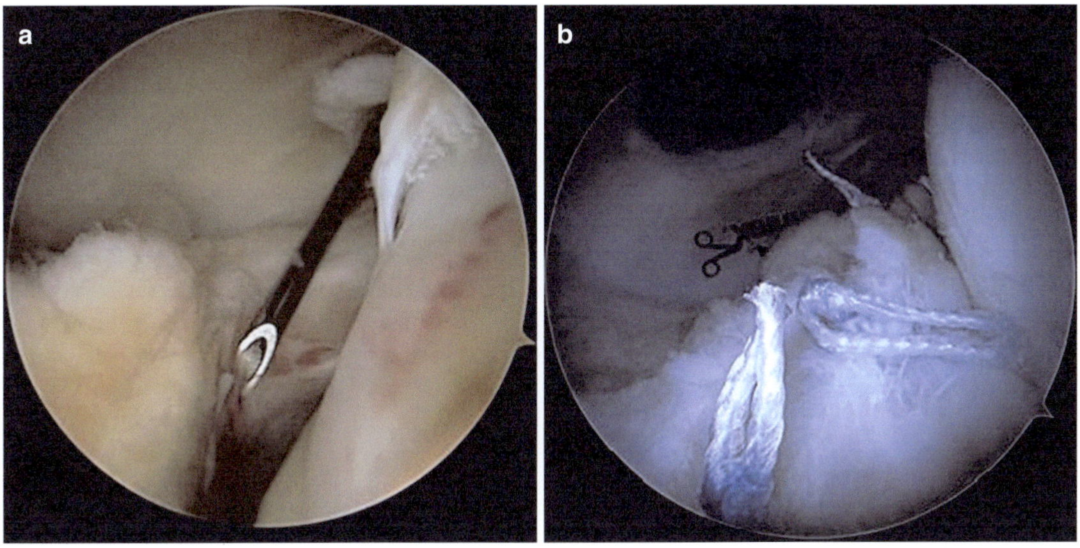

Fig. 12.4 Transcondylar notch view into the posteromedial compartment demonstrating ramp tear (probing with needle) (**a**) and subsequent repair through a cannula with 2-0 vertical mattress sutures placed using a meniscus lasso (**b**)

12.3.3.2 Techniques

Ramp repair has been described using inside-out [77], all-inside [28], and posteromedial portal suture-hook [78] techniques. The inside-out technique requires an open approach for visualization of the exiting needle and prevention of neurovascular injury to the posterior knee. The passing of several sutures is possible and a strong repair construct can be obtained [79]. All-inside repair devices offer a safe alternative, and an additional incision is unnecessary (Fig. 12.4) [80].

The suture-hook technique involves the creation of a posteromedial portal through which a suture is passed across the ramp lesion using a curved suture-passer. The suture-ends are then retrieved and a sliding knot is tied on the posterior aspect of the meniscus. This can be repeated as many times as necessary until the meniscus is reduced and stable [78]. The suture-hook repair utilizes movements that are similar to Bankart repair of the shoulder, and junior surgeons or those who do not also perform shoulder stabilization may find it more technically demanding than the other repair methods [80].

12.3.3.3 Outcomes

There are a limited number of studies reporting long-term outcomes following ramp repair. Despite this, the discussed techniques of ramp repair have shown favorable rates of healing and clinical outcomes [78, 80, 81]. Li et al. followed 23 patients with all-inside fixation of ramp lesions and reported a Lysholm Score improvement from 64.4 ± 4.52 to 91.2 ± 4.60 at a mean follow-up of 14 months [80]. Thaunat et al. reported outcomes on 132 patients who underwent ramp repair using the suture-hook technique with a minimum 2-year follow-up [78]. Cumulative survival rate was reported to be 93.2%, and tears that extended to the midportion of the meniscus had a survival rate of 87.8%.

12.3.4 Discoid Meniscus

12.3.4.1 Indications

Asymptomatic or minimally symptomatic patients with a finding of discoid meniscus on MRI or arthroscopy for other pathology may be followed clinically. All patients with symptoms related to discoid meniscus including:

- Pain
- Snapping
- Popping
- Loss of terminal extension

Patients with above symptoms should be considered for surgery.

12.3.4.2 Techniques

Historically, subtotal or total meniscectomy was performed for discoid meniscus but this resulted in a high rate of early degenerative changes [82–84]. The currently accepted management of discoid meniscus follows two main principles:

- Meniscus saucerization
- Stabilization

During arthroscopic saucerization, shavers and biters are used to achieve a normally shaped meniscus through partial meniscus resection. This procedure aims to recreate not only the appropriate width of meniscal tissue but also the normal triangular wedge shape with a thinner central portion. Care should be taken to leave an adequate meniscal rim of 6–8 mm by not removing too much meniscal tissue [85]. Meniscus stability is then assessed, and tears or congenital instability patterns are stabilized using the standard meniscus repair techniques outlined above.

12.3.4.3 Outcomes

Favorable results have been demonstrated with discoid meniscus saucerization and stabilization of unstable injuries, with worse outcomes associated with more significant meniscal resection procedures [86–88]. After saucerization, if the meniscus is found to be unstable and can be subsequently repaired, outcomes are similar to those who have an isolated saucerization of a stable discoid meniscus [40]. In one level-IV study investigating patient-reported outcome measures following discoid meniscus surgery, age was the only identified variable associated with outcome, with better results seen in younger patients [89].

12.3.5 Biologic Augmentation

Several augmentation techniques have been developed and remain the focus of ongoing research in an effort to improve the healing response of meniscus tears. These include:

- Mechanical stimulation
- Marrow venting procedures
- Fibrin clots
- Platelet-rich-plasma (PRP)
- Stem cell therapies [90].

Two commonly used methods of mechanical stimulation are rasping of the adjacent synovium and trephination (the creation of a channel between low and high vascular zones) [90]. Synovial rasping leads to increases in interleukin-1-alpha, proliferating cell nuclear antigen, transforming growth factor β1, and platelet-derived growth factor, which is believed to promote neovascularization [91]. Trephination has exhibited >90% good to excellent results clinically; however its usefulness must be weighed against the potential negative effects of iatrogenically disrupting the circumferential fibers of the meniscus [92].

The healing rate of meniscal repairs is improved when performed concurrently with ACL reconstruction. It is thought that the ACL tunnel drilling creates a biologic environment that is pro-healing for the meniscus. In an effort to simulate the effects of tunnel drilling, marrow venting procedures are often added to isolated meniscal repair procedures (Fig. 12.5). The addition of this quick procedure has shown healing rates similar to those observed after meniscal repair performed concomitantly with ACL reconstruction [93].

The use of fibrin clot, PRP injections, and stem cell therapies are a topic of ongoing research as current evidence is inconclusive regarding effectiveness. Fibrin clot has demonstrated effectiveness clinically; however comparative studies are needed to confirm and quantify the superiority of its use versus meniscal repair alone [90, 94–96]. Meniscal repairs augmented with PRP injection have shown similar reoperation rates to meniscal repairs without injection [97, 98]. However, pain and function scores were improved at 24 months' follow-up in the PRP injection group in one study [98]. Early results of meniscal repairs augmented with injection of mesenchymal stem cells show promise, but further investigation is needed to better define the role of these augmentation strategies [99].

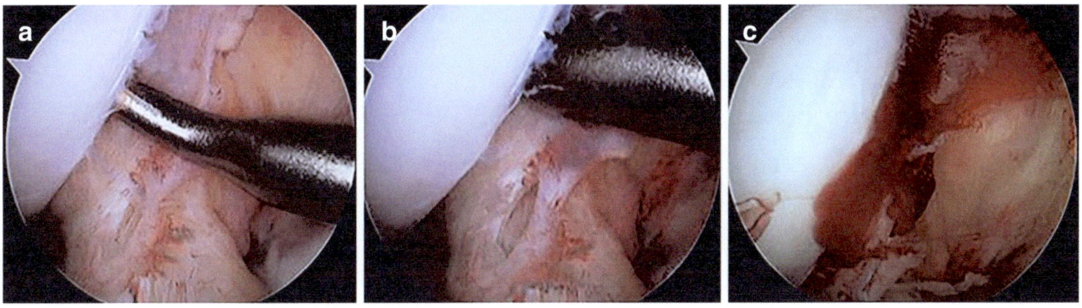

Fig. 12.5 Arthroscopic images demonstrating a marrow venting procedure. An awl is placed against the cortex within the femoral notch (**a**). The awl after mallet-assisted advancement through the outer cortex (**b**). Marrow elements being released after removal of the awl (**c**)

12.3.6 Post-operative Rehabilitation

There is currently no consensus on the optimal post-operative rehabilitation protocol following meniscal repair. Biomechanical testing has found that tear pattern influences the force across the meniscal repair during physiologic loading. For example, while vertical longitudinal tears are reduced and compressed during loading, radial tears experience distraction [100, 101]. Posterior meniscal root repairs are similarly subjected to large tensile forces during weight bearing [102]. The aforementioned accelerated rehabilitation protocols have shown good results for vertical longitudinal meniscal tears [42, 43]; however their utility in the setting of these radial or posterior root repairs has not been established.

Additionally, meniscal tears are often complex, involving more than one tear pattern. For these reasons a standardized rehabilitation protocol should be considered. Patient-specific alterations can then be incorporated as necessary and communicated to the patient and therapist(s) overseeing the post-operative care. Examples of post-operative rehabilitation protocols for meniscus repairs and posterior meniscal root repairs are included in Table 12.1.

12.3.7 Revision Meniscal Repair

The mean failure rate of meniscal repair in the literature is 15% (range 0–43.5%) [103]. Revision meniscal repair can be considered in some patients and has demonstrated good results. Thirty-four patients were retrospectively reviewed after revision repair and 79% reported no pain, mechanical symptoms or revision surgery at a mean final follow-up of 72 months post-operatively [104]. The authors identified younger age as an independent risk factor for failed revision meniscus repair. Another study identified degenerative changes as a potential risk factor for failure of revision repair [105].

12.3.8 Meniscal Deficiency

Meniscal tears or failed meniscal repairs that are judged to be irreparable should undergo partial meniscectomy with an attempt to save as much meniscal tissue as possible [106]. Meniscal allograft transplantation can be considered for patients who develop pain in the involved compartment. Contraindications include arthritis, uncorrected malalignment, or ligamentous instability [107].

12.4 Conclusion

The increased recognition that meniscal preservation is vital to maintain a healthy, functioning knee has led to a better understanding of pathological conditions, expanded surgical indications, constant refinement of repair techniques, and

Table 12.1 Examples of post-operative rehabilitation protocols for meniscus repairs and posterior meniscal root repairs

Protocol	Range of motion (ROM)	Weight bearing (WB)	Additional information
Accelerated rehabilitation [42]	0–90° for 1–2 weeks Full ROM at 3–6 weeks	Toe-Touch WB for 1–2 weeks Progress as tolerated with Full WB at 3–4 weeks	No brace Running permitted at 8 weeks Contact sports permitted at 16 weeks as tolerated
Weight restriction [14]	0–90° for 3–4 weeks	Partial WB with crutches for 3–4 weeks	No squatting or pivoting permitted for 16 weeks post-operative Sports permitted at 16–24 weeks based on clinical progress Often utilized for isolated meniscal tear repair (i.e., bucket-handle tears)
Motion restriction [108]	0–60° for weeks 1–4 0–90° at weeks 5–6 Full ROM after week 6	Full WB with crutches for weeks 1–4 Full WB at week 6	ROM limiting brace applied for 6 weeks post-operative WB restricted to full extension for weeks 1–4 Passive full ROM and isometric closed chain exercises for weeks 1–6 Pain-adapted WB with full ROM after 6 weeks
Dual restriction [109]	0–60° for weeks 1–2 0–90° at week 4 0–120° at week 6 Full ROM after week 8	Partial WB with crutches for weeks 1–4 Progress as tolerated with gradual WB at week 5	Knee extension brace applied for 6 weeks post-operative Often utilized for complex meniscal tear repair (i.e., root or radial tears)

improved patient outcomes. Standardized reporting of long-term results will help further clarify the optimal surgical techniques and better define the role of biologic augmentation methods. Surgeons treating meniscal pathology must therefore maintain a thorough understanding of the evolving literature regarding meniscal repair indications and techniques.

References

1. Makris EA, Hadidi P, Athanasiou KA. The knee meniscus: structure-function, pathophysiology, current repair techniques, and prospects for regeneration. Biomaterials. 2011;32:7411–31.
2. Arnoczky SP, Warren RF. Microvasculature of the human meniscus. Am J Sports Med. 1982;10:90–5.
3. Arnoczky SP, Warren RF. The microvasculature of the meniscus and its response to injury. An experimental study in the dog. Am J Sports Med. 1983;11:131–41.
4. Grant JA, Wilde J, Miller BS, Bedi A. Comparison of inside-out and all-inside techniques for the repair of isolated meniscal tears: a systematic review. Am J Sports Med. 2012;40:459–68.
5. Scott GA, Jolly BL, Henning CE. Combined posterior incision and arthroscopic intra-articular repair of the meniscus. An examination of factors affecting healing. J Bone Joint Surg Am. 1986;68:847–61.
6. Noyes FR, Barber-Westin SD. Arthroscopic repair of meniscus tears extending into the avascular zone with or without anterior cruciate ligament reconstruction in patients 40 years of age and older. Arthroscopy. 2000;16:822–9.
7. Noyes FR, Barber-Westin SD. Arthroscopic repair of meniscal tears extending into the avascular zone in patients younger than twenty years of age. Am J Sports Med. 2002;30:589–600.
8. Barber-Westin SD, Noyes FR. Clinical healing rates of meniscus repairs of tears in the central-third (red-white) zone. Arthroscopy. 2014;30:134–46.
9. Cannon WD, Vittori JM. The incidence of healing in arthroscopic meniscal repairs in anterior cruciate ligament-reconstructed knees versus stable knees. Am J Sports Med. 1992;20:176–81.

10. Warren RF. Meniscectomy and repair in the anterior cruciate ligament-deficient patient. Clin Orthop Relat Res. 1990:55–63.
11. DeHaven KE, Lohrer WA, Lovelock JE. Long-term results of open meniscal repair. Am J Sports Med. 1995;23:524–30.
12. Morgan CD, Wojtys EM, Casscells CD, Casscells SW. Arthroscopic meniscal repair evaluated by second-look arthroscopy. Am J Sports Med. 1991;19:632–7; discussion 637–638.
13. Krych AJ, Pitts RT, Dajani KA, Stuart MJ, Levy BA, Dahm DL. Surgical repair of meniscal tears with concomitant anterior cruciate ligament reconstruction in patients 18 years and younger. Am J Sports Med. 2010;38:976–82.
14. Krych AJ, McIntosh AL, Voll AE, Stuart MJ, Dahm DL. Arthroscopic repair of isolated meniscal tears in patients 18 years and younger. Am J Sports Med. 2008;36:1283–9.
15. Anderson AF, Irrgang JJ, Dunn W, et al. Interobserver reliability of the International Society of Arthroscopy, Knee Surgery and Orthopaedic Sports Medicine (ISAKOS) classification of meniscal tears. Am J Sports Med. 2011;39:926–32.
16. LaPrade CM, James EW, Cram TR, Feagin JA, Engebretsen L, LaPrade RF. Meniscal root tears: a classification system based on tear morphology. Am J Sports Med. 2015;43:363–9.
17. Allaire R, Muriuki M, Gilbertson L, Harner CD. Biomechanical consequences of a tear of the posterior root of the medial meniscus. Similar to total meniscectomy. J Bone Joint Surg Am. 2008;90:1922–31.
18. Padalecki JR, Jansson KS, Smith SD, Dornan GJ, Pierce CM, Wijdicks CA, Laprade RF. Biomechanical consequences of a complete radial tear adjacent to the medial meniscus posterior root attachment site: in situ pull-out repair restores derangement of joint mechanics. Am J Sports Med. 2014;42:699–707.
19. LaPrade CM, Jansson KS, Dornan G, Smith SD, Wijdicks CA, LaPrade RF. Altered tibiofemoral contact mechanics due to lateral meniscus posterior horn root avulsions and radial tears can be restored with in situ pull-out suture repairs. J Bone Joint Surg. 2014;96:471–9.
20. Steineman BD, LaPrade RF, Santangelo KS, Warner BT, Goodrich LR, Haut Donahue TL. Early osteoarthritis after untreated anterior meniscal root tears: an in vivo animal study. Orthop J Sports Med. 2017;5:2325967117702452.
21. Krych AJ, Reardon PJ, Johnson NR, Mohan R, Peter L, Levy BA, Stuart MJ. Non-operative management of medial meniscus posterior horn root tears is associated with worsening arthritis and poor clinical outcome at 5-year follow-up. Knee Surg Sports Traumatol Arthrosc. 2017;25:383–9.
22. Matheny LM, Ockuly AC, Steadman JR, LaPrade RF. Posterior meniscus root tears: associated pathologies to assist as diagnostic tools. Knee Surg Sports Traumatol Arthrosc. 2015;23:3127–31.
23. Krych AJ, Wu IT, Desai VS, Murthy NS, Collins MS, Saris DBF, Levy BA, Stuart MJ. High rate of missed lateral meniscus posterior root tears on preoperative magnetic resonance imaging. Orthop J Sports Med. 2018;6:2325967118765722.
24. Bollen SR. Posteromedial meniscocapsular injury associated with rupture of the anterior cruciate ligament: a previously unrecognised association. J Bone Joint Surg (Br). 2010;92:222–3.
25. Liu X, Feng H, Zhang H, Hong L, Wang XS, Zhang J. Arthroscopic prevalence of ramp lesion in 868 patients with anterior cruciate ligament injury. Am J Sports Med. 2011;39:832–7.
26. DePhillipo NN, Cinque ME, Chahla J, Geeslin AG, Engebretsen L, LaPrade RF. Incidence and detection of meniscal ramp lesions on magnetic resonance imaging in patients with anterior cruciate ligament reconstruction. Am J Sports Med. 2017;45:2233–7.
27. Sonnery-Cottet B, Conteduca J, Thaunat M, Gunepin FX, Seil R. Hidden lesions of the posterior horn of the medial meniscus: a systematic arthroscopic exploration of the concealed portion of the knee. Am J Sports Med. 2014;42:921–6.
28. Stephen JM, Halewood C, Kittl C, Bollen SR, Williams A, Amis AA. Posteromedial meniscocapsular lesions increase tibiofemoral joint laxity with anterior cruciate ligament deficiency, and their repair reduces laxity. Am J Sports Med. 2016;44:400–8.
29. Peltier A, Lording T, Maubisson L, Ballis R, Neyret P, Lustig S. The role of the meniscotibial ligament in posteromedial rotational knee stability. Knee Surg Sports Traumatol Arthrosc. 2015;23:2967–73.
30. DePhillipo NN, Moatshe G, Brady A, Chahla J, Aman ZS, Dornan GJ, Nakama GY, Engebretsen L, LaPrade RF. Effect of meniscocapsular and meniscotibial lesions in ACL-deficient and ACL-reconstructed knees: a biomechanical study. Am J Sports Med. 2018;46:2422.
31. Albertsson M, Gillquist J. Discoid lateral menisci: a report of 29 cases. Arthroscopy. 1988;4:211–4.
32. Ikeuchi H. Arthroscopic treatment of the discoid lateral meniscus. Technique and long-term results. Clin Orthop Relat Res. 1982:19–28.
33. Aichroth PM, Patel DV, Marx CL. Congenital discoid lateral meniscus in children. A follow-up study and evolution of management. J Bone Joint Surg (Br). 1991;73:932–6.
34. Rao SK, Sripathi Rao P. Clinical, radiologic and arthroscopic assessment and treatment of bilateral discoid lateral meniscus. Knee Surg Sports Traumatol Arthrosc. 2007;15:597–601.
35. Klingele KE, Kocher MS, Hresko MT, Gerbino P, Micheli LJ. Discoid lateral meniscus: prevalence of peripheral rim instability. J Pediatr Orthop. 2004;24:79–82.
36. Kini SG, Walker P, Bruce W. Bilateral symptomatic discoid medial meniscus of the knee: a case

report and review of literature. Arch Trauma Res. 2015;4:e27115.
37. Song IS, Kim JB, Lee JK, Park B-S. Discoid medial meniscus tear, with a literature review of treatments. Knee Surg Relat Res. 2017;29:237–42.
38. Rohren EM, Kosarek FJ, Helms CA. Discoid lateral meniscus and the frequency of meniscal tears. Skelet Radiol. 2001;30:316–20.
39. Andrish JT. Meniscal injuries in children and adolescents: diagnosis and management. J Am Acad Orthop Surg. 1996;4:231–7.
40. Carter CW, Hoellwarth J, Weiss JM. Clinical outcomes as a function of meniscal stability in the discoid meniscus: a preliminary report. J Pediatr Orthop. 2012;32:9–14.
41. Watanabe M, Takeda S, Ikeuchi H. Atlas of arthroscopy. 3rd ed. Berlin, Tokyo: Igaku-Shoin, Springer; 1979.
42. Lind M, Nielsen T, Faunø P, Lund B, Christiansen SE. Free rehabilitation is safe after isolated meniscus repair: a prospective randomized trial comparing free with restricted rehabilitation regimens. Am J Sports Med. 2013;41:2753–8.
43. Perkins B, Gronbeck KR, Yue RA, Tompkins MA. Similar failure rate in immediate post-operative weight bearing versus protected weight bearing following meniscal repair on peripheral, vertical meniscal tears. Knee Surg Sports Traumatol Arthrosc. 2018;26:2245–50.
44. Paxton ES, Stock MV, Brophy RH. Meniscal repair versus partial meniscectomy: a systematic review comparing reoperation rates and clinical outcomes. Arthroscopy. 2011;27:1275–88.
45. Nepple JJ, Dunn WR, Wright RW. Meniscal repair outcomes at greater than five years: a systematic literature review and meta-analysis. J Bone Joint Surg Am. 2012;94:2222–7.
46. Lutz C, Dalmay F, Ehkirch FP, et al. Meniscectomy versus meniscal repair: 10 years radiological and clinical results in vertical lesions in stable knee. Orthop Traumatol Surg Res. 2015;101:S327–31.
47. Uzun E, Misir A, Kizkapan TB, Ozcamdalli M, Akkurt S, Guney A. Factors affecting the outcomes of arthroscopically repaired traumatic vertical longitudinal medial meniscal tears. Orthop J Sports Med. 2017;5:2325967117712448.
48. Cho J-H. A modified outside-in suture technique for repair of the middle segment of the meniscus using a spinal needle. Knee Surg Relat Res. 2014;26:43–7.
49. Fillingham YA, Riboh JC, Erickson BJ, Bach BR, Yanke AB. Inside-out versus all-inside repair of isolated meniscal tears: an updated systematic review. Am J Sports Med. 2017;45:234–42.
50. Rankin CC, Lintner DM, Noble PC, Paravic V, Greer E. A biomechanical analysis of meniscal repair techniques. Am J Sports Med. 2002;30:492–7.
51. Bhatia S, Civitarese DM, Turnbull TL, LaPrade CM, Nitri M, Wijdicks CA, LaPrade RF. A novel repair method for radial tears of the medial meniscus: biomechanical comparison of transtibial 2-tunnel and double horizontal mattress suture techniques under cyclic loading. Am J Sports Med. 2016;44:639–45.
52. Kurzweil PR, Lynch NM, Coleman S, Kearney B. Repair of horizontal meniscus tears: a systematic review. Arthroscopy. 2014;30:1513–9.
53. Beamer BS, Masoudi A, Walley KC, et al. Analysis of a new all-inside versus inside-out technique for repairing radial meniscal tears. Arthroscopy. 2015;31:293–8.
54. Cinque ME, Geeslin AG, Chahla J, Dornan GJ, LaPrade RF. Two-tunnel transtibial repair of radial meniscus tears produces comparable results to inside-out repair of vertical meniscus tears. Am J Sports Med. 2017;45:2253–9.
55. Bhatia S, LaPrade CM, Ellman MB, LaPrade RF. Meniscal root tears: significance, diagnosis, and treatment. Am J Sports Med. 2014;42:3016–30.
56. Moon H-K, Koh Y-G, Kim Y-C, Park Y-S, Jo S-B, Kwon S-K. Prognostic factors of arthroscopic pull-out repair for a posterior root tear of the medial meniscus. Am J Sports Med. 2012;40:1138–43.
57. LaPrade RF, LaPrade CM, James EW. Recent advances in posterior meniscal root repair techniques. J Am Acad Orthop Surg. 2015;23:71–6.
58. Raustol OA, Poelstra KA, Chhabra A, Diduch DR. The meniscal ossicle revisited: etiology and an arthroscopic technique for treatment. Arthroscopy. 2006;22:687.e1–3.
59. Kim Y-M, Rhee K-J, Lee J-K, Hwang D-S, Yang J-Y, Kim S-J. Arthroscopic pullout repair of a complete radial tear of the tibial attachment site of the medial meniscus posterior horn. Arthroscopy. 2006;22:795.e1–4.
60. Marzo JM, Kumar BA. Primary repair of medial meniscal avulsions: 2 case studies. Am J Sports Med. 2007;35:1380–3.
61. Nicholas SJ, Golant A, Schachter AK, Lee SJ. A new surgical technique for arthroscopic repair of the meniscus root tear. Knee Surg Sports Traumatol Arthrosc. 2009;17:1433–6.
62. Ahn JH, Wang JH, Lim HC, Bae JH, Park JS, Yoo JC, Shyam AK. Double transosseous pull out suture technique for transection of posterior horn of medial meniscus. Arch Orthop Trauma Surg. 2009;129:387–92.
63. Krych AJ, Johnson NR, Wu IT, Smith PA, Stuart MJ. A simple cinch is superior to a locking loop for meniscus root repair: a human biomechanical comparison of suture constructs in a transtibial pull-out model. Knee Surg Sports Traumatol Arthrosc. 2018;26:2239–44.
64. Mitchell R, Pitts R, Kim Y-M, Matava MJ. Medial meniscal root avulsion: a biomechanical comparison of 4 different repair constructs. Arthroscopy. 2016;32:111–9.
65. Anz AW, Branch EA, Saliman JD. Biomechanical comparison of arthroscopic repair constructs for meniscal root tears. Am J Sports Med. 2014;42:2699–706.

66. Kopf S, Colvin AC, Muriuki M, Zhang X, Harner CD. Meniscal root suturing techniques: implications for root fixation. Am J Sports Med. 2011;39:2141–6.
67. LaPrade RF, Matheny LM, Moulton SG, James EW, Dean CS. Posterior meniscal root repairs: outcomes of an anatomic transtibial pull-out technique. Am J Sports Med. 2017;45:884–91.
68. Chung KS, Noh JM, Ha JK, Ra HJ, Park SB, Kim HK, Kim JG. Survivorship analysis and clinical outcomes of transtibial pullout repair for medial meniscus posterior root tears: a 5- to 10-year follow-up study. Arthroscopy. 2018;34:530–5.
69. Ahn JH, Lee YS, Chang J-Y, Chang MJ, Eun SS, Kim SM. Arthroscopic all inside repair of the lateral meniscus root tear. Knee. 2009;16:77–80.
70. Anderson L, Watts M, Shapter O, Logan M, Risebury M, Duffy D, Myers P. Repair of radial tears and posterior horn detachments of the lateral meniscus: minimum 2-year follow-up. Arthroscopy. 2010;26:1625–32.
71. Pan F, Hua S, Ma Z. Surgical treatment of combined posterior root tears of the lateral meniscus and ACL tears. Med Sci Monit. 2015;21:1345–9.
72. Duchman KR, Westermann RW, Spindler KP, Reinke EK, Huston LJ, Amendola A, MOON Knee Group, Wolf BR. The fate of meniscus tears left in situ at the time of anterior cruciate ligament reconstruction: a 6-year follow-up study from the MOON cohort. Am J Sports Med. 2015;43:2688–95.
73. Pujol N, Beaufils P. Healing results of meniscal tears left in situ during anterior cruciate ligament reconstruction: a review of clinical studies. Knee Surg Sports Traumatol Arthrosc. 2009;17:396–401.
74. Shelbourne KD, Rask BP. The sequelae of salvaged nondegenerative peripheral vertical medial meniscus tears with anterior cruciate ligament reconstruction. Arthroscopy. 2001;17:270–4.
75. Muriuki MG, Tuason DA, Tucker BG, Harner CD. Changes in tibiofemoral contact mechanics following radial split and vertical tears of the medial meniscus an in vitro investigation of the efficacy of arthroscopic repair. J Bone Joint Surg Am. 2011;93:1089–95.
76. Papageorgiou CD, Gil JE, Kanamori A, Fenwick JA, Woo SL, Fu FH. The biomechanical interdependence between the anterior cruciate ligament replacement graft and the medial meniscus. Am J Sports Med. 2001;29:226–31.
77. DePhillipo NN, Cinque ME, Kennedy NI, Chahla J, Geeslin AG, Moatshe G, Engebretsen L, LaPrade RF. Inside-out repair of meniscal ramp lesions. Arthrosc Tech. 2017;6:e1315–20.
78. Thaunat M, Jan N, Fayard JM, Kajetanek C, Murphy CG, Pupim B, Gardon R, Sonnery-Cottet B. Repair of meniscal ramp lesions through a posteromedial portal during anterior cruciate ligament reconstruction: outcome study with a minimum 2-year follow-up. Arthroscopy. 2016;32:2269–77.
79. Chahla J, Dean CS, Moatshe G, Mitchell JJ, Cram TR, Yacuzzi C, LaPrade RF. Meniscal ramp lesions: anatomy, incidence, diagnosis, and treatment. Orthop J Sports Med. 2016;4:2325967116657815.
80. Li W-P, Chen Z, Song B, Yang R, Tan W. The FasT-fix repair technique for ramp lesion of the medial meniscus. Knee Surg Relat Res. 2015;27:56–60.
81. Ahn JH, Lee YS, Yoo JC, Chang MJ, Koh KH, Kim MH. Clinical and second-look arthroscopic evaluation of repaired medial meniscus in anterior cruciate ligament-reconstructed knees. Am J Sports Med. 2010;38:472–7.
82. Washington ER, Root L, Liener UC. Discoid lateral meniscus in children. Long-term follow-up after excision. J Bone Joint Surg Am. 1995;77:1357–61.
83. Räber DA, Friederich NF, Hefti F. Discoid lateral meniscus in children. Long-term follow-up after total meniscectomy. J Bone Joint Surg Am. 1998;80:1579–86.
84. Manzione M, Pizzutillo PD, Peoples AB, Schweizer PA. Meniscectomy in children: a long-term follow-up study. Am J Sports Med. 1983;11:111–5.
85. Hayashi LK, Yamaga H, Ida K, Miura T. Arthroscopic meniscectomy for discoid lateral meniscus in children. J Bone Joint Surg Am. 1988;70:1495–500.
86. Oğüt T, Kesmezacar H, Akgün I, Cansü E. Arthroscopic meniscectomy for discoid lateral meniscus in children and adolescents: 4.5 year follow-up. J Pediatr Orthop B. 2003;12:390–7.
87. Good CR, Green DW, Griffith MH, Valen AW, Widmann RF, Rodeo SA. Arthroscopic treatment of symptomatic discoid meniscus in children: classification, technique, and results. Arthroscopy. 2007;23:157–63.
88. Ahn JH, Kim K-I, Wang JH, Jeon JW, Cho YC, Lee SH. Long-term results of arthroscopic reshaping for symptomatic discoid lateral meniscus in children. Arthroscopy. 2015;31:867–73.
89. Kose O, Celiktas M, Egerci OF, Guler F, Ozyurek S, Sarpel Y. Prognostic factors affecting the outcome of arthroscopic saucerization in discoid lateral meniscus: a retrospective analysis of 48 cases. Musculoskelet Surg. 2015;99:165–70.
90. Woodmass JM, LaPrade RF, Sgaglione NA, Nakamura N, Krych AJ. Meniscal repair: reconsidering indications, techniques, and biologic augmentation. J Bone Joint Surg Am. 2017;99:1222–31.
91. Ochi M, Uchio Y, Okuda K, Shu N, Yamaguchi H, Sakai Y. Expression of cytokines after meniscal rasping to promote meniscal healing. Arthroscopy. 2001;17:724–31.
92. Fox JM, Rintz KG, Ferkel RD. Trephination of incomplete meniscal tears. Arthroscopy. 1993;9:451–5.
93. Dean CS, Chahla J, Matheny LM, Mitchell JJ, LaPrade RF. Outcomes after biologically augmented isolated meniscal repair with marrow venting are comparable with those after meniscal repair with concomitant anterior cruciate ligament reconstruction. Am J Sports Med. 2017;45:1341–8.
94. Ra HJ, Ha JK, Jang SH, Lee DW, Kim JG. Arthroscopic inside-out repair of complete radial

tears of the meniscus with a fibrin clot. Knee Surg Sports Traumatol Arthrosc. 2013;21:2126–30.
95. Jang SH, Ha JK, Lee DW, Kim JG. Fibrin clot delivery system for meniscal repair. Knee Surg Relat Res. 2011;23:180–3.
96. Henning CE, Lynch MA, Yearout KM, Vequist SW, Stallbaumer RJ, Decker KA. Arthroscopic meniscal repair using an exogenous fibrin clot. Clin Orthop Relat Res. 1990:64–72.
97. Griffin JW, Hadeed MM, Werner BC, Diduch DR, Carson EW, Miller MD. Platelet-rich plasma in meniscal repair: does augmentation improve surgical outcomes? Clin Orthop Relat Res. 2015;473:1665–72.
98. Pujol N, Salle De Chou E, Boisrenoult P, Beaufils P. Platelet-rich plasma for open meniscal repair in young patients: any benefit? Knee Surg Sports Traumatol Arthrosc. 2015;23:51–8.
99. Piontek T, Ciemniewska-Gorzela K, Naczk J, Jakob R, Szulc A, Grygorowicz M, Slomczykowski M. Complex meniscus tears treated with collagen matrix wrapping and bone marrow blood injection: a 2-year clinical follow-up. Cartilage. 2016;7:123–39.
100. Richards DP, Barber FA, Herbert MA. Compressive loads in longitudinal lateral meniscus tears: a biomechanical study in porcine knees. Arthroscopy. 2005;21:1452–6.
101. Gao J, Wei X, Messner K. Healing of the anterior attachment of the rabbit meniscus to bone. Clin Orthop Relat Res. 1998:246–58.
102. Stärke C, Kopf S, Lippisch R, Lohmann CH, Becker R. Tensile forces on repaired medial meniscal root tears. Arthroscopy. 2013;29:205–12.
103. Lozano J, Ma CB, Cannon WD. All-inside meniscus repair: a systematic review. Clin Orthop Relat Res. 2007;455:134–41.
104. Krych AJ, Reardon P, Sousa P, Levy BA, Dahm DL, Stuart MJ. Clinical outcomes after revision meniscus repair. Arthroscopy. 2016;32:1831–7.
105. Imade S, Kumahashi N, Kuwata S, Kadowaki M, Ito S, Uchio Y. Clinical outcomes of revision meniscal repair: a case series. Am J Sports Med. 2014;42:350–7.
106. Hede A, Larsen E, Sandberg H. Partial versus total meniscectomy. A prospective, randomised study with long-term follow-up. J Bone Joint Surg (Br). 1992;74:118–21.
107. Noyes FR, Barber-Westin SD. Long-term survivorship and function of meniscus transplantation. Am J Sports Med. 2016;44:2330–8.
108. Stein T, Mehling AP, Welsch F, von Eisenhart-Rothe R, Jäger A. Long-term outcome after arthroscopic meniscal repair versus arthroscopic partial meniscectomy for traumatic meniscal tears. Am J Sports Med. 2010;38:1542–8.
109. Ahn J-H, Kwon O-J, Nam T-S. Arthroscopic repair of horizontal meniscal cleavage tears with marrow-stimulating technique. Arthroscopy. 2015;31:92–8.

Meniscus Allograft Transplantation

13

Davide Reale and Peter Verdonk

13.1 Introduction

Lateral and medial menisci are both "C"-shaped fibrocartilaginous structures placed in the medial and lateral compartments of the knee. The medial meniscus covers approximately one-third of the tibial plateau, and its root attachments are more spaced than those of the lateral meniscus. In contrast, lateral meniscus is more semicircular and covers greater than 50% of the lateral tibial articular surface [1]. The anterior and posterior lateral meniscal insertion horns are closer to the insertion of anterior cruciate ligament (ACL) [2, 3]. In addition, the posterior horn is attached to the tibia in the intercondylar region and to the medial femoral condyle via the ligaments of Humphrey (anterior to the posterior cruciate ligament) and Wrisberg (posterior to the PCL) when present [4, 5]. Despite these attachments, the lateral meniscus is more mobile than the medial meniscus [1]. The semicircular shape of the lateral meniscus, with root attachments in close proximity to each other, differs from the crescent shape of the medial meniscus; this feature plays a role in possible transplantation techniques.

Nowadays it is well known that menisci play an important role in the complex biomechanics and homeostasis of the knee, although once they used to be considered the vestigial remnants of a muscle within the joint. Menisci are well recognized for their key function in shock absorption, load distribution [6–8], joint lubrification [9], proprioception [10], increasing joint congruity [4] and joint stabilization [4, 11, 12]. The medial meniscus also provides secondary constraint to the knee in the antero-posterior direction, while the lateral meniscus is important for rotational control [13, 14]. In the loaded knee, the lateral meniscus transmits 70% and the medial meniscus 50% of the load through the respective compartments of the knee [15].

Unfortunately, meniscus tears are the most common type of intra-articular knee injury, involving about 60–70 per 100,000 inhabitants per year [11, 16]. Although the classical treatment for painful meniscal tears is meniscectomy, in recent times the treatment has shifted from excision to meniscal-repairing surgery. This reflects the widespreading concept that saving meniscal tissue is key to preserve joint integrity [17, 18]. In fact, the loss of meniscal tissue leads to reduced congruency of the articular cartilage surfaces of the tibio-femoral joint, resulting in a decrease of the intra-articular contact area and an increase in loading pressure, some as much as

D. Reale (✉)
IRCCS, Istituto Ortopedico Rizzoli, Clinica Ortopedica e Traumatologica II, Bologna, Italy
e-mail: davide.reale@ior.it

P. Verdonk
Orthoca, Antwerp, Belgium

More Foundation, Antwerp, Belgium

University of Antwerp, Antwerp, Belgium
e-mail: peter.verdonk@azmonica.be

M. Brittberg, K. Slynarski (eds.), *Lower Extremity Joint Preservation*,
https://doi.org/10.1007/978-3-030-57382-9_13

235% after total meniscectomy [19, 20]. The increased intra-articular contact stresses within the knee after meniscectomy lead to "overload" the articular cartilage, leading to early articular cartilage degeneration.

An intact ring structure is essential for proper meniscal function; hence, any damage to the menisci that causes a loss of structural integrity and function leads to altered loading of the chondral bearing surfaces of the knee [21]. This condition can arise even if there is no or very little meniscus tissue loss, as in presence of radial or root tears, and it is important to introduce the concept of "functional meniscus loss".

Despite all these considerations, meniscectomy is still frequently performed, and it is often unavoidable in the case of irreparable meniscal tears or after failure of previous repair.

Meniscal allograft transplantation (MAT) has evolved since the 1980s aiming to limit or even prevent the negative effects of meniscus loss. It is a possible treatment option for the patients with pain after meniscectomy, known as the "post-meniscectomy syndrome", and has been shown to provide predictable symptomatic relief and a return to sporting activity with good long-term survival, and long-term results continue to improve as surgical indications and techniques are evolving. However, there still remains significant variability in how MAT is performed, and as such, there remains opportunity for outcome and graft survivorship to be optimized.

13.2 Evaluation of the Post-meniscectomy Knee

A detailed medical history, a complete physical examination and additional imaging studies (radiographs and MRI) are essential in the evaluation and management of the painful knee after functional meniscus loss.

History taking should focus on determining patient age, characteristics of pain, swelling, loss of motion, instability and mechanical symptoms. In regard to the location of pain, it should be specifically isolated to the meniscal deficient joint line.

A detailed physical examination of the knee should be performed with particular attention given to the axial alignment, presence of effusion, ligamentous stability, range of motion (ROM) and detection of flexion or extension contractures. Coronal alignment should be evaluated in the standing position and during gait.

Radiographic knee evaluation should include weight-bearing antero-posterior (AP) views in full extension, postero-anterior (PA) views at 30° or 45° of flexion (Rosenberg view) and skyline, lateral and full-length bilateral weight-bearing mechanical axis views to determine alignment and joint space changes with narrowing or flattening of the femoral condyles [22, 23]. MRI represents the gold standard for the evaluation of post-meniscectomy pain and concomitant ligamentous pathology. It can also be used to assess the presence of subchondral sclerosis, bony oedema, condylar squaring, osteophytes and cartilage loss, all top be considered as sequelae of meniscus deficiency [24].

13.3 Indications

Successful meniscal transplantation depends on strictly selection for the ideal candidate. Surgery should be considered for symptomatic meniscus-deficient knees only after all non-surgical treatments have been attempted. When conservative therapies fail to provide relief of symptoms or joint space narrowing occurs, meniscal transplantation should be considered.

In 2016, the International Meniscus Reconstruction Expert Forum (IMREF), consisting of 21 international surgeons who are experts in MAT, has established that the primary indication for meniscal allograft transplantation is a patient with unicompartmental pain in a meniscus-deficient knee (or in the presence of total or subtotal "functional" meniscectomy). Symptoms may range from exercise-related pain to constant pain, swelling and/or stiffness [25].

Meniscal transplantation is typically performed in "young" patients who are typically less than 50–55 years old, but it has occasionally been performed in older people [26].

Table 13.1 Indications and contraindications for the meniscal allograft transplantation

Indications	Contraindications
Age <50–55 years	Age >55 years
Persistent unicompartmental pain	Knee instability
Previous total or subtotal meniscectomy	Generalized/grade IV degenerative compartmental cartilage changes
Outerbridge grade <3 articular changes	Marked radiographic changes such as femoral condyle flattening and osteophyte formation
Correct alignment	Varus/valgus malalignment
No ligament laxity	Synovial disease Inflammatory arthritis Obesity

The knee joint should be stable and have normal alignment, with intact articular surfaces (grade I or II). Any grade III or IV lesions should be focal and require concomitant treatment.

Contraindications for meniscal transplantation include diffuse arthritic changes, squaring or flattening of the femoral condyle or tibial plateau and significant osteophyte formation in the involved compartment, untreated knee instability, inflammatory arthritis, synovial disease, previous joint infection, skeletal immaturity or marked obesity (Table 13.1). Although not absolute contraindications, chondral defects, varus/valgus malalignment and ligamentous instability all require consideration for concurrent or staged treatment to ensure that all joint pathology is addressed [27].

13.4 Types of Graft

The choice of graft preservation technique has a potentially significant impact on outcome and survival. In addition, there are potential risks of disease transmission and host immune reactions [28].

Currently, there are four methods of preserving allografts: fresh viable grafts, fresh-frozen grafts, cryopreserved grafts and lyophilized grafts. Of these options, fresh-frozen grafts are the most commonly used.

Fresh viable allografts may be the ideal type of transplant because fresh tissue contains large numbers of viable chondrocytes. Several studies have suggested that these cells result in improved maintenance of the extracellular matrix and the mechanical integrity of the allograft after transplantation [12, 29, 30]. The rationale for maintaining cell viability in meniscal tissue is based on findings in articular cartilage that showed a change in the material properties of nonviable articular cartilage following transplantation [31, 32]. On the other hand, the timing of the procurement and transplantation can be challenging [33]. Fresh allografts can be kept at 4 °C in sterile tissue culture medium for 7 days without loss of viability [34]. However, in clinical practice, the availability of a fresh transplant is limited, and the difficulty of matching the meniscal size of donor and receiver may limit further the applicability of this type of graft. Furthermore, fresh viable grafts have been associated with a higher risk of disease transmission, because serologic testing may not be complete before graft transplantation and chondrocyte preservation strategies preclude sterilization [35].

Non-irradiated deep freezing or fresh freezing is one of the most common conservation methods used in orthopaedics. It can be stored at −80 °C for up to 5 years. This method is technically simple and minimally immunogenic. The menisci, harvested under sterile conditions, are put into physiological solution with an antibiotic agent, followed by rapid freezing [35]. Although donor fibrochondrocytes may be destroyed by the freezing process, it is hypothesized that the same process results in denaturation of the histocompatibility antigens and thus decreases immunogenicity within fresh-frozen menisci [36]. A further advantage is the maintenance of the mechanical properties of the meniscal allograft [37].

It can be stated that the role of cell viability in meniscal allografts is unclear, and to date, no studies have demonstrated a clear advantage between the two methods of storage. Inferior clinical results have been reported with both cryopreserved and lyophilized grafts.

Lyophilization or freeze-drying, which consists in drying tissue under vacuum and freezing conditions, is probably the most convenient method as regards storage, but is no longer a recommended technique due to some change in the mechanical properties of the meniscus and a reduction in graft size [36].

Cryopreservation consists in a deep freezing of the meniscus at −196 °C in a solution with a cryoprotective agent, a culture medium and an antiseptic agent. Theoretically, cryopreservation preserves cell membrane integrity and donor chondrocyte viability [38]. However, the percentage of viable cells decreases with storage time [39]. Furthermore, secondary sterilization techniques that affect cell viability cannot be applied, and this may increase the risk of disease transmission from a donor. Although cryopreservation allows for a more prolonged allograft storage than the fresh-frozen technique, it is a considerably more demanding, difficult and costly technique.

13.5 Sizing of Allograft

MAT should replace the original tissue matching the size of the meniscus to be transplanted with that needed in the recipient, and therefore accurate and reproducible sizing methods are essential to the overall success of the meniscal transplant [13, 40].

Several methods have been proposed to assess recipient meniscal measurements, but it is not clear which methods are the most accurate or reliable.

Meniscal measurements obtained from standard AP and lateral knee radiographs, as proposed by Pollard et al. [41], are the most widely used. According to this method, the coronal width of the medial and lateral menisci roughly equaled the distance from the respective tibial eminence to the periphery of the tibial compartment on AP films. The length of the menisci is then measured on the lateral radiographic view by establishing the size of the tibial plateau, and then a line is drawn at the level of the articular line between the anterior surface of the tibia above the tuberosity and a parallel line that is tangential to the posterior margin of the tibial plateau. The medial meniscus corresponds to 80% and the lateral meniscus to 70% of the measurement of the tibial plateau on the sagittal plane. Calibrators for correction of magnification are needed to correctly calculate the size. However, measurement errors by these predictive criteria showed SDs ranging from 7.4% to 8.4%, showing to be less accurate when sizing the lateral meniscus. To overcome this problem, Yoon et al. proposed a modification of this method based on a mathematical model to increase accuracy [42].

The first studies using MRI reported errors regarding accurately measuring the meniscal size probably because the measurements were taken in the transverse plane. Measurements taken in this plane will be heavily reliant on having the plane of the cuts be exactly parallel to the transverse plane of the menisci, which may be difficult to achieve [9].

A number of more recent studies using MRI have tried to establish a more geometrically accurate allograft size based on specific meniscus measurements [43]. The use of MRI of the contralateral unaffected knee was supported previously by Prodromos et al. [9]. They showed that 97% had sagittal and frontal dimensions within 3 mm of the contralateral meniscus. They concluded that human knee menisci are bilaterally symmetric in size and that direct MRI measurement of the contralateral intact meniscus better predicts the actual meniscal size than estimation of the size indirectly from measurement of the tibial plateau on which it is located. Similar results have been achieved by Yoon et al. [42], which concluded that there were no differences between right and left meniscal measurements according to MRI. Thus, MRI of the contralateral unaffected knee, although costly, may be useful in determining the required size.

Other authors believe that anthropometric data can substitute for MRI in determining meniscal dimensions. Van Thiel et al. [44] have proposed a multivariate regression formula using anthropometric data to establish the meniscal length and width using sex, weight, and height.

13.6 Surgical Technique

Meniscal allograft transplantation may be performed using either open or arthroscopically assisted techniques, or a combination of these, with a mini-arthrotomy to insert the graft and arthroscopic preparation and fixation. Advantages of arthroscopic procedures include decreased morbidity in comparison with open techniques, no disruption of collateral ligaments and early rehabilitation. On the other hand, arthroscopically assisted techniques to implant meniscal allografts are much more technically demanding. Therefore, a considerable learning curve should be considered for the application into clinical practice.

The three main fixation methods that can be used to fix a MAT are suture-only transosseous fixation, bone plug fixation and the keyhole technique. The first one consists of fixing soft tissue graft only using sutures through the body and meniscal horns, while the meniscal roots are fixed using a transtibial suture technique, similar to root lesion repairs. The bone plugs and keyhole techniques are different types of bone fixation. The double plug technique consists in bony fixation to the tibia of the meniscal horns, which are left attached to the allograft bone, and capsular fixation of the peripheral margin of the allograft. In the keyhole or bone bridge technique, the grafts contain a common bone bridge attached to both anterior and posterior horns. This bone bridge is then inserted into a similarly shaped slot in the recipient tibia. It has been recommended that this technique should be used with implantation of a lateral meniscus because the distance between the horns is only 1 cm or less [45]. Both osseous techniques require the preparation of osseous beds in the receptor knee, so the plugs or bridge can fit in it [46].

Concerning medial meniscus, we prefer the use of soft tissue versus bone plug fixation for the meniscal roots as recent biomechanical studies have found no advantage with the addition of bone plugs [47, 48]. A significantly higher cellular viability and collagen organization were found on biopsy of the grafts secured by soft tissue fixation only [49]. This may be related to a higher immunological host response caused by the addition of bone plugs [50].

Surgery is performed under general or regional anaesthesia with appropriate prophylactic antibiotics. The patient is supine on the operating table with a thigh tourniquet, single thigh side support and footrest supporting the knee at 90°.

The meniscus allograft is confirmed to be of the correct side and limb prior to anaesthesia and is thawed to room temperature.

The superior surface of the meniscus is marked to aid in orientation. For the medial meniscus, a point is marked at 40% of the circumference from posterior to anterior. At these points a number 2 non-absorbable suture is placed as an oblique vertical mattress. This represents the middle traction suture.

The meniscus is sharply dissected off the plateau. Number 2 Ultrabraid (S&N, Massachusetts, USA) sutures are placed into the posterior and anterior roots using a modified whip stitch, passing the suture a minimum of three times along the meniscus and back again to ensure a good hold. It is important to ensure the sutures emerge on the inferior aspect of the footprint of the meniscal root. The prepared graft is then wrapped in a vancomycin-soaked swab (Fig. 13.1).

A standard diagnostic arthroscopic procedure was performed, documenting the state of the

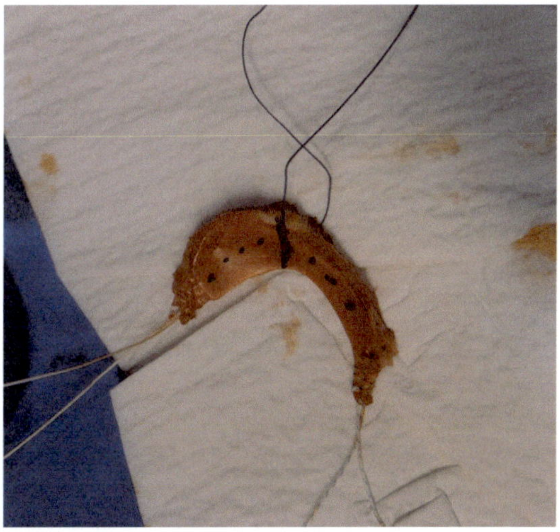

Fig. 13.1 Medial meniscus allograft. The superior surface of the meniscus is marked to aid in orientation

joint surfaces and treating any co-existent pathologies.

The host meniscus is assessed and prepared by resecting the remaining meniscal tissue using a combination of arthroscopic punches and a shaver to leave 1–2 mm peripheral vascular rim of native meniscal tissue that will support the meniscal allograft. A bleeding bed is created at the periphery by passing a Steadman awl (commonly used to perform microfractures) multiple times through the remaining meniscal rim. The tunnel positions for meniscal root attachment points are identified in the knee and prepared using the shaver and punches. For the medial meniscus, posterior horn insertion is just posterior to the medial tibial spine, and the anterior horn insertion point is anterior and medial to the insertion of the ACL on the superior surface of the tibial plateau.

A 2 cm vertical skin incision is made on the proximal tibia on the opposite side of the tibia to the meniscus being transplanted. This is the starting point for the bone tunnels. Depending on previous scars or personal preference, the graft can be inserted from the same side of the knee. The working portal is created by extending the relevant longitudinal arthroscopy portal to 2 cm. The meniscal allograft transplantation drill aimer guide is inserted through the working portal and positioned in the posterior horn insertion point. The drill guide sleeve is then inserted into the handle and positioned onto the tibia through the prepared incision. The posterior horn suture tunnel is drilled with a long 2.4-mm-diameter pin, visualizing the tip emerging through the bone. The guide wire is overdrilled with a cannulated 4.5 mm or 6 mm drill (Fig. 13.2a). The guide wire is removed, leaving the drill bit in situ. A loop of 2/0 Prolene is passed through the drill bit on a suture passer and is retrieved through the working portal using a suture manipulator (Fig. 13.2b). The drill is removed, leaving the suture in situ. The free end of this lead suture is the passed through the loop and clipped so that it hangs unsupported out of the way.

The meniscal transplantation drill aimer guide is reintroduced through the working portal, and the tunnel for the anterior horn is drilled in the centre of the attachment footprint with the same sequence of steps. The suture ends are brought out through the working portal, clipped and hung to the opposite side of the knee. If the size of the graft is considered potentially small, then the anterior tunnel can be drilled after insertion of the meniscus in order to allow for the anterior horn to be fixed in the optimal position. Conversely, if the graft is larger than ideal, then the anterior tunnel can be overdrilled to 6 mm and the anterior

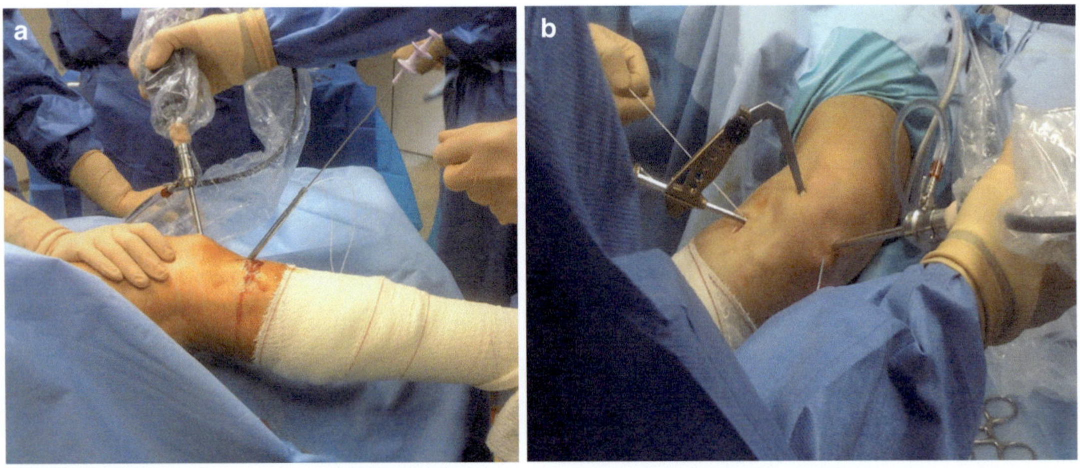

Fig. 13.2 Bone tunnel creation. (**a**) The drill aimer guide is inserted through the working portal and positioned in the posterior and anterior horn insertion points, respectively. (**b**) A loop of 2/0 Prolene is passed through the drill bit on a suture passer, and it is retrieved through the working portal using a suture manipulator

horn pulled into the tunnel slightly after peripheral fixation.

The next stage is insertion of two loops for the middle traction and fixation suture. An 18-gauge needle is used to localize the correct insertion point. For the medial meniscus, it is 40% of the meniscal circumference from the posterior horn insertion. An 18-gauge needle preloaded with a loop of No 1 PDS is used, from outside-in, to position two loops of sutures on the superior and inferior aspect of the meniscal bed. Each loop is the gathered through the working portal and clipped to one side.

Now that all the passing sutures are in place, the graft can be carried through the working portal into the knee joint (Fig. 13.3a). The assistant holds the graft in the correct orientation adjacent to the working portal. Starting with the posterior horn sutures and then working anteriorly, all the meniscal sutures are pulled into position using the pre-placed shuttle suture loops. The graft is delivered into the knee through the working portal by pulling on the posterior and middle traction sutures (Fig. 13.3b). The anterior and posterior horn sutures are then held temporarily over the bone bridge using a single knot throw and a clip. The graft is inspected arthroscopically to assess graft size and position.

The graft is fixed using a hybrid technique of all-inside, inside-out and outside-in suture system. With the arthroscope initially in the ipsilateral portal, the first all-inside meniscal repair device is introduced through the contralateral compartment portal using a slotted cannula. Holding tension on the middle sutures the posterior third is fixed to the prepared meniscal rim, inserting sutures on the superior and inferior surfaces in a stacked vertical mattress pattern. A minimum of two suture devices is recommended.

The middle and anterior thirds of the meniscal graft are secured with inside-out vertical loop sutures that are inserted, preferably achieving at least three loops in the body and anterior third. If there is inadequate suture hold on the anterior 1–2 cm, then outside-in needle suture placement is required, using a needle technique. The inside-out sutures initially emerge directly through the skin. Once the fixation is complete, a 2 cm longitudinal skin incision is made between the sutures which can be seen and retrieved using and arthroscopic hook.

When tying the sutures, it is important to evaluate the position of the meniscus in the knee. Sutures should be tied. In general, the capsule sutures are tied first before the anterior and

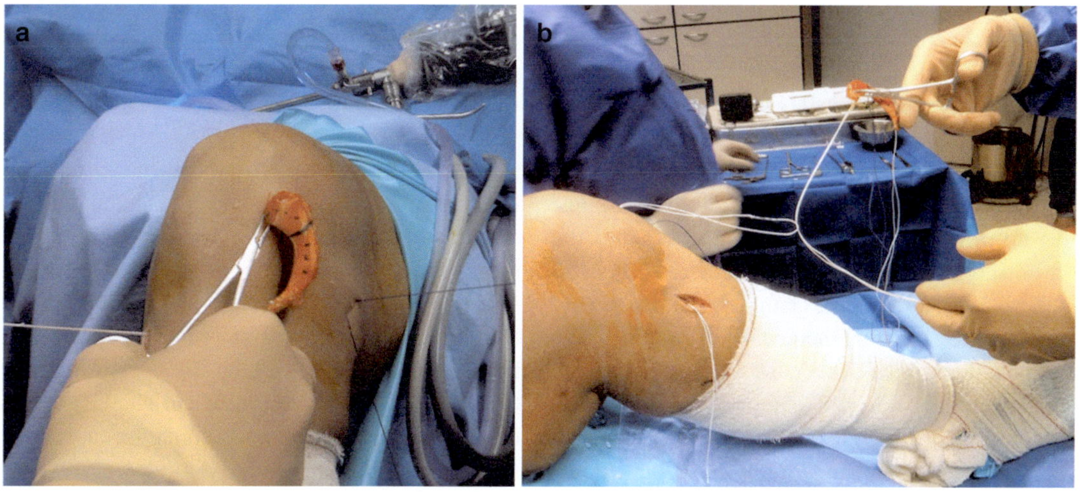

Fig. 13.3 Insertion of the allograft into the knee joint. (**a**) Passing sutures allow the graft to be carried through the working portal into the knee joint. (**b**) The graft is delivered into the knee through the working portal by pulling on the posterior and middle traction sutures

posterior root sutures are tied under strong tension over the bone bridge.

Regarding lateral meniscal allograft transplantation, the bone trough technique is the most commonly used and has shown superior results [51, 52]. However, it is technically demanding and needs perfectly sized graft.

Surgery is performed under general or regional anaesthesia with appropriate prophylactic antibiotics. The patient is supine on the operating table with a thigh tourniquet, single thigh side support and footrest supporting the knee at 90°.

The meniscus allograft is confirmed to be of the correct side and limb prior to anaesthesia and is thawed to room temperature. The meniscal allograft is measured to ensure that it matches with measurement of the tibial plateau. The tibial bone block is cut with an oscillating saw to a width of 10 mm while preserving the meniscal root attachments. The depth is cut to 8 mm to match the tibial through.

The superior surface of the meniscus is marked to aid in orientation, and in the case of lateral meniscus, the most anterior margin of the popliteal hiatus is also marked. At these points a number 2 non-absorbable suture is placed as an oblique vertical mattress. This represents the middle traction suture. Number 2 Ultrabraid (S&N, Massachusetts, USA) sutures are placed into the bone bridge at the midportion and at the portion close to the anterior root, respectively. The prepared graft is then wrapped in a vancomycin-soaked swab (Fig. 13.4).

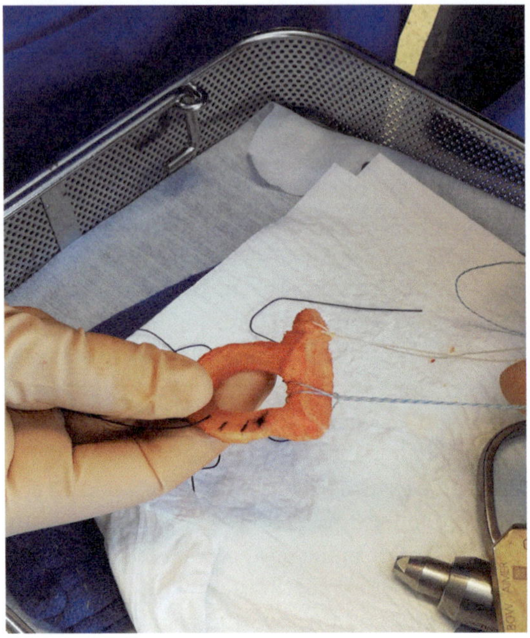

Fig. 13.4 Lateral meniscus allograft with bone bridge

A standard diagnostic arthroscopic procedure is performed, documenting the state of the joint surfaces and treating any co-existent pathologies. An arthroscopic 4.5 shaver is inserted into the knee, and the remnants of the meniscal tissue are debrided to a bleeding rim of approximately 1–2 mm. The residual meniscal rim should not be completely removed because it prevents radial displacement and will support the meniscal allograft [53].

Next, a transpatellar portal is made in the knee flexion position. The tendon is split in line with its fibres to the level of the tibial tubercle, exposing the anterior border of the tibial plateau (Fig. 13.5a). Both meniscal root attachments should be identified arthroscopically. With the aid of an arthroscopic shaver and a curette, a provisional chondral trough is created to the level of subchondral bone aligned with the roots, just lateral to the tibial attachment of the anterior cruciate ligament (ACL).

The hooked trough guide is inserted through the arthrotomy. The guide should contact the subchondral plate at both the anatomic anterior and posterior root positions. Performed correctly, this will direct the guide pin parallel to the meniscal roots, matching their slope, at a depth of 8 mm from the subchondral bone at the insertions. Under direct visualization, the handle/clamp device is advanced on its worm gear until the teeth engage the anterior tibial cortex. After the correct guide wire position was confirmed, an 8-mm-diameter core reamer was used to create a tibial slot without breaching the posterior cortex (Fig. 13.5b). The hook guide and handle are disengaged and removed. A combination of 4.5 mm shaver and a burr is used to debride any residual roof on the trough posteriorly without compromising the back wall. The calibrated trough rasp is inserted under direct visualization and used for final trough preparation. Calibrations confirm

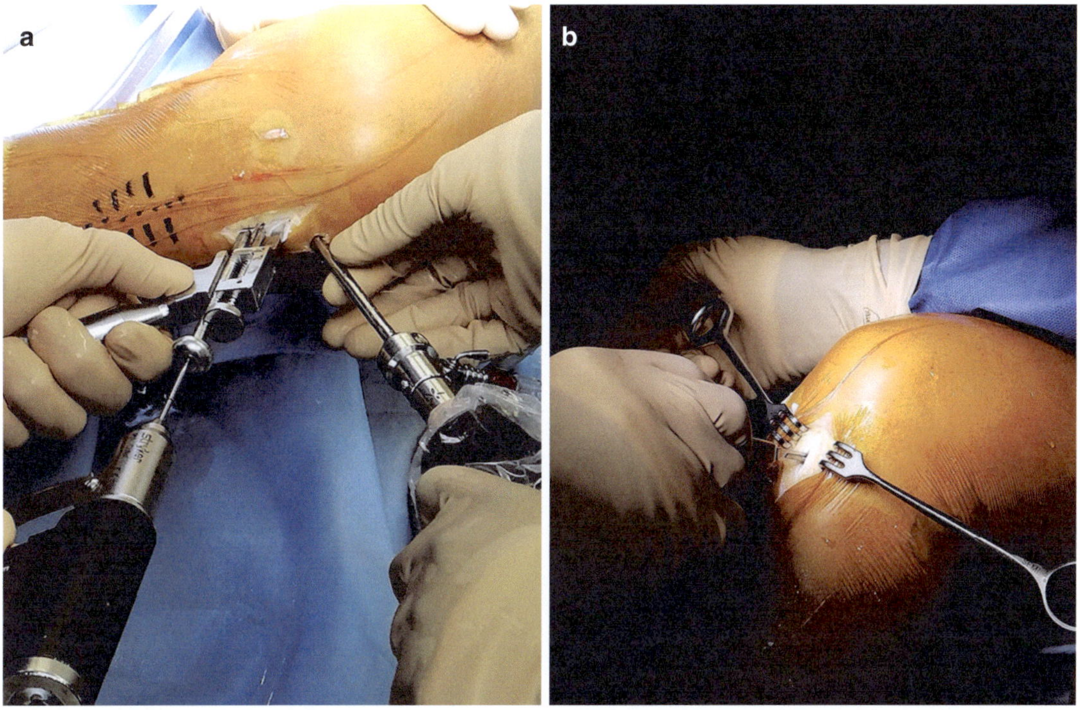

Fig. 13.5 Tibial slot creation. (**a**) Transpatellar portal. (**b**) The hooked trough guide is inserted through the arthrotomy. After the correct guide wire position was confirmed, an 8-mm-diameter core reamer was used to create a tibial slot without breaching the posterior cortex

final trough length, and the graft is measured and truncated accordingly, preferentially removing any excess posterior bone first. The entrance to the trough is evaluated, and obstructing soft tissues are debrided to ensure clear entry.

A 2 cm vertical skin incision is made on the proximal tibia on the opposite side of the tibia to the meniscus being transplanted. This is the starting point for the bone tunnels. The meniscal allograft transplantation drill aimer guide is inserted through the transpatellar portal and positioned in the posterior-middle part horn of the bone slot. The drill guide sleeve is then inserted into the handle and positioned onto the tibia through the prepared incision. The posterior horn suture tunnel is drilled with a long 2.4-mm-diameter pin, visualizing the tip emerging through the bone. The guide wire is overdrilled with a cannulated 4.5 mm drill. The guide wire is removed, leaving the drill bit in situ. A loop of 2/0 Prolene is passed through the 4.5 mm drill bit on a suture passer and is retrieved through the working portal using a suture manipulator. The 4.5 mm drill is removed, leaving the suture in situ. The free end of this lead suture is the passed through the loop and clipped so that it hangs unsupported out of the way. The meniscal transplantation drill aimer guide is reintroduced through the transpatellar portal, and the tunnel for the anterior leading suture is drilled close to the anterior attachment of the meniscus with the same sequence of steps. The suture ends are brought out through the working portal, clipped and hung to the opposite side of the knee. The next stage is insertion of two loops for the middle traction and fixation suture. An 18-gauge needle is used to localize the correct insertion point. For the lateral meniscus, this point is just anterior to the popliteus tendon. An 18-gauge needle preloaded with a loop of No 1 PDS is then used, from outside-in, to position two loops of sutures on the superior and inferior aspect of the meniscal bed. Each loop is the gathered through the working portal and clipped to one side (Fig. 13.6a).

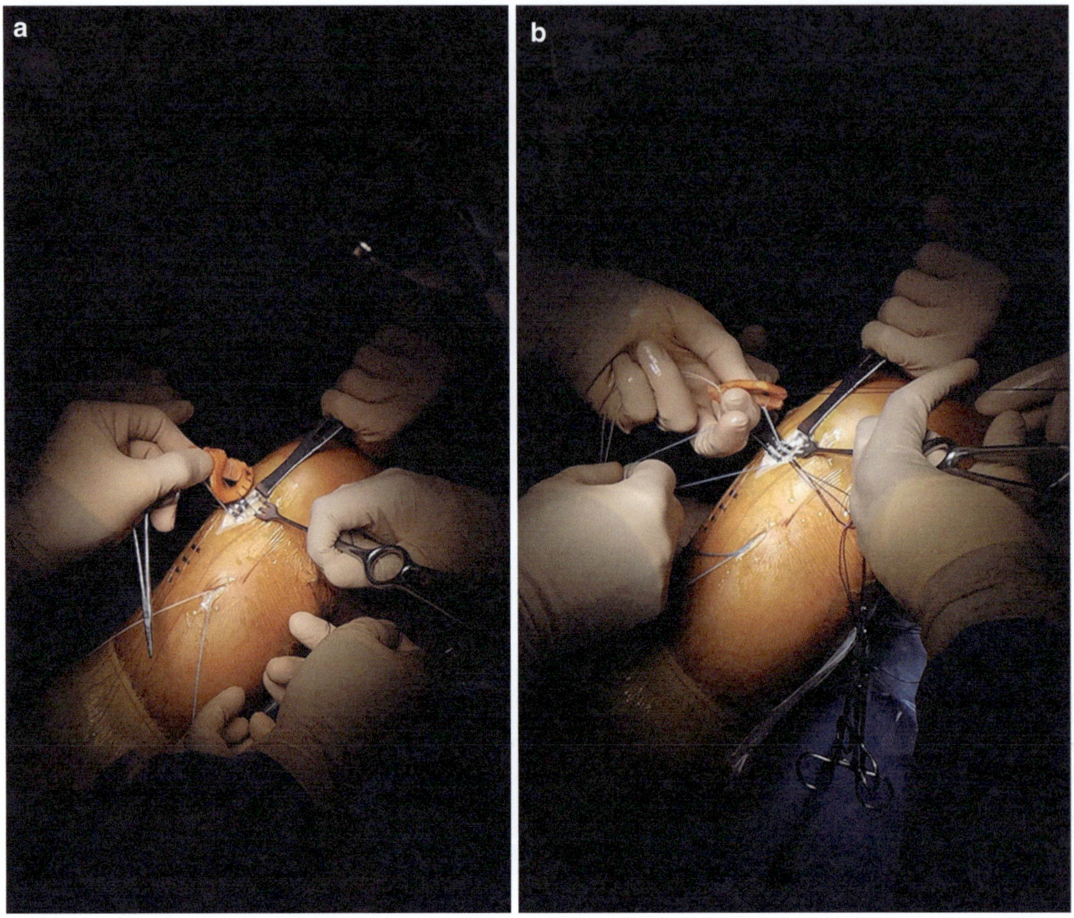

Fig. 13.6 Insertion of the allograft into the knee joint. (**a**) Passing sutures allow the graft to be carried through the transpatellar portal into the knee joint. (**b**) The bone bridge is advanced into the keyhole-shaped slot, and the allograft is manually reduced under the condyle with a finger introduced via the arthrotomy under traction of leading suture through the capsule and the tibial tunnels

Now, the bone bridge is advanced into the keyhole-shaped slot, and the allograft is manually reduced under the condyle with a finger introduced via the arthrotomy under traction of leading suture through the capsule and the tibial tunnels (Fig. 13.6b).

The graft is fixed using a hybrid technique of all-inside, inside-out and outside-in suture system. With the arthroscope initially in the ipsilateral portal, the first all-inside meniscal repair device is introduced through the contralateral compartment portal using a slotted cannula. Holding tension on the middle sutures, the posterior third is fixed to the prepared meniscal rim using all-inside sutures, inserting sutures on the superior and inferior surfaces in a stacked vertical mattress pattern. A minimum of two suture devices is recommended.

The middle and anterior thirds of the meniscal graft are secured with inside-out vertical loop sutures that are inserted, preferably achieving at least three loops in the body and anterior third. If there is inadequate suture hold on the anterior 1–2 cm, then outside-in needle suture placement is required, using a needle technique. The inside-out sutures initially emerge directly through the skin. Once the fixation is complete, a 2 cm longitudinal skin incision is made between the sutures which can be seen and retrieved using and arthroscopic hook.

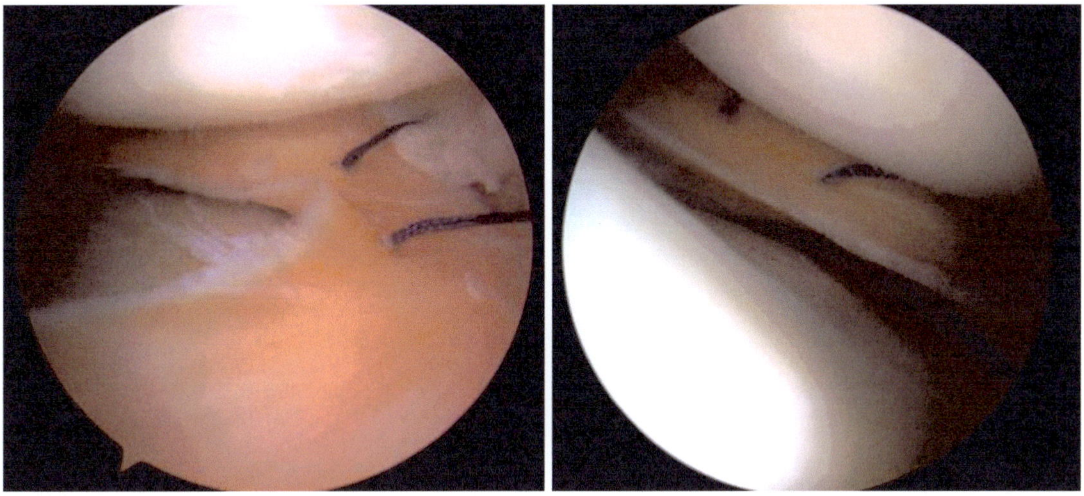

Fig. 13.7 Final arthroscopic look after hybrid fixation technique

When tying the sutures, it is important to evaluate the position of the meniscus in the knee (Fig. 13.7). Sutures should be tied.

13.7 Rehabilitation

The knee is placed in an immobilization brace postoperatively. Weight-bearing is limited to touch weight-bearing for 3 weeks to minimize hoop stress being placed on the graft in the initial phase. Weight-bearing is then gradually increased until full weight-bearing is commenced at 6 weeks. An unloader brace is used for the first 3–6 months during walking and standing activities. Squatting and loading in deep flexion are to be avoided for 6 months. Isometric quads and straight leg raise exercises can commence immediately postoperatively, with closed chain exercises introduced at 6 weeks. By 3 months exercising on a bicycle can be introduced. Running should be avoided for at least 9–12 months, at which time an MRI scan is performed to assess graft integrity.

13.8 Results

Most data published in literature about MAT procedure show generally positive results, in terms of satisfactory clinical outcomes as assessed by significantly increased PROMs at the latest follow-up available after surgery [26, 28, 54].

The Lysholm Knee Scoring Scale, International Knee Documentation Committee Subjective Knee Evaluation Form, Tegner Activity Score (TAS), Visual Analogue Scale and Knee Injury and Osteoarthritis Outcome Score (KOOS) are the most commonly used PROMs to evaluate the outcome following meniscal allograft transplantation. A systematic review of 35 studies, published in 2015, showed an improvement of mean Lysholm score from 55.7 to 81.3, IKDC subjective from 47.8 to 70 and Tegner score from 3.1 to 4.7 [26]. Other measures that have been used to assess the clinical outcomes following MAT include the Short Form (SF-12 and SF-36), Modified Cincinnati Score, Western Ontario and McMaster Universities Osteoarthritis Index and the Hospital for Special Surgery Knee Score. Studies using these PROMs have also shown a consistent improvement in the clinical outcomes at medium- to long-term follow-ups as indicated by Young et al. in a recent review [28]. Similar results have been found in other recent systematic reviews [55, 56].

Return to sport activity after MAT represents a controversial topic with some studies recommending lifelong limits. However, it is more common to allow return to full sports, usually after 6–12 months [26]. In a recent review, Samitier et al. showed how MAT allows return to the same level of competition in 75–85% of patients at short- to mid-term follow-up, but there is a strong limitation about the number of studies and sample size. Moreover, results in competitive sports are very limited [54].

A relatively limited number of studies focused on the radiological outcome following MAT. Joint narrowing is the most commonly radiological outcome measure when assessing the development of osteoarthritic changes. A recent systematic review, across 16 studies, has shown a weighted mean narrowing of 0.03 mm over a follow-up period of 4.5 years [57]. Based on these limited results, available data have shown evidence to support the theory that the MAT is chondroprotective.

Using MRI, graft extrusion has been frequently described following meniscal allograft transplantation, although there are large variations in the timing and method of measurement. A number of studies have looked for a correlation between clinical scores and the amount of extrusion, with most studies finding no correlation [57]. Moreover, meniscal allograft extrusion has been described independent of the surgical fixation technique [56].

In the literature, complications and failure rate are variable across reported case series, and no consensus exists on the criteria for failure or success. The most common definition of failure was conversion to a joint replacement or excision of the allograft. Smith et al. report a mean failure rate across case series as 10.9% at 4.8 years [26]. The most common complication is retear of the allograft; other complications include synovitis or effusion and superficial infection.

References

1. Clark CR, Ogden JA. Development of the menisci of the human knee joint. Morphological changes and their potential role in childhood meniscal injury. J Bone Joint Surg Am. 1983;65(4):538–47.
2. Johnson DL, Swenson TM, Livesay GA, Aizawa H, Fu FH, Harner CD. Insertion-site anatomy of the human menisci: gross, arthroscopic, and topographical anatomy as a basis for meniscal transplantation. Arthroscopy. 1995;11(4):386–94.
3. Nikolic DK. Lateral meniscal tears and their evolution in acute injuries of the anterior cruciate ligament of the knee. Arthroscopic analysis. Knee Surg Sports Traumatol Arthrosc. 1998;6(1):26–30.
4. Heller L, Langman J. The menisco-femoral ligaments of the human knee. J Bone Joint Surg. 1964;46:307–13.
5. LaPrade RF, Ly TV, Wentorf FA, Engebretsen L. The posterolateral attachments of the knee: a qualitative and quantitative morphologic analysis of the fibular collateral ligament, popliteus tendon, popliteofibular ligament, and lateral gastrocnemius tendon. Am J Sports Med. 2003;31(6):854–60.
6. Ahmed AM, Burke DL. In-vitro measurement of static pressure distribution in synovial joints-part I: tibial surface of the knee. J Biomech Eng. 1983;105(3):216–25.
7. Fairbank TJ. Knee joint changes after meniscectomy. J Bone Joint Surg. 1948;30B(4):664–70.
8. Walker PS, Erkman MJ. The role of the menisci in force transmission across the knee. Clin Orthop Relat Res. 1975;109:184–92.
9. Prodromos CC, Joyce BT, Keller BL, Murphy BJ, Shi K. Magnetic resonance imaging measurement of the contralateral normal meniscus is a more accurate method of determining meniscal allograft size than radiographic measurement of the recipient tibial plateau. Arthroscopy. 2007;23:1174–9.
10. Assimakopoulos AP, Katonis PG, Agapitos MV, Exarchou EI. The innervation of the human meniscus. Clin Orthop Relat Res. 1992;275:232–6.
11. Hede A, Jensen DB, Blyme P, Sonne-Holm S. Epidemiology of meniscal lesions in the knee. 1,215 open operations in Copenhagen. Acta Orthop Scand. 1990;61(5):435–7.
12. Siegel MG, Roberts CS. Meniscal allografts. Clin Sports Med. 1993;12:59–80.
13. Lee SR, Kim JG, Nam SW. The tips and pitfalls of meniscus allograft transplantation. Knee Surg Relat Res. 2012;24:137–45.
14. Levy IM, Torzilli PA, Gould JD, Warren RF. The effect of lateral meniscectomy on motion of the knee. J Bone Joint Surg Am. 1989;71(3):401–6.
15. Seedholm B, Dowson D, Wright V. Functions of the menisci: a preliminary study. J Bone Joint Surg (Br). 1974;56(B):381–2.
16. Nielsen AB, Yde J. Epidemiology of acute knee injuries: a prospective hospital investigation. Am J Sports Med. 1991;25(1):7–12.
17. Annandale T. Excision of the internal semilunar cartilage, resulting in perfect restoration of the joint-movements. Br Med J. 1889;1(1467):291–2.
18. Englund M, Roemer FW, Hayashi D, Crema MD, Guermazi A. Meniscus pathology, osteoarthritis and the treatment controversy. Nat Rev Rheumatol. 2012;8(7):412–9. https://doi.org/10.1038/nrrheum.2012.69.
19. Baratz ME, Fu FH, Mengato R. Meniscal tears: the effect of meniscectomy and of repair on intraarticular

contact areas and stress in the human knee. A preliminary report. Am J Sports Med. 1986;14:270–5.
20. Lee SJ, Aadalen KJ, Malaviya P, et al. Tibiofemoral contact mechanics after serial medial meniscectomies in the human cadaveric knee. Am J Sports Med. 2006;34:1334–44.
21. Ode GE, Van Thiel GS, McArthur SA, et al. Effects of serial sectioning and repair of radial tears in the lateral meniscus. Am J Sports Med. 2012;40(8):1863–70.
22. Covall DJ, Wasilewski SA. Roentgenographic changes after arthroscopic meniscectomy: five-years follow-up in patients more than 45 years old. Arthroscopy. 1992;8(2):242–6.
23. Shelbourne KD, Dickens JF. Joint space narrowing after partial medial meniscectomy in the anterior cruciate ligament-intact knee. J Am Acad Orthop Surg. 2007;15(9):519–24.
24. Drobnic M, Ercin E, Gamelas J, Papacostas ET, Slynarski K, Zdanowicz U, Spalding T, Verdonk P. Treatment options for the symptomatic post-meniscectomy knee. Knee Surg Sports Traumatol Arthrosc. 2019;27:1817. https://doi.org/10.1007/s00167-019-05424-3.
25. Getgood A, LaPrade RF, Verdonk P, Gersoff W, Cole B, Spalding T, IMREF Group. International Meniscus Reconstruction Experts Forum (IMREF) 2015 consensus statement on the practice of meniscal allograft transplantation. Am J Sports Med. 2017;45(5):1195–205.
26. Smith NA, MacKay N, Costa M, Spalding T. Meniscal allograft transplantation in a symptomatic meniscal deficient knee: a systematic review. Knee Surg Sports Traumatol Arthrosc. 2015;23(1):270–9. https://doi.org/10.1007/s00167-014-3310-0.
27. Lee AS, Kang RW, Kroin E, Verma NN, Cole BJ. Allograft meniscus transplantation. Sports Med Arthrosc Rev. 2012;20:106–14.
28. Young J, Tudor F, Mahmoud A, Meyers P. Meniscal transplantation: procedures, outcomes and rehabilitation. Orthop Res Rev. 2017;15(9):35–43.
29. Arnoczky SP, Milachowski KA. Meniscal allografts: where do we stand? In: Ewing JW, editor. Articular cartilage and knee joint function: basic science and arthroscopy. New York, NY: Raven; 1990. p. 129–36.
30. Verdonk R, van Daele P, Claus B, et al. Viable meniscus transplantation [in German]. Orthopade. 1994;23(29):153–9.
31. Black J, Shadle CA, Parsons JR, Brighton CT. Articular cartilage preservation and storage. II. Mechanical indentation of viable, stored articular cartilage. Arthritis Rheum. 1979;22:1102–8.
32. Brighton CT, Shadle CA, Jimenez SA, Irwin JT, Lane JM, Lipton M. Articular cartilage preservation and storage. I. Application of tissue culture techniques to the storage of viable articular cartilage. Arthritis Rheum. 1979;22:1093–101.
33. Verdonk PC, Demurie A, Almqvist KF, Veyes EM, Verbruggen G, Verdonk R. transplantation of viable meniscal allograft: survivorship analysis and clinical outcome of one hundred cases. J Bone Joint Surg Am. 2005;87(4):715–24.
34. Garrett JC. Meniscal transplantation. In: Aichroth PC, Canon WD, Patel DV, editors. Knee surgery: current practice. New York, NY: Raven; 1992. p. 95–103.
35. Rijik PC. Meniscal allograft transplantation, part I: background, results, graft selection and preservation, and surgical considerations. Arthroscopy. 2004;20(7):728–43.
36. Binnet MS, Akan B, Kaya A. Lyophilised medial meniscus transplantation in ACL-deficient knees. A 19-years follow-up. Knee Surg Sports Traumatol Arthrosc. 2012;20(1):109–13.
37. Sekiya JK, Ellingson CI. Meniscal allograft transplantation. J Am Acad Orthop Surg. 2006;14(3):164–74.
38. Kuhn JE, Wojtis EM. Allograft meniscal transplantation. Clin Sports Med. 1996;15:537–56.
39. Arnoczky SP, McDevitt CA, Schmidt MB, Mow VC, Warren RF. The effect of cryopreservation in canine menisci. A biochemical morphologic and biochemical evaluation. J Orthop Res. 1988;6:1–12.
40. Berhouet J, Marty F, Rosset P, Favard L. Evaluation of direct anatomical, indirect radiographic and photographic methods in 10 cadaver knee. Orthop Traumatol Surg Res. 2013;99:291–7.
41. Pollard ME, Kang Q, Berg EE. Radiographic sizing for meniscal transplantation. Arthroscopy. 1995;11(6):684–7.
42. Yoon JR, Jeong HI, Seo MJ, et al. The use of contralateral knee magnetic resonance imaging to predict meniscal size during meniscal allograft transplantation. Arthroscopy. 2014;30(10):1287–93.
43. Haut TL, Hull ML, Howell SM. Use of roentgenography and magnetic resonance imaging to predict meniscal geometry determined with a three-dimensional coordinate digitizing system. J Orthop Res. 2000;18(2):228–37.
44. Van Thiel GS, Verma N, Yanke A, Basu S, Farr J, Cole B. Meniscal allograft size can be predicted by height, weight, and gender. Arthroscopy. 2009;25(7):722–7.
45. Cole BJ, Carter TR, Rodeo SA. Allograft meniscal transplantation. Background, techniques and results. J Bone Joint Surg Am. 2002;84:1236–50.
46. Verdonk R. Alternative treatment for meniscal injuries. J Bone Joint Surg Am. 1997;79:866–73.
47. Hunt SS, et al. Bone plug versus suture fixation of the posterior horn in medial meniscal allograft transplantation: a biomechanical study. Bull NYU Hosp Jt Dis. 2008;66(1):22–6.
48. McDermott ID, et al. The effects of lateral meniscal allograft transplantation techniques on tibiofemoral contact pressure. Knee Surg Sports Traumatol Arthrosc. 2008;16(6):553–60.
49. Rodeo SA, et al. Histological analysis of human meniscal allografts. A preliminary report. J Bone Joint Surg. 2000;82-A(8):1071–82.
50. Von Lewinski G, et al. The influence of nonanatomical insertion and incongruence of meniscal transplants on the articular cartilage in an ovine model. Am J Sports Med. 2008;36(5):841–50.

51. Rodeo SA. Meniscal allografts-Where do we stand? Am J Sports Med. 2001;29:246–61.
52. Sekiya JK, West RV, Groff YJ, Irrgang JJ, Fu FH, Harner CD. Clinical outcomes following isolated lateral meniscal allograft transplantation. Arthroscopy. 2006;22:771–80.
53. Chahla J, Olivetto J, Dean CS, Serra Cruz R, LaPrade RF. Lateral meniscal allograft transplantation: the bone trough technique. Arthrosc Tech. 2016;5(2):e371–7.
54. Samitier G, Alentorn-Geli E, Taylor DC, Rill B, Lock T, Moutzouros V, Kolowich P. Meniscal allograft transplantation. Part 2: systematic review of transplant timing, outcomes, return to competition, associated procedures, and prevention of osteoarthritis. Knee Surg Sports Traumatol Arthrosc. 2015;23(1):323–33.
55. Rosso F, Bisicchia S, Bonasia DE, Amendola A. Meniscal allograft transplantation: a systematic review. Am J Sports Med. 2014;43(4):998–1007.
56. Verdonk R, Volpi P, Verdonk P, Van der Bracht H, Van Laer M, Alqvist KF, Vander Eecken S, Prospero E, Quaglia A. Indications and limits of meniscal allografts. Injury. 2013;44(Suppl 1):S21–7.
57. Smith NA, Parkinson B, Hutchinson CE, Costa ML, Spalding T. Is meniscal allograft transplantation chondroprotective? A systematic review of radiological outcomes. Knee Surg Sports Traumatol Arthrosc. 2015;24(9):2923–35.

14 Biomaterials in Meniscus Repair

Tomasz Piontek, Kinga Ciemniewska-Gorzela, and Paweł Bąkowski

14.1 Introduction

Meniscal injuries located in the low or nonvascularized zones (red-white and white-white zones) are often treated with partial or total meniscectomy. Although meniscectomy is a relatively simple and quick surgery with good immediate postoperative clinical outcomes, the long-term results are less good. It has been accepted that surgeons should preserve as much meniscal tissue as possible. Both complete and partial meniscectomies are associated with early degenerative osteoarthritis. To preserve the function of the knee joint, it is now suggested that meniscal tears should be treated by meniscus repair instead of meniscectomy whenever possible. Among the methods currently used to repair the meniscus, the ideal solution has not yet been found [1–7].

Biological augmentation techniques and meniscus tissue engineering strategies are being devised to enhance the likelihood and rate of healing in meniscus repair. Preclinical and clinical studies have shown that the introduction of cellular elements of blood, bone marrow, and related growth factors has the potential to enhance meniscus repair [8–16].

Tissue adhesives hold great potential to replace, or support, sutures and staples. Many new adhesive materials, with a good prognosis for use in a variety of applications, have been developed. However, most of them have not been sufficiently characterized to be able to be qualified for meniscus repair. Nevertheless, chemically cross-linked adhesives seem the most versatile as these are based on existing natural or synthetic polymers and can be readily modified. Their properties can be adjusted by careful molecular design and chemical functionalization to make them suitable for the intended application. Standardized relevant biomechanical and biological models need to be defined to compare different available and developed tissue adhesives and to be able to address their suitability for the repair of meniscal tears. In clinical practice, the most successful treatment modality remains the use of sutures. Nevertheless, there is a great need for a suitable meniscus tissue adhesive. Such an adhesive should be easily applied in a meniscal tear, bound strongly to meniscal tissue, hold the torn region together, facilitate its healing, and then gradually degrade into nontoxic products [17, 18].

T. Piontek (✉)
Spine Disorders and Pediatric Orthopedics Department, University of Medical Science, Poznań, Poland

Rehasport Clinic, Poznań, Poland
e-mail: tomasz.piontek@rehasport.pl

K. Ciemniewska-Gorzela · P. Bąkowski
Rehasport Clinic, Poznań, Poland
e-mail: kinga@rehasport.pl; pawel.bakowski@rehasport.pl

M. Brittberg, K. Slynarski (eds.), *Lower Extremity Joint Preservation*,
https://doi.org/10.1007/978-3-030-57382-9_14

The next area where the biomaterials play a main role in meniscus repair is partial and total meniscal replacement with 3D scaffolds. One of the main targets in this research area is to create biomaterials or formulations that are able to mimic as much as possible the meniscus native extracellular matrix. In the last few years, the characteristics and behaviors of different biomaterials have been explored, and several processing routes have been attempted to obtain an adequate architecture for proper cell adhesion, ingrowths, proliferation, and differentiation. The panoply of biomaterials that has been tested as a meniscus substitute/scaffold can be divided into two different categories, i.e., the non-resorbable polymers and resorbable polymers. A non-resorbable polymer is used as a permanent implant with biomechanical properties similar to the native tissue. The resorbable polymers, which can be natural or synthetic, are used in strategies which form new meniscal tissue while a slow degradation of the scaffold occurs [19, 20].

The number of biomaterials that has been used in meniscus tissue engineering strategies is presented in Fig. 14.1.

14.2 Biomaterials in Clinical Practice of Meniscus Repair Technique

14.2.1 Augmentation of Meniscus Repair with Fibrin/Blood Clots [21–25]

14.2.1.1 Indication

- Younger patients with a stable knee with a degenerative horizontal cleavage tear (Figs. 14.2 and 14.3a)
- Isolated and symptomatic painful horizontal grade 2 meniscal lesions (intrasubstance meniscal lesions)
- Posterolateral aspect of the lateral meniscus
- Complete radial tear of the meniscus

14.2.1.2 Techniques

Technique 1

Fibrin Clot Preparation I

Once the tear is deemed reparable, the patient's blood is collected and placed through a series of centrifugations using the Cascade Autologous

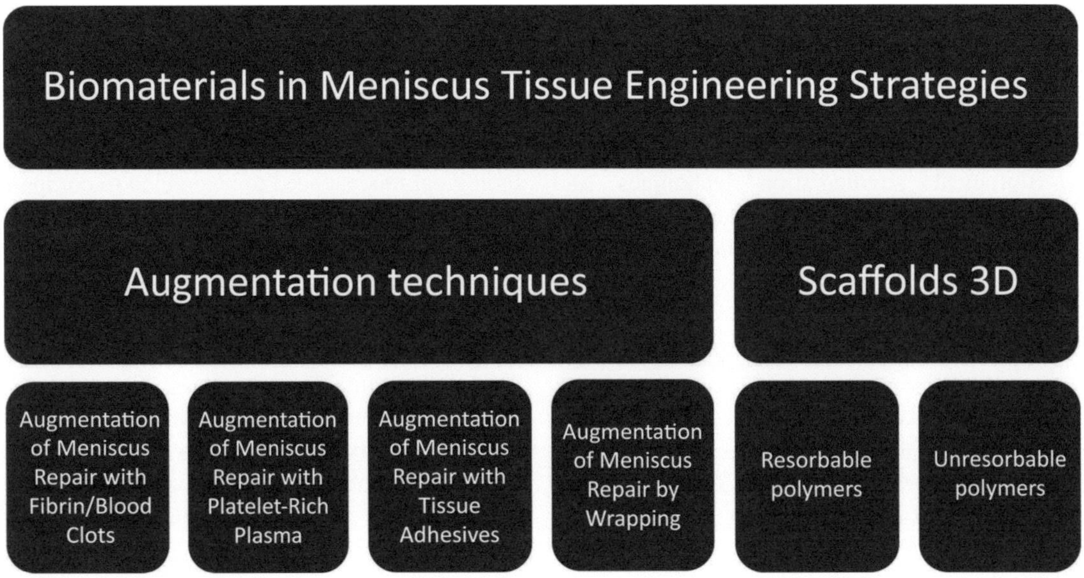

Fig. 14.1 The panoply of biomaterials that has been used in meniscus tissue engineering strategies

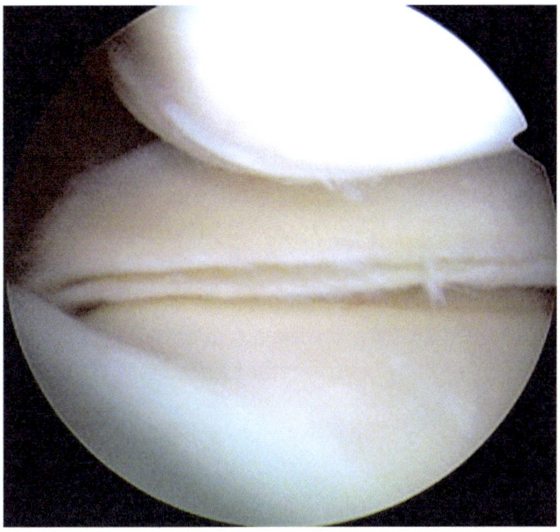

Fig. 14.2 The arthroscopic viewing of right knee medial meniscus—cleavage tear

Platelet System (Cascade Medical Enterprises, 20 Greenup Court, Wayne Nu, USA). The first centrifugation, which lasts 6 min, separates the PRP from the blood cells. The PRP is transferred into another tube and is spun in the centrifuge for 15–20 min to create the fibrin clot. A longer duration of centrifugation time produces a more reliable and rigid clot. The clot is aseptically removed from the vial and placed onto the surgical field.

Absorbable polyfilament sutures of different colors, for example, dyed and undyed 0 Vicryl sutures (Ethicon, Somerville, NJ, USA), are carefully passed through each end of the clot in a locking pattern.

Implantation of the Graft to the Meniscal Defect

While the blood sample is being processed, the meniscal tear can be prepared. An 18-gauge

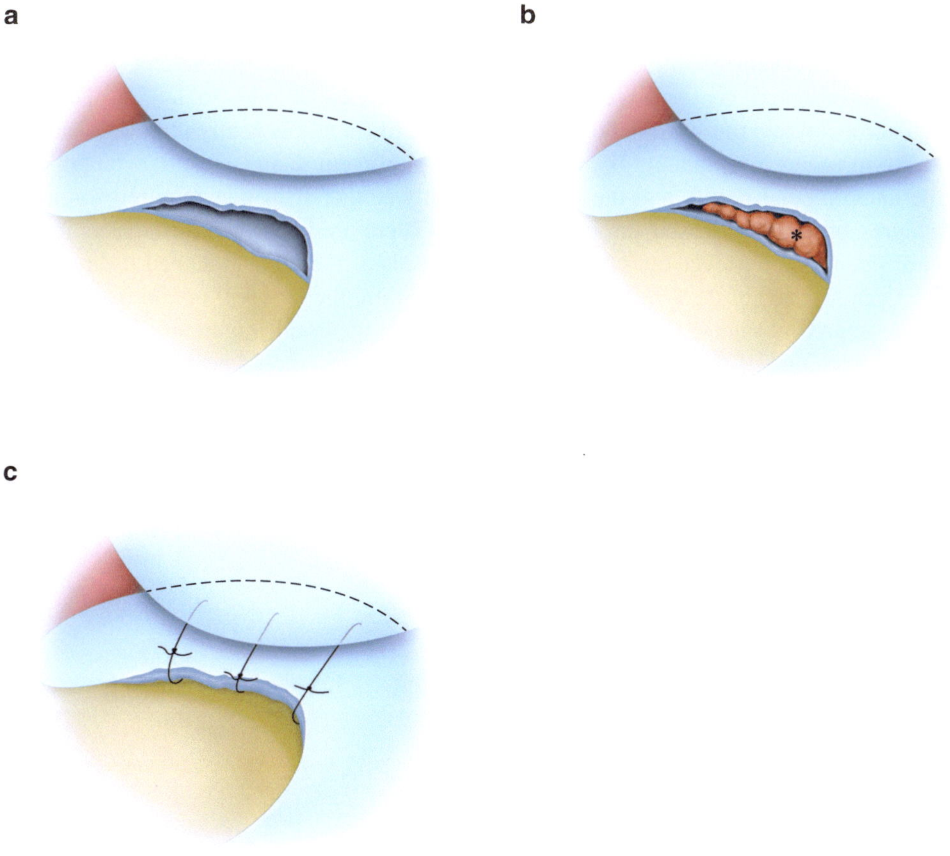

Fig. 14.3 Schematic draft of arthroscopic viewing of right knee medial meniscus. (**a**) Cleavage tear of medial meniscus. (**b**) The fibrin clot (*) is in the horizontal meniscal cleft. (**c**) The meniscal cleft is closed by sutures (MFC, medial femoral condyle)

spinal needle is inserted through the skin overlying the posteromedial skin. The needle should be directed at the anterior extent of the tear and should enter the knee between the superior and inferior leaflets of the tear. Once the needle has been adequately positioned at the anterior extent of the tear, a 0 monofilament suture (Prolene, Ethicon) is passed through the needle and grasped using an arthroscopic grasper. Before retrieving the suture out from the anteromedial portal, the needle is retracted from the joint to prevent the tip of the needle from lacerating the suture. A second monofilament suture is shuttled through the posterior extent of the tear using a similar technique.

The meniscal tissue is prepared to create an adequate bed for healing. A meniscal rasp is used to debride the degenerative tissue often found within the tear. Debridement of the degenerative meniscal tissue occurs between the two sutures and should proceed until bleeding is encountered within the base of the lesion.

The joint is prepared for passage of the platelet-rich fibrin clot into the apex of the meniscal tear. A 5.0-mm-diameter cannula is inserted through the anteromedial portal, and the monofilament sutures previously passed through the meniscus are again each retrieved out of the joint through the cannula. Each of these monofilament suture tails is secured to one of the suture pairs passed through each end of the clot. The monofilament sutures will be used to position the platelet-rich fibrin clot into the center of the meniscal tear. Each monofilament suture is sequentially removed from the joint by pulling on the suture limb exiting the skin overlying the posteromedial knee, and thus, the clot is slowly manipulated into the tear one end at a time. Once all polyfilament suture limbs are passed through the meniscus and out the posteromedial knee, tension is applied to both polyfilament sutures, and the graft is further entrenched into position between the two leaflets of the tear (Fig. 14.3b).

The meniscus can now be repaired. A self-capturing suture passing device (Knee Scorpion, Arthrex, Naples, FL) is used to pass a high-strength braided suture (2-0 FiberWire, Arthrex) through both superior and inferior meniscal leaflets at the tear's midpoint and 2–3 mm from the central edge of the tear. The suture limbs are secured using a series of half-hitch knots on the meniscus' superior surface. Additional sutures are placed anteriorly and posteriorly to the initial suture until the edges of the tear are re-approximated (Fig. 14.3c) with the platelet-rich fibrin clot firmly entrapped within the repaired meniscus. The polyfilament sutures passed through the clot are resected as they exit the skin overlying the posteromedial knee.

Technique 2

Fibrin Clot Preparation II

Approximately 25 mL of blood is collected from the patient's arm into a sterile glass syringe. The blood is stirred in the glass syringe for 10 min using a stainless steel swizzle stick measuring approximately 4 mm in diameter. The elastic fibrin clot adheres to the swizzle stick, resulting in a tubular-shaped fibrin clot that measured approximately 60 mm in length. The tubular-shaped fibrin clot is gently removed using Adson forceps and cut to an appropriate length which is slightly longer than that required for implantation. There are individual differences in the wall thickness of the tubular-shaped fibrin clot. If the wall is thin, the clot will be too fragile for packaging the meniscal fragments. Therefore, a tube with two layers should be made.

The meniscal fragments are inserted into the tubular-shaped fibrin clot using a rongeur, and both ends of the tube are tied with 4-0 absorbable sutures. This creates a construct that resembles a piece of candy (Fig. 14.4). A repair suture is pre-

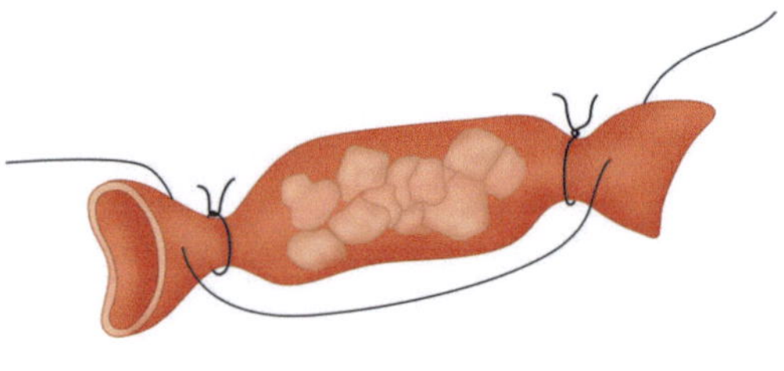

Fig. 14.4 Schematic of graft preparation. The meniscal fragments are inserted into the tubular-shaped fibrin clot

pared using the inside-out device, including straight needle-suture combination, such as Henning meniscal suture kit (Stryker, Kalamazoo, MI), and woven through the open ends of the packaged graft.

Implantation of the Graft to the Meniscal Defect

A lateral skin incision is made over the repair site, and the superficial fascia and iliotibial band are divided to allow the sutures to be retrieved later. The arthroscope is then inserted into the joint space from the infrapatellar lateral portal, and a larger cylindrical guide is inserted from the medial portal in the standard approach for an inside-out lateral meniscus repair technique. The prepared graft is positioned using the guide, and horizontal sutures are placed across both edges of the meniscal defect. The repair suture is tied to the lateral capsule through the lateral incision. The graft implant is secured with a supplemental vertical suture and applied with an all-inside meniscal repair device (FAST-FIX; Smith & Nephew Endoscopy, Andover, MA, USA). The graft position is confirmed (Fig. 14.5), and the iliotibial band, fascia, and soft tissues are then closed.

Fibrin Clot Preparation III

Thirty milliliters of venous blood is collected by anesthesia, and the blood is delivered by sterile technique into a stainless steel 50-mL bowl, and a frosted glass syringe rod (routinely obtained from a generic spinal tap set) is used to stir the clot slowly and create the fibrin clot. It can take several minutes for the clot to develop on the frosted rod. Once it develops, the clot is carefully delivered off the rod and then placed on a 4/4 gauze.

Implantation of the Graft to the Meniscal Defect

Switching portals, an arthroscopic grasper is then used to deliver this no. 0 PDS initially through the viewing portal. This will help limit entangling the suture shuttle and the placed circumferential sutures. Viewing once again from the primary viewing portal, a generic 7-mm cannula that can easily have the external fluid valve removed is placed through the primary working portal, still keeping the valve in place at this time. Using a self-capture single-use suture passer, Ceterix NovoStitch device (Ceterix, Fremont, CA, USA), through the working portal, a 2-0 UHMPE suture is passed circumferentially from the inferior to the superior leaflets in

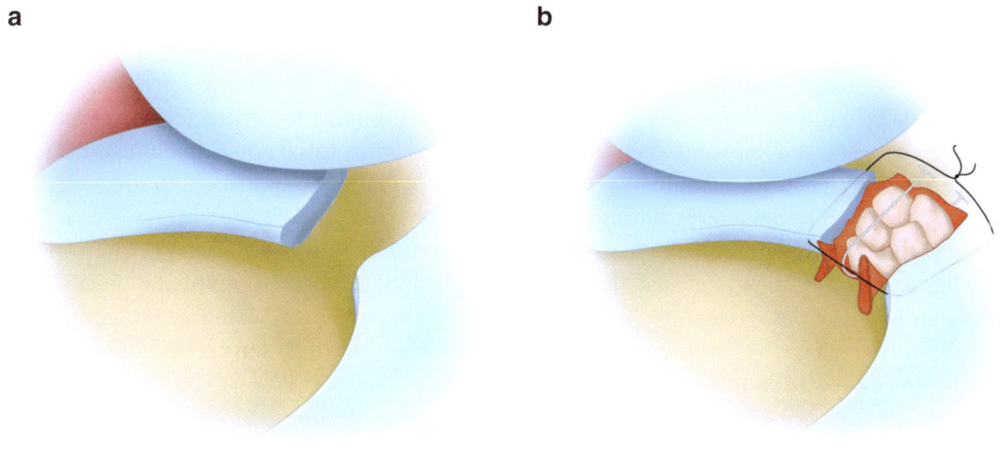

Fig. 14.5 Intraoperative schematic arthroscopic view of the lateral meniscal defect. (**a**) The large radial defect is observed extending from the middle to the posterior segment of the lateral meniscus with degenerative flaps. (**b**) Schematic of the technique showing implantation of the graft into the meniscal defect

the peripheral zone of the tear. The suture is retrieved through the same portal. Given the all-inside all-suture use of this device and self-capture ability, sutures can be placed circumferentially at the meniscocapsular intersection, or even at the popliteal hiatus without capturing the popliteus tendon, unlike many of the all-inside meniscal repair implantable devices. This is done as many times as required working anteriorly and spacing out the sutures every 5 mm. Should the most anterior suture not be available to be placed by this all-inside all-suture technique, then an 18-gauge spinal needle can be used from outside-in with the needle visualized to enter the superior aspect of the anterior meniscal tissue at the red-red zone and exiting on the tibial articular side of the inferior surface. A no. 0 PDS is then passed and retrieved through the working portal, and a corresponding 2-0 suture is shuttled through the tissue. An atraumatic ring grasper is then used to retrieve the superior aspect of the shuttled suture end through the working portal. This can be tied arthroscopically at the end of the case.

Fibrin Clot Shuttling/Suture Tying

Next, the previously placed no. 0 PDS suture, which passes through the midsubstance of the tear, is retrieved through the working cannula, and the fluid valve is removed from the cannula, so there is no obstacle to shuttle the fibrin clot. The no. 0 PDS is then placed through the fibrin clot by using a size-appropriate eyelet straight Keeth needle. Two stacked knots are then tied in the PDS, effectively creating a mulberry knot. The clot is shuttled from outside-in through the cannula into the joint by pulling on the no. 0 PDS suture, at which time it is seated into the cleft of the horizontal cleavage tear and adjusted with use of an atraumatic ring grasper as needed. After the fibrin clot has been fully delivered into the meniscal defect, then each previously passed suture which has a limb inferior and superior to the meniscus and thus the fibrin clot is tied in successive fashion. The PDS suture shuttle is then removed. This can be done either before or after the sutures have been tied, but it is recommended to have at least one suture tied so that it aids in the maintenance of clot reduction. When tying great care is taken to ensure the knots are on the inferior tibial articular surface of the meniscus and as peripheral as possible. The final adjustments are made to the clot as needed as the sutures are each individually tied and the construct is probed.

There are two other techniques to treat posterior medial horn and anterior lateral horn which are carefully described by Laidlaw and Gwathmey [24].

Post-op Rehab

Postoperatively, all patients with an isolated meniscal tear remain with non-weight bearing for 4–6 weeks. Physical therapy emphasizes early quadriceps muscle activation and knee flexion from 0° to 90° within the first 2 weeks with continuous progress after. Six weeks postoperatively, weight bearing is initiated. Also at this time, patients may begin the use of a stationary bike with low resistance settings and 25% body weight leg presses to a maximum of 70° of knee flexion. All increases in low-impact knee exercises are permitted as tolerated starting at 12 weeks postoperatively. Patients are recommended to avoid deep squatting, sitting cross leg, and performing any heavy lifting or squatting activities for a minimum of 4 months following surgical procedure. After 4 months, full flexion, squatting, and return to daily activities or sports are allowed.

Expected Outcomes

Early results have been promising regarding the healing properties of biologics; however, much more research and long-term follow-up are needed.

Complete healing had occurred in 70–100% depending on the technique and number of cases included.

14.2.2 Augmentation of Meniscus Repair with Platelet-Rich Plasma [26, 27]

14.2.2.1 Indication

- **Technique 1**
  - Symptomatic horizontal cleavage (Grade II or III) of the meniscus
  - Young patients—younger than 40 years old
- **Technique 2**
  - Unstable complete vertical longitudinal tears in Cooper Zone 2

14.2.2.2 Techniques

Technique 1

Anteromedial and anterolateral portals are created and a diagnostic arthroscopy is performed. The meniscal tear is identified in cases of Grade 3 lesions. If present in Grade 3 lesions, unstable meniscal fragments and fibrous tissue are removed using a motorized shaver or basket forceps. To repair the medial meniscal tear, a posteromedial mini-arthrotomy is performed. To repair the lateral meniscal tear, a posterolateral mini-arthrotomy is performed. The capsule is open on the upper side of the meniscus, and the meniscosynovial intersection is detached vertically in order to create access to the horizontal cleavage. The lesion is abraded with a rasp and a curette. Meniscus repair is performed by vertical sutures with type No. 0 polydioxanone (PDS; Ethicon, Somerville, NJ, USA), in order to close the two layers (Fig. 14.1). The capsule is then closed. 5 mL of PRP is obtained using the GPS®III system (Biomet, Warsaw, Indiana, USA) and injected directly into the repaired lesion before the closure of the wound. No drainage is used.

Technique 2

The PRP preparation procedure involved drawing 120 mL of venous blood before surgery and centrifuging the blood using a refrigerated centrifuge in a two-step process. Autologous thrombin is obtained by recalcification of a patient's platelet poor plasma (PPP) with 120-mm calcium chlorate ratio 5:1. Thrombin is recovered after centrifugation and PRP/activator ratio 9:1 is used to induce gel formation. This method allows for isolation of leukocyte- and platelet-rich plasma (L-PRP).

The menisci are repaired using standard procedures (rasping, reduction, and fixation). Fixation is performed via the all-inside technique using a FAST-FIX device (Smith and Nephew, Cordova, TN, USA). In patients with a tear extending from the posterior horn to zone 2b (middle body), additional sutures are placed via the outside-in technique using Prolene suture material (Ethicon, Somerville, NJ, USA). Outside-in technique is used for middle body repair. All sutures are placed in an oblique manner with spacing every 5 mm. PRP is activated using 20-mM $CaCl_2$ (Teva, Basel, Israel) and 25-IU/mL autologous thrombin by the operative team. This double activation system is used to abolish the anticoagulative effect of the citrate present in the pre-donation blood bag. It is then injected into the repair site of the meniscus with a double-chamber syringe. Needle localization is confirmed with arthroscopic visualization. Clot formation is observed around the repair site. No drainage is applied to the operated knee joint.

Post-op Rehab

In the first week postoperatively, a passive range of motion from 0° to 90° is initiated, allowing partial weight bearing for 4 weeks. For the first 4 weeks, a hinged knee brace locked in full extension is used. Jogging is not permitted until 3 months postoperatively. Return to pivoting sports is allowed 6–7 months after surgery.

Expected Outcomes

The global failure rate is 12% for horizontal tear and 15% for vertical group.

Both meniscus repair and PRP augmentation are effective at midterm follow-up in young patients. Although encouraging, no recommendation can be made. These techniques should be further evaluated in larger studies with a longer follow-up.

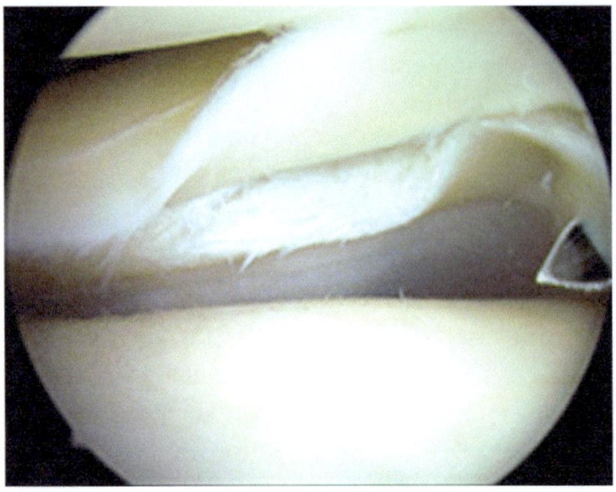

Fig. 14.6 The full-thickness, combined medial meniscal tear

14.2.3 Augmentation of Meniscus Repair by Wrapping [28, 29]

14.2.3.1 Indication

- Full-thickness, combined meniscal tear greater than 20 mm in length (Fig. 14.6)
- Horizontal and radial tear
- Tear location reaching more than 6 mm from the meniscocapsular intersection including the avascular zone
- Both degenerative and non-degenerative meniscus (i.e., horizontal and radial tears, involving the white-white and red-white zones, as well as extensive tears of the bucket-handle type)
- Anterior cruciate ligament (ACL) deficiencies stabilized at the time of the index surgery

14.2.3.2 Techniques

A diagnostic knee arthroscopy is performed to identify other pathologies, such as ligament or cartilage lesions. All cartilage and ligament lesions were repaired during surgery. The extent and type of meniscal lesion are evaluated to determine whether or not the meniscal lesion meets the inclusion criteria of treatment procedure.

Lesions are stabilise and meniscal fragments are fixed with a meniscal fixing device (FAST-FIX, Smith & Nephew, Andover, MA, USA), or the outside-in technique using Prolene suture material (Ethicon, Somerville, NJ, USA) and the inside-out technique using Arthrex Protector Meniscus Suturing depend on the place of meniscal lesions.

The matrix, usually of the size 30 × 20 mm, is prepared by addition of nonabsorbable suture loops (Ethibond, Ethicon, Inc.), passing through the surface of the matrix on both sides. The matrix is then inserted into an applicator. By using direct arthroscopic vision, the loops of threads running through the meniscal posterior horn and the meniscal body are passed with a special suture shuttle (Accupass, Smith & Nephew, Andover, MA, USA) at the level of the anterior border of the tear.

Ethibond 2, matrix-passing sutures are inserted to the meniscal posterior horn and to the anterior part of the lesion. The applicator with the collagen matrix is introduced into the knee joint. The matrix is inserted into the knee joint with smooth surface facing cartilaginous surfaces of the tibia and femur and with porous part directed to the meniscal surface.

After assuring that the matrix adhered to the meniscus from the tibial side, the scaffold is fixed to the meniscus, with arthroscopic simple knotted sutures. As a result, the meniscus is wrapped by the collagen matrix on both sides, and the matrix is fixed into the meniscus in a stable way. Additionally, 1–4 (3 on average, depending on the extension of the tear) FAST-FIX sutures are inserted into the meniscus and wrapped with the matrix for a better stabilization of the meniscal tear and for an increased tightness between the meniscus and the matrix.

An example of suture placement and meniscus wrapping with collagen matrix is shown in Fig. 14.7 and as a schematic drawing in Fig. 14.8.

The bone marrow aspirate is obtained from the tibial proximal epiphysis of the operated knee or from the internal part of the femoral condyles through the anteromedial portal. Approximately 5 mL of liquid bone marrow is aspirated. The bone marrow aspirate is injected between the Chondro-Gide matrix and the meniscus (Fig. 14.8b), under direct arthroscopic control and carried out in “dry arthroscopy” conditions.

The surgery is completed by closing the wounds without draining the knee joint. No knee-stabilizing orthosis is used.

Post-op Rehab

Patients began postoperative treatment from toe touch crutch walking and a range of motion exercises on the first postoperative day, for a period of 4 weeks. Over the next 2–4 weeks, the patients are allowed to walk with partial weight bearing. The patients are encouraged to return to their daily activity by 12 weeks. Sports activity is possible after 6 months postoperatively.

Expected Outcomes

The success rate is about 95% in 2 years of follow-up. The surgical technique is still developed for more simplified technique. Further studies are needed to confirm the usefulness of AMMR technique in basic clinical practice.

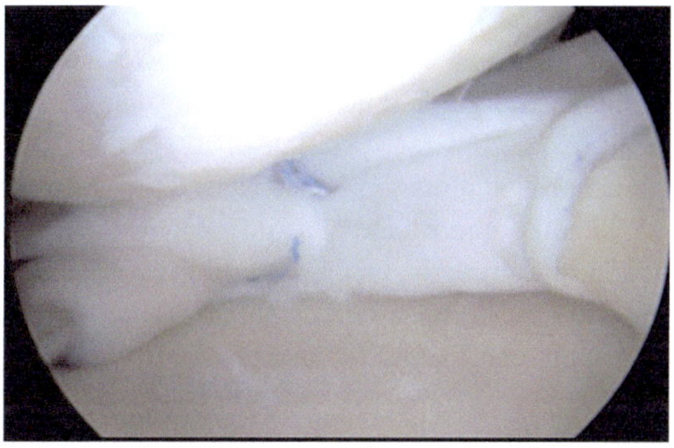

Fig. 14.7 An example of suture placement and meniscus wrapping with collagen matrix

14.2.4 CMI: Collagen Meniscus Implant [30–33]

Resorbable collagen meniscus scaffolds are made from processed bovine Achilles tendon tissue from which type I collagen fibers are extracted and later cross-linked with glutaraldehyde to form a matrix-like scaffold material. The resulting product is a flexible disk that can be trimmed and shaped to fit a meniscal defect.

14.2.4.1 Indication

- Irreparable acute meniscal tears requiring partial meniscectomy or chronic prior loss of meniscal tissue (traumatic or degenerative) greater than 25%.
- Intact anterior and posterior attachments of the meniscus.
- Intact rim (1 mm or greater) over the entire circumference of the involved meniscus.
- Anterior cruciate ligament (ACL) deficiencies stabilized at the time of the index surgery.
- Participant between 15 and 60 years of age.

14.2.4.2 Techniques

Diagnostic arthroscopy is performed through standard portals and verification that a correct diagnosis is made. The CMI is then dipped in physiological

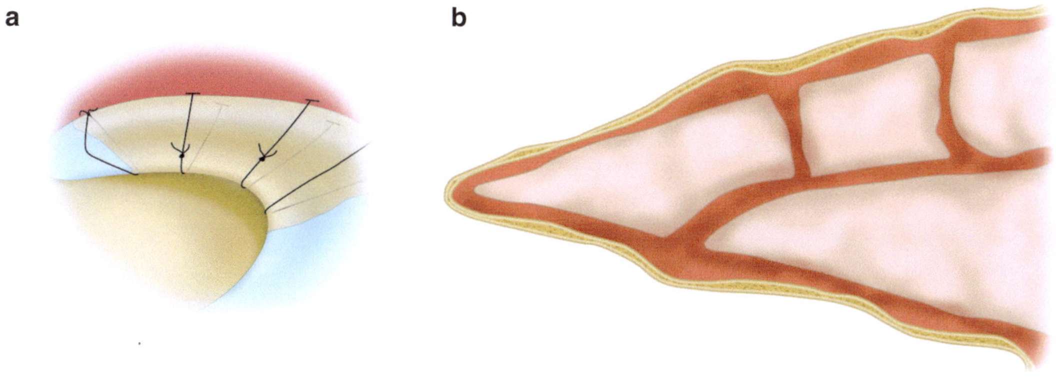

Fig. 14.8 Schematic drawing of a suture placement and meniscus wrapping (**a**), the bone marrow aspirate injected between the collagen matrix and the meniscus (**b**)

saline solution. Partial resection of the medial meniscus leaves a stable outer rim in the white-red or red-red zone (Fig. 14.9). Trepanation of the meniscal rim in inside-out or outside-in technique, until bleeding occurs at scattered sites across the base of the meniscus, is performed.

Insertion of the measuring gauge with a scale through the anteromedial portal and measurement of the defect size is done. On a side table, the required size of the implant is cut out from the hydrogenated CMI. A temporary holding loop made from thread size 0 USP is positioned using the inside-out technique in the region of the pars intermedia of the medial meniscus. The transparent plastic sleeve is armed with the customized CMI. The plastic sleeve is inserted into the anteromedial portal so that transfer of the implant into the joint can be achieved without difficulty. The CMI is then pushed out of the transparent plastic sleeve into the joint and passed through the previously positioned suture loop. Correct positioning of the CMI is carried out in the implant area with a probe and careful tightening of the suture loop around the implant. In this way, the implant can be held in the correct position against the outer rim of the meniscus. The suture loop should only be tightened carefully and slightly; otherwise, the thread will cut into the soft tissue of the CMI and will destroy it. Definitive fixation of the CMI with non-resorbable threads using the inside-out technique is then performed. The sutures may be placed in a horizontal or vertical U-shape. The distance between the U-sutures should be approximately 5 mm (Fig. 14.10). A transverse skin incision about 2 cm long is done, just distal to the medial joint line and division of the subcutis to the joint capsule. This aims to prevent later damage to the saphenous nerve and its infrapatellar branch when the threads are knotted. The U-shaped sutures are knotted consecutively directly onto the joint capsule under arthroscopic view. The medial skin incision is extended in a posterior direction for fixation of the CMI in the region of the posterior horn. Then division of the subcutaneous tissue to the capsule and insertion of a ster-

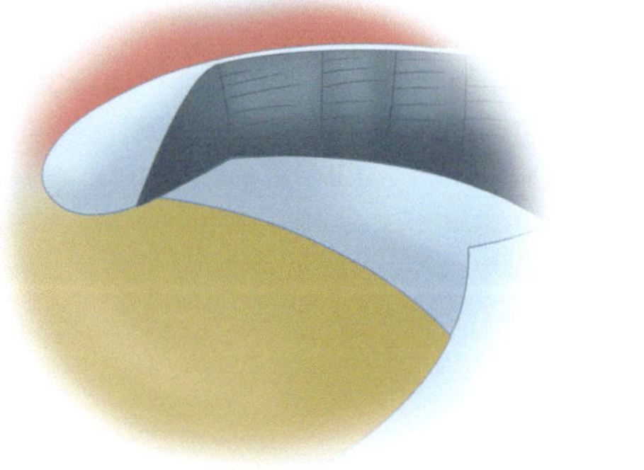

Fig. 14.9 Resection of the medial meniscus leaving a stable outer rim in the white-red or red-red zone

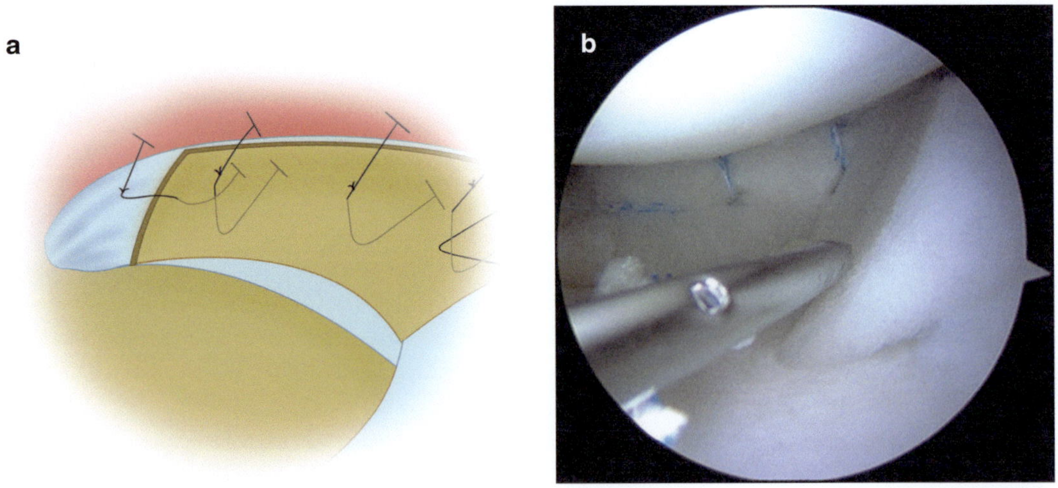

Fig. 14.10 Schematic draft (**a**) and arthroscopic viewing (**b**) of definitive fixation of the CMI with threads

ile meniscus retractor is performed. The latter is used in the inside-out technique to divert the needle in an anteromedial direction as it exits posteriorly from the capsule, thus avoiding damage to the neurovascular structures in the popliteal fossa. Each pair of threads is secured with a small clip outside the joint. After positioning all threads, the adaptation of the CMI to the outer rim can be assessed arthroscopically and tested by pulling on the threads. Arthroscopic monitoring of the implant is when the threads are being knotted and is indispensable to avoid too strong tightening which would cause the threads to cut into the tissue of the CMI. It is only necessary to give a careful and measured pull on the threads to achieve adaptation. Adaptive subcutaneous sutures with resorbable thread size 3-0 USP and skin closure with non-resorbable interrupted reverse sutures are performed. Finally, sterile dressing and elastic compression bandage is applied.

Post-op Rehab

Knee brace with restriction of motion to extension/flexion of 0/0/60° until the fourth postoperative week, and then 0/0/90° until the sixth postoperative week, is applied.

Continuous passive motion (CPM) within the permitted range of motion is started from the first postoperative day. Actively assisted physiotherapy is necessary. No weight bearing on the operated limb is started for 6 weeks. Increased weight bearing over a period of 2 weeks, until full weight bearing, is achieved. Thromboembolism prophylaxis with low molecular heparin until full weight bearing is achieved. Cycling can commence from the third month. Full sports are poseable activities after 6 months.

Expected Outcomes

The improvements in pain relief, activity level, general health, and radiological outcomes had been documented with the use of MCMI at a minimum 10-year follow-up. On the basis of available results, 87% of the patients benefited from this scaffold implantation.

14.2.5 Actifit: Polyurethanes (PU) (Orteq Ltd, London, UK) [34, 35]

Polyurethane is a polymer that is formed by reacting a diisocyanate or a polymeric isocyanate (hard segment) with a polyol (soft segment) in the presence of suitable catalysts and additives.

14.2.5.1 Indication

- 18–50 years old—skeletally mature patient.
- Partial lesion with stable rim (NB intact popliteal bridge in the lateral indication).
- Both horns present.
- Stable, well-aligned knee.
- ICRS classification <3.
- Patient understands the importance of, and commits to adhere to, rehabilitation program.

14.2.5.2 Techniques

The surgical procedure of scaffold implantation is performed through an arthroscopic approach. After preparing the implant site and making a full-thickness meniscal defect without degenerative tissue, the anterior and posterior meniscal attachment points are trimmed square for the scaffold to fit in precisely. After measuring the prepared meniscal defect, the polyurethane scaffold Actifit is trimmed to fill the defect. The implant is inserted into the defect and secured to the host meniscus remnant with all-inside sutures (nonabsorbable ULTRABRAID no. 0 wire and poly-L-lactide bioabsorbable ULTRA FAST-FIX implants, Smith & Nephew, Andover, Massachusetts). Vertical/oblique stitches are placed every 5 mm, while horizontal stitches are used only in the posterior and anterior junctions.

Post-op Rehab

After the operation, a knee brace is immediately applied and locked in full extension. The brace is continuously worn by the patient for 4 weeks but removed four times daily to allow continuous passive motion (CPM): CPM from 0° to 60° is allowed for the first 2 weeks and then increased to 90° of flexion, and after another 2 weeks, complete passive motion is allowed. Weight bearing is not allowed for the first 2 weeks and ambulation is permitted only using crutches. Then, progressive weight bearing is allowed toward full weight bearing. Early isometric exercises are performed. Voluntary muscular contraction and neuromuscular electrical stimulation (NMES) are indicated and could be started at patient discharge. Elastic resistance and isotonic strengthening programs are started in the fourth postoperative week. The rehabilitation protocol is peculiarly adapted to the patients according to concurrent procedures and postoperative clinical trends. Patients are allowed to return to full unrestricted activity after 6 months if asymptomatic and with regained neuromuscular control. For contact sports, return to full activity is usually allowed after 9 months.

Expected Outcomes

In accordance with the current literature, a significant improvement of the patient-reported outcome scores is seen up to 24 months post surgery. The 23% failure rate in Leroy's [34] study and 38% failure rate in Dhollander et al.'s [36] report are high, and we should always consider it before choosing the treatment option.

14.3 Biomaterials in Preclinical Study of Meniscus Repair Technique

14.3.1 Augmentation of Meniscus Repair with Tissue Adhesives

Tissue adhesives are attractive biomaterials to be used for treating meniscal tears. They have already been used in clinical practice for various applications. Cyanoacrylates are used clinically for gluing skin lacerations, fibrin glue for pulmonary leaks and repair of cardiovascular defects, and Tissue Glu for abdominoplasty. However, these materials are not suitable for the repair of meniscal tears either due to their cytotoxicity or their insufficient mechanical and adhesive properties. Therefore, there is a growing interest in the development of new tissue adhesives, which are strong, nontoxic, biodegradable, and fast-curing. Further studies are needed to confirm the biocompatibility of these systems with cells and tissues in vitro and in vivo.

14.3.2 Non-resorbable Polymers and Resorbable Polymers

There are still many synthetic and natural products in preclinical studies presented by many authors. Polyethylene terephthalate (PET), polytetrafluorethylene terephthalate (PTFE), polycarbonate-urethane (PCU), poly(vinyl alcohol) hydrogel (PVA-H), poly(a-hydroxy acids) (PHAs), silk, and gelatin, on the animal models present in meniscus tissue engineering, were addressed as a potential meniscus substitute/scaffold with promising results in preclinical stages. Regarding synthetic non-resorbable materials, the most important aspect is that the implant is biocompatible, intrinsically stable, and safe and mimics the biomechanical properties of the native meniscus. Concerning synthetic resorbable materials, it is important to access the tissue ingrowth and the degradation profile of the material.

References

1. Paxton EP, Stock MV, Brophy RH. Meniscal repair versus partial meniscectomy: a systematic review comparing reoperation rates and clinical outcomes. Arthroscopy. 2011;27:1275–88.
2. Rangger C, Klestil T, Gloetzer W, Kemmler G, Benedetto KP. Osteoarthritis after arthroscopic partial meniscectomy. Am J Sports Med. 1995;23:240–4.
3. Anetzberger H, Mayer A, Glaser C, Lorenz S, Birkenmaier C, Muller-Gerbl M. Meniscectomy leads to early changes in the mineralization distribution of subchondral bone plate. Knee Surg Sports Traumatol Arthrosc. 2014;22:112–9.
4. Chatain F, Robinson AH, Adeleine P, Chambat P, Neyret P. The natural history of the knee following arthroscopic medial meniscectomy. Knee Surg Sports Traumatol Arthrosc. 2001;9:15–8.
5. Hede A, Larsen E, Sandberg H. The long term outcome of open total and partial meniscectomy related to the quantity and site of the meniscus removed. Int Orthop. 1992;16:122–5.
6. Verdonk R, Madry H, Shabshin N, Dirisamer F, Peretti GM, Pujol N, Spalding T, Verdonk P, Seil R, Condello

V, Di Matteo B, Zellner J, Angele P. The role of meniscal tissue in joint protection in early osteoarthritis. Knee Surg Sports Traumatol Arthrosc. 2016;24:1763. https://doi.org/10.1007/s00167-016-4069-2.
7. Lee D-Y, Park Y-J, Kim H-J, Nam D-C, Park J-S, Song S-Y, Kang D-G. Arthroscopic meniscal surgery versus conservative management in patients aged 40 years and older: a meta-analysis. Arch Orthop Trauma Surg. 2018;138:1731. https://doi.org/10.1007/s00402-018-2991-0.
8. Chen M, Guo W, Gao S, Hao C, Shen S, Zhang Z, Wang Z, Wang Z, Xu L, Jing X, Zhang X, Yuan Z, Wang M, Zhang Y, Peng J, Wang A, Wang Y, Sui X, Liu S, Guo Q. Biochemical stimulus-based strategies for meniscus tissue engineering and regeneration. Biomed Res Int. 2018;2018:8472309. https://doi.org/10.1155/2018/8472309. 15 pages.
9. Kim S-H, An Y-H, Kim HD, Kim K, Lee S-H, Yim H-G, Kim B-G, Hwang NS. Enzyme - mediated tissue adhesive hydrogels for meniscus repair. Int J Biol Macromol. 2018;110:479. https://doi.org/10.1016/j.ijbiomac.2017.12.053.
10. Pillai MM, Gopinathan J, Selvakumar R, Bhattacharyya A. Human knee meniscus regeneration strategies: a review on recent advances. Curr Osteopor Rep. 2018;16:224. https://doi.org/10.1007/s11914-018-0436-x.
11. Zhang Z, Guo W, Gao S, Chen M, Li X, Zhang X, Jing X, Wang M, Zhang Y, Shen S, Wang Z, Sun B, Chai Y, Zhou C, Liu S, Guo Q. Native tissue-based strategies for meniscus repair and regeneration. Cell Tissue Res. 2018;37:337. https://doi.org/10.1007/s00441-017-2778-6.
12. Zadeh LG, Chevrier A, Farr J, Rodeo SR, Buschmann MD. Augmentation techniques for meniscus repair. J Knee Surg. 2018;31:99–116.
13. Bilgen B, Jayasuriya CT, Owens BD. Current concepts in meniscus tissue engineering and repair. Adv Healthcare Mater. 2018;2018:1701407. https://doi.org/10.1002/adhm.201701407.
14. Mauck RL, Burdick JA. From repair to regeneration: biomaterials to reprogram the meniscus wound microenvironment. Ann Biomed Eng. 2015;43(3):529–42. https://doi.org/10.1007/s10439-015-1249-z.
15. Jülke H, Mainil-Varlet P, Jakob RP, Brehm W, Schäfer B, Nesic D. The role of cells in meniscal guided tissue regeneration: a proof of concept study in a goat model. Cartilage. 2015;6(1):20–9.
16. Qu F, Lin J-MG, Esterhai JL, Fisher MB, Mauck RL. Biomaterial-mediated delivery of degradative enzymes to improve meniscus integration and repair. Acta Biomater. 2013;9:6393–402.
17. Bochynska AI, Hannink G, Grijpma DW, Buma P. Tissue adhesives for meniscus tear repair: an overview of current advances and prospects for future clinical solutions. J Mater Sci Mater Med. 2016;27:85.
18. Kean CO, Brown RJ, Chapman J. The role of biomaterials in the treatment of meniscal tears. PeerJ. 2017;5:e4076. https://doi.org/10.7717/peerj.4076.
19. Koch M, Achatz FP, Lang S, Pfeifer CG, Pattappa G, Kujat R, Nerlich M, Angele P, Zellner J. Tissue engineering of large full-size meniscus defects by a polyurethane scaffold: accelerated regeneration by mesenchymal stromal cells. Stem Cells Int. 2018;2018:8207071. https://doi.org/10.1155/2018/8207071. 11 pages.
20. Chen Y, Chen J, Zhang Z, Lou K, Zhang Q, Wang S, Ni J, Liu W, Fan S, Lin X. Current advances in the development of natural meniscus scaffolds: innovative approaches to decellularization and recellularization. Cell Tissue Res. 2017;370:41–52. https://doi.org/10.1007/s00441-017-2605-0.
21. Kowalski C, Gallo RA. Platelet-rich fibrin clote augmented repair of horizontal cleavage meniscal tear. Arthrosc Tech. 2017;6(5):e2047–51.
22. Kamimura T, Kimura M. Repair of a chronic large meniscal defect with implantation of autogenous meniscal fragments using a tubular-shaped fibrin clot. Arthrosc Tech. 2018;7(3):e257–63.
23. Ra HJ, Ha JK, Jang SH, Lee DW, Kim JG. Arthroscopic inside-out repair of complete radial tears of the meniscus with a fibrin clot. Knee Surg Sports Traumatol Arthrosc. 2013;21:2126. https://doi.org/10.1007/s00167-012-2191-3.
24. Laidlaw MS, Gwathmey FW. Circumferential suture repair of isolated horizontal meniscal tears augmented with fibrin clot. Arthrosc Tech. 2017;6(5):e1567–72.
25. van Trommel MF, Simonian PT, Potter HG, Wickiewicz TL. Arthroscopic meniscal repair with fibrin clot of complete radial tears of the lateral meniscus in the avascular zone. Arthroscopy. 1998;14(4):360–5.
26. Pujol N, De Chou ES, Boisrenoult P, Beaufils P. Platelet-rich plasma for open meniscal repair in young patients: any benefit? Knee Surg Sports Traumatol Arthrosc. 2015;23:51–8. https://doi.org/10.1007/s00167-014-3417-3.
27. Kaminski R, Kulinski K, Kozar-Kaminska K, Wielgus M, Langner M, Wasko MK, Kowalczewski J, Pomianowski S. A prospective, randomized, double-blind, parallel-group, placebo-controlled study evaluating meniscal healing, clinical outcomes, and safety in patients undergoing meniscal repair of unstable, complete vertical meniscal tears (bucket handle) augmented with platelet-rich plasma. Biomed Res Int. 2018;2018:9315815. https://doi.org/10.1155/2018/9315815. 9 pages.
28. Piontek T, Ciemniewska-Gorzela K, Szulc A, Słomczykowski M, Jakob RP. All-arthroscopic technique of biological meniscal tear therapy with collagen matrix. Polish Orthop Traumatol. 2012;77:39–45.
29. Piontek T, Ciemniewska-Gorzela K, Naczk J, Jakob R, Szulc A, Grygorowicz M, Slomczykowski M. Complex meniscus tears treated with collagen matrix wrapping and bone marrow blood injection: a 2-year clinical follow-up. Cartilage. 2016;7(2):123–39.

30. Rodkey WG, Steadman JR, Li ST. A clinical study of collagen meniscus implants to restore the injured meniscus. Clin Orthop. 1999;367(Suppl):S281–92.
31. Linke RD, Ulmer M, Imhoff AB. Replacement of the meniscus with a collagen implant (CMI). Eur J Trauma Emerg Surg. 2007;33:435–40.
32. Linke RD, Ulmer M, Imhoff AB. Replacement of the meniscus with a collagen implant (CMI). Oper Orthop Traumatol. 2006;18:453–62.
33. Zaffagnini S, Muccioli GMM, Lopomo N, Bruni D, Giordano G, Ravazzolo G, Molinari M, Marcacci M. Prospective long-term outcomes of the medial collagen meniscus implant versus partial medial meniscectomy: a minimum 10-year follow-up study. Am J Sports Med. 2011;39:977.
34. Leroy A, Beaufils P, Faivre B, Steltzlen C, Boisrenoult P, Pujol N. Actifit® polyurethane meniscal scaffold: MRI and functional outcomes after a minimum follow-up of 5 years. Orthop Traumatol Surg Res. 2017;103:609. https://doi.org/10.1016/j.otsr.2017.02.012.
35. Schüttler KF, Haberhauer F, Gesslein M, Heyse TJ, Figie J, Lorbach O, Efe T, Roessler PP. Midterm follow-up after implantation of a polyurethane meniscal scaffold for segmental medial meniscus loss: maintenance of good clinical and MRI outcome. Knee Surg Sports Traumatol Arthrosc. 2016;24:1478. https://doi.org/10.1007/s00167-015-3759-5.
36. Dhollander A, Verdonk P, Verdonk R. Treatment of painful, irreparable partial meniscal defects with a polyurethane scaffold: midterm clinical outcomes and survival analysis. Am J Sports Med. 2016;44(10):2615–21.

15 Internal Bracing of the Anterior Cruciate Ligament and Posterior Cruciate Ligament with Suture Tape Augmentation

Graeme P. Hopper and Gordon M. Mackay

15.1 Introduction

Internal bracing involves the augmentation of a ligament repair with suture tape which reinforces the ligament and acts as a secondary stabiliser. This promotes natural healing by protecting the ligament during the healing phase and allowing early mobilisation. Additionally, autograft is not required thereby the unnecessary morbidity of graft harvest is avoided. The suture tape is FiberTape® (Arthrex) which is a ultra-high strength 2 mm-width tape, consisting of a long-chain ultra-high molecular weight polyethylene (UHMWPE), and acts as an internal brace.

We first described the concept of internal bracing and its various uses in our review paper [1]. In addition, the paper outlined the early results of repair of the anterior cruciate ligament (ACL) using internal bracing. The technique has also been utilised for the medial and lateral ankle ligaments, the syndesmosis complex, all of the ligaments around the knee and the ulnar collateral ligament of the elbow [2–9]. Additionally, the concept of internal bracing has been applied to repair of the acromioclavicular joint, the patellar tendon, and the Achilles tendon [10–13]. This chapter describes internal bracing of the anterior and posterior cruciate ligaments.

G. P. Hopper (✉)
College of Medical, Veterinary & Life Sciences, University of Glasgow, Glasgow, Scotland
e-mail: graemehopper@nhs.net

G. M. Mackay
University of Stirling, Stirling, Scotland

15.2 Anterior Cruciate Ligament Internal Bracing

The anterior cruciate ligament (ACL) is one of the main stabilisers of the knee and is the primary restraint to anterior tibial translation of the knee [14]. ACL rupture is a common injury in the young adult population, and ACL reconstruction with hamstring or patellar tendon autograft has been the gold standard surgical option for many years. However, it has been reported that only 63–65% of the patients return to their previous level of sporting activity, and 10.3% have a graft failure after 10 years [15]. In addition, ACL reconstruction does not protect patients from developing post-traumatic osteoarthritis [16–19]. As a result, there has been a renewed interest in primary repair of the ACL.

Indeed, primary repair of the ACL was the gold standard treatment for ACL ruptures in the 1970s and 1980s [20–22]. However, high failure rates were described at mid-term follow-up [23–25]. As a result, ACL reconstruction became the gold standard treatment in the 1990s [26, 27]. Nevertheless, advancements in arthroscopic instrumentation, suture materials, imaging, and rehabilitation protocols should theoretically lead to improved out-

M. Brittberg, K. Slynarski (eds.), *Lower Extremity Joint Preservation*,
https://doi.org/10.1007/978-3-030-57382-9_15

comes with primary repair of the ACL when compared to these historic techniques.

ACL repair with internal bracing uses FiberTape® (Arthrex) which bridges the ligament and is fixed on the femur with a button (Retrobutton® or TightRope RT®, Arthrex) and a knotless bone anchor (SwiveLock®, Arthrex) on the tibia. A looped suture (FiberLink®, Arthrex) secures the distal ACL stump to its femoral attachment. Internal bracing of the ACL acts as a secondary stabiliser which promotes natural healing of the ligament by protecting it during the healing phase and supporting early mobilisation. In addition, graft harvest is not required which avoids muscle atrophy leading to an accelerated recovery. Moreover, the native ACL is spared thereby providing proprioceptive properties.

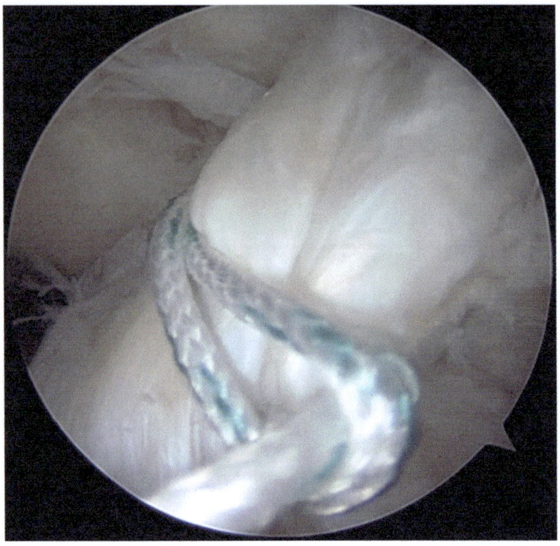

Fig. 15.1 The FiberLink® forms a lasso around the distal ACL stump

15.2.1 Surgical Technique

Standard anterolateral and anteromedial portals are used, and a passport cannula (Arthrex) is placed in the anteromedial portal. The ACL is probed to assess its suitability for primary repair. Proximal ruptures of the ACL are repaired with internal bracing. On the other hand, mid-substance or distal ruptures and ruptures where the ACL remnant is retracted are not suitable for repair. We previously used a standard ACL reconstruction procedure for these cases, but this has since progressed to the use of a hybrid ACL reconstruction with internal bracing similar to that described by Smith et al. [28].

The ACL remnant is left intact, and a standard tibial ACL guide is placed at the centre of the footprint. A small skin incision is made above the pes anserinus and a 3.5 mm tibial tunnel is drilled. The drill is subsequently exchanged for a FiberStick™ (Arthrex); then a suture grasper is used to take the FiberWire suture (Arthrex) out of the FiberStick™ and through the medial portal. A FiberLink® is passed through the mid-substance of the ACL stump using a Scorpion™ suture passer (Arthrex) and retracted through the medial portal, forming a lasso around the distal ACL stump (Fig. 15.1). A second FiberLink® can be added if there is any doubt about the grip on the distal stump.

The femoral attachment is then identified, microfracturing is performed, and then a 3.5 mm femoral tunnel is drilled. The FiberLink® suture and the FiberWire suture are then passed through the femoral tunnel. A femoral button (Retrobutton® or TightRope RT®, Arthrex) loaded with FiberTape® is subsequently transported proximally through the tibial tunnel, the centre of the ACL, and the femoral tunnel. The button is flipped on the femoral cortex and the FiberTape® is advanced in the femoral tunnel by pulling the two tensioning strands. The suture tape is fixed distally, just below the tibial tunnel, using a 4.75 mm SwiveLock® loaded with both ends of the FiberTape®. Prior to insertion, the FiberTape® is marked at the laser line and repositioned in the eye of the SwiveLock® to avoid overtensioning (Fig. 15.2). Finally, the ACL is gently tensioned using the cinch to approximate the distal stump to the femoral footprint; then the FiberLink® is tied on the femoral button with the appropriate tension on the ACL (Fig. 15.3).

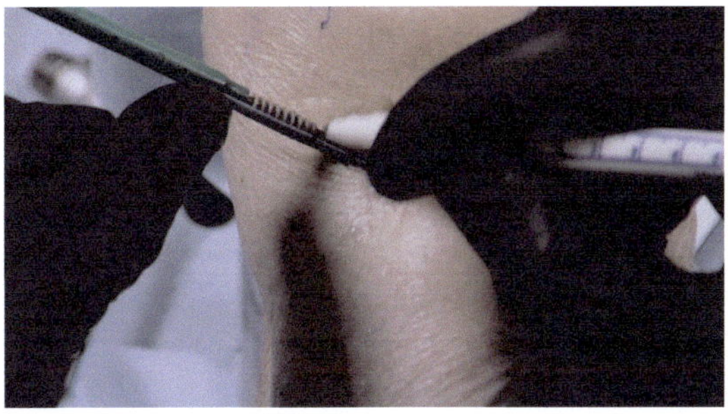

Fig. 15.2 The FiberTape® is marked at the laser line to avoid overtensioning

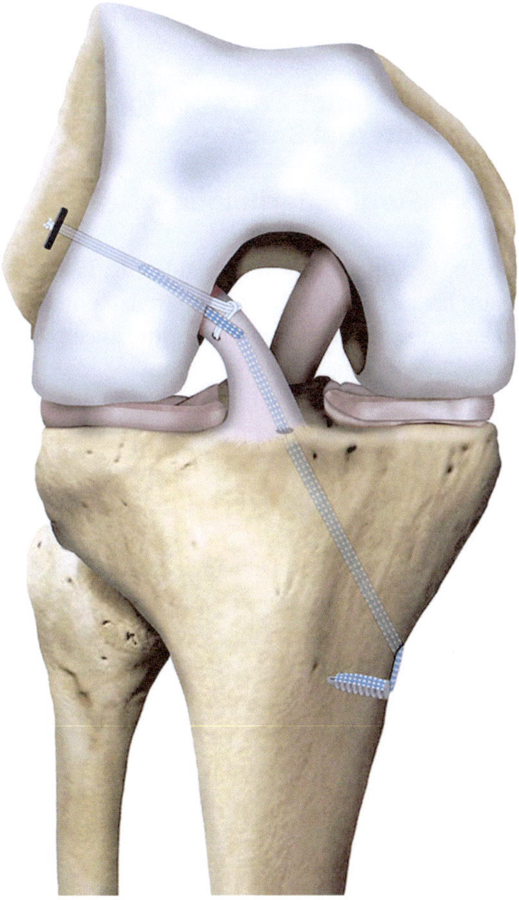

Fig. 15.3 Final construct demonstrates internal bracing of the ACL with suture tape augmentation

15.2.2 Rehabilitation

Patients are allowed to fully weight bear with crutches as required during the first weeks, and physical therapy focuses on early range of movement, muscle control, and restoration of function. This is enabled by the limited pain and swelling, allowing accelerated early phase rehabilitation. Most patients are able to perform pivoting sports around 5 months postoperatively.

15.2.3 Expected Outcomes and Discussion

ACL reconstruction became the gold standard treatment for ACL ruptures in the 1990s when primary repair of the ACL was found to be associated with high failure rates [23–25]. This combined with improved results with ACL reconstructions and enhanced arthroscopic techniques led to the abandonment of primary repair of the ACL [26, 27]. However, ACL reconstruction techniques are not without their own problems including the loss of proprioception, graft harvest morbidity, post-traumatic osteoarthritis and graft failure. These drawbacks alongside modern advancements in arthroscopic instrumentation and suture materials, in addition to an enhanced understanding of ACL healing, have resulted in a renewed interest in ACL repair.

ACL repair with internal bracing retains the proprioceptive fibres of the ACL which is invaluable postoperatively as it is thought that the loss of these fibres leads to a lack of confidence in the knees of those who have underwent ACL reconstruction [29–31]. Furthermore, less than 50% of patients of patients return to playing sport at their preinjury level following ACL reconstruction, and it is thought that a lot of this is due to the lack of proprioception and confidence in the knee [32].

Internal bracing of the ACL avoids the need for an autograft. Graft harvest in patients undergoing ACL reconstruction is associated with a number of donor site morbidities. Knee flexor weakness with hamstring grafts and anterior knee pain with patellar tendon grafts are commonly reported [33–35]. In addition, Kowalk et al. [36] demonstrated that ACL reconstruction with patellar tendon grafts restores knee stability, but there is a reduction in knee power and work performed post-operatively.

Evidence suggests that ACL reconstruction does not prevent future osteoarthritis. A systematic review by Ajuied et al. [19] evaluated 596 patients with an ACL rupture across nine studies and showed 20% of these patients have moderate or severe radiological changes at 10 years postinjury. In addition, they determined that patients treated nonoperatively would develop osteoarthritis quicker; however, 23% of the patients undergoing ACL reconstruction still had moderate or severe osteoarthritis at 10 years. Furthermore, a recent systematic review by Poehling-Monaghan et al. [37] evaluated ten studies to compare patellar tendon and hamstring autografts outcomes and found a number of studies demonstrated a significantly increased rate of osteoarthritis with patellar tendon grafts. Moreover, one of the studies they reviewed by Leys et al. [38] indicated that 69% of patients undergoing ACL reconstruction with hamstring autograft had radiologically detectable osteoarthritis 15 years postoperatively. We hypothesise that internal bracing with ACL repair will reduce rates of osteoarthritis due to the reduced morbidity associated with the technique, namely, not requiring autograft, retaining proprioceptive fibres and smaller bone tunnels. However, long-term follow-up studies in the future are required to support this hypothesis.

The high failure rates (>50%) associated with primary repairs of the ACL in the 1970s and 1980s was one of the reasons behind ACL reconstruction becoming the gold standard surgical option [23–25]. However, ACL reconstructions remain associated with high failure rates when using hamstring autografts and allografts and, in particular, in younger age groups [39–41]. Internal bracing of the ACL reinforces the ligament and acts as a secondary stabiliser allowing for early mobilisation. Hypothetically this should reduce the high failure rates (>50%) and associated pain and stiffness that accompanied the historic primary repairs. These patients had a large arthrotomy as well as cast immobilisation postoperatively which are essentially the opposite of our technique using arthroscopic surgery and early mobilisation postoperatively. Importantly, the tunnels associated with internal bracing are situated in the same position as the larger tunnels used for hamstring or patellar tendon autografts in ACL reconstruction. As a result, any failures of our ACL repair technique would have a routine primary ACL reconstruction using autograft without compromise of the knee joint and the additional complications associated with revision surgery [41].

15.2.4 Conclusion

We have had excellent clinical results with internal bracing of the ACL with suture tape augmentation. However, further clinical studies are needed to outline the overall outcomes of this procedure.

15.3 Posterior Cruciate Ligament Internal Bracing

15.3.1 Surgical Technique

The posterior cruciate ligament (PCL) is the primary restraint to posterior tibial translation of the knee and is a crucial stabiliser of the knee [42]. It originates on the medial femoral condyle and inserts on the posterior intercondylar area of the tibia [43]. The PCL is composed of two bundles, an anterolateral bundle and a posteromedial bundle [44]. PCL injury accounts for up to 20% of injuries to the ligaments around the knee [45]. The most common mechanism of injury is a direct blow to the anterior tibia with the knee flexed which is classically associated with motor vehicle accidents and soccer injuries [46]. However, isolated injuries to the PCL are rare, and they are more likely to represent one aspect of a multiligament knee injury [44].

An increased incidence of osteoarthritis in patients with posterior cruciate ligament deficiency has been reported in the literature [47]. Consequently, one of the main aims in patients with a PCL injury is to restore the function of the ligament as close to normal as possible. Surgery is therefore recommended in patients with Grade III PCL tears, symptomatic chronic tears and PCL tears associated with other ligamentous knee injuries. Several procedures have been described in the literature, but no technique has been shown to be superior to any other.

15.3.2 Rehabilitation

Standard anteromedial and anterolateral portals are used with the addition of an accessory posteromedial portal. The first step is to elevate the PCL and track it down to its tibial insertion. The residual PCL fibres are retained and pushed posteriorly with the other posterior structures allowing for a safe and adequate exposure. An anteromedial incision is made over the proximal tibia, then a standard PCL guide is used to drill a 3.5 mm tunnel. The drill is advanced under direct vision to minimize any risk of complication. The anterior tibial cortex is tapped, and the drill is switched for a FiberStick™ (Arthrex). The FiberWire® (Arthrex) is grasped out of the FiberStick™ and taken through the anteromedial portal.

The insertion point of the PCL on the femur is then identified and marked using electrosurgery which guarantees accuracy when the guide pin is passed. Reaming allows easier passage of the femoral button (Retrobutton® or TightRope RT®, loaded with FiberTape®, Arthrex) when it is shuttled from the anterolateral port directly through the tunnel (Fig. 15.4). The suture tape is then secured 1 cm distal to the tibial tunnel using a 4.75 mm SwiveLock® (Arthrex) with the knee in 90° of flexion and an assistant providing anterior translation to hold the tibia in a reduced position with adequate tension on the PCL. Prior to insertion, the laser line is marked which indicates the anatomical length of the PCL. If there are any reservations, the knee should be put through a full range of movement in the reduced position prior to marking as excessive tensioning can result in difficulty achieving full extension. Securing the suture tape distally is an essential step as this restores the length of the anatomical PCL (Fig. 15.5).

15.3.3 Expected Outcomes and Discussion

Patients fully weight bear with crutches as required during the first weeks after surgery. The limited pain and swelling of this procedure in comparison to other techniques allows accelerated early phase rehabilitation with a focus on early range of movement and restoration of function. Most patients will return to pivoting sports around 5–6 months following surgery when neuromuscular function has recovered.

15.3.4 Conclusion

Numerous techniques have been described in the literature for the surgical management of patients with PCL ruptures [9, 42, 43, 48, 49]. Even with all of the techniques described, no single technique has been shown to outdo any of the others. Historically, primary PCL repair was the most common surgical option; however, PCL reconstruction procedures are now more commonly performed.

PCL repair was originally performed as an open procedure with inconsistent results [50–52]. Hughston et al. [52] evaluated the outcomes of 29 PCL repairs demonstrating good objective results in 65% of patients. On the other hand, Strand et al. [51] established the results of 32 patients undergoing PCL repair with more than 50% of patients having posterior instability, postoperatively. Moreover, Pournaras et al. [50] described the results of 20 patients undergoing PCL repair and found that 100% of cases had posterior instability postoperatively. More recently, arthroscopic PCL repair has been described using a number of different techniques. Wheatley et al. [53] reported satisfactory patient-reported outcome scores at a mean follow-up of 51 months in patients who underwent repair following PCL soft tissue avulsions. DiFelice et al. [49] described a variation of this technique in a small case series of three patients. They used suture anchors to repair soft tissue peel off injuries to the PCL with satisfactory outcomes at 64 months. In addition, Van Der List et al. [9] described a similar technique to ours with PCL repair and augmentation with an internal brace. However, there are no clinical outcome results of arthroscopic PCL repair in the literature.

PCL reconstruction techniques are more commonly performed; therefore several clinical out-

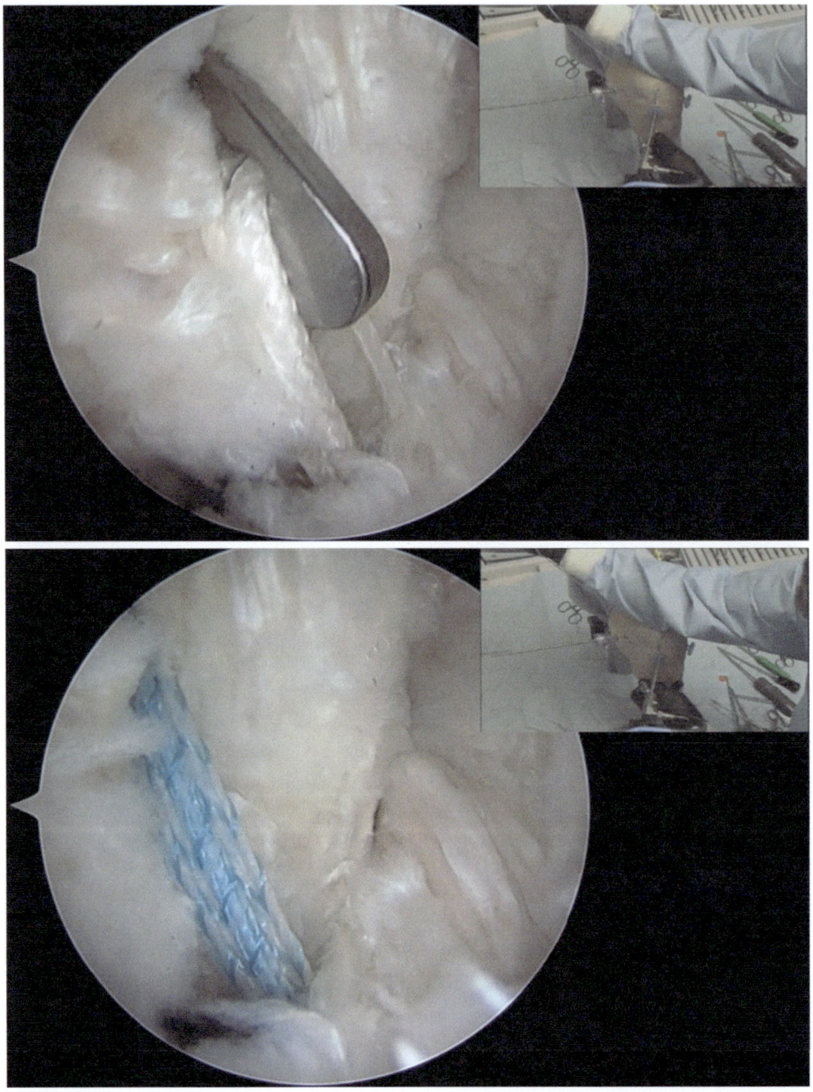

Fig. 15.4 The femoral button (Retrobutton® or TightRope RT®, loaded with FiberTape®, Arthrex) is shuttled from the anterolateral port directly through the tunnel

comes studies have been published. Chahla et al. [42] reviewed 441 patients in 11 studies in a systematic review and meta-analysis which compared single-bundle versus double-bundle PCL reconstructions. They conveyed significantly improved posterior stability and IKDC scores in the double-bundle group. Belk et al. [43] analysed 132 patients in five studies in a systematic review and meta-analysis comparing PCL reconstruction with allograft versus autograft. This review demonstrated improved clinical outcomes in each group with no differences between the groups. Another study by Del Buono et al. [54] reviewed 34 papers with patients undergoing PCL reconstruction or PCL augmentation. This review found comparable results in each group. The augmentation procedures analysed in the paper included a remnant posterior cruciate ligament-augmenting stent procedure and double-bundle augmentation with Achilles allograft [55, 56].

Internal bracing of the PCL with suture tape augmentation reinforces the ligament and acts as a secondary stabiliser. This augment protects the ligament during the healing phase allowing natural healing while allowing early mobilisation.

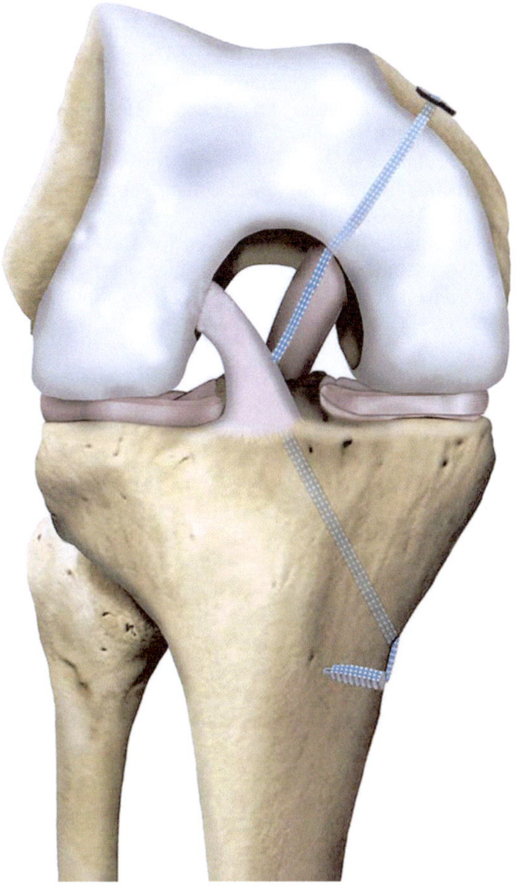

Fig. 15.5 Final construct demonstrates internal bracing of the PCL with suture tape augmentation

Additionally, the morbidity associated with graft harvest is avoided leading to a reduction in muscle atrophy postoperatively thereby accelerating rehabilitation. Moreover, the proprioceptive properties that are retained in the native PCL could also contribute to an accelerated rehabilitation period and benefit long-term recovery and return to sporting activity.

15.3.5 Conclusion

We have observed excellent clinical results with internal bracing of the PCL with suture tape augmentation. However, further clinical studies are required to define the overall outcomes of this procedure.

Acknowledgements Professor Mackay is a consultant for, and receives royalties from, Arthrex, Inc. Mr. Hopper has no *conflict of interest* to disclose.

References

1. Mackay GM, Blyth MJ, Anthony I, Hopper GP, Ribbans WJ. A review of ligament augmentation with the InternalBrace™: the surgical principle is described for the lateral ankle ligament and ACL repair in particular, and a comprehensive review of other surgical applications and techniques is presented. Surg Technol Int. 2015;26:239.
2. Regauer M, Mackay G, Lange M, Kammerlander C, Syndesmotic BW. World J Orthop. 2017;8(4):301.
3. Urch E, DeGiacomo A, Photopoulos CD, Limpisvasti O, ElAttrache NS. Ulnar collateral ligament repair with suture bridge augmentation. Arthrosc Tech. 2018;7(3):e219.
4. Trofa DP, Lombardi JM, Noticewala MS, Ahmad CS. Ulnar collateral ligament repair with suture augmentation. Arthrosc Tech. 2018;7(1):e53.
5. Coetzee JC, Ellington JK, Ronan JA, Stone RM. Functional results of open Broström ankle ligament repair augmented with a suture tape. Foot Ankle Int. 2018;39(3):304.
6. Acevedo J, Vora A. Anatomical reconstruction of the spring ligament complex: "internal brace" augmentation. Foot Ankle Spec. 2013;6(6):441.
7. Lubowitz JH, MacKay G, Gilmer B. Knee medial collateral ligament and posteromedial corner anatomic repair with internal bracing. Arthrosc Tech. 2014;3(4):e505.
8. Hirahara AM, Mackay G, Andersen WJ. Ultrasound-guided suture tape augmentation and stabilization of the medial collateral ligament. Arthrosc Tech. 2018;7(3):e205.
9. van der List JP, DiFelice GS. Arthroscopic primary posterior cruciate ligament repair with suture augmentation. Arthrosc Tech. 2017;6(5):e1685.
10. Hopper GP, Mackay GM. Achilles tendon repair using the InternalBrace principle. Surg Technol Int. 2017;30:325.
11. Byrne PA, Hopper GP, Wilson WT, Mackay GM. Knotless repair of achilles tendon rupture in an elite athlete: return to competition in 18 weeks. J Foot Ankle Surg. 2017;56(1):121.
12. Sanchez G, Ferrari MB, Sanchez A, Moatshe G, Chahla J, DePhillipo N, Provencher MT. Proximal patellar tendon repair: internal brace technique with unicortical buttons and suture tape. Arthrosc Tech. 2017;6(2):e491.
13. Byrne PA, Hopper GP, Wilson WT, Mackay GM. Acromioclavicular joint stabilisation using the internal brace principle. Surg Technol Int. 2018;33:294–8.
14. Butler DL, Noyes FR, Grood ES. Ligamentous restraints to anterior-posterior drawer in the human

knee. A biomechanical study. J Bone Joint Surg Am. 1980;62(2):259.
15. Anderson MJ, Browning WM, Urband CE, Kluczynski MA, Bisson LJ. A systematic summary of systematic reviews on the topic of the anterior cruciate ligament. Orthop J Sports Med. 2016;4(3):2325967116634074.
16. Lohmander LS, Ostenberg A, Englund M, Roos H. High prevalence of knee osteoarthritis, pain, and functional limitations in female soccer players twelve years after anterior cruciate ligament injury. Arthritis Rheum. 2004;50(10):3145.
17. Leiter JR, Gourlay R, McRae S, de Korompay N, MacDonald PB. Long-term follow-up of ACL reconstruction with hamstring autograft. Knee Surg Sports Traumatol Arthrosc. 2014;22(5):1061.
18. von Porat A, Roos EM, Roos H. High prevalence of osteoarthritis 14 years after an anterior cruciate ligament tear in male soccer players: a study of radiographic and patient relevant outcomes. Ann Rheum Dis. 2004;63(3):269.
19. Ajuied A, Wong F, Smith C, Norris M, Earnshaw P, Back D, Davies A. Anterior cruciate ligament injury and radiologic progression of knee osteoarthritis: a systematic review and meta-analysis. Am J Sports Med. 2014;42(9):2242.
20. England RL. Repair of the ligaments about the knee. Orthop Clin North Am. 1976;7(1):195.
21. Weaver JK, Derkash RS, Freeman JR, Kirk RE, Oden RR, Matyas J. Primary knee ligament repair—revisited. Clin Orthop Relat Res. 1985;199:185.
22. Sherman MF, Bonamo JR. Primary repair of the anterior cruciate ligament. Clin Sports Med. 1988;7(4):739.
23. Feagin JA, Curl WW. Isolated tear of the anterior cruciate ligament: 5-year follow-up study. Am J Sports Med. 1976;4(3):95.
24. Lysholm J, Gillquist J, Liljedahl SO. Long-term results after early treatment of knee injuries. Acta Orthop Scand. 1982;53(1):109.
25. Engebretsen L, Benum P, Sundalsvoll S. Primary suture of the anterior cruciate ligament. A 6-year follow-up of 74 cases. Acta Orthop Scand. 1989;60(5):561.
26. Engebretsen L, Benum P, Fasting O, Mølster A, Strand T. A prospective, randomized study of three surgical techniques for treatment of acute ruptures of the anterior cruciate ligament. Am J Sports Med. 1990;18(6):585.
27. Andersson C, Odensten M, Gillquist J. Knee function after surgical or nonsurgical treatment of acute rupture of the anterior cruciate ligament: a randomized study with a long-term follow-up period. Clin Orthop Relat Res. 1991;264:255.
28. Smith PA, Bley JA. Allograft anterior cruciate ligament reconstruction utilizing internal brace augmentation. Arthrosc Tech. 2016;5(5):e1143.
29. Barrett DS. Proprioception and function after anterior cruciate reconstruction. J Bone Joint Surg Br. 1991;73(5):833.
30. Co FH, Skinner HB, Cannon WD. Effect of reconstruction of the anterior cruciate ligament on proprioception of the knee and the heel strike transient. J Orthop Res. 1993;11(5):696.
31. Fridén T, Roberts D, Ageberg E, Waldén M, Zätterström R. Review of knee proprioception and the relation to extremity function after an anterior cruciate ligament rupture. J Orthop Sports Phys Ther. 2001;31(10):567.
32. Ardern CL, Taylor NF, Feller JA, Webster KE. Return-to-sport outcomes at 2 to 7 years after anterior cruciate ligament reconstruction surgery. Am J Sports Med. 2012;40(1):41.
33. Setuain I, Izquierdo M, Idoate F, Bikandi E, Gorostiaga EM, Aagaard P, Cadore EL, Alfaro-Adrián J. Differential effects of 2 rehabilitation programs following anterior cruciate ligament reconstruction. J Sport Rehabil. 2017;26(6):544.
34. Konrath JM, Vertullo CJ, Kennedy BA, Bush HS, Barrett RS, Lloyd DG. Morphologic characteristics and strength of the hamstring muscles remain altered at 2 years after use of a hamstring tendon graft in anterior cruciate ligament reconstruction. Am J Sports Med. 2016;44(10):2589.
35. Xie X, Xiao Z, Li Q, Zhu B, Chen J, Chen H, Yang F, Chen Y, Lai Q, Liu X. Increased incidence of osteoarthritis of knee joint after ACL reconstruction with bone-patellar tendon-bone autografts than hamstring autografts: a meta-analysis of 1,443 patients at a minimum of 5 years. Eur J Orthop Surg Traumatol. 2015;25(1):149.
36. Kowalk DL, Duncan JA, McCue FC, Vaughan CL. Anterior cruciate ligament reconstruction and joint dynamics during stair climbing. Med Sci Sports Exerc. 1997;29(11):1406.
37. Poehling-Monaghan KL, Salem H, Ross KE, Secrist E, Ciccotti MC, Tjoumakaris F, Ciccotti MG, Freedman KB. Long-term outcomes in anterior cruciate ligament reconstruction: a systematic review of patellar tendon versus hamstring autografts. Orthop J Sports Med. 2017;5(6):2325967117709735.
38. Leys T, Salmon L, Waller A, Linklater J, Pinczewski L. Clinical results and risk factors for reinjury 15 years after anterior cruciate ligament reconstruction: a prospective study of hamstring and patellar tendon grafts. Am J Sports Med. 2012;40(3):595.
39. Gifstad T, Foss OA, Engebretsen L, Lind M, Forssblad M, Albrektsen G, Drogset JO. Lower risk of revision with patellar tendon autografts compared with hamstring autografts: a registry study based on 45,998 primary ACL reconstructions in Scandinavia. Am J Sports Med. 2014;42(10):2319.
40. Persson A, Fjeldsgaard K, Gjertsen JE, Kjellsen AB, Engebretsen L, Hole RM, Fevang JM. Increased risk of revision with hamstring tendon grafts compared with patellar tendon grafts after anterior cruciate ligament reconstruction: a study of 12,643 patients from the Norwegian Cruciate Ligament Registry, 2004–2012. Am J Sports Med. 2014;42(2):285.

41. Lind M, Menhert F, Pedersen AB. Incidence and outcome after revision anterior cruciate ligament reconstruction: results from the Danish registry for knee ligament reconstructions. Am J Sports Med. 2012;40(7):1551.
42. Chahla J, Moatshe G, Cinque ME, Dornan GJ, Mitchell JJ, Ridley TJ, LaPrade RF. Single-bundle and double-bundle posterior cruciate ligament reconstructions: a systematic review and meta-analysis of 441 patients at a minimum 2 years' follow-up. Arthroscopy. 2017;33(11):2066.
43. Belk JW, Kraeutler MJ, Purcell JM, McCarty EC. Autograft versus allograft for posterior cruciate ligament reconstruction: an updated systematic review and meta-analysis. Am J Sports Med. 2017;46(7):1752–7.
44. LaPrade CM, Civitarese DM, Rasmussen MT, LaPrade RF. Emerging updates on the posterior cruciate ligament: a review of the current literature. Am J Sports Med. 2015;43(12):3077.
45. Smith C, Ajuied A, Wong F, Norris M, Back D, Davies A. The use of the ligament augmentation and reconstruction system (LARS) for posterior cruciate reconstruction. Arthroscopy. 2014;30(1):111.
46. Kannus P, Bergfeld J, Järvinen M, Johnson RJ, Pope M, Renström P, Yasuda K. Injuries to the posterior cruciate ligament of the knee. Sports Med. 1991;12(2):110.
47. Van de Velde SK, Bingham JT, Gill TJ, Li G. Analysis of tibiofemoral cartilage deformation in the posterior cruciate ligament-deficient knee. J Bone Joint Surg Am. 2009;91(1):167.
48. Lee DY, Park YJ. Single-bundle versus double-bundle posterior cruciate ligament reconstruction: a meta-analysis of randomized controlled trials. Knee Surg Relat Res. 2017;29(4):246.
49. Difelice GS, Lissy M, Haynes P. Surgical technique: when to arthroscopically repair the torn posterior cruciate ligament. Clin Orthop Relat Res. 2012;470(3):861.
50. Pournaras J, Symeonides PP. The results of surgical repair of acute tears of the posterior cruciate ligament. Clin Orthop Relat Res. 1991;267:103.
51. Strand T, Mølster AO, Engesaeter LB, Raugstad TS, Alho A. Primary repair in posterior cruciate ligament injuries. Acta Orthop Scand. 1984;55(5):545.
52. Hughston JC, Bowden JA, Andrews JR, Norwood LA. Acute tears of the posterior cruciate ligament. Results of operative treatment. J Bone Joint Surg Am. 1980;62(3):438.
53. Wheatley WB, Martinez AE, Sacks T, Schurhoff MR, Uribe JW, Hechtman KS, Zvijac JE. Arthroscopic posterior cruciate ligament repair. Arthroscopy. 2002;18(7):695.
54. Del Buono A, Radmilovic J, Gargano G, Gatto S, Maffulli N. Augmentation or reconstruction of PCL? A quantitative review. Knee Surg Sports Traumatol Arthrosc. 2013;21(5):1050.
55. Yoon KH, Bae DK, Song SJ, Lim CT. Arthroscopic double-bundle augmentation of posterior cruciate ligament using split Achilles allograft. Arthroscopy. 2005;21(12):1436.
56. Jung YB, Jung HJ, Song KS, Kim JY, Lee HJ, Lee JS. Remnant posterior cruciate ligament-augmenting stent procedure for injuries in the acute or subacute stage. Arthroscopy. 2010;26(2):223.

Anterior Cruciate Ligament Reconstruction

16

John Dabis and Adrian Wilson

16.1 Introduction

16.1.1 Anatomy

Detailed understanding of the anterior cruciate ligament (ACL) anatomy is the basis for an anatomical ACL reconstruction. Many authors understood the tibial ACL insertion to be oval, with the insertion of the anteromedial (AM) bundle in the AM aspect and in direct relation to the medial tibial spine, whereas the posterolateral (PL) bundle was defined as inserting into the PL aspect of the ACL footprint in close relation to the lateral tibial spine directly anterior to the posterior root of the lateral meniscus. Siebold et al. [1] performed an anatomical cadaveric study to investigate the macroscopic appearance of the mid-substance ACL and tibial insertion in fresh frozen and paraffined knee specimens. The tibial insertion is "C" shaped from along the medial tibial spine to the anterior aspect of the anterior root of the lateral meniscus around a central and PL area. There are no centrally inserting ACL fibres and no PL tibial ACL insertion. The outer fibres of the anterior and posterior horns of the lateral meniscus blend with the "C"-shaped ACL insertion. The ACL forms a "ring"-like structure with the lateral meniscus. The ACL has direct and indirect tibial insertions with the direct insertion being the narrow but long "C"-shaped attachment, whereas the indirect fibres extend from the mid-substance fibres and broadly spread underneath the transverse ligament towards the anterior rim of the tibial plateau in a "fanlike extension." Both insertions together form a "duck-foot-like" bony ACL footprint. Smigielski et al. [2] evaluated the macroscopic appearance of the ACL from the femoral origin to the mid-substance. In all the fresh frozen cadaveric knees, the intra-ligamentous part of the ACL from close to its femoral insertion to mid-substance was observed to have a ribbon-like structure. The femoral bony insertion of the ribbon was in exact continuity of the posterior femoral cortex. This confirmed earlier reports, by Mochizuki et al. [3], that the configuration of the fibres in the mid-substance to be "rather flat like, looking like lasagne." Like the tibia, the femur has a direct femoral ACL insertion in which dense collagen fibres are connected to the bone by a fibrocartilaginous layer. This direct insertion is located in a depression between the lateral intercondylar ridge and 7–10 mm anterior to the articular cartilage margin. The indirect attachment of the thin fibrous tissue extends from the mid-substance fibres and broadly spreads out like a fan on the posterior condyle.

J. Dabis (✉)
Brisbane Orthopaedic & Sports Medicine Centre, Spring Hill, QLD, Australia
e-mail: J.dabis@nhs.net

A. Wilson
Queen Anne Medical Centre & The Wellington Hospital, London, UK

M. Brittberg, K. Slynarski (eds.), *Lower Extremity Joint Preservation*,
https://doi.org/10.1007/978-3-030-57382-9_16

16.1.2 Biomechanics

When the ACL is subjected to tensile loading, the resulting load-elongation curve represents the structural properties of the ACL. The fibres within the ACL have an initial toe region. The stress decreases with increased strain due to the uncoiling of the crimped fibres. Stress is proportional to strain in the linear region, and the area under the linear region represents energy. Dips herald the end of the linear region and represent plastic deformation. As there is very little plastic deformation for ligaments, the dips occur because of sequential fibre failure with increased strain. The ligament structure also expresses viscoelastic properties such as creep and stress relaxation. Definitions of the former; under sustained constant stress there is time-dependant deformation and the latter; under constant sustained strain there is a time-dependant reduction in stress. The ACL is the primary restraint against anterior tibial translation in relation to the femur. In the native ACL, there is no true isometry due to the different kinematic properties of its individual fibres and bundles and its complex geometry. The secondary role of the ACL is to resist internal tibial rotation, which is most pronounced in knee extension. As far as the bundles are concerned, the AM bundle is orientated more vertically in the intercondylar notch in the coronal plane. It therefore has very little ability to restrain rotation as it is located close to the vertical axis of rotation. The PL bundle, however, has a more horizontal orientation and is more distant to the axis of rotation. Taylor et al. investigated the length and relative strain of the ACL during the gait cycle using a combination of marker-based motion capture, MR imaging and biplanar fluoroscopy. The ACL length and knee flexion were inversely related. Maximum relative strain levels correlated to instances when flexion angles were at their lowest; the relative strain in the ACL was highest at mid-stance with the knee near full extension [4].

16.1.3 Operative Techniques

16.1.3.1 Timing

The optimal timing for ACL reconstruction remains controversial [5]. Persistent instability and delayed reconstruction will increase the risk of chondral and meniscal injury [6, 7].

Several studies have attempted to ascertain the optimal time frame for intervention, some studies quoting a duration as short as 6 weeks and some as long as 12 months; however there is no consensus. The landmark publication by Shelbourne et al. recommended delaying surgery for at least 3 weeks to reduce the incidence of arthrofibrosis. Recent evidence has suggested there is no difference in clinical outcome between patients who underwent early and delayed ACL reconstruction [8]. Mok et al. investigated the correlation between times of surgery with the prevalence of concomitant intra-articular injuries detected on arthroscopy during ACL reconstruction. Over 650 ACL reconstructions were retrospectively reviewed; univariate and multivariate logistic regression analysis was performed. 39.7% of the study population had a medial meniscal tear which was detected on arthroscopy. The presence of medial meniscal tears was significantly associated with increasing time to surgery, >12 months compared to <3 months after index injury [9].

16.1.3.2 Graft Options

Graft selection can be divided into three broad categories:

- Autograft.
- Allograft.
- Synthetics.

The most commonly used are the hamstring tendon autografts (HT) and bone-patellar tendon-bone (BPTB) autografts. Grafts used for ACL reconstruction should recreate the anatomical and biomechanical properties of the native ligament, guarantee safe fixation, provide rapid biological integration, and reduce donor site morbidity [10]. BPTB grafts have long been considered the gold standard surgical graft option. However, in order to minimize donor site morbidity associated with the harvest, HT grafts are being increasingly used. Literature has quoted the intact ACL ultimate tensile load (UTL) to be 2160 N. The doubled semitendinosus and gracilis tendon grafts have greater mechanical strength (UTL 4090 N) than a BTB (UTL 2977 N).

There are a few ways to form a single-bundle quadruple hamstring autograft:

- By doubling the semitendinosus and gracilis tendons.
- Quadrupling semitendinosus.

One main concern, with graft preparation, is if the diameter of the graft is less than 8 mm, there is an increased risk of graft revision [11, 12]. However, by utilising the whole HT length, five- or six-strand HT autografts can reliably provide grafts with diameters greater than or equal to 8 mm [13].

After HT harvest, the ST and G can be left attached the pes insertion. The ST and G are doubled over a high-resistance #2 suture. Constant tension is maintained on the high-resistance suture. A ruler then measures 8 cm of graft from the pes, and the high-resistance suture is moved to this position. A curved haemostat now anchors the base of the HT at the pes to the HT ensuring 8 cm of graft is maintained. The distal end of the HT, whether it be one or two strands, is then attached to a curved clip, and this is manoeuvred to be enveloped by the ST and G folded over the high-resistance suture. 2–0 high-resistance non-resorbable sutures are then whip stitched on the proximal and distal ends of the graft. This triplicating procedure achieves a strong six-folded graft. The best method of incorporating the tripled strand into the construct of a suspensory fixation is unknown.

Historically quadriceps tendon (QT) autografts had inferior biomechanical properties compared with the native ACL and was associated with high rates of rotatory knee laxity and quadriceps weakness. QT autograft has been shown to have a significantly larger cross-sectional area than BPTB autografts (91.2 ± 10 mm^2 vs. 48.4 ± 8 mm^2) and greater ultimate load to failure (2186.9 ± 758 N vs. 1580 ± 479 N). The QT is very versatile and can be harvested in different lengths, widths and thicknesses and can be used with or without a bone block. MRI can also assess tendon thickness. QT harvest is safe and is associated with minimum donor site morbidity. Various series have published results suggesting QT autograft may be preferable to BPTB with respect to post-operative knee stability, range of motion and functional outcomes. Several recent comparative studies have investigated the difference in clinical outcome between HT and QT autografts. Cavaignac et al. performed a retrospective comparative review assessing the functional outcome differences between QT and HT autografts.

- There were no significant differences in reoperation rates between the two groups.
- The functional outcome scores (Lysholm, KOOS symptoms and KOOS sport) were all significantly better in the QT group.
- The QT group had significantly better mean side-to-side differences based on the KT-1000 compared to the HT group (1.1 ± 0.9 mm vs. 3.1 ± 1.3 mm, respectively) [14].

Runer et al. [15] demonstrated no difference at any follow-up until 2 years in any of the patient-reported outcome measures. They found the QT to be a reliable graft alternative to HT for primary ACL reconstruction.

16.1.3.3 Techniques

Single-Bindle ACL Reconstruction

There remains controversy in the optimal tunnel positioning. There has been an evolution of ACL reconstruction techniques over the last few decades with a decline in femoral tunnel drilling through a transtibial technique with an increase in lateral "outside-in" retrosockets and medial portal femoral socket preparation. With transtibial femoral preparation, the femoral socket placement is dictated by the tibial tunnel which invariably results in a relatively vertical position of the graft. Although good early clinical outcomes, the procedure is shown to be non-anatomic. Alternative methods for femoral tunnel preparation are anteromedial (AM) portal drilling in which independent tunnel preparation is performed. Exact appreciation of the intra-articular bony anatomy on the medial face of the lateral femoral condyle, including the intercondylar and bifurcate ridges, is required. Anatomic footprint ACL reconstruction, in its current form, utilises an accessory medial portal which allows simultaneous medial viewing and preparation of the femoral tunnel. Despite improved visualisation, issues with overcrowding can occur especially with the knee in hyperflexion. The trans-lateral technique can avoid these issues as femoral tunnel preparation is performed with the knee in 90° of flexion. The portals in the trans-lateral techniques are lower and more central than conventional techniques, and all the femoral preparation is carried out through the lateral portal. Other advantages of the trans-lateral technique include being able to place the femoral tunnel in an anatomic position without the pitfalls of creating an accessory medial portal. This technique can be employed to utilise the standard hamstring graft preparation in which semitendinosus and gracilis are doubled to make a four-strand hamstring graft. Alternatively, a single semitendinosus hamstring tendon can be harvested and quadrupled to perform an "all-inside" ACL reconstruction [16]. The gracilis tendon can be preserved and will serve as a secondary stabiliser or for use as further graft.

- The patient is positioned supine with the knee flexed to 90°.
- A side support and foot rest are used.
- A thigh tourniquet is used.
- The modified anterolateral portal is used.
- Following a single semitendinosus tendon harvest, the quadrupled HT is prepared on two adjustable cortico-suspensory devices (TightRope RT, Arthrex) to make a GraftLink.
- The medial wall of the lateral femoral condyle wall is prepared with a curved radiofrequency probe to preserve the bifurcate and intercondylar ridges. This allows the native footprint to be preserved and the femoral position to be marked out.
- The femoral and tibial tunnels are created by the retrograde "outside in" approach; the femoral guide is inserted through the modified AL portal and positioned at the pre-marked anatomic femoral origin.
- With the knee flexed to 90°, a 3.5 mm femoral pilot hole is created with the flipcutter by an outside-in drilling method. A retrosocket is created to a depth of 20 mm.
- A stiffened plastic tube containing high-tensile strength loop of suture is passed through the femoral tunnel, and this is retrieved in the knee joint.
- The tibial tunnel is prepared in the same way. A tibial retrosocket of 35 mm is ideally created.
- A semitendinosus HT harvest of 26–27 cm is ideal; after quadrupling the tendon, a graft of 68–70 mm should be prepared.
- One end of each tunnel suture is retrieved through the AM portal simultaneously to avoid soft tissue bridging.
- Pull through loops are fashioned at the end of each socket sutures. Firstly, the GraftLink is docked and bottomed out into the femoral tunnel, and the button is flipped on the lateral cortex of the femur.
- The tibial cortical suspensory device is shuttled through the tibial tunnel, and the button is flipped. The knee is cycled, and final tensioning of the graft by synching the adjustable loops is the final stage.

Double-Bundle ACL Reconstruction

Despite successful short-term clinical outcomes with traditional reconstructions techniques, poor long-term outcomes with early onset degenerative arthrosis have been reported.

Inadequate restoration of normal knee kinematics is possibly the most important cause for this accelerated change. A move away from conventional techniques, such as transtibial drilling, which put the graft in a non-anatomic position, led to a move towards "anatomic" reconstruction focusing on locating the graft within the native ACL footprint. Double-bundle ACL reconstruction was developed to improve the procedure with a more anatomic restoration of both the anteromedial (AM) and posterolateral (PL) bundles. The aim was to recreate the two individual bundles to restore normal knee biomechanics [17, 18]. Each bundle has different insertion sites and different tension patterns. Double-bundle reconstruction (DBR) was thought to replicate native ACL closer than conventional single-bundle reconstructions. The diameter of the AM bundle is usually in the range between 6 and 7 mm and for the PL bundle between 5 and 6 mm. Therefore the size of the knee may be the most important factor which may influence the decision to proceed with a single-bundle or double-bundle reconstruction. DBR involves four tunnels and passage of two grafts which can be technically challenging leading to increased complications and high patient morbidity rates with no added benefit in clinical outcome [19, 20]. For these reasons, DBR lost popularity; however, long-term studies showing reduced graft failure rates with DBR have recently been published [21, 22].

DBR is said to be indicated in high-level athletes as well as pivoting sports. DBR may restore knee kinematics during pivot shift testing better than single-bundle reconstruction in patients with ACL ruptures associated with meniscal injury [23]. The drilling of the femoral tunnels may be performed with special aimers or freehand technique.

- The AM and PL bone tunnel positions are marked with an awl. It is critical to maintain sufficient distance between the markings to preserve a bony bridge between the two tunnels.
- The use of fluoroscopy can be used to prevent incorrect positions; a guide pin is placed to the marked AM position and drilled through the femoral condyle at 120° of knee flexion.
- A tunnel depth of 25–35 mm is created with a diameter of the HT harvest.
- The PL femoral tunnel is drilled in a similar fashion in a flexion angle between 90° and 130°.
- Both grafts are deployed from distal to proximal and seated into the femoral tunnels.
- The PL graft is passed first. The tibial tunnels are prepared with a tibial drill guide.
- The AM tunnel is prepared first and placed on the AM aspect of the ACL footprint.
- The PL tunnel position is on the PL aspect of the tibial footprint, and new studies have suggested the tibial insertion sight to be at the posteromedial aspect of the ACL footprint.
- Both angles on the tibial guide are set to 55°.
- The PL tibial tunnel position is more medial than the standard tibial tunnel.
- An osseous bridge of 1–2 cm between the two tibial tunnels should be preserved.

16.1.4 Anterolateral Complex (ALC) Reconstruction

Even with a well-performed single- or double-bundle reconstruction, rotatory laxity can persist. The ACL has an oblique orientation close to the centre of rotation so its lever arm to control rotation is limited. Lateral extra-articular procedures were promoted as having a biomechanical advantage over intra-articular reconstructions in terms of rotational control [24, 25]. Combined ACL reconstruction and ALC reconstruction is associated with a significantly lower rate of failure of medial meniscal repairs when compared with those performed at the time of isolated ACL reconstruction [26]. Slocum and Larson first recognised the importance of rotational instability in the ACL deficient knee [27]. There are numerous techniques to address anterolateral extra-articular stabilisation. Lemaire was one of the first described techniques where a strip of iliotibial band is harvested [28]. It is detached proximally and left attached to Gerdy's, and the strip is routed under the LCL before passing through a bone tunnel proximal and posterior to the lateral epicondyle. The graft is then passed under the LCL again before being secure in a second bony tunnel at Gerdy's tubercle. Macintosh described a similar procedure; however, no bone tunnels were used. The ITB strip is passed under the LCL and passed through a subperiosteal tunnel behind the origin of the LCL and looped behind the insertion of the lateral intermuscular septum, before passing under the LCL. Macintosh also described a combined intra- and extra-articular reconstruction passing the ITB graft over the top behind the lateral femoral condyle into the joint.

More anatomical-based anterolateral ligament (ALL) reconstructions use the gracilis tendon to recreate the anterolateral ligament complex. There are several techniques which have been described addressing the ALL [29]. A hamstring graft can either be fashioned in a triangular shape, by creating two tibial tunnels, to mimic the wider anatomy of the distal ALL or by a single-bundle reconstruction [30, 31]. It is essential to perform an isometry test before ALL reconstruction to avoid over constraint of the lateral compartment. Physiological non-isometric ALL graft reconstruction is the aim. The suture isometry test should be tight in extension and loose in flexion. The femoral tunnel is located proximal and posterior to the lateral epicondyle.

Following the ALC consensus group meeting in October 2017, several aims were discussed including developing a consensus in terms of the anatomical terminology utilised for structures with in the ALC, to produce position statements as to the kinematic role of key structures in the knee, pertaining specifically to anterolateral rotatory laxity and ACL deficiency and providing clinical guidance on when to utilise an anterolateral procedure in the ACL deficient knee. Appropriate indications include revision ACL reconstructions, high-grade pivot shift, generalised ligamentous laxity and genu recurvatum and young patients returning to pivoting activities [32]. A well-designed multicentre randomized clinical trial comparing anterior cruciate ligament reconstruction with and without lateral extra-articular tenodesis in individuals who are at high risk of graft failure is currently being undertaken. The results are yet to be published and, however, will be of interest to the orthopaedic community dealing with these complex injuries.

16.1.4.1 Outcomes

Claes et al. [33] performed a meta-analysis assessing the long-term outcome after autologous ACL reconstruction. The definition of osteoarthritis was based on the IKDC radiological grading system. Many of the included reports mentioned a subpopulation of meniscectomised patients at final follow-up; therefore, the radiographic outcome of this subset of patients was studied separately to evaluate the impact of meniscectomy on the prevalence of osteoarthritis. Two hundred and eleven articles were isolated as part of the meta-analysis; however, only five prospective studies and 11 retrospective studies, culminating in 1554 subject, fulfilled the search criteria. The combined estimate for the prevalence of OA, i.e. IKDC C or D, was 27.9%. The subgroup analysis revealed patients who did not undergo meniscectomy had an OA prevalence of 16.4%; however, patients undergoing meniscectomy had an OA prevalence of 50.4%. The results demonstrate the prevalence of knee OA after ACL reconstruction is significantly lower than commonly perceived.

16.1.4.2 Rehabilitation

Initial and early phase rehabilitation focuses on pain relief, anti-inflammatories, restoration of free range of movement and neuromuscular control. Bracing following ACL reconstruction was once thought to improve the outcomes by improving extension and decreasing pain and graft strain and provides protection from excessive force. Evidence now has been published refuting this, and a systematic review of 12 level 1 randomised controlled trials failed to find any evidence that pain, range of motion and graft stability were any different in the braced groups [34]. The first two weeks should consist of:

- Knee extensor muscle training.
- Isometric closed kinetic chain exercises as these avoid increased tension on the graft.

Closed chain exercises, with the distal segment fixed, produce co-contraction of the hamstrings and quadriceps causing contraction within the joint.

Open-chain exercises without additional weight are safe after 2 weeks following the reconstruction. Open-chain exercises are essential in the rehabilitation after ACL reconstruction as these exercises address quadriceps strength.

To prevent flexion deformities, early active and passive range of movement with an emphasis on full extension is critical. It is important to resume full weight bearing for cartilage nutrition and facilitation of collagen reorganisation during healing. During the first 4 postoperative weeks, stair climbing is recommended with the healthy leg up first and with the operated leg down, to avoid overload on the graft.

The intermediate phase should concentrate on normalizing lower extremity muscle strength for performing activities of daily living. Manual therapy and patella mobilisations are encouraged. Closed chain kinetic exercises are further emphasized in this phase to increase joint stability. An example of a lower leg strengthening exercise which has low loads on the graft is leg press. Another example is the double-leg squat and single-leg squat. The double-leg squat should be optimised before undertaking the single-leg squat. Neuromuscular training is especially important to avoid abnormal joint translation. Static balance exercises such as single- or double-leg stance on flat surfaces with progression to unstable surfaces are examples of this. Progression to dynamic balance exercises help to keep the knee stable during the landing phase.

The late phase of rehabilitation focuses on regaining dynamic joint stability to allow functional movement patterns which are needed both for low-level and high-level sport activities. Plyometric exercises with increased resistance muscle strength training also occur in this phase. Sport-specific training should be the main focus.

References

1. Siebold R, Schuhmacher P, Fernandez F, Śmigielski R, Fink C, Brehmer A, Kirsch J. Flat midsubstance of the anterior cruciate ligament with tibial "C"-shaped insertion site. Knee Surg Sports Traumatol Arthrosc. 2015;23(11):3136–42.
2. Śmigielski R, Zdanowicz U, Drwięga M, Ciszek B, Ciszkowska-Łysoń B, Siebold R. Ribbon like appearance of the midsubstance fibres of the anterior cruciate ligament close to its femoral insertion site: a cadaveric study including 111 knees. Knee Surg Sports Traumatol Arthrosc. 2015;23(11):3143–50.
3. Mochizuki T, Fujishiro H, Nimura A, Mahakkanukrauh P, Yasuda K, Muneta T, Akita K. Anatomic and histologic analysis of the mid-substance and fan-like extension fibres of the anterior cruciate ligament during knee motion, with special reference to the femoral attachment. Knee Surg Sports Traumatol Arthrosc. 2014;22(2):336–44.
4. Taylor KA, Cutcliffe HC, Queen RM, Utturkar GM, Spritzer CE, Garrett WE, DeFrate LE. In vivo measurement of ACL length and relative strain during walking. J Biomech. 2013;46(3):478–83.
5. Smith TO, Davies L, Hing CB. Early versus delayed surgery for anterior cruciate ligament reconstruction: a systematic review and meta-analysis. Knee Surg Sports Traumatol Arthrosc. 2010;18(3):304–11.
6. Manandhar RR, Chandrashekhar K, Kumaraswamy V, Sahanand S, Rajan D. Functional outcome of an early anterior cruciate ligament reconstruction in comparison to delayed: are we waiting in vain? J Clin Orthop Trauma. 2018;9(2):163–6.
7. Kay J, Memon M, Shah A, Yen YM, Samuelsson K, Peterson D, Simunovic N, Flageole H, Ayeni OR. Earlier anterior cruciate ligament reconstruction is associated with a decreased risk of medial meniscal and articular cartilage damage in children and adolescents: a systematic review and meta-analysis. Knee Surg Sports Traumatol Arthrosc. 2018;26(12):3738–53.
8. Kwok CS, Harrison T, Servant C. The optimal timing for anterior cruciate ligament reconstruction with respect to the risk of postoperative stiffness. Arthroscopy. 2013;29(3):556–65.
9. Mok YR, Wong KL, Panjwani T, Chan CX, Toh SJ, Krishna L. Anterior cruciate ligament reconstruction performed within 12 months of the index injury is associated with a lower rate of medial meniscus tears. Knee Surg Sports Traumatol Arthrosc. 2019;27:117–23.
10. Lord BR, El-Daou H, Sabnis BM, Gupte CM, Wilson AM, Amis AA. Biomechanical comparison of graft structures in anterior cruciate ligament recon-

struction. Knee Surg Sports Traumatol Arthrosc. 2017;25(2):559–68.
11. Magnussen RA, Lawrence JT, West RL, Toth AP, Taylor DC, Garrett WE. Graft size and patient age are predictors of early revision after anterior cruciate ligament reconstruction with hamstring autograft. Arthroscopy. 2012;28(4):526–31.
12. Conte EJ, Hyatt AE, Gatt CJ Jr, Dhawan A. Hamstring autograft size can be predicted and is a potential risk factor for anterior cruciate ligament reconstruction failure. Arthroscopy. 2014;30(7):882–90.
13. Tutkus V, Kluonaitis K, Silove S, Tutkuviene J. ACL reconstruction using 5- or 6-strand hamstring autograft provides graft's diameter bigger than 8 mm. Knee Surg Sports Traumatol Arthrosc. 2018;26(5):1349–56.
14. Cavaignac E, Coulin B, Tscholl P, Nik Mohd Fatmy N, Duthon V, Menetrey J. Is quadriceps tendon autograft a better choice than hamstring autograft for anterior cruciate ligament reconstruction? a comparative study with a mean follow-up of 3.6 years. Am J Sports Med. 2017;45(6):1326–32.
15. Runer A, Wierer G, Herbst E, Hepperger C, Herbort M, Gföller P, Hoser C, Fink C. There is no difference between quadriceps- and hamstring tendon autografts in primary anterior cruciate ligament reconstruction: a 2-year patient-reported outcome study. Knee Surg Sports Traumatol Arthrosc. 2018;26(2):605–14.
16. Wilson AJ, Yasen SK, Nancoo T, Stannard R, Smith JO, Logan JS. Anatomic all-inside anterior cruciate ligament reconstruction using the translateral technique. Arthrosc Tech. 2013;2(2):e99–e104.
17. Maeyama A, Hoshino Y, Kato Y, Debandi A, Lertwanich P, Wang JH, Smolinski P, Fu FH. Anatomic double bundle ACL reconstruction outperforms any types of single bundle ACL reconstructions in controlling dynamic rotational laxity. Knee Surg Sports Traumatol Arthrosc. 2018;26(5):1414–9.
18. Svantesson E, Sundemo D, Hamrin Senorski E, Alentorn-Geli E, Musahl V, Fu FH, Desai N, Stålman A, Samuelsson K. Double-bundle anterior cruciate ligament reconstruction is superior to single-bundle reconstruction in terms of revision frequency: a study of 22,460 patients from the Swedish National Knee Ligament Register. Knee Surg Sports Traumatol Arthrosc. 2017;25(12):3884–91.
19. Aga C, Risberg MA, Fagerland MW, Johansen S, Trøan, Heir S, Engebretsen L. No difference in the KOOS quality of life subscore between anatomic double-bundle and anatomic single-bundle anterior cruciate ligament reconstruction of the knee: a prospective randomized controlled trial with 2 years' follow-up. Am J Sports Med. 2018;46(10):2341–54.
20. El-Sherief FAH, Aldahshan WA, Wahd YE, Abdelaziz AM, Soliman HAG, Hassan TG, Elbehairy HF, Awadallah AH. Double-bundle anterior cruciate ligament reconstruction is better than single-bundle reconstruction in terms of objective assessment but not in terms of subjective score. Knee Surg Sports Traumatol Arthrosc. 2018;26(8):2395–400.
21. Järvelä T. Double-bundle versus single-bundle anterior cruciate ligament reconstruction: a prospective, randomize clinical study. Knee Surg Sports Traumatol Arthrosc. 2007;15(5):500–7.
22. Järvelä S, Kiekara T, Suomalainen P, Järvelä T. Double-bundle versus single-bundle anterior cruciate ligament reconstruction: a prospective randomized study with 10-year results. Am J Sports Med. 2017;45(11):2578–85.
23. Musahl V, Bedi A, Citak M, O'Loughlin P, Choi D, Pearle AD. Effect of single-bundle and double-bundle anterior cruciate ligament reconstructions on pivot-shift kinematics in anterior cruciate ligament- and meniscus-deficient knees. Am J Sports Med. 2011;39(2):289–95.
24. Kittl C, Inderhaug E, Williams A, Amis AA. Biomechanics of the anterolateral structures of the knee. Clin Sports Med. 2018;37(1):21–31.
25. Mathew M, Dhollander A, Getgood A. Anterolateral ligament reconstruction or extra-articular tenodesis: why and when? Clin Sports Med. 2018;37(1):75–86.
26. Sonnery-Cottet B, Saithna A, Blakeney WG, Ouanezar H, Borade A, Daggett M, Thaunat M, Fayard JM, Delaloye JR. Anterolateral ligament reconstruction protects the repaired medial meniscus: a comparative study of 383 anterior cruciate ligament reconstructions from the SANTI Study Group with a minimum follow-up of 2 years. Am J Sports Med. 2018;46(8):1819–26.
27. Slocum DB, Larson RL. Rotatory instability of the knee: its pathogenesis and a clinical test to demonstrate its presence. Clin Orthop Relat Res. 2007;454:5–13.
28. Lemaire M. Chronic knee instability. Technics and results of ligament plasty in sports injuries. J Chir (Paris). 1975;110(4):281–94. (French).
29. Claes S, Vereecke E, Maes M, Victor J, Verdonk P, Bellemans J. Anatomy of the anterolateral ligament of the knee. J Anat. 2013;223(4):321–8.
30. Sonnery-Cottet B, Thaunat M, Freychet B, Pupim BH, Murphy CG, Claes S. Outcome of a combined anterior cruciate ligament and anterolateral ligament reconstruction technique with a minimum 2-year follow-up. Am J Sports Med. 2015;43(7):1598–605.
31. Smith JO, Yasen SK, Lord B, Wilson AJ. Combined anterolateral ligament and anatomic anterior cruciate ligament reconstruction of the knee. Knee Surg Sports Traumatol Arthrosc. 2015;23(11):3151–6.
32. Getgood A, Brown C, Lording T, Amis A, Claes S, Geeslin A, Musahl V, ALC Consensus Group. The anterolateral complex of the knee: results from the International ALC Consensus Group Meeting. Knee Surg Sports Traumatol Arthrosc. 2018;27(1):166–76.
33. Claes S, Hermie L, Verdonk R, Bellemans J, Verdonk P. Is osteoarthritis an inevitable consequence of anterior cruciate ligament reconstruction? A meta-analysis. Knee Surg Sports Traumatol Arthrosc. 2013;21(9):1967–76.
34. Wright RW, Fetzer GB. Bracing after ACL reconstruction: a systematic review. Clin Orthop Relat Res. 2007;455:162–8. Review.

Preservation of the Anterior Cruciate Ligament: Arthroscopic Primary Repair of Proximal Tears

17

Jelle P. van der List, Anne Jonkergouw, and Gregory S. DiFelice

17.1 Introduction

Injury to the anterior cruciate ligament (ACL) is relatively common with an estimated incidence of over 200,000 cases per year in the United States [1–3]. Surgical treatment is the main choice of treatment for younger and more active patients, who wish to maintain an active lifestyle and/or participate in sports. The current gold standard of surgical treatment for ACL injuries consists of ACL reconstruction, in which the native tissue is removed and replaced by either autograft or allograft tissue in an attempt to simulate the native ACL.

Over the last decade, there has been a renewed interest in preservation of the ACL (mainly using primary repair) in which the torn ligament is preserved rather than removed and replaced. This has several advantages: native biology and proprioception are preserved, the procedure has significantly lower morbidity, and the knee function is potentially better restored at short and longer-term follow-up. In this book chapter, we will discuss the (1) history of primary repair, (2) rationale of modern-day primary repair, (3) patient selection, (4) surgical technique, (5) rehabilitation, and (6) outcomes of modern primary ACL repair. Finally, we will discuss the future clinical and research directions of primary ACL repair.

17.2 History of Primary Repair

The first documented surgical treatment of an ACL injury was performed over 120 years ago when Mayo Robson primarily repaired a proximally avulsed ACL and posterior cruciate ligament (PCL) back to the femur with a good outcome at 6-year follow-up [4]. In the twentieth century, the concept of primary repair was further developed by Palmar [5, 6] and O'Donoghue [7, 8] who both suggested better outcomes were achieved when performing early open repair when compared to the gold standard of that time that consisted of conservative treatment.

Open primary repair became the main surgical treatment in the 1970s, and several authors reported very good short-term (2-year) outcomes of this technique [9–11]. In 1976, however, Feagin and Curl were the first to report a

J. P. van der List (✉)
Orthopaedic Sports Medicine and Trauma Service, Department of Orthopaedic Surgery, Hospital for Special Surgery, New York-Presbyterian, Weill Medical College of Cornell University, New York, NY, USA

Department of Orthopaedic Surgery, Spaarne Gasthuis Hospital, Hoofddorp, The Netherlands

A. Jonkergouw · G. S. DiFelice
Orthopaedic Sports Medicine and Trauma Service, Department of Orthopaedic Surgery, Hospital for Special Surgery, New York-Presbyterian, Weill Medical College of Cornell University, New York, NY, USA
e-mail: difeliceg@hss.edu

M. Brittberg, K. Slynarski (eds.), *Lower Extremity Joint Preservation*, https://doi.org/10.1007/978-3-030-57382-9_17

deterioration of open primary repair outcomes at mid-term (5-year) follow-up [12]. In the following years, others also noted this deterioration of outcomes with longer follow-up [13–15]. As a result, several prospective trials comparing open primary repair with reconstruction and conservative treatment were performed [16–21] that noted that the outcomes of primary repair were inconsistent and could not be recommended as routine surgical treatment for ACL injury. These findings and studies ultimately led to the abandonment of the open primary repair technique at the early 1990s and the gold standard of treatment shifted toward ACL reconstruction for all patients, which is still the case today [22].

17.3 Rationale for Modern-Day Repair

The awareness of historical limitations along with several modern-day technological developments has resulted in a different assessment regarding the risks and benefits of primary ACL repair. We will first discuss the limitations of traditional open repair that contributed to the disappointing results in the historical literature and that are no longer limitations in the modern-day surgical treatment. Then we will discuss the advantages of primary repair over the current gold standard of ACL reconstruction in certain clinical situations and discuss why there is a place for ACL preservation and primary ACL repair in the current treatment algorithm of ACL injuries.

17.3.1 Limitations of Traditional Open Repair

When critically reviewing the historical literature of open primary repair, it becomes clear that several biases are present and that there may be a role for primary repair in the modern-day era. Firstly, and most importantly, the aforementioned studies in the open repair era did not take ACL tear location into account. In 1991, when Sherman et al. aimed to understand in 1991 the reasons for the deterioration of outcomes of open primary repair at mid-term follow-up, in what was considered a landmark paper by Feagin [15], they noted that patients with proximal avulsion (type I) tears and with good tissue quality had less deterioration of outcomes when compared to patients with midsubstance tears and poor tissue quality. Recently, our group performed a systematic review of historical studies on open primary repair and stratified the results by tear location: better outcomes were indeed found in studies that only performed primary repair in proximal tears, as opposed to studies repairing all tears or only midsubstance tears [23]. The difference in outcome between both tear locations could be explained by the fact that a proximally torn ACL can be reattached to the femoral wall and has been described to have similar healing capacities to the medial collateral ligament (MCL) [24], whereas midsubstance tears have been described to not heal as a result of the fibrin clot being washed away by the synovial fluid [25]. Reviewing these studies, it makes sense that there may be a role for primary repair in proximally avulsed tears with good tissue quality that are of sufficient length for reattachment to the femoral footprint.

Secondly, primary repair in the historical studies was performed via arthrotomy, whereas modern-day knee ligament surgery is routinely performed arthroscopically. Many patients complained of knee stiffness following open primary repair (and following open reconstruction), which could partially be explained by the invasiveness of the arthrotomy [26–28]. With modern-day arthroscopic surgery, the surgical morbidity of the procedure is dramatically less, and therefore one can expect less stiffness and knee pain following arthroscopic primary repair with resultant better outcomes.

Thirdly, most historical studies relied on prolonged long-time joint immobilization following ACL surgery, keeping patients for up to 6 weeks in a cast [15, 19, 29–31], which lasted until the pioneering work of Shelbourne et al. in the early 1990s [32, 33]. Prolonged joint immobilization can cause decreased range of motion (ROM), decreased function, and pain [34, 35], and one can expect better results for patients when an early ROM protocol is adopted.

When these points are taken into consideration, the rationale of why modern-day primary repair works as opposed to the disappointing historical outcomes can be explained, in large part, by the modern-day technical and scientific developments: good outcomes can be expected when only performing primary repair in patients with proximal tears and when using an arthroscopic approach and early motion rehabilitation protocol. In our opinion, this changes the current gold standard from a "one size fits all" reconstructive surgery to an individualized approach in which preservation depends critically on patient characteristics such as the tear type and tissue quality of the injured ACL.

17.3.2 Advantages of ACL Preservation

There are several (theoretical) advantages of preserving the ACL and rather performing primary repair than ACL reconstruction. Firstly, the native ligament and biology of the knee are preserved when repairing the ACL that consists of several nerve fibers that are thought to contribute to knee joint proprioception [36–38]. It has been reported that joint awareness (measured by the Forgotten Joint Score (FJS)) is relatively high following ACL reconstruction indicating that patients are aware of their knee joint following ACL reconstruction [39]. The designers of this score hypothesized that removing the remnant with its proprioception lowers this score and expect that there is less joint awareness for patients following ACL preservation surgery [39]. We noticed in our cohort that indeed patients following primary repair had signficantly less daily awareness of their operated knee when compared to patients following ACL reconstruction https://doi.org/10.1016/j.arthro.2019.09.041.

Secondly, the morbidity of arthroscopic primary ACL repair is significantly lower when compared to ACL reconstruction, as no grafts need to be harvested and no tunnels need to be drilled. Many patients following patellar tendon reconstruction complain of anterior knee pain and kneeling pain, whereas patients have decreased hamstring strength following hamstring tendon reconstruction [40, 41]. Anecdotally, it is not uncommon for patients being in seen in our offices for contralateral ACL injury or for revision ACL evaluation to describe having gone through ACL reconstruction as the worst experience of their lives. This is in dramatic distinction to the experience with arthroscopic primary repair where the morbidity of the surgery is similar to that of an arthroscopic meniscectomy and patients only use pain medications for a few days. As a result, patients usually have an easier recovery and pass rehabilitation milestones quicker, which will be discussed later in this chapter.

Thirdly, several studies have assessed the incidence of osteoarthritis following ACL reconstruction and have reported very high incidence (up to 78%) of radiographic osteoarthritis at 14-year follow-up [42–46], which might be explained by the fact that ACL reconstruction does not restore native kinematics and is a relatively invasive surgery in which a significant second trauma is induced [47–49]. Some long-term and experimental studies have suggested that primary repair results in a lower incidence of osteoarthritis when compared to reconstruction surgery [50, 51] although modern-day comparative long-term studies are needed to confirm these findings.

Finally, in the case that the patient experiences a reinjury and the primary ACL repair fails, no bridges have been burned for future primary ACL reconstruction surgery as no grafts have been harvested nor tunnels drilled. Furthermore, ACL reconstruction following failed ACL repair is similar to primary reconstruction https://doi.org/10.23736/S0394-3410.19.03924-9. This is very different from ACL reconstruction, where revision surgery can be fraught with difficulties that arise from pre-existing hardware, malpositioning of tunnels, and the fact that the optimal graft has oftentimes already been used. Not surprisingly, the outcomes of revision reconstruction surgery have been reported to be inferior compared to outcomes of primary reconstruction [52–54].

17.4 Patient Selection

Learning from the aforementioned historical studies, primary ACL repair should only be performed in a select group of patients. In this section, we discuss the tear type and tissue quality that characterize candidates for primary repair, the incidence of potential candidates, the timing in which to perform surgery, and other patient characteristics that predict the possibility of primary repair.

17.4.1 Tear Type and Tissue Quality

Recently, our group has developed a classification system for the different ACL tear types [55, 56], which consist of five tear types that depend on the location of the tear: proximal avulsion tears (tear in top 10% of ligament length), proximal tears (tear in top 10–25%), midsubstance tears (tear in middle 25–75%), distal tears (tear in bottom 75–90%), and distal avulsion tears (tear in bottom 10% of ligament) (Table 17.1). These tear types are based on different preservation techniques that can be used for each of these tears. The interobserver and intra-observer reliability of this classification system on MRI was good with 0.670 (95% confidence interval 0.505–0.836) and 0.741–0.934, respectively. In this chapter, we mainly discuss proximal avulsion type tears (Type 1) and proximal tears (Type 2) as these have the highest likelihood of being repairable (this is further discussed in Sect. 17.4.2. These tear types are often of sufficient length to be reapproximated to the femoral wall. Distal avulsion tears can also be repaired but remain out of the scope of this chapter as they are very rare (3% in adults) and more common in children (especially under age 11) [57–59] (Table 17.1).

In a previous study of 353 consecutive MRIs of adult patients with acute (<1 month) isolated complete ACL tears, our group has assessed the incidence of these different tear types [57] (Table 17.1). It was noted that 43% of all patients had a tear in the proximal quarter of which 16% had proximal avulsion type tears and 27% proximal tears that the majority of patients (52%) had midsubstance tears and only a minority had distal (1%) or distal avulsion type tears (3%). Furthermore, no femoral bony avulsion tears were seen, whereas most of the distal avulsion type tears were bony avulsions (2.5% of 3.1%). Our group has also assessed the tear types in pediatric and adolescent patients and noted that nearly all pediatric patients (92%) (<11 years of age) had bony avulsion type tears and that 32% of patients 11–13 years of age had proximal avulsion type tears, 16% proximal tears, and 32% midsubstance tears, whereas adolescent patients (aged 14–17 years) had a similar tear type distribution as adult patients [58] (Table 17.1).

Tissue quality has not been extensively researched and classified but is often referred to as the possibility to withhold sutures or not. In a previous MRI study [60], our group preoperatively assessed the tissue quality as "good," "fair," or "poor" depending on the direction of the fibers on MRI, and the signal intensity on T1 and T2

Table 17.1 Tear types of the anterior cruciate ligament with the incidence of different tear types on MRI in different age groups

Tear type	Description	Tear location, %	Incidence of tear types in different age groups <11 years [58], %	11–14 years [58], %	15–17 years [58], %	18–35 years [57], %	>35 years [57], %
Type I	Proximal avulsion	>90	7	32	14	8	23
Type II	Proximal	75–90	0	16	25	25	30
Type III	Midsubstance	25–75	0	32	57	60	45
Type IV	Distal	10–25	0	4	1	1	1
Type V	Distal (bony) avulsion	<10	93	16	2	6	1

MRI magnetic resonance imaging

images, but did not assess the interobserver and intra-observer reliability of this classification.

17.4.2 Incidence of Primary Repair

In a recent study, our group assessed the possibility of primary repair based on the preoperative MRI tear type classification [60]. It was noted that 90% of type I tears, 46% of type II tears, and 14% of type III tears were found repairable intraoperatively if surgery was performed within 3 months. When combining these numbers with the previously reported incidence of the different tear types, it can be estimated that 34% of all acute (<1 month) ACL tears can be repaired. The senior author utilizes an ACL preservation approach in which primary repair was performed when possible (depending on intraoperative tear type and tissue quality) and otherwise ACL reconstruction is performed. In fact, when utilizing this preservation approach, 44% of the last 380 patients underwent repair of the ACL. This discrepancy can likely be explained by the fact that patients with potentially repairable tears are commonly referred to the senior author in light of his pioneering experience in ACL preservation surgery.

17.4.3 Timing

Primary repair is generally performed in the relatively acute setting as better tissue quality is often seen in the acute setting, and several authors have described retraction of the ligament after several weeks [7, 8, 61–63]. However, in most cases of proximal tears, the ligament reattaches to the PCL or to the notch rather than being reabsorbed [64–66]. The senior author has even been able to primarily repair a chronic 11-year-old proximal ACL tear that had scarred to the PCL. Given that the ligament had maintained its length over the years, the ACL was dissected off of the PCL and then reattached to the femoral footprint with good outcomes at 2-year follow-up [67].

When reviewing the case series of the senior author (approximately 200 complete ACL tears that were repaired), the time of surgery ranges from 4 days to 13 years. In a currently submitted study in which our group assessed predictors of the intraoperative (successful) possibility of primary repair, a cut-off of 4 weeks was found, indicating that the surgery should be performed within 4 weeks of injury to increase the chance of a successful primary repair. This data point should be interpreted with nuance as it does not mean that the ACL cannot be repaired after 4 weeks but merely that a significantly better chance of repair exists if the patient can be brought to surgery within the first month after injury.

17.4.4 Patient Characteristics

Generally, patients of all ages and activity levels can be treated with arthroscopic primary ACL repair. Recently, it has been noticed that the likelihood of a repairable proximal tear is increased when patients are above 35 years of age [57]. Although the reason for this remains unclear to us, it may be partially explained by the fact that some mucoid degeneration in the proximal part of ligaments is often seen in older patients and that this leads to a weaker proximal part of the ligament with a higher chance of tearing when compared to the rest of the ligament. A reason for this might be decreased vascularity in the proximal part of the ACL leading to a weaker point of the ligament, but this has not been extensively examined [68]. To date, no clear correlation between the likelihood of repair and gender, injury mechanism, or concomitant injuries has been found.

17.5 Surgical Technique

17.5.1 Surgical Setup

The surgery is started with the patient placed in supine position and prepped and draped as for standard knee arthroscopy. Equipment and implants from the standard knee arthroscopy and the shoulder arthroscopy set are used.

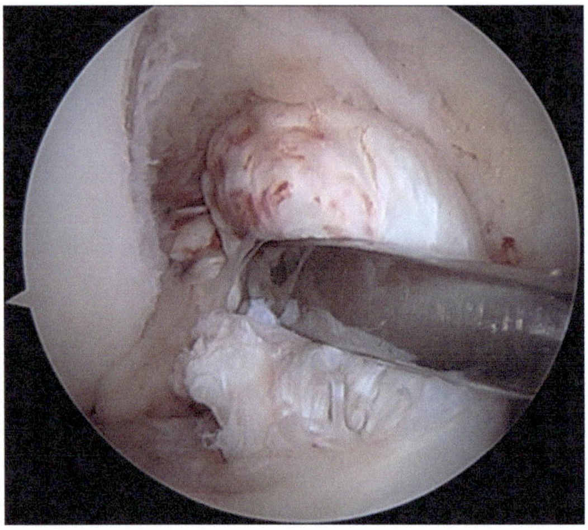

Fig. 17.1 This patient was operated 23 days following a non-contact basketball injury. Intraoperatively, a femoral avulsion tear of the ACL can be noted

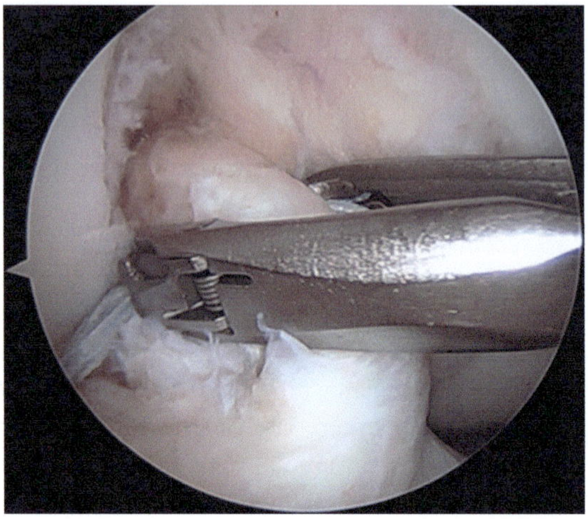

Fig. 17.2 Using a suture passer, a No. 2 FiberWire suture is passed through the anteromedial bundle of the ACL

Anteromedial and anterolateral portals are created, and the knee joint is inspected. The ligament is visualized, and with a probe, the tear type and tissue quality of the ligament are assessed (Fig. 17.1). If the distal part of the ligament remnant has sufficient length to be reapproximated to the femoral wall (a grasper can be used to assess this) and sufficient tissue quality is present, the decision is made to repair the ACL. A malleable PassPort cannula (Arthrex, Naples, FL) is now placed in the anteromedial portal to facilitate suture passage, suture management, and the repair.

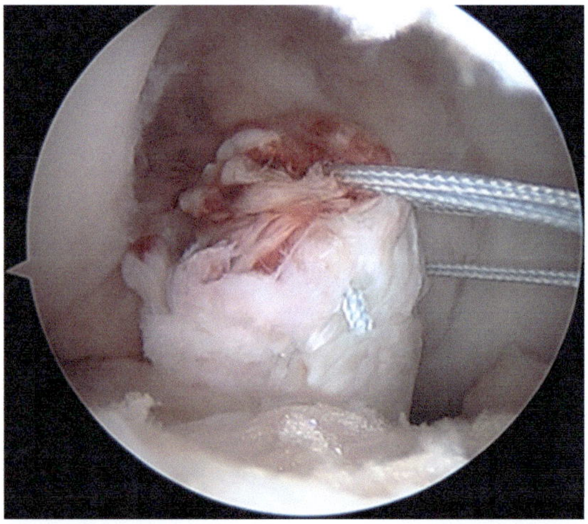

Fig. 17.3 The final pass of the anteromedial bundle should exit to the avulsed end toward the femoral wall

17.5.2 Ligament Suturing

The anteromedial (AM) and posterolateral (PL) bundles of the ACL are identified. First, the AM bundle is sutured from as distal as possible toward the proximal end using No. 2 FiberWire sutures in an alternating, interlocking Bunnell-type pattern with a Scorpion Suture Passer (Arthrex, Naples, FL) (Fig. 17.2). If possible it is preferred that the last pass should exit the avulsed femoral end toward the femoral wall (Fig. 17.3). An accessory portal above the anteromedial portal can be created with a stab incision to insert a grasper and place tension on the ligament remnant to facilitate suture passage while avoiding splaying of the ligament. The portal can also be helpful after suture passage to park the sutures away and keep them out of harm's way. The same process is now repeated for the PL bundle using No. 2 TigerWire sutures (Fig. 17.4). Careful, gentle traction on the AM bundle sutures can help to visualize the PL bundle and facilitate suture passage. Care should be taken to not transect previously passed sutures, and the Suture Passer

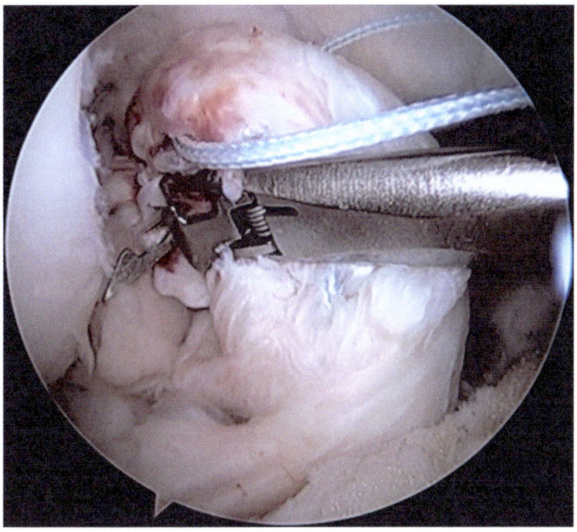

Fig. 17.4 No. 2 TigerWire suture is passed through the posterolateral bundle

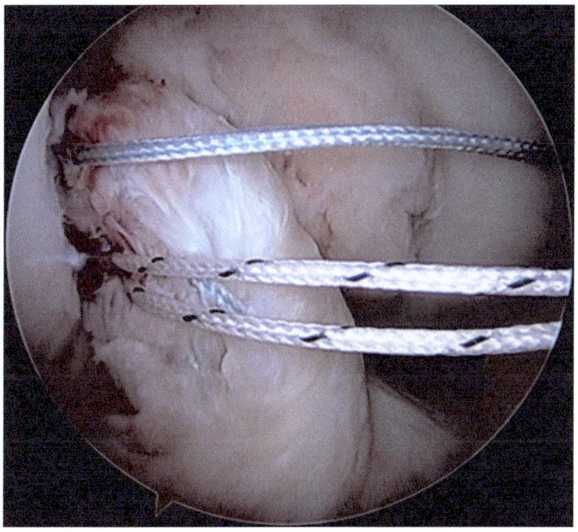

Fig. 17.5 Both sutures have been passed through the anteromedial and posterolateral bundle and exit the avulsed ligament toward the femoral footprint

should therefore be repositioned when great resistance is felt. The PL bundle sutures are also parked away via the accessory portal (Fig. 17.5). Traction on both sutures can visualize the femoral footprint, and a small notchplasty can now be safely performed in order to improve visualization and enable bleeding for an optimal healing environment.

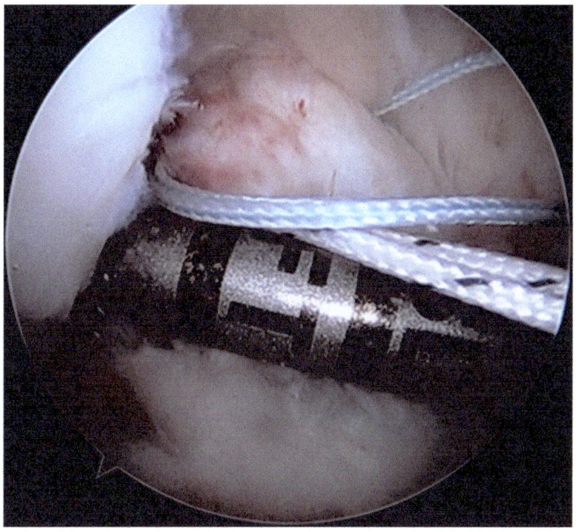

Fig. 17.6 A hole is punched in the posterolateral footprint from an accessory medial portal prior to suture anchor placement

17.5.3 Ligament Fixation

With the knee in 90° flexion, a 4.5 × 20 mm hole is punched, tapped, or drilled (only in very high-density bone) into the origin of the anteromedial bundle within the femoral footprint. The AM FiberWire sutures are then retrieved from the accessory portal and passed through the eyelet of a 4.75 mm Vented BioComposite SwiveLock suture anchor (Arthrex, Naples, FL). With the knee in 90° flexion, the first suture anchor is then deployed into the femur while tensioning the AM remnant toward the femoral wall, with care taken to make sure that no gap is visual (Fig. 17.6). The same procedure is then performed for the PL bundle with tapping a hole in the PL footprint (Fig. 17.7) and inserting the ligament with the TigerWire sutures, with the knee at 115° of flexion in order to ensure an optimal angle of approach to the femoral PL footprint and to avoid perforation of the posterior condyle. It should be noted that the order of tensioning and fixing the bundles will vary on a case to case basis.

Once the anchors are fully deployed and are flush with the femoral footprint, the core stitches are unloaded, and the sutures are cut short using an open-ended Suture Cutter (Arthrex, Naples,

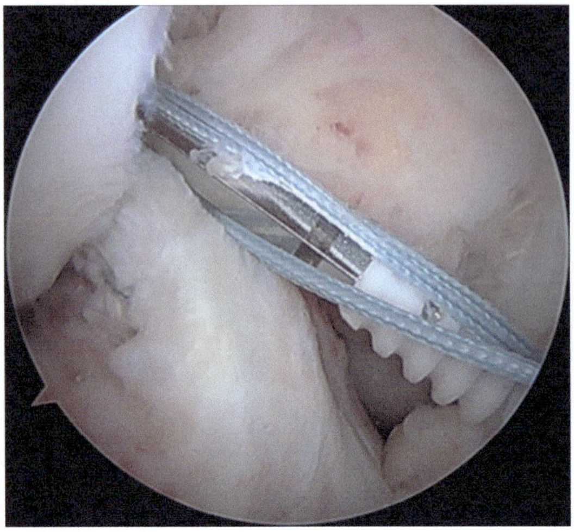

Fig. 17.7 After the posterolateral bundle is reattached to the femur and a hole is punched in the anteromedial femoral footprint, a BioComposite SwiveLock suture anchor is placed in the femoral footprint while tensioning the anteromedial bundle

FL). At times, when the tissue quality is good enough, the core stitches from the PL anchor will be passed from lateral to medial through the ACL using the Scorpion and then tied down tight using a knot pusher and alternating half hitches. This provides a compressive force vector at the footprint to optimize contact with the femoral bone. The repair is now complete, and the ligament is tested for stiffness using a probe and for impingement by moving the knee through full ROM (Fig. 17.8). A Lachman examination is performed to confirm the elimination of anterior laxity.

17.5.4 Additional Internal Brace Augmentation

In patients with a higher risk for rerupture (e.g., high laxity patients, valgus knees, young (female) patients, suboptimal tissue quality), an InternalBrace (Arthrex, Naples, FL) can be easily added to the repair construct in order to protect the repaired ligament and potentially decrease the rerupture rate. With the procedure, the AM suture anchor is preloaded with FiberTape (Arthrex, Naples, FL), which functions as an internal suture augmentation. The FiberTape will be channeled down along the anterior third of the ligament. To accomplish this, an ACL guide is used to facilitate drilling a drill pin up from the anteromedial tibial cortex to the anteromedial tibial ACL footprint. A Straight MicroSutureLasso (Arthrex, Naples, FL) is then used to retrieve the FiberTape out of the knee through this drill hole (Fig. 17.9), where it is then fixed into the anteromedial tibial cortex using a 4.75 mm BioComposite SwiveLock. Prior to fixation the knee is cycled multiple times with tension on the Fiber Tape. Care

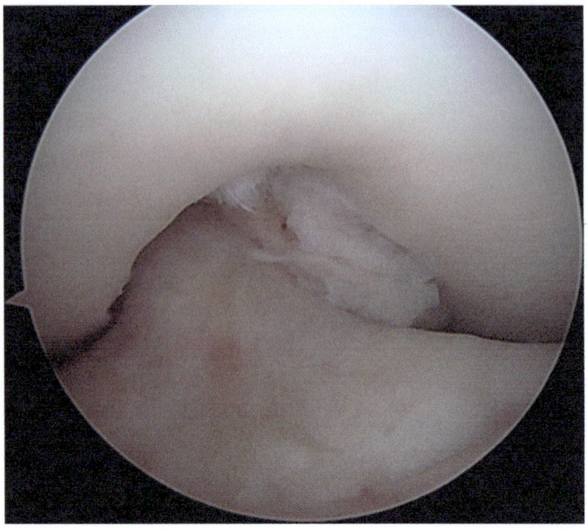

Fig. 17.8 By fully extending the knee, it can be noted that no impingement is seen of the ACL

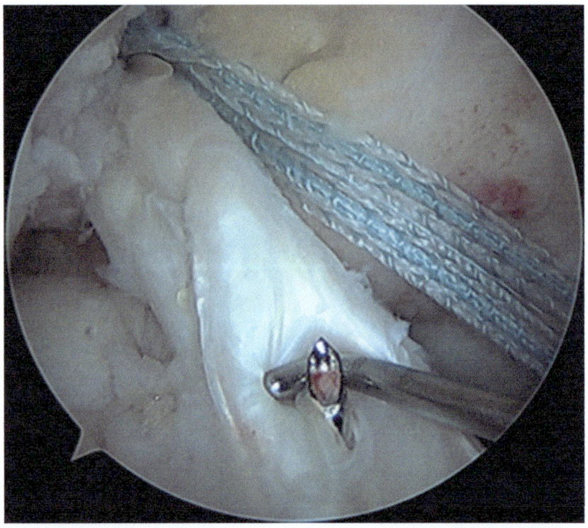

Fig. 17.9 Using a drill guide a straight MicroSutureLasso with a nitinol wire is used to retrieve the InternalBrace that has been preloaded at the anteromedial suture anchor (different patient)

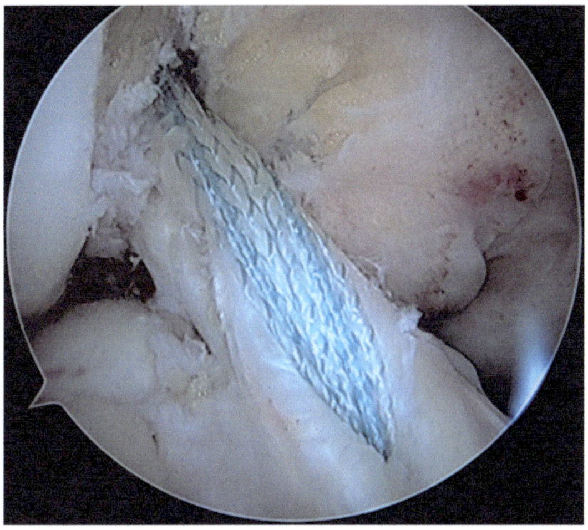

Fig. 17.10 The InternalBrace is tensioned along the ACL and fixed at the anteromedial tibial cortex

should be taken to tension the InternalBrace at near full extension to prevent an extension deficit, and the SwiveLock should be flush with the anteromedial cortex in order to prevent hardware irritation. The augmented repair is now complete (Fig. 17.10).

17.6 Rehabilitation

The main initial goals of rehabilitation are controlling edema and regaining early ROM. Early ROM exercises are started the day after surgery, although a brace is worn during ambulation for the first weeks until full volitional quadriceps muscle control is regained. The preference of the senior author is to drain any hemarthrosis within 1 week postoperatively in order to decrease pain, improve ROM and prevent reactive quadriceps muscle atrophy. Formal physical therapy is started after the first week consisting mainly of swelling control, ROM, and regaining quadriceps control. The rehabilitative course after ACL primary repair is generally dramatically easier than after reconstruction and quite commonly will shock the inexperienced practitioner. Patients generally progress quickly, and in general, after one month gentle strengthening and a standard ACL rehabilitation protocol are begun.

In a previously published study, our group has compared the postoperative milestones following arthroscopic primary ACL repair and ACL reconstruction [69]. It was noted that patients following primary repair had more ROM at 1 week, 1 month, and 3 months postoperatively and sooner regained full ROM when compared to ACL reconstruction. Furthermore, fewer complications were noted following primary ACL repair, which can likely be explained by the shorter surgery and the minimal invasiveness when compared to ACL reconstruction [69].

17.7 Outcomes of Primary ACL Repair

The first study reporting outcomes of modern-day arthroscopic primary repair of proximal ACL tears was reported by our group [70]. In a pilot study of the first 11 patients, excellent outcomes with one failure (9%) and high functional outcomes scores (Table 17.1) were found at short-term, average 3.5-year, follow-up. Shortly after, Achtnich et al. reported the outcomes of 20 repair patients versus 20 reconstruction patients and reported a 15% failure rate and good functional outcomes with primary ACL repair that did not differ significantly from ACL reconstruction [71]. Smith et al. [72] and Bigoni et al. [73] then reported good outcomes of arthroscopic primary repair of proximal tears in small cohorts of pediatric patients (three and five patients, respectively). Recently, the short-term outcomes of the first 56 consecutive patients that were treated with primary ACL repair have been presented by our group [74], and a failure rate of 10.7% and reoperation rate of 7.1% were noted along with excellent functional outcomes (Table 17.2).

As already discussed in the section on the historical outcomes of primary repair, the mid-term outcomes are of critical importance as the outcomes of open primary repair deteriorated at around 5-year follow-up in the historical studies. Our group has recently published the mid-term outcomes of our initial pilot study of 11 patients and noted no deterioration of outcomes at mid-

Table 17.2 Outcomes of recent studies performing arthroscopic primary repair of proximal ACL tears

Authors	Techn.	Year	Pts	Age (year)	FU (year)	Fail., %	Reop., %	KT-1000*	IKDC (%) A, %	IKDC (%) B, %	IKDC (%) C, %	IKDC (%) D, %	IKDC subj	Lysh.	Mod. Cinc.	SANE	KOOS
DiFelice et al. [70]	2 SA	2015	11	37	3.5	9	0	88%	82	9	9	0	86.4	93.2	91.5	91.5	
DiFelice and Van der List [76]	2 SA	2018	11	37	6.0	9	9		82	9	9	0	92.3	96.0	95.4	95.4	
Jonkergouw et al. [74]	2 SA ± IB	2018	56	33	3.2	11	7		73	15	12		90.0	94.2	89.7	89.7	
Achtnich et al. [71]	1 SA	2016	20	30	2.3	15	5	2 mm	65	20	15	0					
Hoffmann et al. [77]	1 SA	2017	11	43	6.6	18	0	82%	73	9	18	0	87.3	85.3			
Nyland et al. [82]	? + IB	2018	30	27	3.0	11											94.7
Bigoni et al. [73]	1 SA	2017	5	9	3.6	0	0		0	100	0	0		93.6			
Smith et al. [72]	TOT + IB	2016	5	6	1.6	0	0							100			95.5
Anthony and Mackay [83]	TOT + IB	2016	68	34	1.6	2	4										80.4

*KT-1000 indicates either number of patients with <3 mm side-to-side difference (in %) or the absolute side-to-side difference (in mm)

Studies using a dynamic spring device or biological scaffold have not been included in this overview

Tech. surgical technique, *SA* suture anchor, *IB* internal brace, *TOT* transosseous tunnels in femur and tibia, *pts.* number of patients in study, *FU* follow-up in years, *fail.* failure, *reop* reoperation for other reasons than failure/reconstruction, *Lysh.* Lysholm score, *Mod. Cinc.* modified Cincinnati score, *SANE* Single assessment numeric evaluation

term follow-up with still one failure (9%), one reoperation (9%), and excellent functional outcomes [75, 76]. A recent study of Hoffmann et al. confirmed these findings by also reporting good mid-term outcomes and concluding primary repair is an excellent treatment for proximal ACL tears, despite having a higher failure rate (25%) (which they partially contributed to concomitant injuries or illnesses such as a patellar tendon rupture and rheumatoid arthritis, respectively) [77]. The difference between the deterioration of mid-term outcomes in the historical studies and the fact that the excellent outcomes are maintained at mid-term follow-up in modern-day studies can likely be explained by the appropriate patient selection (i.e., proximal tears and good tissue quality rather than all tears) and modern-day surgery (i.e., arthroscopy rather than arthrotomy) and rehabilitation (i.e., focus on early ROM rather than prolonged joint immobilization).

17.8 Future Directions

Future studies on the topic of arthroscopic primary repair should first assess the outcomes of primary repair in larger cohorts of patients in order to assess the failure rates, return to sports rates, and assess which patients benefit from the surgery and which patients are at a higher risk of failure of primary ACL repair. Furthermore, more studies with larger cohorts are needed to assess the mid-term and long-term outcomes in order to assess if the outcomes are maintained at longer-term follow-up. These studies are also important to examine the incidence of osteoarthritis with the suggested lower incidence with this less invasive and more preserving surgical treatment. In addition, studies assessing outcomes of primary repair of other knee ligaments, such as the PCL [78, 79], MCL [80], LCL, or multiligamentous injured knee [81], are also needed.

Ultimately, higher level of evidence (prospective) studies is needed in order to decrease potential bias in literature. The final step is to perform a randomized clinical trial in which patients with proximal tears are randomized between preservation surgery consisting of arthroscopic primary ACL repair and the current gold standard of ACL reconstruction.

An additional focus of research could investigate the potential role of adding biologic augmentation to the repair construct. This is a relatively new area of orthopedic research and could potentially improve the healing potential of the native ligament. Finally, the potential addition of procedures to address the anterolateral ligament (ALL) in conjunction with ACL repair could improve outcomes for higher risk patients with proximal ACL tears that are amenable to repair.

17.9 Conclusions

The historical outcomes of open primary repair have been reported as disappointing, which could partially be attributed to inappropriate patient selection, relatively invasive surgery, and prolonged postoperative joint immobilization. Better results of primary repair can, however, be expected with modern advances in patient selection (i.e., only treating proximal tears), less invasive surgery (i.e., arthroscopy), and modern-day rehabilitation (i.e., focus on early ROM). ACL preservation consisting of primary ACL repair has the advantages of preserving native biology, does not need graft harvesting or tunnel drilling, and does not burn any bridges for future reconstruction, if necessary.

Recent studies have carefully assessed patient selection, postoperative rehabilitation, and short-term outcomes of arthroscopic primary ACL repair and have noted that a quicker and less morbid rehabilitation is seen following primary repair with excellent short-term outcomes similar to ACL reconstruction. Future larger studies are needed to assess the outcomes of primary repair in specific patient populations (e.g., young patients, high-level athletes), the mid-term outcomes in larger cohorts and assess the incidence of osteoarthritis at long-term follow-up. Ultimately, randomized controlled trials comparing arthroscopic primary repair with the current gold standard of reconstruction of proximal ACL tears are needed.

References

1. Lyman S, Koulouvaris P, Sherman S, Do H, Mandl LA, Marx RG. Epidemiology of anterior cruciate ligament reconstruction: trends, readmissions, and subsequent knee surgery. J Bone Joint Surg Am. 2009;91(10):2321–8.
2. Sanders TL, Maradit Kremers H, Bryan AJ, Larson DR, Dahm DL, Levy BA, Stuart MJ, Krych AJ. Incidence of anterior cruciate ligament tears and reconstruction: a 21-year population-based study. Am J Sports Med. 2016;44(6):1502–7.
3. Gianotti SM, Marshall SW, Hume PA, Bunt L. Incidence of anterior cruciate ligament injury and other knee ligament injuries: a national population-based study. J Sci Med Sport. 2009;12(6):622–7.
4. Robson AW. VI. Ruptured crucial ligaments and their repair by operation. Ann Surg. 1903;37(5):716–8.
5. Palmer I. On the injuries to the ligaments of the knee joint. Acta Orthop Scand. 1938;53:17.
6. Palmer I. On the injuries to the ligaments of the knee joint: a clinical study. Clin Orthop Relat Res. 2007;454:17–22.
7. O'Donoghue DH. Surgical treatment of fresh injuries to the major ligaments of the knee. J Bone Joint Surg Am. 1950;32A(4):721–38.
8. O'Donoghue DH. An analysis of end results of surgical treatment of major injuries to the ligaments of the knee. J Bone Joint Surg Am. 1955;37(1):1–13.
9. Liljedahl SO, Lindvall N, Wetterfors J. Early diagnosis and treatment of acute ruptures of the anterior cruciate ligament; a clinical and arthrographic study of forty-eight cases. J Bone Joint Surg Am. 1965;47(8):1503–13.
10. Feagin JA, Abbott HG, Rokous JR. The isolated tear of the anterior cruciate ligament. J Bone Joint Surg Am. 1972;54(6):1340–1.
11. England RL. Repair of the ligaments about the knee. Orthop Clin North Am. 1976;7(1):195–204.
12. Feagin JA Jr, Curl WW. Isolated tear of the anterior cruciate ligament: 5-year follow-up study. Am J Sports Med. 1976;4(3):95–100.
13. Straub T, Hunter RE. Acute anterior cruciate ligament repair. Clin Orthop Relat Res. 1988;227:238–50.
14. Kaplan N, Wickiewicz TL, Warren RF. Primary surgical treatment of anterior cruciate ligament ruptures. A long-term follow-up study. Am J Sports Med. 1990;18(4):354–8.
15. Sherman MF, Lieber L, Bonamo JR, Podesta L, Reiter I. The long-term follow-up of primary anterior cruciate ligament repair. Defining a rationale for augmentation. Am J Sports Med. 1991;19(3):243–55.
16. Odensten M, Hamberg P, Nordin M, Lysholm J, Gillquist J. Surgical or conservative treatment of the acutely torn anterior cruciate ligament. A randomized study with short-term follow-up observations. Clin Orthop Relat Res. 1985;198:87–93.
17. Harilainen A, Myllynen P. Treatment of fresh tears of the anterior cruciate ligament. A comparison of primary suture and augmentation with carbon fibre. Injury. 1987;18(6):396–400.
18. Andersson C, Odensten M, Good L, Gillquist J. Surgical or non-surgical treatment of acute rupture of the anterior cruciate ligament. A randomized study with long-term follow-up. J Bone Joint Surg Am. 1989;71(7):965–74.
19. Engebretsen L, Benum P, Fasting O, Molster A, Strand T. A prospective, randomized study of three surgical techniques for treatment of acute ruptures of the anterior cruciate ligament. Am J Sports Med. 1990;18(6):585–90.
20. Jonsson T, Peterson L, Renstrom P. Anterior cruciate ligament repair with and without augmentation. A prospective 7-year study of 51 patients. Acta Orthop Scand. 1990;61(6):562–6.
21. Andersson C, Odensten M, Gillquist J. Knee function after surgical or nonsurgical treatment of acute rupture of the anterior cruciate ligament: a randomized study with a long-term follow-up period. Clin Orthop Relat Res. 1991;264:255–63.
22. van der List JP, DiFelice GS. Primary repair of the anterior cruciate ligament: a paradigm shift. Surgeon. 2017;15(3):161–8.
23. van der List JP, DiFelice GS. Role of tear location on outcomes of open primary repair of the anterior cruciate ligament: a systematic review of historical studies. Knee. 2017; https://doi.org/10.1016/j.knee.2017.05.009.
24. Nguyen DT, Ramwadhdoebe TH, van der Hart CP, Blankevoort L, Tak PP, van Dijk CN. Intrinsic healing response of the human anterior cruciate ligament: an histological study of reattached ACL remnants. J Orthop Res. 2014;32(2):296–301.
25. Murray MM. Current status and potential of primary ACL repair. Clin Sports Med. 2009;28(1):51–61.
26. Cameron SE, Wilson W, St Pierre P. A prospective, randomized comparison of open vs arthroscopically assisted ACL reconstruction. Orthopedics. 1995;18(3):249–52.
27. Laffargue P, Delalande J, Maillet M, Vanhecke C, Decoulx J. Anterior cruciate ligament reconstruction: arthrotomy versus arthroscopy. Rev Chir Orthop Reparatrice Appar Mot. 1999;85(4):367–73.
28. Yip DK, Wong JW, Chien EP. Arthroscopic surgery in the posterior compartment of the knee: suture fixation of anterior and posterior cruciate ligament avulsions. Arthroscopy. 2003;19(3):23e.
29. Genelin F, Trost A, Primavesi C, Knoll P. Late results following proximal reinsertion of isolated ruptured ACL ligaments. Knee Surg Sports Traumatol Arthrosc. 1993;1(1):17–9.
30. Marshall JL, Warren RF, Wickiewicz TL. Primary surgical treatment of anterior cruciate ligament lesions. Am J Sports Med. 1982;10(2):103–7.
31. Warren RF. Primary repair of the anterior cruciate ligament. Clin Orthop Relat Res. 1983;172:65–70.
32. Shelbourne KD, Wilckens JH, Mollabashy A, DeCarlo M. Arthrofibrosis in acute anterior cruciate ligament reconstruction. The effect of timing of

reconstruction and rehabilitation. Am J Sports Med. 1991;19(4):332–6.
33. Shelbourne KD, Nitz P. Accelerated rehabilitation after anterior cruciate ligament reconstruction. J Orthop Sports Phys Ther. 1992;15(6):256–64.
34. Enneking WF, Horowitz M. The intra-articular effects of immobilization on the human knee. J Bone Joint Surg Am. 1972;54(5):973–85.
35. Millett PJ, Wickiewicz TL, Warren RF. Motion loss after ligament injuries to the knee. Part I: causes. Am J Sports Med. 2001;29(5):664–75.
36. Raunest J, Sager M, Burgener E. Proprioceptive mechanisms in the cruciate ligaments: an electromyographic study on reflex activity in the thigh muscles. J Trauma. 1996;41(3):488–93.
37. Georgoulis AD, Pappa L, Moebius U, Malamou-Mitsi V, Pappa S, Papageorgiou CO, Agnantis NJ, Soucacos PN. The presence of proprioceptive mechanoreceptors in the remnants of the ruptured ACL as a possible source of re-innervation of the ACL autograft. Knee Surg Sports Traumatol Arthrosc. 2001;9(6):364–8.
38. Dhillon MS, Bali K, Vasistha RK. Immunohistological evaluation of proprioceptive potential of the residual stump of injured anterior cruciate ligaments (ACL). Int Orthop. 2010;34(5):737–41.
39. Behrend H, Zdravkovic V, Giesinger JM, Giesinger K. Joint awareness after ACL reconstruction: patient-reported outcomes measured with the Forgotten Joint Score-12. Knee Surg Sports Traumatol Arthrosc. 2016; https://doi.org/10.1007/s00167-016-4357-x.
40. Kraeutler MJ, Bravman JT, McCarty EC. Bone-patellar tendon-bone autograft versus allograft in outcomes of anterior cruciate ligament reconstruction: a meta-analysis of 5182 patients. Am J Sports Med. 2013;41(10):2439–48.
41. Biau DJ, Tournoux C, Katsahian S, Schranz PJ, Nizard RS. Bone-patellar tendon-bone autografts versus hamstring autografts for reconstruction of anterior cruciate ligament: meta-analysis. BMJ. 2006;332(7548):995–1001.
42. Ajuied A, Wong F, Smith C, Norris M, Earnshaw P, Back D, Davies A. Anterior cruciate ligament injury and radiologic progression of knee osteoarthritis: a systematic review and meta-analysis. Am J Sports Med. 2014;42(9):2242–52.
43. Luc B, Gribble PA, Pietrosimone BG. Osteoarthritis prevalence following anterior cruciate ligament reconstruction: a systematic review and numbers-needed-to-treat analysis. J Athl Train. 2014;49(6):806–19.
44. Oiestad BE, Engebretsen L, Storheim K, Risberg MA. Knee osteoarthritis after anterior cruciate ligament injury: a systematic review. Am J Sports Med. 2009;37(7):1434–43.
45. Kessler MA, Behrend H, Henz S, Stutz G, Rukavina A, Kuster MS. Function, osteoarthritis and activity after ACL-rupture: 11 years follow-up results of conservative versus reconstructive treatment. Knee Surg Sports Traumatol Arthrosc. 2008;16(5):442–8.
46. von Porat A, Roos EM, Roos H. High prevalence of osteoarthritis 14 years after an anterior cruciate ligament tear in male soccer players: a study of radiographic and patient relevant outcomes. Ann Rheum Dis. 2004;63(3):269–73.
47. Imhauser C, Mauro C, Choi D, Rosenberg E, Mathew S, Nguyen J, Ma Y, Wickiewicz T. Abnormal tibiofemoral contact stress and its association with altered kinematics after center-center anterior cruciate ligament reconstruction: an in vitro study. Am J Sports Med. 2013;41(4):815–25.
48. Logan MC, Williams A, Lavelle J, Gedroyc W, Freeman M. Tibiofemoral kinematics following successful anterior cruciate ligament reconstruction using dynamic multiple resonance imaging. Am J Sports Med. 2004;32(4):984–92.
49. Ristanis S, Stergiou N, Patras K, Vasiliadis HS, Giakas G, Georgoulis AD. Excessive tibial rotation during high-demand activities is not restored by anterior cruciate ligament reconstruction. Arthroscopy. 2005;21(11):1323–9.
50. Strand T, Molster A, Hordvik M, Krukhaug Y. Long-term follow-up after primary repair of the anterior cruciate ligament: clinical and radiological evaluation 15–23 years postoperatively. Arch Orthop Trauma Surg. 2005;125(4):217–21.
51. Murray MM, Fleming BC. Use of a bioactive scaffold to stimulate anterior cruciate ligament healing also minimizes posttraumatic osteoarthritis after surgery. Am J Sports Med. 2013;41(8):1762–70.
52. Lind M, Menhert F, Pedersen AB. Incidence and outcome after revision anterior cruciate ligament reconstruction: results from the Danish registry for knee ligament reconstructions. Am J Sports Med. 2012;40(7):1551–7.
53. Lefevre N, Klouche S, Mirouse G, Herman S, Gerometta A, Bohu Y. Return to sport after primary and revision anterior cruciate ligament reconstruction. Am J Sports Med. 2017;45(1):34–41.
54. Kamath GV, Redfern JC, Greis PE, Burks RT. Revision anterior cruciate ligament reconstruction. Am J Sports Med. 2011;39(1):199–217.
55. van der List JP, DiFelice GS. Preservation of the anterior cruciate ligament: a treatment algorithm based on tear location and tissue quality. Am J Orthop (Belle Mead NJ). 2016;45(7):E393–405.
56. van der List JP, DiFelice GS. Preservation of the anterior cruciate ligament: surgical techniques. Am J Orthop (Belle Mead NJ). 2016;45(7):E406–14.
57. van der List JP, Mintz DN, DiFelice GS. The location of anterior cruciate ligament tears: a prevalence study using magnetic resonance imaging. Orthop J Sports Med. 2017;5(6):2325967117709966.
58. van der List JP, Mintz DN, DiFelice GS. The location of anterior cruciate ligament tears in pediatric and adolescent patients: a magnetic resonance imaging study. J Pediatr Orthop. 2017; https://doi.org/10.1097/BPO.0000000000001041.
59. van der List JP, DiFelice GS. The role of primary repair in pediatric anterior cruciate ligament injuries. In: Parikh SN, editor. The pediatric anterior cruciate liga-

ment, vol. 1. New York, NY: Springer; 2018. p. 227–39. https://doi.org/10.1007/978-3-319-64771-5_22.
60. van der List JP, DiFelice GS. Preoperative magnetic resonance imaging predicts eligibility for arthroscopic primary anterior cruciate ligament repair. Knee Surg Sports Traumatol Arthrosc. 2017; https://doi.org/10.1007/s00167-017-4646-z.
61. O'Donoghue DH, Rockwood CA Jr, Frank GR, Jack SC, Kenyon R. Repair of the anterior cruciate ligament in dogs. J Bone Joint Surg Am. 1966;48(3):503–19.
62. Magarian EM, Fleming BC, Harrison SL, Mastrangelo AN, Badger GJ, Murray MM. Delay of 2 or 6 weeks adversely affects the functional outcome of augmented primary repair of the porcine anterior cruciate ligament. Am J Sports Med. 2010;38(12):2528–34.
63. Murray MM, Martin SD, Martin TL, Spector M. Histological changes in the human anterior cruciate ligament after rupture. J Bone Joint Surg Am. 2000;82-A(10):1387–97.
64. Crain EH, Fithian DC, Paxton EW, Luetzow WF. Variation in anterior cruciate ligament scar pattern: does the scar pattern affect anterior laxity in anterior cruciate ligament-deficient knees? Arthroscopy. 2005;21(1):19–24.
65. Fowler PJ, Regan WD. The patient with symptomatic chronic anterior cruciate ligament insufficiency. Results of minimal arthroscopic surgery and rehabilitation. Am J Sports Med. 1987;15(4):321–5.
66. Vahey TN, Broome DR, Kayes KJ, Shelbourne KD. Acute and chronic tears of the anterior cruciate ligament: differential features at MR imaging. Radiology. 1991;181(1):251–3.
67. van der List JP, DiFelice GS. Successful arthroscopic primary repair of a chronic anterior cruciate ligament tear 11 years following injury. HSS J. 2017;13(1):90–5.
68. Petersen W, Hansen U. Blood and lymph supply of the anterior cruciate ligament: Cadaver study by immunohistochemical and histochemical methods. J Orthop Sci. 1997;2(5):313–8.
69. van der List JP, DiFelice GS. Range of motion and complications following primary repair versus reconstruction of the anterior cruciate ligament. Knee. 2017;24(4):798–807.
70. DiFelice GS, Villegas C, Taylor SA. Anterior cruciate ligament preservation: early results of a novel arthroscopic technique for suture anchor primary anterior cruciate ligament repair. Arthroscopy. 2015;31(11):2162–71.
71. Achtnich A, Herbst E, Forkel P, Metzlaff S, Sprenker F, Imhoff AB, Petersen W. Acute proximal anterior cruciate ligament tears: outcomes after arthroscopic suture anchor repair versus anatomic single-bundle reconstruction. Arthroscopy. 2016;32(12):2562–9.
72. Smith JO, Yasen SK, Palmer HC, Lord BR, Britton EM, Wilson AJ. Paediatric ACL repair reinforced with temporary internal bracing. Knee Surg Sports Traumatol Arthrosc. 2016;24(6):1845–51.
73. Bigoni M, Gaddi D, Gorla M, Munegato D, Pungitore M, Piatti M, Turati M. Arthroscopic anterior cruciate ligament repair for proximal anterior cruciate ligament tears in skeletally immature patients: surgical technique and preliminary results. Knee. 2017;24(1):40–8.
74. Jonkergouw A, van der List JP, DiFelice GS. Arthroscopic primary repair of proximal anterior cruciate ligament tears: with or without additional suture augmentation? Orthop J Sports Med. 2018;6(7_Suppl 4):2325967118S2325960006. https://doi.org/10.1177/2325967118s00063.
75. van der List J, DiFelice G. Arthroscopic primary repair of proximal anterior cruciate ligament tears: no deterioration at mid-term follow-up. Arthroscopy. 2017;33(6):e7.
76. DiFelice GS, van der List JP. Clinical outcomes of arthroscopic primary repair of proximal anterior cruciate ligament tears are maintained at midterm follow-up. Arthroscopy. 2018; https://doi.org/10.1016/j.arthro.2017.10.028.
77. Hoffmann C, Friederichs J, von Ruden C, Schaller C, Buhren V, Moessmer C. Primary single suture anchor re-fixation of anterior cruciate ligament proximal avulsion tears leads to good functional mid-term results: a preliminary study in 12 patients. J Orthop Surg Res. 2017;12(1):171.
78. DiFelice GS, van der List JP. Arthroscopic primary repair of posterior cruciate ligament injuries. Oper Tech Sports Med. 2015;23(4):307–14.
79. van der List JP, DiFelice GS. Arthroscopic primary posterior cruciate ligament repair with suture augmentation. Arthrosc Tech. 2017;6(5):e1685–90. https://doi.org/10.1016/j.eats.2017.06.024.
80. van der List JP, DiFelice GS. Primary repair of the medial collateral ligament with internal bracing. Arthrosc Tech. 2017;6(4):e933–7.
81. Jonkergouw A, van der List JP, DiFelice GS. Multiligament repair with suture augmentation in a knee dislocation with medial-sided injury. Arthrosc Tech. 2018; https://doi.org/10.1016/j.eats.2018.04.006.
82. Nyland J, Caborn DN, Wheeldon B, Kalloub AACL. Femoral avulsion reapproximation with internal bracing and PRP augmentation: excellent return to sports outcomes and low re-injury rates at 3 year follow-up. Glasgow: Annual meeting of ESSKA; 2018.
83. Anthony IC, Mackay GM. Anterior cruciate ligament repair revisited. preliminary results of primary repair with internal brace ligament augmentation: a case series. Orthop Muscul Syst. 2015;4:2. https://doi.org/10.4172/2161-0533.1000188.

18 The Anterolateral Ligament

Stijn Bartholomeeusen and Steven Claes

18.1 Introduction

In 1879, Dr. Paul Segond was the first to describe the existence of a "pearly, resistant, fibrous band" at the anterolateral aspect of the human knee. In the following decades, other authors described a ligamentous structure in the same anatomical region of the knee, but this ligament was described rather confusingly and was referred to by many different names [1]. In 1976, Hughston reported about the "mid-third lateral capsular ligament"; this name was later adopted by Johnson in 1979 and by Laprade in 2005 [2–4]. In 1987, Irvine described a similar structure as "the anterior band of the lateral collateral ligament" [5], and between 2002 and 2012, other authors reported about the "anterior oblique band" and the "anterolateral ligament" [6–8]. In 2013, a profound analysis of these papers inspired the first thorough anatomical study of this enigmatic knee structure, thenceforth unanimously called the "anterolateral ligament" (ALL) of the knee [9] (Fig. 18.1).

By characterizing precise anatomical landmarks of the ALL and suggesting an important influence on rotational stability of the ACL-injured knee, this chapter has provoked a shockwave of anatomical, biomechanical, and clinical publications in recent literature. It also created a lot of controversy especially in the first couple of years, as some authors denied the existence and/or importance of this structure. This initial controversy is now abate, and in 2018, an extensive review of literature, together with cadaveric dissection sessions, by a group of 33 international expert knee surgeons and scientists resulted in a consensus paper which confirms the existence and biomechanical importance of the ALL [1].

By now, the ALL has been consistently demonstrated to attach posterior and proximal to the lateral femoral epicondyle and the origin of the LCL, and it runs superficial to the LCL and attaches on the tibia midway between the anterior border of the fibular head and the posterior border of Gerdy's tubercle [1] (Fig. 18.2).

The initial hypothesis regarding the biomechanical properties of the ALL suggested an effect of controlling internal rotation and anterior translation together with the anterior cruciate ligament (ACL) [9]. Different biomechanical studies have confirmed this, and the ALL is now known to be an important restraint restricting tibial internal rotation [10–13]. Furthermore, injuries to the ALL have been shown to induce high-grade results of the pivot shift test in ACL-deficient knees [14].

For many decades, even before the characterization of the ALL, lateral extra-articular tenodesis (LET) techniques were used in order to

S. Bartholomeeusen (✉) · S. Claes
Department of Orthopaedic Surgery, General Hospital of Herentals, Herentals, Belgium
e-mail: stijn.bartholomeeusen@azherentals.be; Steven.Claes@azherentals.be

M. Brittberg, K. Slynarski (eds.), *Lower Extremity Joint Preservation*, https://doi.org/10.1007/978-3-030-57382-9_18

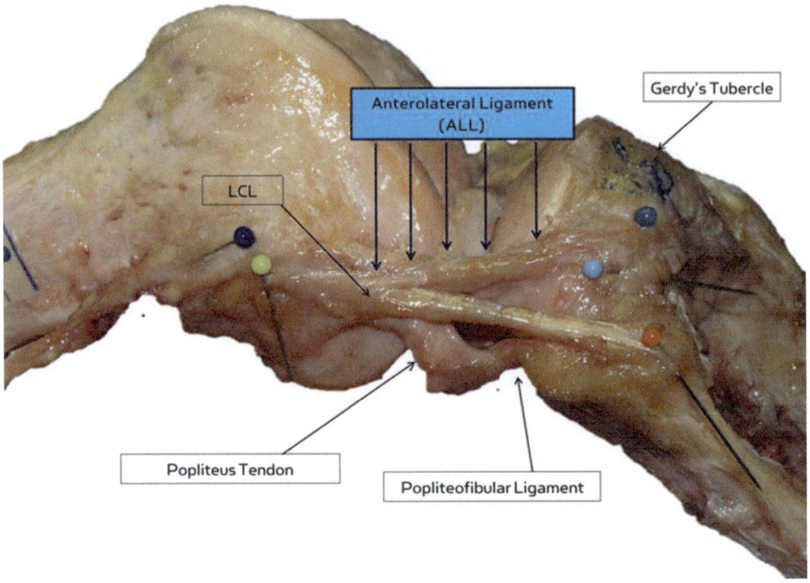

Fig. 18.1 Photograph of a right knee after complete dissection of the anterolateral ligament (ALL), popliteus tendon, popliteo-fibular ligament, and lateral collateral ligament as originally published by Claes et al. in the *Journal of Anatomy* [8] (From "Anatomy of the anterolateral ligament of the knee" by S. Claes et al., 2013, Journal of Anatomy, 223 p. 321–328. Copyright (2013) by Anatomical Society. Reprinted with permission. [with permission from first author S. Claes])

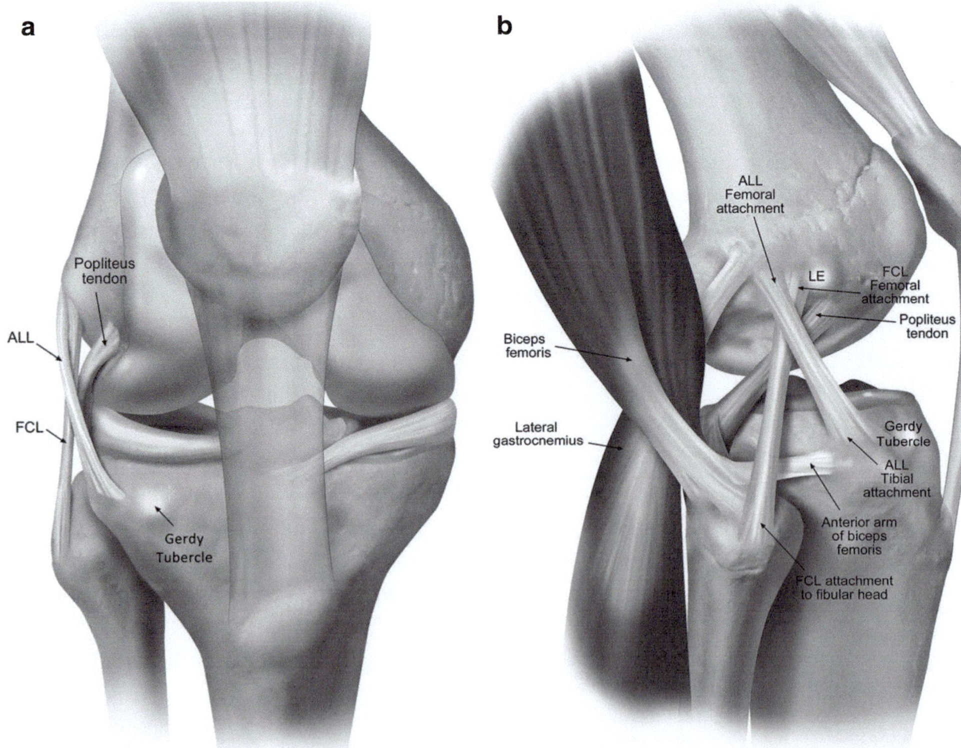

Fig. 18.2 Illustration of topographic location of the anterolateral ligament (ALL) and its relations to bony landmarks and ligamentous structures (From "The Anterolateral Ligament" by M. Kennedy et al., 2015, Am J Sports Med 43:1606–1615 [with permission from second author S. Claes])

eliminate rotational laxity and the pivot shift witnessed in many ACL-injured patients. However, about 20 years ago, with the advent of arthroscopic surgery and the quest for minimal invasive techniques, interest in LET was lost by many surgeons. The recent anatomical and biomechanical characterization of the ALL has not only renewed interest in these LET techniques but has also led to the development of new surgical techniques for anatomical reconstruction of the ALL (Fig. 18.3).

This chapter discusses current indications for ALL reconstruction, describes the most common surgical techniques, has a brief review of historical lateral tenodesis techniques, and discusses outcomes of both older and newer techniques.

18.1.1 Indications

Original concerns about lateral over constraining and stiffness have led to an initial reserved attitude toward new anatomic ALL reconstruction and lateral extra-articular tenodesis techniques [15–18]. However, as these concerns are now fading, a gain of interest for these techniques is

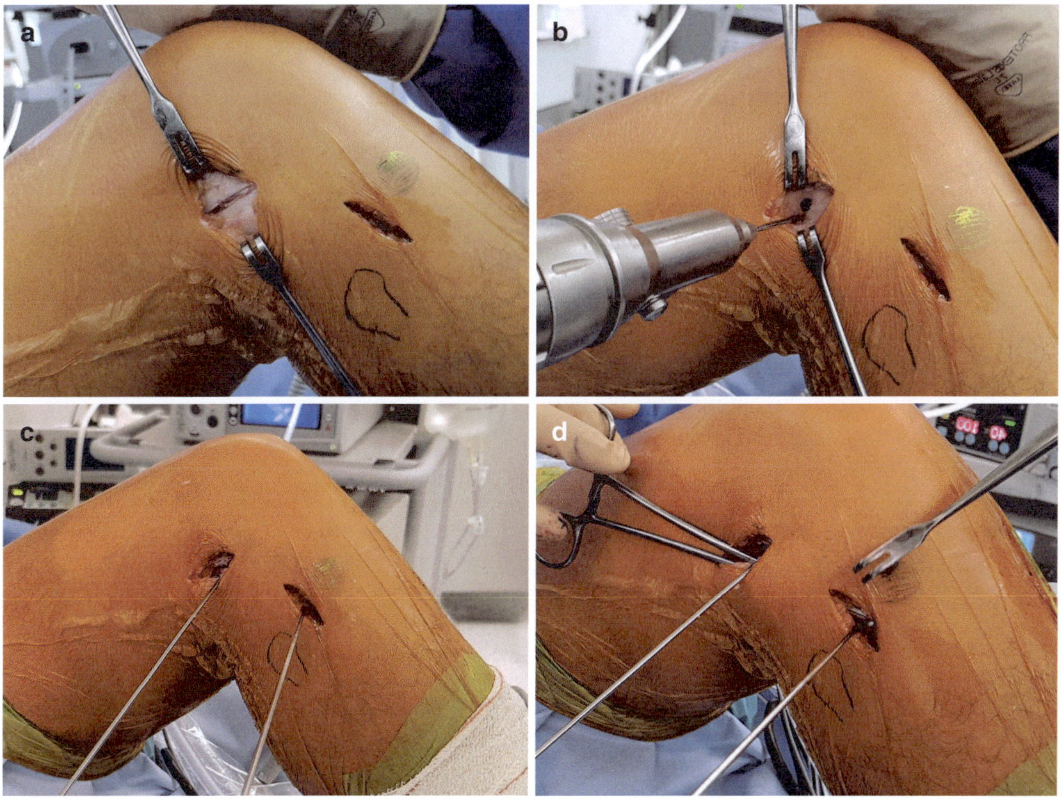

Fig. 18.3 Anatomic ALL reconstruction—single-limb technique (lateral view, right knee). (**a**) Proximal skin incision at lateral epicondyle with ITB split. Distal skin incision between Gerdy's and the fibular head. (**b**) Insertion of femoral guide pin, 5 mm posterior and 5 mm superior to lateral epicondyle. (**c**) Tibial guide pin 7 mm below cartilage edge. (**d**) Instrument tunneled under the ITB from distal to proximal, used to pass suture wire. (**e**) Proximally the suture wire is wrapped around the guide pin and used for testing isometry. (**f**) Both bony tunnels are drilled and the proximal part of the graft is secured with an anchor. The suture wire is used to guide the graft from the proximal to the distal incision. (**g**) Final fixation with anchor in full extension and neutral rotation. Excessive length is cut after fixation distally. (**h**) ALL graft in situ

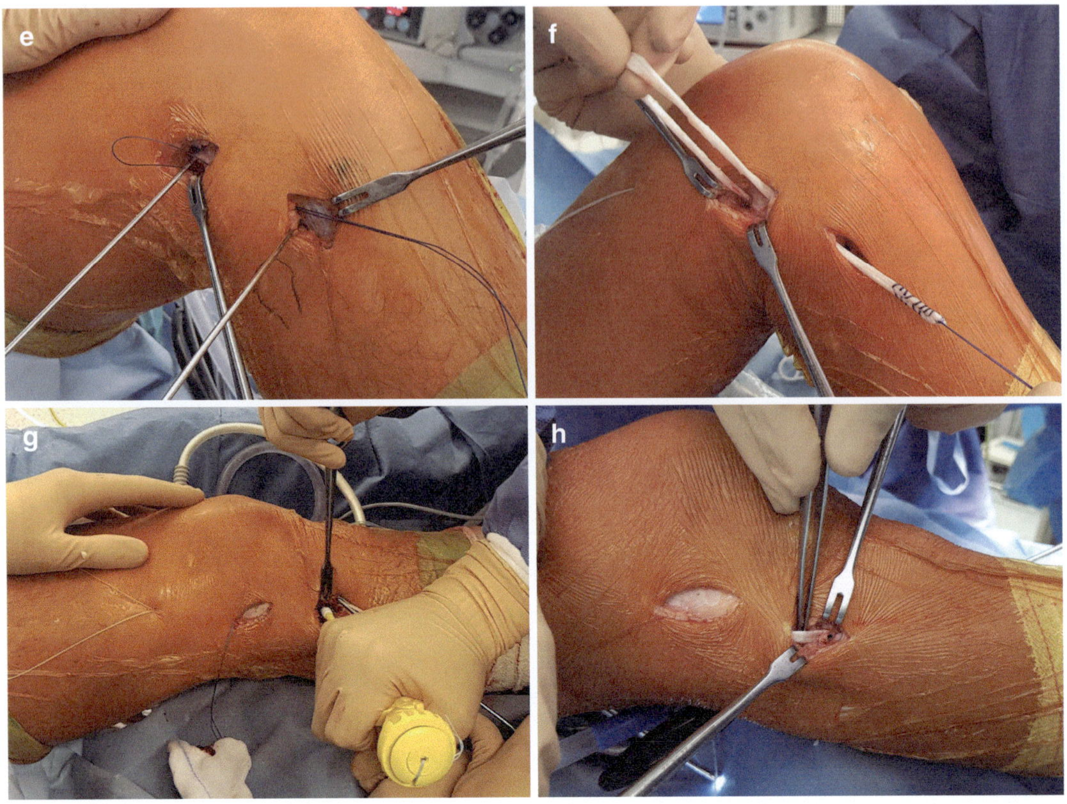

Fig. 18.3 (continued)

marked, and numerous indications are now being proposed. In the process of defining the right indications, it is important to keep in mind the outcomes of ALL reconstruction as described in the section "Outcomes" below, and even though anatomic ALL reconstruction and LET are now both considered safe techniques [19–22], it is important to select patients who will benefit most from adding it to ACL surgery. Indications are summarized in Table 18.1.

Table 18.1 Summary of indications for ALL reconstruction

Indications for the reduction of ACL re-rupture rate:
Young patients (<25 years)
High-level athletes
Participation pivoting sports
Grade 3 Lachman test
Grade 3 pivot shift test
Revision ACL surgery
Other indications:
Chronic ACL injuries (>12 months)
Meniscal repair
Persisting rotational instability after isolated ACL repair
Segond fracture

As extensively discussed below in the section "Outcomes," the rather high risk of re-injury (ACL graft re-ruptures) is an important issue in ACL surgery. The substantial risk reduction of graft re-rupture rates associated with ALL reconstruction is the most important driver of majority of current indications [21, 23–26]. Re-rupture rates are known to be highest in young patients (<25 years), high-level athletes, and patients participating pivoting sports, as well as in patients presenting with high grade preoperative laxity, shown by high-grade Lachman (grade 3) and high-grade pivot shift test (grade 3). In these cases, an additional lateral procedure is advised. In case of revision ACL surgery, it is recommended to perform ALL reconstruction (LET technique) in order to minimize the risk for repeated re-rupture of the revised ACL repair.

Additional indications are mainly based on the positive influence of ALL reconstruction other than graft re-rupture rates. We advise to perform ALL reconstruction in chronic ACL injuries (more than 12 months), as it was shown this improves postoperative subjective outcome scores [19]. In ACL injuries with concomitant meniscal injuries amendable for repair, it has shown to have higher meniscal repair success rates; therefore, in these cases, an additional lateral procedure is also recommended [20].

Furthermore, in case of persisting clinical significant rotational instability after isolated ACL repair, ALL reconstruction could be used. These patients often present with very subtle complaints of instability withholding them to return to pre-injury levels of sport, and by our experience, these complaints can be redressed by performing ALL reconstruction without the need for a full ACL revision. Rehabilitation is often fast, and return to sports is possible after a couple of weeks.

Finally, ALL reconstruction is recommended in Segond fractures. Although still under debate, the anterolateral ligament is believed to be the anatomic ligamentous substrate for these avulsion type of fractures [27–29]. Initially it was thought that primary fixation of the avulsed fragment would effect clinical improvements similar to ALL reconstruction; however, it has been shown that Segond fracture fixation is not effective in reducing graft re-rupture rates and does not improve subjective or objective outcome scores [30–32]. Hence, it is recommended is to reconstruct the ALL and not to fixate the Segond fracture.

18.2 Surgical Techniques

In general, reconstruction of ALL injuries can be classified into two main categories. First, the anatomical reconstruction techniques, in which the main goal is to reconstruct the anatomical properties of the ALL using a tendinous graft. Second, the lateral extra-articular tenodesis (LET) techniques in which a strip of the Iliotibial band (ITB) is secured to the lateral femur in order to mimic the function and anatomy of the ALL.

18.2.1 Anatomical ALL Reconstruction

Several different techniques for anatomical ALL reconstructions are described in literature, generally in each of these techniques, a tendinous auto- or allograft is used to reconstruct the anterolateral ligament and is secured to its original femoral and tibial anatomical origin. The main differences between different techniques are found in the method of fixation to the bone (type of anchor which is used) and the use of a single- or double-limb fixation on the tibia.

The *single-limb anatomic reconstruction* is performed percutaneous by the use of two incisions. The first incision on the femoral side is centered posterior and proximal to the lateral epicondyle. The iliotibial band is then split in a longitudinal fashion along its fibers. Through this incision, the femoral origin of the lateral collateral ligament (LCL) is visualized. A guide pin is placed about 5 mm proximal and posterior to the origin of the LCL [33]. The second incision is made between the middle of Gerdy's tubercle and the anterior margin of the fibular head, just below the level of the joint line. The deeper fascial layer is split in a longitudinal fashion and a guide pin in drilled about 7 mm below the level of the articular cartilage. These pins now mark the femoral and tibial origin of the ALL. Isometry is tested by using a suture wire wrapped around both the pins. The ALL reconstruction should be isometric or may show a little slackening in flexion when compared to extension (no more than 5 mm slackening in flexion, if more than 5 mm, you should consider a too proximal or too posterior pin positioning). If the suture on the other hand is tensed in flexion and slack in extension, a too distal or too anterior femoral pin position should be considered. It is important to avoid this kind of isometry, as it induces the risk of over constraining the lateral compartment.

After correct isometry has been confirmed, the gracilis tendon autograft is tunneled from proximal to distal through the skin incisions, and it should lie superficially from the synovial and capsular layer but underneath the ITB (between Seebacher layers 2 and 3). The suture wire used to test isometry can now be used to shuttle the graft. Final fixation of the ALL is performed after ACL fixation (as this will reduce possible anterior subluxation of the tibia) and should be done in full extension with neutral rotation, again to avoid over-constraining the lateral compartment and to attain favorable ligament isometry.

A technical consideration performing this technique combined with ACL reconstruction with femoral suspensory fixation is the risk of tunnel convergence of the femoral ALL socket and the femoral ACL socket. It can cause failure of the ACL femoral suspensory fixation wires by drilling the ALL guidewire (or cannulated drill) through these wires. Therefore, it is advised to drill femoral and tibial guidewires and sockets before deploying the femoral suspensory fixation mechanism of the ACL.

The *double-limb anatomical reconstruction* is very similar to the previously described technique. The major difference of this technique is the use of two strands of tendinous graft to reconstruct the ALL. The femoral fixation is the same as in single-limb reconstruction; however, at the tibia, each separate limb is fixed in a separate bony socket. Different locations of these sockets are suggested, mostly one tunnel is situated at the posterior border of Gerdy's tubercle and the other at least 1 cm more posterior, often just anterior to the fibular head [34]. It creates a broader tibial insertion and is based on the findings of anatomical studies, demonstrating a fan-shaped ALL toward its tibial insertion.

A modification to this technique is the use of a looped graft through a bony tunnel at the tibia. This technique is performed by using the same femoral incision as described above, but making two stab incisions at the level of the tibia. The first one is situated at the superolateral corner of Gerdy's tubercle, the second more proximally and laterally, just anterior of the fibular head. A 3.2- or 4.5-mm drill is used to create a bony tunnel between these landmarks. A suture wire is passed through both stab incisions and the bony tunnel. This wire is can be used for testing isometry and thus correct femoral tunnel position. The graft is passed under the ITB from the proximal femoral incision to the most anterior distal tibial incision. The suture wire is used to pass the graft through the tunnel from anterior to posterior. The remaining end of the graft is again passed deep from the ITB, from the more posterior tibial stab incision to proximal, and finally can be anchored in the femoral tunnel joining the other free graft end [22, 35].

In case of combined ALL and ACL reconstruction, these techniques (double and single limb) can be modified in order to prevent the need for two different femoral tunnels. In this modification, the femoral ACL tunnel is drilled by use of an outside-in femoral ACL drill guide, the guide is positioned at the outer border of the lateral femoral condyle in such a way that the guide pin and cannulated drill pierce the anatomical femoral origin of the ALL and debouche the notch intra-articularly at the femoral attachment of the ACL. A tripled semitendinosus (ST) tendon graft and single gracilis tendon graft are used, they are both pulled (inside-out) in the femoral tunnel, and the triple loop ST should not protrude the lateral cortex, though the single gracilis tendon is pulled through. Both are secured in the femoral tunnel by use of an interference screw. The protruding end of the gracilis tendon, now located at the anatomical origin of the ALL, can thus be fixed at the tibia as described above (single or double limb depending on the remaining length of the graft) [22, 35]. The looped graft technique described above was specially designed to capacitate double-limb reconstruction combined with the femoral tunnel reduction technique.

18.2.2 Lateral Extra-articular Tenodesis (LET)

Before the introduction of the arthroscopically assisted intra-articular ACL reconstruction in the late 1980s, lateral extra-articular tenodesis (LET) was a widespread technique for treating an ACL injury, and throughout history, many different techniques were described [36]. In 1967, Lemaire described the first lateral extra-articular tenodesis technique for stabilizing an ACL-deficient knee [37]. He used a long strip of the ITB attached to Gerdy's tubercle, which was passed under the lateral collateral ligament (LCL). This was followed by femoral fixation through an anteroposterior orientated bony tunnel just proximal to the lateral epicondyle. The strip was again passed under the LCL and secured in a bony tunnel at Gerdy's tubercle. In 1979, Elison described a different technique in which the entire width of the ITB was isolated and detached from the proximal tibia (together with a bony part of Gerdy's tubercle), without sectioning or cutting the proximal part of the ITB. The ITB together with the bony part was passed under the LCL, and the bone of Gerdy's tubercle was reattached with a staple, just slightly anterior to its original insertion. This was performed in forced external rotation and 90° of flexion [38]. Around the same time, in the mid-1970s, MacIntosh described his variant of the LET [39]. He used a long strip of the ITB in the same way as Lemaire and passed it under the LCL. Proximally, it is sutured to a periosteal flap at the lateral femoral condyle and passed through the distal attachment of the intermuscular septum. The ITB strip is routed distally again, under the LCL and secured at Gerdy's tubercle [40]. This technique was later simplified by Arnold and Coker, often called the modified MacIntosh procedure. In this technique, which is still commonly used today, an ITB strip is first passed under the popliteus tendon and LCL and then simply looped around the LCL to be reattached at Gerdy's tubercle [41].

After the description of the ALL in 2013 and in particular the characterization of the femoral origin, most of these techniques were abandoned or at least modified to obtain a precise anatomical femoral fixation of the LET. Many techniques now use an incision over the lateral side of the knee, running from the Gerdy's tubercle just proximal to the lateral epicondyle [42]. The ITB is dissected and a portion of the ITB of approximately 1 cm wide and 10–15 cm long is used. Several authors suggest using the mid-part of the ITB, others prefer to use the posterior part. The tibial attachment to Gerdy's tubercle is typically kept as tibial insertion for the ALL reconstruct. The strip is mostly passed underneath the LCL and fixed to the lateral femoral condyle at the anatomical origin of the ALL, very similar to the anatomical reconstruction techniques. The gap in the ITB is often closed side-to-side after the procedure. The main difference to the anatomical reconstruction techniques can be found in the tibial fixation, as the ITB is not detached from Gerdy's tubercle, the tibial insertion of this tenodesis lies approximately 1 cm more anteriorly compared to the anatomical ALL insertion, which hypothetically could induce an improper isometry. Moreover, a portion of the ITB is sacrificed when LET is performed, which could adversely affect the restraint on internal rotation of the ITB shown by Laprade [10].

In deciding whether one should perform an anatomical ALL reconstruction or a lateral extra-articular tenodesis, no clear advice can be given. At this moment, there is no proven difference between both techniques if technically well performed. The authors of this chapter prefer the anatomical ALL reconstruction in cases with available ipsilateral gracilis tendons as we believe the perfect anatomical reconstruction should lead to the best clinical short- and long-term results. However, in revision cases when gracilis tendons already were harvested, a LEAT procedure is performed. Future research might show us advantages of one technique over another but until that moment one should perform the technique he is most familiar with, so the technique can be technically well performed.

Postoperative rehabilitation protocol of ALL reconstruction, whether an anatomical reconstruction or a LET is used, does not differ from that of isolated ACL reconstruction. Even though it might facilitate more aggressive rehabilitation, allowing earlier pivoting maneuvers or earlier return to sport hence the protective effect of the ALL reconstruction on the forces transmitted to the ACL graft [21, 43].

18.3 Outcomes

18.3.1 Biomechanical Outcomes

As described above, a long history of non-anatomical lateral extra-articular tenodesis (LET) techniques exists. Generalized outcomes of these different procedures did not prove to be consistent and although some authors showed improved biomechanical results concerning rotational control and significant decrease of re-rupture rates, other studies showed no significant improvement of combined ACL and LET compared to ACL reconstruction alone. It should be noticed that these studies report outcomes of LET before current insights in the anatomical landmarks of the ALL and especially location of femoral fixation showed a wide variance in different techniques. The non-anatomical nature of the femoral fixation could explain the inconsistent results of these empirical, experience-based techniques.

After adapting techniques allowing for improved anatomic graft fixation at the lateral femoral condyle, reports on biomechanical outcomes of combined ACL and ALL reconstruction have shown a significant positive effect of combined reconstruction compared to ACL reconstruction alone. The maximum internal rotation is reduced in all degrees of flexion to a value not significantly different from the non-injured side. Furthermore, during a pivot shift test, both anterior translation and internal rotation are significantly reduced by combining ACL and ALL reconstruction to a value not significantly different from the non-injured side [12, 44]. Anterior tibial translation in different degrees of flexion is not influenced by adding an ALL reconstruction.

Thus, in vitro ALL reconstruction is an effective technique in controlling residual rotational instability and pivot shift after ACL reconstruction leading to rotational stability similar to a pre-injury state.

18.3.2 Clinical Outcomes

18.3.2.1 Effect on Subjective Outcome Scores

Subjective outcomes of older LET techniques with non-anatomical femoral fixation show inconclusive results regarding patient-reported subjective outcome scores. Even though most studies comparing (non-anatomical) LET + ACL reconstruction and ACL reconstruction alone showed at least similar results concerning subjective outcome scores, some already showed significantly results [45–47]. Reports on subjective outcome scores of the effect of newer ALL reconstruction techniques are still scarce, but recent literature seems to be in favor of combining ALL + ACL reconstruction. In a selected population of chronic (>12 months old) ACL lesions, significantly better results concerning residual pivot-shift, IKDC, and Lysholm scores were reported, if ALL reconstruction was performed [19]. These results could not yet be confirmed in a general population, even though no reduced scores have been reported [21, 48].

As current results show significantly improved subjective outcomes for patients with chronic ACL tears if treated with combined ALL and ACL repair, it is suggested to routinely address the ALL in this specific population.

18.3.2.2 Effect on Graft Re-rupture Rates

One of the most common problems after ACL reconstruction is the event of re-rupture of the ACL graft. Rates in a young and active population are reported to be as high as 15–18%, with a significant increased risk for patients participating pivoting sports [26, 49, 50]. Furthermore, the risk of re-rupture is increased in patients showing a high grade of laxity in the preoperative status

[51]. The combination of ALL and ACL reconstruction has an indisputable impact on these re-rupture rates. Anatomical ALL reconstruction combined with Hamstring tendon (HT) ACL reconstruction has shown to cause a risk reduction of 3.1 times when compared to HT ACL reconstruction alone and a 2.5 times risk reduction when compared to Bone–Patellar Tendon–Bone (BTB) ACL reconstruction alone [21]. Similar results were found for different types of older LET procedures in long-term follow-up studies (5–25 years), showing re-rupture rates of only 2–4% [23–26]. These results could be explained by the protective effect of a lateral extra-articular tenodesis on ACL strains, and in biomechanical tests, up to 43% less forces were measured in the ACL graft when combined with lateral tenodesis [43].

As it is known that subjective outcomes after ACL revision surgery are significantly worse than those after primary ACL repair [52], together with the burden of re-operation including demanding rehabilitation for the patient, this powerful reduction of ACL graft re-rupture is considered to be the most important outcome of additional ALL reconstruction in ACL surgery.

18.3.2.3 Effect on Medial Meniscus Repair

Meniscal injuries are associated with ACL rupture, and incidences are reported to be 16–82% for acute injuries and 96% for chronic injuries [53]. The important role of the medial meniscus in the prevention of medial osteoarthritis is well known [54, 55], and its role in the stabilization of the knee has been shown in several cadaveric studies [56–58]. This has led to an important trend to save the meniscus whenever possible. Even though meniscal repair has shown to be more successful in case of concomitant ACL reconstruction, failure rates are still reported to be as high as 26% [59]. Concerning meniscal repair failure rates, a risk reduction of two times was noted when combining anatomical ALL reconstruction and ACL reconstruction when compared to meniscal repair and ACL reconstruction alone [20].

18.3.3 Complications

The main concern when introducing new surgical techniques to be performed on regular basis is the manifestation of technique-related complications. Results of different older lateral tenodesis techniques raised many concerns about these techniques. The first concern was that of possible early lateral osteoarthritis, related to an increase in lateral compartment stresses [15–18]. One must however remember that these results date from the time before precise anatomical knowledge of the ALL, and therefore, in the most older LET techniques, a non-anatomical femoral fixation point was used. Furthermore, through history, fixation of the tenodesis was advised to be completed in 90° of flexion and forced tibial external rotation, which could form an explanation for the issue of lateral overconstraining. The second concern is that of historical poor clinical results after lateral tenodesis with loss of range of motion and marked stiffness; however, in postoperative rehabilitation protocols of these older techniques, a plaster immobilization for several weeks was used after surgery, which could explain these adverse effects [60]. In recent studies using more anatomical LET techniques, concerns of lateral over constraining and stiffness are not confirmed, and these techniques are trusted to be safe [45, 61], and thus far, no study could demonstrate an increased risk of lateral or patellofemoral osteo-arthritis associated with any ALL reconstruction technique [1]. Furthermore, no signs of increased early complication rate of any concern were shown in numerous studies, thus the anatomical ALL reconstruction and LET technique are considered to be safe procedures [19–22].

References

1. Getgood A, Brown C, Lording T, Amis A, Claes S, Geeslin A, Musahl V, ALC Consensus Group. The anterolateral complex of the knee: results from the International ALC Consensus Group Meeting. Knee Surg Sport Traumatol Arthrosc. 2018; https://doi.org/10.1007/s00167-018-5072-6.

2. Hughston JC, Andrews JR, Cross MJ, Moschi A. Classification of knee ligament instabilities. Part II. The lateral compartment. J Bone Joint Surg Am. 1976;58:173–9.
3. Moorman CT, LaPrade RF. Anatomy and biomechanics of the posterolateral corner of the knee. J Knee Surg. 2005;18:137–45.
4. Johnson LL. Lateral capsular ligament complex: anatomical and surgical considerations. Am J Sports Med. 1979;7:156–60.
5. Irvine GB, Dias JJ, Finlay DB. Segond fractures of the lateral tibial condyle: brief report. J Bone Joint Surg Br. 1987;69:613–4.
6. Campos JC, Chung CB, Lektrakul N, Pedowitz R, Trudell D, Yu J, Resnick D. Pathogenesis of the Segond fracture: anatomic and MR imaging evidence of an iliotibial tract or anterior oblique band avulsion. Radiology. 2001;219:381–6.
7. Vincent J-P, Magnussen RA, Gezmez F, et al. The anterolateral ligament of the human knee: an anatomic and histologic study. Knee Surg Sports Traumatol Arthrosc. 2012;20:147–52.
8. Vieira ELC, Vieira EA, da Silva RT, Berlfein PA dos S, Abdalla RJ, Cohen M. An anatomic study of the iliotibial tract. Arthroscopy. 2007;23:269–74.
9. Claes S, Vereecke E, Maes M, Victor J, Verdonk P, Bellemans J. Anatomy of the anterolateral ligament of the knee. J Anat. 2013;223:321–8.
10. Vap AR, Schon JM, Moatshe G, Cruz RS, Brady AW, Dornan GJ, Turnbull TL, LaPrade RF. The role of the peripheral passive rotation stabilizers of the knee with intact collateral and cruciate ligaments: a biomechanical study. Orthop J Sport Med. 2017;5:2325967117708190.
11. Sonnery-Cottet B, Lutz C, Daggett M, Dalmay F, Freychet B, Niglis L, Imbert P. The involvement of the anterolateral ligament in rotational control of the knee. Am J Sports Med. 2016;44:1209–14.
12. Rasmussen MT, Nitri M, Williams BT, Moulton SG, Cruz RS, Dornan GJ, Goldsmith MT, LaPrade RF. An in vitro robotic assessment of the anterolateral ligament, part 1. Am J Sports Med. 2016;44:585–92.
13. Parsons EM, Gee AO, Spiekerman C, Cavanagh PR. The biomechanical function of the anterolateral ligament of the knee. Am J Sports Med. 2015;43:669–74.
14. Monaco E, Sonnery-Cottet B, Daggett M, Saithna A, Helito CP, Ferretti A. Elimination of the pivot-shift sign after repair of an occult anterolateral ligament injury in an ACL-deficient knee. Orthop J Sport Med. 2017;5:2325967117728877.
15. Schon JM, Moatshe G, Brady AW, Serra Cruz R, Chahla J, Dornan GJ, Turnbull TL, Engebretsen L, LaPrade RF. Anatomic anterolateral ligament reconstruction of the knee leads to overconstraint at any fixation angle. Am J Sports Med. 2016;44:2546–56.
16. Strum GM, Fox JM, Ferkel RD, Dorey FH, Del Pizzo W, Friedman MJ, Snyder SJ, Markolf K. Intraarticular versus intraarticular and extraarticular reconstruction for chronic anterior cruciate ligament instability. Clin Orthop Relat Res. 1989;245:188–98.
17. Roth JH, Kennedy JC, Lockstadt H, McCallum CL, Cunning LA. Intra-articular reconstruction of the anterior cruciate ligament with and without extra-articular supplementation by transfer of the biceps femoris tendon. J Bone Joint Surg Am. 1987;69:275–8.
18. O'Brien SJ, Warren RF, Pavlov H, Panariello R, Wickiewicz TL. Reconstruction of the chronically insufficient anterior cruciate ligament with the central third of the patellar ligament. J Bone Joint Surg Am. 1991;73:278–86.
19. Helito CP, Camargo DB, Sobrado MF, Bonadio MB, Giglio PN, Pécora JR, Camanho GL, Demange MK. Combined reconstruction of the anterolateral ligament in chronic ACL injuries leads to better clinical outcomes than isolated ACL reconstruction. Knee Surg Sport Traumatol Arthrosc. 2018; https://doi.org/10.1007/s00167-018-4934-2.
20. Sonnery-Cottet B, Saithna A, Blakeney WG, Ouanezar H, Borade A, Daggett M, Thaunat M, Fayard J-M, Delaloye J-R. Anterolateral ligament reconstruction protects the repaired medial meniscus: a comparative study of 383 anterior cruciate ligament reconstructions from the SANTI Study Group with a minimum follow-up of 2 years. Am J Sports Med. 2018;46:1819–26.
21. Sonnery-Cottet B, Saithna A, Cavalier M, Kajetanek C, Temponi EF, Daggett M, Helito CP, Thaunat M. Anterolateral ligament reconstruction is associated with significantly reduced ACL graft rupture rates at a minimum follow-up of 2 years: a prospective comparative study of 502 patients from the SANTI Study Group. Am J Sports Med. 2017;45:1547–57.
22. Thaunat M, Clowez G, Saithna A, Cavalier M, Choudja E, Vieira TD, Fayard J-M, Sonnery-Cottet B. Reoperation rates after combined anterior cruciate ligament and anterolateral ligament reconstruction: a series of 548 patients from the SANTI Study Group with a minimum follow-up of 2 years. Am J Sports Med. 2017;45:2569–77.
23. Marcacci M, Zaffagnini S, Iacono F, Vascellari A, Loreti I, Kon E, Presti M. Intra- and extra-articular anterior cruciate ligament reconstruction utilizing autogeneous semitendinosus and gracilis tendons: 5-year clinical results. Knee Surg Sport Traumatol Arthrosc. 2003;11:2–8.
24. Marcacci M, Zaffagnini S, Giordano G, Iacono F, Lo PM. Anterior cruciate ligament reconstruction associated with extra-articular tenodesis: a prospective clinical and radiographic evaluation with 10- to 13-year follow-up. Am J Sports Med. 2009;37:707–14.
25. Ferretti A, Monaco E, Ponzo A, Basiglini L, Iorio R, Caperna L, Conteduca F. Combined intra-articular and extra-articular reconstruction in anterior cruciate ligament-deficient knee: 25 years later. Arthroscopy. 2016;32:2039–47.
26. Morgan MD, Salmon LJ, Waller A, Roe JP, Pinczewski LA. Fifteen-year survival of endoscopic anterior cru-

ciate ligament reconstruction in patients aged 18 years and younger. Am J Sports Med. 2016;44:384–92.
27. Klos B, Scholtes M, Konijnenberg S. High prevalence of all complex Segond avulsion using ultrasound imaging. Knee Surg Sports Traumatol Arthrosc. 2017;25:1331–8.
28. Cavaignac E, Faruch M, Wytrykowski K, Constant O, Murgier J, Berard E, Chiron P. Ultrasonographic evaluation of anterolateral ligament injuries: correlation with magnetic resonance imaging and pivot-shift testing. Arthroscopy. 2017;33:1384–90.
29. Claes S, Luyckx T, Vereecke E, Bellemans J. The Segond fracture: a bony injury of the anterolateral ligament of the knee. Arthroscopy. 2014;30:1475–82.
30. Gaunder CL, Bastrom T, Pennock AT. Segond fractures are not a risk factor for anterior cruciate ligament reconstruction failure. Am J Sports Med. 2017;45:3210–5.
31. Fernandes LR, Ouanezar H, Saithna A, Sonnery-Cottet B. Combined ACL reconstruction and Segond fracture fixation fails to abolish anterolateral rotatory instability. BMJ Case Rep. 2018;2018:bcr–2018-224457.
32. Melugin HP, Johnson NR, Wu IT, Levy BA, Stuart MJ, Krych AJ. Is treatment of Segond fracture necessary with combined anterior cruciate ligament reconstruction? Am J Sports Med. 2018;46:832–8.
33. Kennedy MI, Claes S, Fuso FAF, Williams BT, Goldsmith MT, Turnbull TL, Wijdicks CA, LaPrade RF. The anterolateral ligament. Am J Sports Med. 2015;43:1606–15.
34. Zein AMN, Elshafie M, Elsaid ANS, Elrefai MAE. Combined anatomic anterior cruciate ligament and double bundle anterolateral ligament reconstruction. Arthrosc Tech. 2017;6:e1229–38.
35. Sonnery-Cottet B, Thaunat M, Freychet B, Pupim BHB, Murphy CG, Claes S. Outcome of a combined anterior cruciate ligament and anterolateral ligament reconstruction technique with a minimum 2-year follow-up. Am J Sports Med. 2015;43:1598–605.
36. Slette EL, Mikula JD, Schon JM, Marchetti DC, Kheir MM, Turnbull TL, LaPrade RF. Biomechanical results of lateral extra-articular tenodesis procedures of the knee: a systematic review. Arthroscopy. 2016;32:2592–611.
37. Lemaire M. Rupture ancienne du ligament croisé antérieur du genou. J Chir. 1967;93:311–20.
38. Ellison AE. Distal iliotibial-band transfer for anterolateral rotatory instability of the knee. J Bone Joint Surg Am. 1979;61:330–7.
39. Maclntosh DL, Darby TA. Lateral substitution reconstruction. J Bone Jointt Surg. 1976;58B:142.
40. Ireland J, Trickey EL. Macintosh tenodesis for anterolateral instability of the knee. J Bone Joint Surg Br. 1980;62:340–5.
41. Arnold JA, Coker TP, Heaton LM, Park JP, Harris WD. Natural history of anterior cruciate tears. Am J Sports Med. 1979;7:305–13.
42. Ntagiopoulos P, Dejour D. Extra-articular plasty for revision anterior cruciate ligament reconstruction. Clin Sports Med. 2018;37:115–25.
43. Engebretsen L, Lew WD, Lewis JL, Hunter RE. The effect of an iliotibial tenodesis on intraarticular graft forces and knee joint motion. Am J Sports Med. 1990;18:169–76.
44. Nitri M, Rasmussen MT, Williams BT, Moulton SG, Cruz RS, Dornan GJ, Goldsmith MT, LaPrade RF. An in vitro robotic assessment of the anterolateral ligament, part 2. Am J Sports Med. 2016;44:593–601.
45. Ferretti A, Monaco E, Ponzo A, Basiglini L, Iorio R, Caperna L, Conteduca F. Combined intra-articular and extra-articular reconstruction in anterior cruciate ligament–deficient knee: 25 years later. Arthroscopy. 2016;32:2039–47.
46. Rezende FC, de Moraes VY, Martimbianco ALC, Luzo MV, da Silveira Franciozi CE, Belloti JC. Does combined intra- and extraarticular ACL reconstruction improve function and stability? A meta-analysis. Clin Orthop Relat Res. 2015;473:2609–18.
47. Vadalà AP, Iorio R, De Carli A, Bonifazi A, Iorio C, Gatti A, Rossi C, Ferretti A. An extra-articular procedure improves the clinical outcome in anterior cruciate ligament reconstruction with hamstrings in female athletes. Int Orthop. 2013;37:187–92.
48. Ibrahim SA, Shohdy EM, Marwan Y, Ramadan SA, Almisfer AK, Mohammad MW, Abdulsattar WS, Khirat S. Anatomic reconstruction of the anterior cruciate ligament of the knee with or without reconstruction of the anterolateral ligament: a randomized clinical trial. Am J Sports Med. 2017;45:1558–66.
49. Persson A, Fjeldsgaard K, Gjertsen J-E, Kjellsen AB, Engebretsen L, Hole RM, Fevang JM. Increased risk of revision with hamstring tendon grafts compared with patellar tendon grafts after anterior cruciate ligament reconstruction: a study of 12,643 patients from the Norwegian Cruciate Ligament Registry, 2004–2012. Am J Sports Med. 2014;42:285–91.
50. Kamath GV, Murphy T, Creighton RA, Viradia N, Taft TN, Spang JT. Anterior cruciate ligament injury, return to play, and reinjury in the elite collegiate athlete: analysis of an NCAA Division I cohort. Am J Sports Med. 2014;42:1638–43.
51. Magnussen RA, Reinke EK, Huston LJ, et al. Effect of high-grade preoperative knee laxity on anterior cruciate ligament reconstruction outcomes. Am J Sports Med. 2016;44:3077–82.
52. Grassi A, Ardern CL, Marcheggiani Muccioli GM, Neri MP, Marcacci M, Zaffagnini S. Does revision ACL reconstruction measure up to primary surgery? A meta-analysis comparing patient-reported and clinician-reported outcomes, and radiographic results. Br J Sports Med. 2016;50:716–24.
53. Kilcoyne KG, Dickens JF, Haniuk E, Cameron KL, Owens BD. Epidemiology of meniscal injury associated with ACL tears in young athletes. Orthopedics. 2012;35:208–12.
54. Claes S, Hermie L, Verdonk R, Bellemans J, Verdonk P. Is osteoarthritis an inevitable consequence of anterior cruciate ligament reconstruction? A meta-analysis. Knee Surg Sport Traumatol Arthrosc. 2013;21:1967–76.

55. Pernin J, Verdonk P, Si Selmi TA, Massin P, Neyret P. Long-term follow-up of 24.5 years after intra-articular anterior cruciate ligament reconstruction with lateral extra-articular augmentation. Am J Sports Med. 2010;38:1094–102.
56. Levy IM, Torzilli PA, Warren RF. The effect of medial meniscectomy on anterior-posterior motion of the knee. J Bone Joint Surg Am. 1982;64:883–8.
57. Shoemaker SC, Markolf KL. The role of the meniscus in the anterior-posterior stability of the loaded anterior cruciate-deficient knee. Effects of partial versus total excision. J Bone Joint Surg Am. 1986;68:71–9.
58. Seon JK, Gadikota HR, Kozanek M, Oh LS, Gill TJ, Li G. The effect of anterior cruciate ligament reconstruction on kinematics of the knee with combined anterior cruciate ligament injury and subtotal medial meniscectomy: an in vitro robotic investigation. Arthroscopy. 2009;25:123–30.
59. Nepple JJ, Dunn WR, Wright RW. Meniscal repair outcomes at greater than five years. J Bone Joint Surg Am. 2012;94:2222–7.
60. Dodds AL, Gupte CM, Neyret P, Williams AM, Amis AA. Extra-articular techniques in anterior cruciate ligament reconstruction. J Bone Joint Surg Br. 2011;93B:1440–8.
61. Devitt BM, Bell SW, Ardern CL, Hartwig T, Porter TJ, Feller JA, Webster KE. The role of lateral extra-articular tenodesis in primary anterior cruciate ligament reconstruction: a systematic review with meta-analysis and best-evidence synthesis. Orthop J Sport Med. 2017;5:232596711773176.

ACL and Cartilage Lesions

19

Philippe Landreau

19.1 Introduction

Cartilage lesions are frequently observed at the time of an anterior cruciate ligament (ACL) reconstruction. Some of them are asymptomatic, but we do not know how they can affect the short-term clinical outcomes, the return to sport, and the future potential of osteoarthritis [1]. It is not well-known if these lesions can change the outcome in short- and long-term after ACL reconstruction. Therefore, it is not certain if and how these lesions must be treated during the same surgical procedure.

19.1.1 Epidemiology

It is important to mention that cartilage lesions do not occur only in combination with ACL rupture. The overall prevalence of full-thickness focal chondral defects in athletes have been estimated around 36%, according to a systematic review reported by Flanigan et al. [2], including 931 subjects. Fourteen percentage of these athletes were asymptomatic at the time of the diagnosis. Therefore, when an ACL tear occurs, it is sometimes difficult to identify whether the cartilage lesion is recent or not.

The presence of cartilage and meniscal lesions in ACL tears is well recognized. It has been shown that severe cartilage injuries combined with ACL tears occur between 16% and 46%, in comparison with meniscal injuries which are present between 55% and 65% of knees [3, 4].

Rotterud et al. [5] reported the cartilage and meniscal lesions observed in a large population of patients registered in the Norwegian and the Swedish National Knee Ligament Registry from 2005 to 2008, a total of 8476 knees. They found that 27% of the patients had at least one cartilage lesion at the time of the ACL reconstruction. As a comparison, in the same population, they found 43% of meniscal lesions, 20% of the patients had an ICRS grades 1–2 cartilage lesion, and 7% had a grades 3–4 cartilage lesion. The main localization was the medial femoral condyle (34–51%), and approximately half of the lesion had a surface area less than 2 cm^2.

For Tandogan et al. [6], 19.1% of patients with ACL tear had at least one chondral injury observed during an arthroscopy, 60% were observed in the medial compartment, mainly on the weight-bearing area of the medial condyle, and 67% of the chondral lesions were ICRS grades 1 and 2 and 33% grades 3 and 4. The mean surface was 219 ± 175 mm^2. There was a correlation between the presence of grade 3/4, in the age and the time between the injury and the arthroscopy.

P. Landreau (✉)
Aspetar, Orthopaedic and Sports Medicine Hospital, Doha, Qatar

M. Brittberg, K. Slynarski (eds.), *Lower Extremity Joint Preservation*,
https://doi.org/10.1007/978-3-030-57382-9_19

19.2 Cartilage Lesion and Timing of the ACL Surgery

The cartilage injury can occur at the time of the initial trauma or in chronic ACL injuries, as a consequence of a variety of factors, including alteration of tibiofemoral biomechanics and recurrent knee injuries resulting from episodes of instability. The literature supports the increase of cartilage lesions incidences in chronic cases in comparison with acute cases. Shelbourne [7] found respectively 23% and 54% of articular damage in knees with acute ACL tear and those with chronic ACL laxity. Joseph et al. [8] demonstrated that both athletes and non-athletes are equally susceptible for long-term cartilage injuries if ACL reconstruction is not performed early. They found a significant increase of meniscal and cartilage injuries after 1 year of evolution following ACL tear if the ACL reconstruction was not carried out.

In Tandogan's study [6], the odds of having a grade 3 or 4 lesion were 2.7 times greater if time from injury was 2–5 years versus 1 year, and these odds increased to 4.7 when patients at more than 5 years' time from injury were compared to those in the 2–5 years category. In this study, multivariate analysis validated that time from injury and age were equally important predictors of grade 3 or 4 chondral lesions.

Yuksel et al. [9] evaluated arthroscopically the type, localization, and prevalence of the meniscal and chondral lesions accompanying complete rupture of the anterior cruciate ligament in patients who elected not to restrict their daily activities after the initial trauma. They compared three groups according to time from injury until treatment: acute (0–6 weeks), subchronic (6 weeks to 12 months), and chronic (more than 12 months). Chondral lesions were noted at a rate of 8.9%, 25.9%, and 69.9%, respectively, in each group, with a significant increase in the chronic group.

For Michalitsis et al. [10], in a series of 109 consecutive patients with ACL rupture, the presence of high-grade cartilage lesion significantly increased in an ACL-deficient knee when reconstruction was performed more than 12 months after injury.

Anderson et al. [11] demonstrated that delayed ACL reconstruction increased the risks of secondary meniscal and chondral injuries in the population of pediatric patients.

More recently, Taketomi et al. [12], about a retrospective study involving 226 patients, concluded that ACL reconstruction should be performed within 6 months after the injury if we want to prevent associated cartilage and meniscus lesions.

Bambrilla et al. [13], in 2015, already found that ACL reconstruction within 12 months of injury can significantly reduce the risk of meniscal tears and chondral lesions. In their study, older age and increased BMI were risk factors for the occurrence of at least one associated lesion.

Therefore, it seems that attention should be paid to patients with an elevated BMI and older age when considering the timing of ACL reconstruction surgery.

Very few studies have evaluated the incidence of cartilage injuries in case of ACL revision. Wyatt et al. [4] have shown on a case series of 261 patients that the prevalence of cartilage injuries increased from 14.9% at primary ACLR to 31.8% at revision ACLR. Interestedly, in the same series, they observed that the prevalence of meniscal lesions decreased between the two surgeries.

19.2.1 Effect of Cartilage Injuries on ACL Reconstruction Outcomes

Among the predictors of poor outcome at 5–15 years after ACL reconstruction, cartilage damage is important, along with the medial meniscectomy and the lateral meniscectomy.

Rotterud et al. [5] evaluated the effect of articular cartilage lesions on patient-reported outcome 2 years after an ACL reconstruction. They showed that concomitant full-thickness cartilage lesion (grades 3–4) in ACL reconstruction have negative effects on knee function (KOOS) at 2 years follow-up.

Janssen et al. [14] conducted a prospective study of 100 patients who sustained an ACL reconstruction using four-strand hamstring tendon autograft. They have shown that, at 10 years follow-up, radiological signs of osteoarthritis were present in 53.5% of the cases. They demonstrated in their study that the risk factors for osteoarthritis were meniscectomy prior or during the ACL reconstruction and cartilage lesions observed at the time of the ACL surgery.

In the study performed by Kowalchuk [15] (402 subjects who had undergone primary single-bundle arthroscopic ACL reconstruction at a mean follow-up of 6.3 years), the lower International Knee Documentation Committee (IKDC) score was correlated to chondral injuries observed at the time of ACL reconstruction.

Cox et al. [16], in a 6-year multicenter cohort study, concluded that both articular cartilage injury (grades 3 and 4) and meniscus tears/treatment at the time of ACLR were significant predictors of lower IKDC and KOOS scores 6 years after ACLR.

However, other studies [7, 17–19] have found that cartilage lesion didn't affect the outcomes after ACL reconstruction. Shelbourne [7] found no difference after 8.7 years. Widuchowski [19] showed in a study at 10 and 15 years follow-up that the presence of a deep cartilage injury found during ACL reconstruction, left with no treatment, does not appear to affect the Lysholm, Tegner, and IKDC scores after ACL reconstruction in comparison with a control group.

In a systematic review including 37 studies, Filardo et al. [20] concluded that most of the studies in the literature showed a correlation between lesions of the articular surface and a poorer outcome after ACL reconstruction. Only few studies did not find any correlation.

With the above discrepancy and the absence of consensus, it is difficult to define an accurate algorithm to guide the surgeon in the decision whether or not to repair the cartilage lesions during ACL reconstruction. However, knowing that isolated grade 3/4 cartilage knee injuries can cause pain and effusion and affect the return to sport, it is difficult to ignore the cartilage lesions observed during an ACL surgery.

Despite this lack of literature support, it seems appropriate to manage high-grade focal chondral defects simultaneously with ACL surgical treatment, particularly if a meniscus lesion is present.

19.2.2 Results of Cartilage Repair and ACLR

Few series have shown that the treatment of cartilage injuries in the same time as the ACL reconstruction has resulted in acceptable outcomes.

Imade et al. [21] found no differences in IKDC scores in patients with concomitant ACL reconstruction and osteochondral lesions treated by drilling or autologous osteochondral grafting at a minimum follow-up of 1 year, regardless of the differences at arthroscopic grading of the ICRS classification, but only 40 patients were included in this case-control study.

It is accepted that there is a potential of spontaneous healing process after cartilage injuries. During ACL reconstruction, intra-articular enrichment in growth factors and progenitor cells might be involved in the repair processes of injured cartilage like it has been observed in meniscal repair. Nakamura et al. [22] demonstrated that at second-look arthroscopy, after ACL reconstruction without any intervention to the articular cartilage, there was a significant recovery of chondral lesions by Outerbridge grading on both the medial and lateral femoral condyles. Conversely, there was no significant recovery of chondral lesions observed at the patellofemoral joint or tibial plateaus. They concluded that there was a location-specific difference in the natural healing response of chondral injury.

In a nationwide prospective cohort study from Norway and Sweden of 368 patients with 5-year follow-up, comparing simple debridement, microfracture, and no surgical treatment of concomitant full-thickness cartilage lesions after anterior cruciate ligament reconstruction, Ulstein et al. [23] showed no difference on KOOS scores.

19.2.3 Which Cartilage Lesion Must Be Repaired at the Time of ACL Reconstruction?

There is little evidence whether the full-thickness cartilage should be repaired at the time of ACL reconstruction. However, in Rotterud study [5], the difference in outcomes between absence of cartilage lesion or partial lesion and full-thickness lesion suggests to perform a cartilage repair in the same time as the ACL reconstruction, especially in case of grade 3 or 4 ICRS cartilage lesions.

In addition, according to the literature already discussed above in this chapter, it should be recommended to prevent the cartilage lesion by shortening the time between the injury and the ACL reconstruction to decrease the risk of additional cartilage lesion.

19.2.4 Influence on Physiotherapy Protocol

The presence of concomitant cartilage lesions, treated or not, in the setting of ACL reconstruction represents a challenge in terms of postoperative physiotherapy management. Most of the authors would recommend prudence in the rehabilitation protocol. However, there is little evidence in the literature to recommend a specific protocol. Thrush et al. [24] published a systematic review of the studies describing the management of concomitant ACL rupture and chondral injury and the postoperative rehabilitation regimen. Only six studies were selected. They showed very little uniformity, and no strong recommendations could be concluded regarding the most appropriate rehabilitation. Particularly, the use of aggressive rehabilitation, early weight-bearing, no immobilization, and immediate range of motion did not compromise outcomes compared to more conservative protocols. The authors mentioned themselves that due to the limitation of the current available studies, it is difficult to make strong recommendations. Then, the good sense should be used for a case-by-case management until more robust evidence will be available in the future.

19.3 Technical Considerations

The purpose of this chapter is not to describe the cartilage repair techniques that are used in the setting of ACL ruptures. They are treated elsewhere in this book, and they do not differ in their realization. Nevertheless, their choice and selection can be influenced by the fact that they are performed during the reconstruction of the ACL.

A simple debridement, a microfracture procedure, or even a mosaicplasty are quick and simple techniques that will not require postoperative immobilization of the knee. But performing more sophisticated procedures, such as scaffolds or chondrocyte implantation, requires usually a postoperative period of immobilization. This can compromise the rehabilitation of the ACL based on early mobilization. The choice of the cartilage repair technique will have to be adapted to each situation. In our experience, only grade 3 and 4 ICRS lesions are treated at the same time as ACL surgery. Microfractures and mosaicplasty procedures are performed for the lesions inferior to 3 cm^2 [Fig. 19.1]. In condyle cartilage lesions, if the cartilage damage has a significant surface, the mosaicplasty has our preference, especially as the literature shows better results for sport recovery [25]. Above 3–4 cm^2, osteochondral allograft is a good option, if available, because it allows to start an early mobilization after the combined surgery.

19.3.1 Patient Information

Patient should be informed at the time of ACL surgery about the possible outcome if there is a full-thickness cartilage lesion observed during the surgery, whether the treatment is conservative or not. It is particularly important in athletic population where the expectation of an ACL

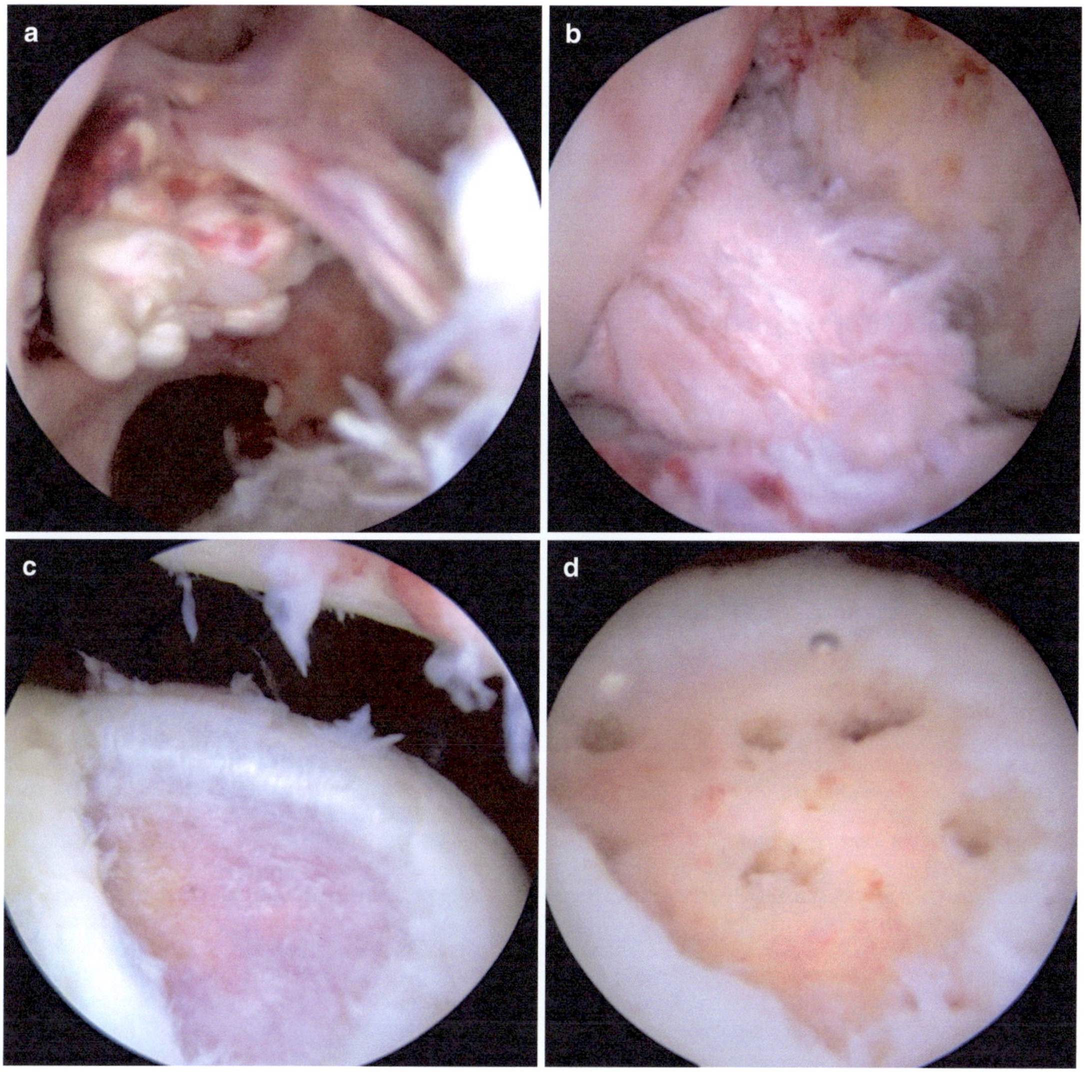

Fig. 19.1 Right knee ACL graft tear (**a**). Revision with bone patellar tendon bone graft (**b**). Trochlear grade 4 cartilage lesion (**c**). Microfracture procedure allowing the usual ACL postoperative physiotherapy protocol without any restriction (**d**)

reconstruction could be disappointed if the cartilage lesion led to residual pain, swelling, and limitation to return to sport.

19.4 Conclusion

The presence of full-thickness cartilage injury in conjunction with ACL tear leads to worse outcomes after ACL reconstruction than those with absence of cartilage lesion or even partial thickness cartilage lesion. These results have been noticed in short time follow-up and should be confirmed at longer follow-up. There is a lack of knowledge and evidence concerning the benefit of cartilage repair combined with ACL reconstruction. However, the current literature suggests that a full-thickness cartilage injury observed during an ACL reconstruction should be treated in the same time. Microfracture procedure, chondrocyte implantation, or the use of scaffolds will be decided based on the experience of the surgeon and on the surface of the cartilage damage.

Currently there is no evidence to support the treatment of partial cartilage lesion (grades 1–2) during an ACL reconstruction, and there are still some questions concerning the potential morbidity of this combined procedure.

The literature suggests that the severe cartilage lesions (grades 3 and 4) should be treated at the same time as the ACL reconstruction. The results of these concomitant surgeries are encouraging and could hope to decrease the incidence of future osteoarthritis. More studies should be set up in the future to determine evidence and true recommendation which type of cartilage lesions (depth, size, and localization) should be treated and which specific techniques should be performed.

References

1. Øiestad BE, Engebretsen L, Storheim K, Risberg MA. Knee osteoarthritis after anterior cruciate ligament injury: a systematic review. Am J Sports Med. 2009;37(7):1434–43.
2. Flanigan DC, Harris JD, Trinh TQ, Siston RA, Brophy RH. Prevalence of chondral defects in athletes' knees: a systematic review. Med Sci Sports Exerc. 2010;42(10):1795–801.
3. Brophy RH, Zeltser D, Wright RW, Flanigan D. Anterior cruciate ligament reconstruction and concomitant articular cartilage injury: incidence and treatment. Arthroscopy. 2010;26(1):112–20.
4. Wyatt RW, Inacio MC, Liddle KD, Maletis GB. Prevalence and incidence of cartilage injuries and meniscus tears in patients who underwent both primary and revision anterior cruciate ligament reconstructions. Am J Sports Med. 2014;42(8):1841–6.
5. Røtterud JH, Sivertsen EA, Forssblad M, Engebretsen L, Arøen A. Effect of meniscal and focal cartilage lesions on patient-reported outcome after anterior cruciate ligament reconstruction: a nationwide cohort study from Norway and Sweden of 8476 patients with 2-year follow-up. Am J Sports Med. 2013;41(3):535–43.
6. Tandogan RN, Taşer O, Kayaalp A, et al. Analysis of meniscal and chondral lesions accompanying anterior cruciate ligament tears: relationship with age, time from injury, and level of sport. Knee Surg Sports Traumatol Arthrosc. 2004;12:262–70.
7. Shelbourne KD, Jari S, Gray T. Outcome of untreated traumatic articular cartilage defects of the knee: a natural history study. J Bone Joint Surg Am. 2003;85-A(Suppl 2):8–16.
8. Joseph C, Pathak SS, Aravinda M, Rajan D. Is ACL reconstruction only for athletes? A study of the incidence of meniscal and cartilage injuries in an ACL-deficient athlete and non-athlete population: an Indian experience. Int Orthop. 2008;32(1):57–61.
9. Yüksel HY, Erkan S, Uzun M. The evaluation of intraarticular lesions accompanying ACL ruptures in military personnel who elected not to restrict their daily activities: the effect of age and time from injury. Knee Surg Sports Traumatol Arthrosc. 2006;14(11):1139–47.
10. Michalitsis S, Vlychou M, Malizos KN, Thriskos P, Hantes ME. Meniscal and articular cartilage lesions in the anterior cruciate ligament-deficient knee: correlation between time from injury and knee scores. Knee Surg Sports Traumatol Arthrosc. 2015;23(1):232–9.
11. Anderson AF, Anderson CN. Correlation of meniscal and articular cartilage injuries in children and adolescents with timing of anterior cruciate ligament reconstruction. Am J Sports Med. 2015;43(2):275–81.
12. Taketomi S, Inui H, Yamagami R, Kawaguchi K, Nakazato K, Kono K, Kawata M, Nakagawa T, Tanaka S. Surgical timing of anterior cruciate ligament reconstruction to prevent associated meniscal and cartilage lesions. J Orthop Sci. 2018;23(3):546–51.
13. Brambilla L, Pulici L, Carimati G, Quaglia A, Prospero E, Bait C, Morenghi E, Portinaro N, Denti M, Volpi P. Prevalence of associated lesions in anterior cruciate ligament reconstruction: correlation with surgical timing and with patient age, sex, and body mass index. Am J Sports Med. 2015;43(12):2966–73.
14. Janssen RP, du Mée AW, van Valkenburg J, Sala HA, Tseng CM. Anterior cruciate ligament reconstruction with 4-strand hamstring autograft and accelerated rehabilitation: a 10-year prospective study on clinical results, knee osteoarthritis and its predictors. Knee Surg Sports Traumatol Arthrosc. 2013;21(9):1977–88.
15. Kowalchuk DA, Harner CD, Fu FH, Irrgang JJ. Prediction of patient-reported outcome after single-bundle anterior cruciate ligament reconstruction. Arthroscopy. 2009;25(5):457–63.
16. Cox CL, Huston LJ, Dunn WR, Reinke EK, Nwosu SK, Parker RD, Wright RW, Kaeding CC, Marx RG, Amendola A, McCarty EC, Spindler KP. Are articular cartilage lesions and meniscus tears predictive of IKDC, KOOS, and Marx activity level outcomes after anterior cruciate ligament reconstruction? A 6-year multicenter cohort study. Am J Sports Med. 2014;42(5):1058–67.
17. Hjermundrud V, Bjune TK, Risberg MA, Engebretsen L, Arøen A. Full-thickness cartilage lesion do not affect knee function in patients with ACL injury. Knee Surg Sports Traumatol Arthrosc. 2010;18(3):298–303.
18. Spindler KP, Warren TA, Callison JC Jr, Secic M, Fleisch SB, Wright RW. Clinical outcome at a minimum of five years after reconstruction of the anterior cruciate ligament. J Bone Joint Surg Am. 2005;87(8):1673–9.
19. Widuchowski W, Widuchowski J, Koczy B, Szyluk K. Untreated asymptomatic deep cartilage lesions

associated with anterior cruciate ligament injury: results at 10- and 15-year follow-up. Am J Sports Med. 2009;37(4):688–92.

20. Filardo G, de Caro F, Andriolo L, Kon E, Zaffagnini S, Marcacci M. Do cartilage lesions affect the clinical outcome of anterior cruciate ligament reconstruction? A systematic review. Knee Surg Sports Traumatol Arthrosc. 2017;25(10):3061–75.
21. Imade S, Kumahashi N, Kuwata S, Kadowaki M, Tanaka T, Takuwa H, Uchio Y. A comparison of patient-reported outcomes and arthroscopic findings between drilling and autologous osteochondral grafting for the treatment of articular cartilage defects combined with anterior cruciate ligament injury. Knee. 2013;20(5):354–9.
22. Nakamura N, Horibe S, Toritsuka Y, Mitsuoka T, Natsu-ume T, Yoneda K, Hamada M, Tanaka Y, Boorman RS, Yoshikawa H, Shino K. The location-specific healing response of damaged articular cartilage after ACL reconstruction: short-term follow-up. Knee Surg Sports Traumatol Arthrosc. 2008;16(9):843–8.
23. Ulstein S, Årøen A, Engebretsen L, Forssblad M, Lygre SHL, Røtterud JH. A controlled comparison of microfracture, debridement, and no treatment of concomitant full-thickness cartilage lesions in anterior cruciate ligament-reconstructed knees: a nationwide prospective cohort study from Norway and Sweden of 368 patients with 5-year follow-up. Orthop J Sports Med. 2018;6(8):2325967118787767.
24. Thrush C, Porter TJ, Devitt BM. No evidence for the most appropriate postoperative rehabilitation protocol following anterior cruciate ligament reconstruction with concomitant articular cartilage lesions: a systematic review. Knee Surg Sports Traumatol Arthrosc. 2018;26(4):1065–73.
25. Krych AJ, Harnly HW, Rodeo SA, Williams RJ III. Activity levels are higher after osteochondral autograft transfer mosaicplasty than after microfracture for articular cartilage defects of the knee: a retrospective comparative study. J Bone Joint Surg Am. 2012;94:971–8.

Repair and Reconstruction of the Medical Collateral Ligament

20

Martin Lind

20.1 Anatomy

The primary structures involved in medial knee stabilization are the superficial MCL, (POL) and the deep MCL [9]. The sMCL, also named the tibial collateral ligament, is the largest structure of the medial aspect of the knee. This structure has one femoral and two tibial attachments. The femoral attachment is oval and is located just posterior to the medial epicondyle. Distally the sMCL has two tibial attachments. The proximal tibial attachment of is a soft tissue attachment over the termination of the anterior arm of the semimembranosus tendon located 10–12 mm distal to the tibial joint line. The distal tibial attachment has a broad attachment directly to bone at an average of 60 mm distal to the tibial joint line located just anterior to the posteromedial crest of the tibia. The POL is a fibrous extension off the distal aspect of the semimembranosus, which blends with and reinforces the posteromedial joint capsule. It consists of three facial attachments at the knee joint, with the most important portion being the central arm. On average, the central arm of the POL attaches on the femur just posterior to femoral sMCL insertion. The sMCL and the POL are separate structures [9]. The deep medial collateral ligament is comprised of the thickened medial joint capsule, which is deep to the sMCL. It is divided into meniscofemoral and meniscotibial components. The meniscofemoral ligament portion has an attachment 12 mm distal and deep to the sMCL's femoral attachment [9].

20.2 Biomechanical Properties of the Medial Knee Structures

The primary valgus stabilizing structure is the sMCL, which is an almost isometric structure with a strength of 550 N. The POL is tight in extension and becomes lax in flexion and contributes to external rotatory stability. POL lesion can result in anteromedial instability where the tibial plateau subluxates anteromedially during external rotation load [16].

The biomechanical properties of anatomical reconstruction of the MCL and posteromedial corner on valgus and rotatory stability have been investigated in a cadavers study [4]. The anatomical reconstruction technique involved single tendon strand reconstruction of the superficial MCL and POL with interference screw fixation at their anatomical femoral and tibial insertion sites. The reconstruction was supplied with an anchor fixation at the proximal tibial insertion of the superficial MCL.

M. Lind (✉)
Department of Orthopedics, Aarhus University Hospital, Aarhus, Denmark
e-mail: Martinlind@dadlnet.dk

M. Brittberg, K. Slynarski (eds.), *Lower Extremity Joint Preservation*,
https://doi.org/10.1007/978-3-030-57382-9_20

The study found a significant increase in valgus angulation and external rotation after sectioning the medial knee structures at all tested knee flexion angles. This was recovered following the anatomical medial knee reconstruction. The study concluded that an anatomic medial knee reconstruction could restore pre-injury stability to a knee with a complete sMCL and posterior oblique ligament injury, while avoiding overconstraining the reconstructed ligament grafts. Another study by Petersen et al. tested the importance of the POL in PCL deficient knees. In their study sectioning of the sMCL and deep MCL did not increase posterior instability, whereas sectioning of the POL resulted in significant increased posterior instability [15].

20.3 Injury Classifications (Table 20.1)

The most widely utilized medial knee injury grading scale is the American Medical Association Standard Nomenclature of Athletic Injuries in which medial collateral injuries are graded from I to III. Grade I or first-degree tear, presents with localized tenderness along the ligament with no valgus laxity. Grade II or second-degree tears, present with broadened tenderness and an increased joint gapping. This represents partially torn medial collateral and posterior oblique fibers. Grade III or third-degree tears, with a clear laxity without any resistance to an applied valgus stress. Grade III injury represents a complete disruption of all medial structures. Isolated medial knee injuries have also been classified in accordance to the amount of laxity observed at 30° of knee flexion with a valgus applied moment. These are Grade 1+, 2+, and 3+, which have been reported to correspond to 3–5 mm, 6–10 mm, and greater than 10 mm of subjective medial joint line gapping laxity respectively when compared to the noninjured contralateral side [6].

Table 20.1 Clinical evaluation of anteromedial knee instability

	Isolated superficial MCL lesion	Combined superficial MCL and posteromedial injury
Manual valgus testing 0°	No gapping	Increased gapping
Manual valgus testing 20–30°	Increased gapping without endpoint	Increased gapping without endpoint
Positive anterior drawer test	No	Yes
Positive dial test	No	Yes
Stress radiography 0°	>1.7 mm	>6.5 mm
Stress radiography 20–30°	>3.2 mm	>9.8 mm

The table presents the clinical findings of both manual examinations and stress radiography in case of isolated superficial MCL lesion and combined superficial MCL and posteromedial injury. The stress radiography thresholds are based on biomechanical studies from LaPrade et al. [8]

20.4 Clinical Evaluation of Valgus Instability

Examination of the superficial MCL is performed by valgus stress tests, which should be performed at both 0 and 20–30° of flexion. With the American Medical Association Standard Nomenclature of Athletic Injuries for grades I–III. Grade I injury has no valgus gapping, grade II, has clearly increased medial joint gapping but with a clear endpoint. Grade III, has clear laxity without any endpoint to an applied valgus stress. Isolated medial knee injuries have also been classified in accordance to the amount of laxity observed at 30° of knee flexion with a valgus applied moment. These are Grade 1+, 2+, and 3+, which have been reported to correspond to 3–5 mm, 6–10 mm, and greater than 10 mm of subjective medial joint line gapping laxity respectively when compared to the noninjured contralateral side [6].

A finding of valgus laxity at 0° indicates a concomitant cruciate ligament injury [19] but can also represent an injury and laxity of the posteromedial structures including the POL.

20.4.1 Stress Radiography

Valgus stress radiographs can be useful for quantitative grading of medial knee instability and to identify the insufficient structures that result in the medial compartment gapping. One study reported that compared to the intact knee, medial joint gapping increases of 1.7 and 3.2 mm were produced at 0° and 20° flexion, respectively, by a clinician-applied load when isolated grade III superficial MCL injury was present. A complete medial knee injury involving sectioning of the superficial and deep MCL and POL resulted in gapping increases of 6.5 mm and 9.8 mm at 0° and 20°, respectively [8].

20.4.2 Anteromedial Instability and Posteromedial Injury Assessment (Table 20.1)

Anteromedial instability is characterized by combined lesion of the superficial MCL and POL and the posteromedial capsule. The anteromedial drawer test and the dial test can evaluate this combined lesion.

The anteromedial drawer test is performed by flexing the knee to approximately 90° while externally rotating the foot 10–15° and applying an anteromedial rotational force to the knee. An anteromedial tibial plateau subluxation is a positive test and is indicative of POL and posteromedial capsule injury.

Also a complete injury to the medial structures will cause increased external rotation at both 30° and 90° of knee flexion resulting in a positive Dial test [17]. However it is important to palpate the tibial plateau in relation to the femoral condyle while performing the dial test. If the tibial plateau performs an anteromedial subluxation it is indicative of anteromedial instability whereas a posterolateral subluxation is a sign of posterolateral instability [13].

20.5 Indications for Surgical Treatment of MCL Lesion (Table 20.2)

20.5.1 Indication for Medial Repair

Acute surgical intervention by repair technique is to be indicated with the presence of the so-called Stener-type lesion of the distal MCL where the distal tibial insertion fibers are overlying the pes anserine attachment or in case of an avulsion fracture with sizeable osseous fragment. These lesions have a poor ability to healing frequently resulting in chronic medial instability.

Table 20.2 Treatment algorithm for MCL injuries

Injury type	Nonoperative management	Operative management
MCL grade 1 injury	RICE	No
MCL grade 2 injury	Hinged brace with free ROM for 6 weeks	No
MCL grade 3 injury	Hinged brace with free ROM for 6 weeks	MCL reconstruction if there is continued valgus instability after brace treatment If combined valgus and posteromedial instability use full anatomical reconstruction
MCL grade 3 injury with distal avulsion		Acute distal MCL insertion repair
MCL grade 3 injury + ACL injury	Initial hinged brace with free ROM for 6 weeks	ACL and MCL if there is continued medial instability reconstruction. If combined valgus and posteromedial instability use full anatomical reconstruction
MCL grade 3 injury in knee dislocation		Early or delayed full anatomical medial reconstruction and cruciate reconstruction
MCL grade 3 injury in knee dislocation with impinged medial tissue intraarticular		Acute reduction of impinged tissue and MCL insertion repair. Likely need for later reconstruction

20.5.2 Indication for Medial Reconstruction

In case of failed nonoperative treatment of a grade III injury resulting in continued excessive medial joint gapping or valgus laxity after the brace treatment medial reconstruction is indicated. In case of valgus instability without signs of POL lesion (rotational instability and/or valgus instability at full extension) and isolated sMCL reconstruction can be performed.

In multiligament injuries including grade III MCL injuries brace treatment of the medial injury have a higher failure rate than in cases of isolated grade III MCL injuries. Therefore in multiligament cases an acute approach with reconstruction of all injures structures (cruciates and collaterals) can be attempted. But also a staged principle with initial brace treatment for 2 months with free ROM and active muscle exercises and subsequent reconstruction of the ligaments that have not responded to the brace treatment with sufficient reestablishment of stability. In knee dislocation type injuries the capsular lesions are always significant resulting in the need to perform full anatomical medial reconstructions including both the sMCL and POL structures. In the rare cases of knee dislocation with impinged medial tissue intraarticular acute open reduction of this tissue is necessary in order to avoid necrosis. Medial repair can be done at the same time to optimize MCL healing, but delayed reconstruction of all involved ligaments in the knee dislocation is typically necessary [11].

20.6 Surgical Techniques

20.6.1 MCL Repair Techniques

Operative techniques which have been reported for acute direct repair of the superficial medial collateral ligament and posterior oblique ligament are numerous: such as primary repair with augmentation, advancement of the superficial medial collateral ligament tibial insertion site, pes anserinus transfer, advancement of the superficial medial collateral ligament with pes anserinus transfer. As there is very little literature to define the indication for acute repair treatment, it is beyond the scope of this chapter to present all these possible surgical techniques.

However, in the setting of combined grade III MCL and bicruciate injuries, a more aggressive approach with repair or reconstruction of all clinically insufficient structures can be considered [3]. Another acute setting where repair should be considered is when the superficial MCL is torn from its tibial insertion and become displaced outside the pes anserinus tendons. In these cases the ligament is unable to reattach to its insertion on the tibia with insufficient healing and increased risk of chronic instability as a result. The surgical technique is the following in for distal MCL avulsions. Expose the distal aspects of the tibial MCL insertion by opening the pes anserinus bursa as for standard hamstring graft harvest. Identify the avulsed MCL structures. Reinsert MCL fibers anatomically by 2–3 suture anchors.

Also tibial-sided injuries to the meniscal attachment to the deep MCL and posteromedial capsule can be considered restored by placing suture anchors along the peripheral rim of the tibia and bringing them through the deep MCL [7].

20.7 Anatomical MCL Reconstruction Techniques

Medial knee ligament reconstruction techniques that address both the superficial MCL and the posterior oblique ligament have only been described in few studies. In this section the main surgical techniques are described including the clinical data supporting the techniques. These techniques use hamstring tendon autografts. However other MCL reconstruction techniques have been described using allografts or autografts for typically isolated reconstruction of the superficial MCL [1, 14].

20.7.1 LaPrade–Engebretsen MCL Reconstruction Technique

This anatomic technique consists of a reconstruction of the sMCL and posterior oblique ligament using two separate grafts with four reconstruction tunnels [10]. The approach can be performed with either one large medial knee incision or by using three smaller medial knee incisions to access the anatomic attachment points of the ligaments. The sartorius muscle fascia is then incised and the gracilis and semitendinosus tendons were exposed. The semitendinosus is then harvested using a hamstring stripper and sectioned into two parts, one measuring 16 cm for subsequent sMCL reconstruction and the other 12 cm for subsequent POL reconstruction. Each portion of the tendon is tubularized on both ends using No. 2 nonabsorbable sutures to fit into 7 mm tunnels. Alternatively, allograft tendon may be used.

Attention is turned to the distal tibial attachment of the superficial MCL, approximately six cm distal to the joint line. Careful dissection is performed to identify the sartorial branch of the saphenous nerve through this incision. To protect the sartorial branch of the saphenous nerve, which usually courses posterior to the sartorius muscle belly and tendon at this level, the fascia anterior to the sartorius muscle tendon is incised, and the sartorius tendon is retracted distally. At this point, the attachment site of the central arm of the POL is identified at the posteromedial tibia near the direct arm of the semimembranosus tendon. After isolating the attachment locations of the superficial medial collateral and posterior oblique ligaments, attention is returned to drilling the reconstruction tunnels. Using an eyelet pin 7 diameter and 30 mm deep sockets are drilled at the femoral attachment of the sMCL and the posterior oblique ligament. The 16 and 12 cm sections of semitendinosus tendon that was previously tubularized are then passed into the tunnels and using an eyelet pin, and is recessed 25 mm into the tunnel and fixed with 7 mm cannulated bioabsorbable screws.

The tibial tunnels for the distal sMCL and posterior oblique ligament anatomic attachment points are reamed in similar fashion next. The distal superficial MCL tunnel is reamed first through the center of the distal superficial MCL anatomic attachment point located 6 cm distal to the joint line. Next, an eyelet pin is drilled through the center of the tibial attachment of the central arm of the POL, which exited just distal and medial to Gerdy's tubercle. A 7 × 30 mm socket is reamed. The superficial MCL graft is then passed under the fascia to the distal superficial MCL tunnel recessed to a depth of 25 mm. The knee is placed in 30° of knee flexion, in neutral rotation, and a varus force is applied to reduce any gapping of the medial compartment. The superficial MCL reconstruction graft is then tensioned and secured in place with a 7 mm bioabsorbable screw at the distal aperture of the tunnel. The knee is then placed through a full passive range of motion to verify proper positioning of the superficial MCL graft. The proximal tibial attachment point of the superficial MCL, which is primarily to soft tissues and located just distal to the joint line is recreated by suturing the sMCL graft to the anterior arm of the semimembranosus muscle with a suture anchor. Finally, the POL graft is passed into the tibial tunnel and recessed. The graft is tensioned secured with a 7-mm bioabsorbable screw.

20.7.2 Danish MCL Reconstruction Technique (Fig. 20.1)

This anatomic MCL reconstruction technique consists of a reconstruction of the sMCL and posterior oblique ligament using the semitendinosus tendon placed in one femoral tunnel and two tibial tunnels [12]. The approach can be performed with either one large medial knee incision or by using three smaller medial knee incisions to access the anatomic attachment points of the ligaments. The semitendinosus tendon is harvested at the pes anserinus and the insertion at pes anserinus is kept intact. The medial femoral epicondyle is exposed through a longitudinal incision. The femoral MCL insertion site is identified just posterior to the medial epicondyle and anterior to adductor tubercle. An eyelet pin K-wire is drilled

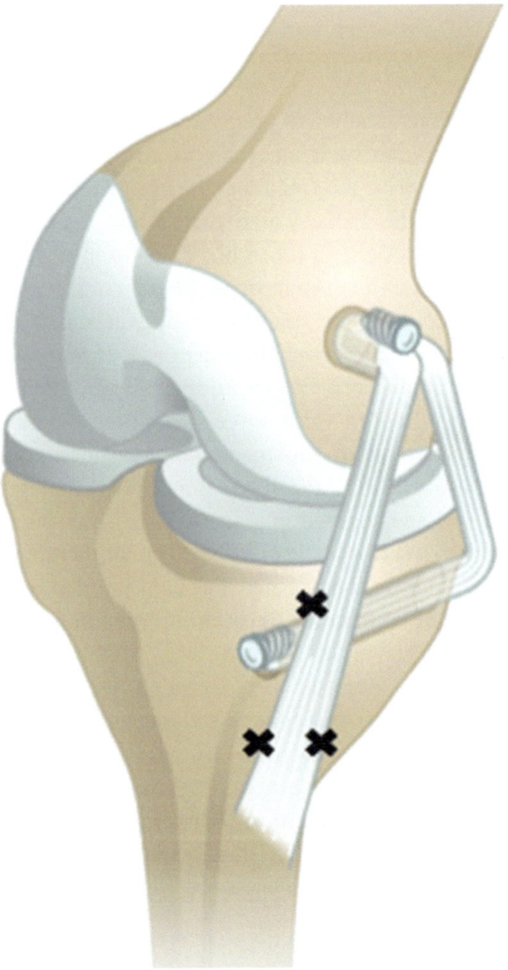

Fig. 20.1 The Danish anatomical MCL reconstruction with semitendinosus autograft. The tibial insertion is left intact and the tendon is redirected anatomically over the tibial MCL insertion with two suture anchors (xx). The tendon is then looped into at femoral drill hole at the femoral MCL insertion to reconstruct the sMCL. The posterior graft strand is taken into a drill at the upper aspects of the semimembranosus tibial insertion to reconstruct the POL. Finally the proximal tibial insertion of sMCL is established with a suture anchor (x)

in the proximal center of femoral MCL insertion. An 8 × 30 mm tunnel is drilled sized according to the measured diameter of the double looped tendon. Now the released semitendinosus tendon is pulled along the K-wire and folded to create a tendon loop that will enable the loop to be recessed 25 mm into the femoral drillhole and fitted with No 2 Fiberwire baseball suture. The semitendinosus tendon is then passed under the fascia to the femoral drill tunnel. The sutured loop is then passed into the tunnel with pull-through technique and fixed with an 8 × 25 interference screw to reconstruct the superficial MCL. The reconstruction is tightened at 10° of flexion and neutral rotation. The non-fixated free end of the tendon is now used to for the posterior oblique ligament reconstruction. A tibial tunnel is then drilled at the posterior corner of the medial tibial condyle just proximal to tibial insertion of semimembranosus tendon. Tunnel diameter is the size of semitendinosus graft, which typically was 6 mm. The free end of graft is passed under the fascia from the femoral condyle to the tibial posterior oblique ligament tunnel. The graft is tensioned at 10° of flexion and fixed with an interference screw with the same diameter as the drill tunnel to reconstruct the posteromedial corner. The reconstruction will appear as an inverted V on the medial aspect of the knee.

20.8 Post-op Rehab

For isolated MCL reconstruction procedures a hinged brace is used for 6 weeks to protect the reconstruction from excessive valgus load. During the first two weeks and partial weight bearing and 0–90° of motion can be allowed. From week 3 to 6, free range of motion and free weight bearing during standing and walking are allowed. After 6 weeks free activity was allowed without brace. Controlled sports activities after 3 months and contact sports after 6 months were allowed. For MCL reconstruction in combination with ACL reconstruction a similar rehabilitation protocol can be but return to contact sports was delayed to 12 months postoperatively. For MCL reconstruction in combination med PCL reconstruction the rehabilitation protocol need to be more restrictive with a PCL support hinged brace with 0–90° of motion and no weight bearing for 6 weeks followed by another 6 weeks in with free ROM and full weight bearing. Return to contact sports was then delayed to 12 months postoperatively.

20.9 Expected Outcomes

20.9.1 Clinical Outcome After MCL Repair Surgery

The literature on clinical outcome after isolated MCL repair is limited with no level one evidence for clinical efficiency of isolated repair procedures. A recent systematic review has looked at the outcome with different MCL repair procedures in case series [2]. The study found acceptable clinical outcome with repair procedures with 75% of patients achieving good valgus stability and 90% good subjective outcome. However these results are comparable with nonoperative treatment for isolated MCL injury.

There is level one evidence for MCL repair in combination with ACL reconstruction in patients with combined ACL and MCL lesion. In a randomized study in which patients with combined ACL and MCL lesions where randomized to either ACL reconstruction combined with MCL repair or isolated ACL. MCL repair was not found to improve MCL stability and clinical outcome over no repair [5].

MCL repair outcome in knee dislocation multiligament injuries have been investigated by Stannard et al. [18] This study compared the outcomes of surgical repair versus reconstruction in knee dislocation patients who have sustained injury to the posteromedial corner of the knee. A total of 25 repair patients had five failures (20%), whereas 48 patients reconstruction of the PMC had two failures (4%) indicating that repair had poorer outcome than reconstruction in knee dislocation injuries.

20.9.2 Clinical Outcome After Anatomical MCL Reconstruction

The LaPrade–Engebretsen technique has been investigated in a case series of 28 patients (19 male, nine females). The average age was 32.4 years (range, 16–56 years). There were eight acute and 20 chronic injuries. All patients presented with subjective and objective valgus instability limiting activities of daily living and sports activities. Minimum follow-up was 6 months (average, 1.5 years; range, 0.5–3 years). It was found that subjective outcome evaluated by International Knee Documentation Committee (IKDC) subjective outcome scores improved from preoperative 43.5 (range, 14–66) to final postoperative values of 76.2 (range, 54–88). Preoperative valgus stress radiographs averaged 6.2 mm of medial compartment gapping compared with the contralateral normal knee, whereas postoperative stress radiographs averaged 1.3 mm [10].

The Danish technique has been investigated in a case series 61 patients with grade 3 or 4 medial instability were treated with MCL reconstruction. Thirteen patients had isolated MCL reconstructions, 34 were combined with ACL reconstruction and 14 were multiple ligament reconstructions. All had reconstruction of the medial collateral ligament and the POL with a semitendinosus autograft. Fifty patients were available for follow-up more than 24 months postoperatively and were examined by an independent observer using objective IKDC measures and subjective Knee Osteoarthritis Outcome Score (KOOS). Objective IKDC medial stability at follow-up was in 98% of patients normal or nearly normal (grade A or B). The overall objective IKDC score patients improved from 5% grade A or B preoperatively to 74%. Ninety-one per cent were satisfied or very satisfied with the result and 88% would go through surgery again. KOOS score improved primarily for sports and quality of life subscales with approximately 10 point improvements. It was concluded that MCL reconstruction with combined collateral and POL reconstruction technique resulted in good clinical outcome in patients suffering from chronic valgus instability [12].

References

1. Borden PS, Kantaras AT, Caborn DN. Medial collateral ligament reconstruction with allograft using a double-bundle technique. Arthroscopy. 2002;18(4):E19.
2. DeLong JM, Waterman BR. Surgical repair of medial collateral ligament and posteromedial corner

injuries of the knee: a systematic review. Arthroscopy. 2015;31(11):2249–55.
3. Engebretsen L, Risberg MA, Robertson B, Ludvigsen TC, Johansen S. Outcome after knee dislocations: a 2–9 years follow-up of 85 consecutive patients. Knee Surg Sports Traumatol Arthrosc. 2009;17(9):1013–26.
4. Griffith CJ, LaPrade RF, Johansen S, Armitage B, Wijdicks C, Engebretsen L. Medial knee injury: part 1, static function of the individual components of the main medial knee structures. Am J Sports Med. 2009;37(9):1762–70.
5. Halinen J, Lindahl J, Hirvensalo E, Santavirta S. Operative and nonoperative treatments of medial collateral ligament rupture with early anterior cruciate ligament reconstruction: a prospective randomized study. Am J Sports Med. 2006;34(7):1134–40.
6. Hughston JC. Acute knee injuries in athletes. Clin Orthop. 1962;23:114–33.
7. Jacobson KE, Chi FS. Evaluation and treatment of medial collateral ligament and medial-sided injuries of the knee. Sports Med Arthrosc. 2006;14(2):58–66.
8. LaPrade RF, Bernhardson AS, Griffith CJ, Macalena JA, Wijdicks CA. Correlation of valgus stress radiographs with medial knee ligament injuries: an in vitro biomechanical study. Am J Sports Med. 2010;38(2):330–8.
9. LaPrade RF, Engebretsen AH, Ly TV, Johansen S, Wentorf FA, Engebretsen L. The anatomy of the medial part of the knee. J Bone Joint Surg Am. 2007;89(9):2000–10.
10. LaPrade RF, Wijdicks CA. Surgical technique: development of an anatomic medial knee reconstruction. Clin Orthop Relat Res. 2012;470(3):806–14.
11. Levy BA, Fanelli GC, Whelan DB, Stannard JP, MacDonald PA, Boyd JL, Marx RG, Stuart MJ, Knee Dislocation Study G. Controversies in the treatment of knee dislocations and multiligament reconstruction. J Am Acad Orthop Surg. 2009;17(4):197–206.
12. Lind M, Jakobsen BW, Lund B, Hansen MS, Abdallah O, Christiansen SE. Anatomical reconstruction of the medial collateral ligament and posteromedial corner of the knee in patients with chronic medial collateral ligament instability. Am J Sports Med. 2009;37(6):1116–22.
13. Lubowitz JH, Bernardini BJ, Reid JB III. Current concepts review: comprehensive physical examination for instability of the knee. Am J Sports Med. 2008;36(3):577–94.
14. Marx RG, Hetsroni I. Surgical technique: medial collateral ligament reconstruction using Achilles allograft for combined knee ligament injury. Clin Orthop Relat Res. 2012;470(3):798–805.
15. Petersen W, Loerch S, Schanz S, Raschke M, Zantop T. The role of the posterior oblique ligament in controlling posterior tibial translation in the posterior cruciate ligament-deficient knee. Am J Sports Med. 2008;36(3):495–501.
16. Robinson JR, Bull AM, Thomas RR, Amis AA. The role of the medial collateral ligament and posteromedial capsule in controlling knee laxity. Am J Sports Med. 2006;34(11):1815–23.
17. Slocum DB, Larson RL. Rotatory instability of the knee: its pathogenesis and a clinical test to demonstrate its presence. 1968. Clin Orthop Relat Res. 2007;454:5–13; discussion 13–4.
18. Stannard JP, Black BS, Azbell C, Volgas DA. Posteromedial corner injury in knee dislocations. J Knee Surg. 2012;25(5):429–34.
19. Torg JS, Conrad W, Kalen V. Clinical diagnosis of anterior cruciate ligament instability in the athlete. Am J Sports Med. 1976;4(2):84–93.

The Posterolateral Ligament Complex of the Knee

21

Jon Karlsson, Louise Karlsson, Eric Hamrin Senorski, and Eleonor Svantesson

21.1 Introduction

The posterolateral corner (PLC), including the lateral (fibular) collateral ligament (LCL/FCL), has been referred to as "the dark side of the knee". The LCL/FCL is one of the four main stabilising ligaments of the knee, but, even though it is important in its stabilising role, the literature is scarce when it comes to descriptions of its anatomy and function [2]. The main reason for this is thought to be that the lateral ligaments are not injured as frequently as the other ligaments of the knee.

The LCL/FCL is taut in extension and slackens in flexion in order to allow tibial rotation of the flexed knee. This ligament is the main structure responsible for resisting lateral laxity, and it also plays a major role in limiting the external rotation of the flexed knee. The involvement of limiting internal rotation is much less, or negligible. Taken together, the LCL/FCL is the main restraint to primary varus rotation in all positions of knee flexion. The isolated sectioning of the LCL/FCL results in a small yet significant increase in varus rotation at all angles of knee flexion. The synergistic function of the LCL/FCL and the posterolateral structures also control the axial rotation of the tibia. Studies have also shown that the posterolateral structures, such as the LCL/FCL and popliteus, act as secondary restraints to posterior tibial translation [2, 4, 7].

The lateral knee structures can be divided into three distinct layers. The deepest layer, which is the lateral part of the capsule, divides into two thin layers just posterior to the overlying iliotibial tract. There are three ligaments, the LCL/FCL, the fabello-fibular and the arcuate ligaments. The main contributors to the static stabilisation of the PLC are the LCL/FCL, the popliteal tendon and the popliteo-fibular ligament. The main functional contributions of these ligaments are varus restraint, external rotation and external rotation, coupled with the posterior translation of the tibia relative to the femur [7].

It has been shown that an isolated lateral ligament injury elicits abnormal knee laxity, with functional instability and limitations. An LCL injury results in a varus thrust gait pattern with the development of medial meniscal tears and subsequent medial compartment osteoarthritis due to the excessive compressive forces on the medial tibio-femoral compartment. Moreover, varus laxity, which is mainly due to a deficient LCL/FCL (sometimes as a part of a non-diagnosed and non-treated posterolateral knee injury), will cause a significant increase in force on both the anterior cruciate ligament (ACL) and

J. Karlsson · L. Karlsson · E. Hamrin Senorski (✉)
E. Svantesson
Department of Orthopaedics, Sahlgrenska University Hospital, Institute of Clinical Sciences, Sahlgrenska Academy, University of Gothenburg, Gothenburg, Sweden, Mölndal, Sweden
e-mail: eric.hamrin.senorski@gu.se

M. Brittberg, K. Slynarski (eds.), *Lower Extremity Joint Preservation*,
https://doi.org/10.1007/978-3-030-57382-9_21

posterior cruciate ligament (PCL) and may result in the failure of ACL and PCL reconstructive grafts. Accordingly, reconstructive techniques to address both the ACL/PCL and LCL at the same time are of major importance [4, 7].

Despite major advances in terms of diagnostic evaluation and treatment algorithms, lateral and posterolateral laxity/instability is difficult to diagnose and treat. It is also noteworthy that, unlike medial knee ligament injuries, grade III lateral injuries rarely heal by themselves and usually require surgical repair and/or reconstruction.

It is also important to recognise that lateral and posterolateral injuries rarely occur in isolation; in other words, surgeons should always look for combined injuries, especially intraoperatively. Failure to recognise posterolateral lesions when performing an ACL or PCL reconstruction is an important cause of failure in these reconstructions (Figs. 21.1 and 21.2).

21.2 Anatomy

The complex anatomy of the lateral aspect of the knee is arranged in static and dynamic stabilising structures [4]. The primary role of the static structures, i.e. the ligaments, is to restrain abnormal motion. The LCL is between 55 and 73 mm long (with a mean of 63–70 mm) and has a semicircular attachment on the femoral epicondyle. The average length differs by only a few mm between studies. The attachment is slightly proximal and slightly posterior to the lateral epicondyle. There is a small bony depression just posterior to the lateral epicondyle, where the main ligament attachment is located (Fig. 21.1). There are also fibres that extend proximally and anteriorly over the lateral epicondyle in a fanlike fashion. The distance between the ligament and the popliteal tendon on the femur is less than 2 cm. The cross-sectional area is 0.43–0.48 cm^2.

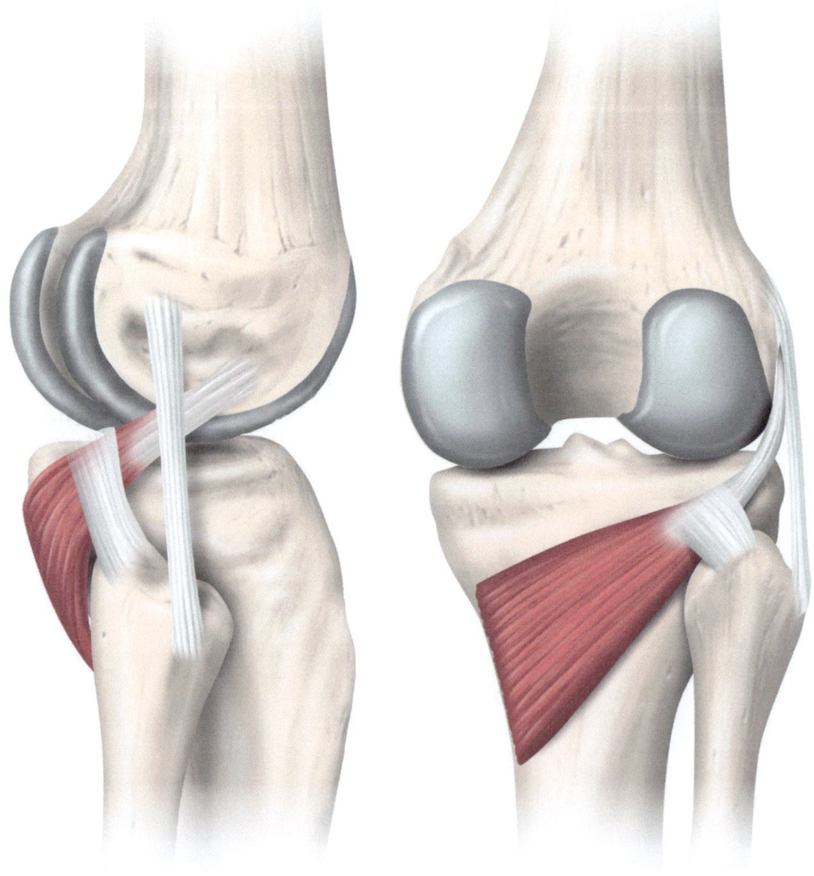

Fig. 21.1 Normal anatomy of the lateral aspect of the knee, showing the attachment sites of the fibular collateral ligament (FCL) on the femur and fibula, the popliteal tendon (PLT) in the popliteal sulcus of the femur and the popliteo-fibular ligament. Lateral view (left) and posterior view (right)

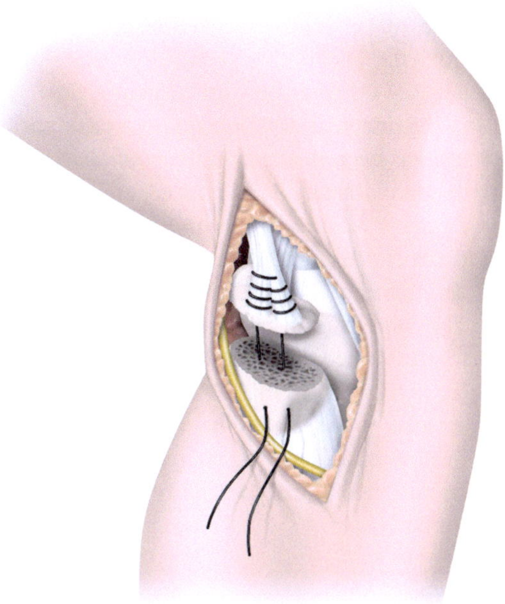

Fig. 21.2 Repair (reinsertion) of the distal aspect of the biceps femoris tendon with drill holes through the proximal fibula. Note the small fracture of the proximal fibula

The attachment is fairly constant from knee to knee [16].

The LCL is attached distally on the lateral aspect of the fibular head, where the attachment is approximately 8 mm posterior to the anterior margin of the fibular head. It is located approximately 28 mm distal to the tip of the fibular styloid process. The fibular attachment is fan shaped where the most lateral fibres act as a reinforcement of the fascia of the peroneus longus muscle in the lateral compartment of the lower leg. The fibular attachment is in a bony depression that extends more or less to the distal third of the lateral aspect of the fibular head [4].

The popliteus muscle courses anteriorly and laterally over the posterolateral aspect of the knee. The attachment is on the postero-medial tibia, and, in the lateral third of the popliteal fossa, the muscle becomes the popliteal tendon (Fig. 21.2). An important ligament – often overlooked at injury—is the popliteo-fibular ligament, which is attached to the popliteus complex at the musculotendinous junction. The popliteal tendon is partially intra-articular, running anterolaterally around the posterior aspect of the lateral femoral condyle and medial to the LCL/FCL, attaching to the popliteal sulcus. The attachment of the popliteal tendon is always anterior to the femoral attachment of the LCL. The average length of the popliteal tendon is approximately 55 mm [10].

The third important posterolateral stabilising structure is the popliteo-fibular ligament. It originates at the musculotendinous junction from the popliteus muscle. It consists of two bundles, one anterior and one posterior. Proximally and medially, the anterior bundle is attached to the popliteal tendon at the musculotendinous junction. The posterior bundle is attached at the postero-medial aspect of the styloid process of the fibular head. The posterior bundle is always larger than the anterior bundle, approximately 6 mm wide [10].

Finally, the lateral gastrocnemius tendon originates at the supracondylar process of the distal femur. There is a fabello-fibular ligament, which can be defined as the distal edge of the capsular part of the biceps femoris short head. The attachment of the lateral gastrocnemius tendon is approximately 15 mm posterior to the LCL attachment on the femur. The average distance between the lateral gastrocnemius attachment of the femur to the popliteal tendon attachment is approximately 30 mm [10].

Moreover, secondary stabilisers are the lateral capsular thickening of the mid-lateral capsular ligament, plus the coronary ligament, with an attachment on the posterior aspect of the lateral meniscus to the tibia, the fabello-fibular ligament, which is a thickening of capsular part of the biceps femoris short head, the long head of the biceps femoris and the iliotibial band (ITB).

21.3 Epidemiology

Lateral ligament injuries are less common than medial injuries; they constitute less than 10% of all knee ligament injuries. In a recent meta-analysis, it was reported that 60% of PLC injuries are combined with PCL injuries, while 23% had combined ACL injuries, 6% had combined ACL and PCL injuries and 12% had an isolated PLC injury.

21.4 Evaluation

Most PLC injuries are due to hyperextension and non-contact varus stress. In many cases, posterolateral injuries are associated with ACL and/or PCL injuries, which underlines the necessity for a thorough PLC examination of all cruciate ligament injuries. There is a probability that PLC injuries are often overlooked. The patient typically complains of pain, side-to-side instability (often close to extension) and difficulty walking on uneven ground or up- and downstairs. In most cases, swelling and haemarthrosis are profound. Varus thrust gait is noted, especially at the initiation of the stance phase. A complaint of paraesthesia from the common peroneal nerve is frequent, and injury to the nerve occurs in approximately one third of all cases.

The clinical tests include:

- *Varus stress testing*: performed in full extension and 20–30° of flexion. The lateral compartment gap is compared with the contralateral side. With an increased gap at 30°, both the LCL and the secondary stabilisers of the PLC are injured, while an isolated injury to the LCL is diagnosed if laxity is restored in full extension. With varus laxity persisting in full extension, a diagnosis of LCL, PLC and cruciate ligament injury is established.
- *The dial test*: this test measures external rotation of the tibia relative to the femur. The patient is in a prone position and the knee is flexed at 30°; with the femur fixed, the ankle and foot are externally rotated. An increase of more than 10° of external rotation suggests an injury to the PLC. The knee is then flexed at 90°. If the PLC is intact, the external rotation of the tibia will decrease, but, with an increase in external rotation—as compared with 30°, the diagnosis of a combined PCL and PLC injury is established.
- *Reverse pivot shift test*: this test is essential in a PLC evaluation. The patient is in a supine position, with the knee flexed, close to 90°. As valgus load is applied through the knee, an external rotation force is applied to the tibia and the knee is slowly extended. A positive test is shown by a reduction in the subluxated lateral tibia plateau at 35–40° of flexion. This is due to ITB changes from the knee flexor to knee extensor at this angle. A comparison with the contralateral knee is important. It is worth noting that a positive test has been reported in the contralateral knee in approximately 35% of all cases.
- *External rotation recurvatum test*: the value of this test is difficult to understand, but it can be an important part of the diagnostic evaluation. The patient is in a supine position, with the legs extended. The big toe is grasped and the leg is lifted from the table, while the femur is secured to the table. The height of the heel is then measured and compared with the contralateral side. The specificity of this test is limited [3].

21.5 Imaging

In most cases, imaging is necessary to determine PLC injuries. Standard anteroposterior, patellar and bent knee patellofemoral views on plain radiographs are frequently normal. In chronic injuries, a standing long-leg anteroposterior image is always necessary, due to the risk of malalignment, which often needs to be corrected by osteotomy, either a two-stage procedure or one stage at the time of PLC/PCL reconstruction.

Varus stress radiographs are essential for diagnostic purposes and to plan surgical reconstruction. Varus stress radiographs have been reported to be reliable when securely evaluating the severity of lateral and posterolateral lesions. Stress radiographs should be taken bilaterally, with the knee in 20° of flexion. This method has been reported to be valid, reliable, clinically relevant and useful. The gap in the lateral compartment is determined by measuring the shortest distance between the subchondral bone surfaces of the distal femur and proximal tibia, respectively. A comparison with the contralateral side is obligatory. A side-to-side difference of 2.7–4.0 mm indicates an isolated complete LCL rupture, while a difference of 4.0 mm or more indicates a grade III PLC injury and is thereby an indication for surgical intervention.

Magnetic resonance imaging (MRI) should always be performed in order to evaluate soft-tissue injuries (especially in terms of acute injuries) and to assess concurrent injuries.

21.6 Treatment

Grade I and II PLC injuries are usually treated non-surgically. However, scientific knowledge of the outcome after grade I and II injuries is very limited. The treatment protocol usually includes bracing for up to 6 weeks or early mobilisation and early weight-bearing. With regard to grade III PLC injuries, poor functional outcomes have been reported after non-surgical treatment. Outcomes include persistent instability, limited functional recovery and osteoarthritis at the medium-term follow-up. If PLC injuries are not addressed, there is major risk of further injury to the ACL and/or PCL or graft failure [11, 12].

Primary repair or reconstruction poses a difficult question [11, 12]. Primary repair is possible if it is performed within 2–3 weeks after injury, but thereafter it is technically difficult or even impossible [17]. Primary repairs of complete LCL/FCL and/or popliteus avulsions have therefore been performed and are technically feasible. A rupture of the biceps femoris tendon may be involved as well (Fig. 21.2). However, several studies have reported a poor outcome after repair, and the general treatment rationale is reconstruction rather than repair, even in the acute phase [17]. This means that repair is possible, but, in addition to the repair, reconstruction is indicated. Several studies have shown poor results after repair in only approximately 40% of cases, but fewer than 10% in the reconstructive group [18].

The timing of surgery is important. Several studies have reported better outcomes if treatment is undertaken within 3 weeks, instead of at 3 weeks or more, when the injury is regarded as chronic [8, 11, 12].

In terms of the treatment of chronic injuries, the alignment should always be carefully evaluated. In the event of malalignment, osteotomy (often biplanar) is the treatment of choice. Alignment must always be corrected before ligament reconstruction is performed. Failure to address malalignment will inevitably lead to increased stress on the reconstructed grafts and ultimate failure [9, 11, 12].

There are several reconstructive techniques, based on either isometry or anatomic landmarks (footprints). Surgeons need to restore the native knee biomechanics, as much as possible at the very least [1, 12, 18]. The anatomic reconstruction of all three static stabilisers of the PLC is therefore preferred. After a lateral curved skin incision, deep dissection is made between the tubercle of Gerdy and the fibular head. The next step is always to identify the common peroneal nerve. Neurolysis is performed and the nerve is well protected throughout the procedure [13–15]. The remnant of the LCL/FCL is located and secured with sutures. Either an autograft or an allograft can be used to reconstruct the torn ligaments. A 7 mm tunnel in the fibular head is reamed from the footprint of the LCL/FCL to the posteromedial aspect of the fibular head where the popliteo-fibular ligament is located and attaches. A 9 mm tunnel is then reamed from distal to medial to the tubercle of Gerdy, through the lateral tibia. The graft is trimmed and passed into the tunnel from posterior to anterior. The popliteal tendon is then addressed. It is located approximately 18 mm anterior and distal to the attachment of the LCL/FCL [14, 15]. Two tunnels are drilled in the femoral condyle, in the anatomic location of the ligament and the popliteal tendon, respectively. The grafts are fixed in the femoral tunnels and the popliteus graft is then passed through the popliteal hiatus, while the LCL graft is passed distally over the popliteus graft and under the superficial ITB. The graft is passed through the fibular tunnel and fixed on the fibula with a screw, with the knee in 20° of flexion. Finally, both grafts are passed from posterior to anterior through the tibia and secured with a screw, in 60° of knee flexion. A bioabsorbable ligament screw is frequently used (Figs. 21.3, 21.4, 21.5, 21.6, 21.7, and 21.8) [5, 6, 8, 11, 12, 18].

The knee is usually immobilised for 6–8 weeks, non-weight-bearing. However, rehabilitation begins directly after surgery, with progress to full range of motion as tolerated. Closed

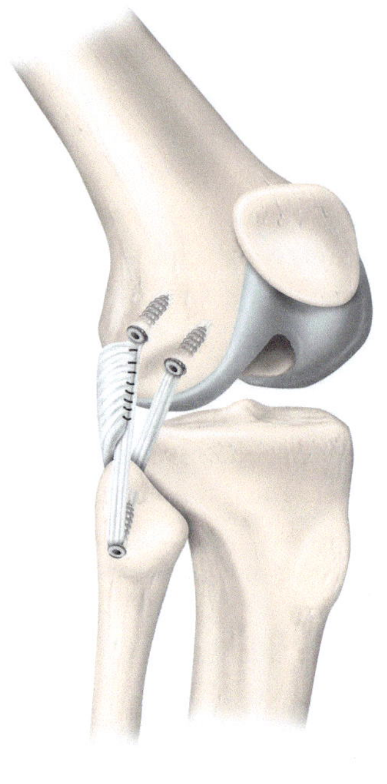

Fig. 21.3 Posterolateral capsular shift. The capsular shift attaches the posterolateral capsule to the fibular collateral ligament (LCL/FCL) graft. Note that there are two tunnels in the distal femur, but one graft only

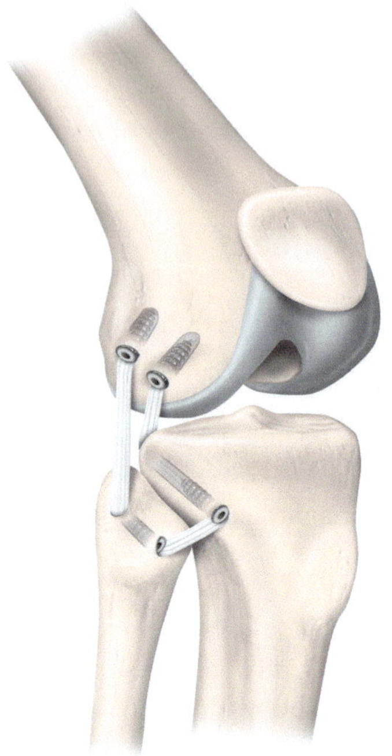

Fig. 21.5 Posterolateral corner reconstruction using one graft to reconstruct the fibular collateral ligament (FCL), popliteal tendon and popliteo-fibular ligament

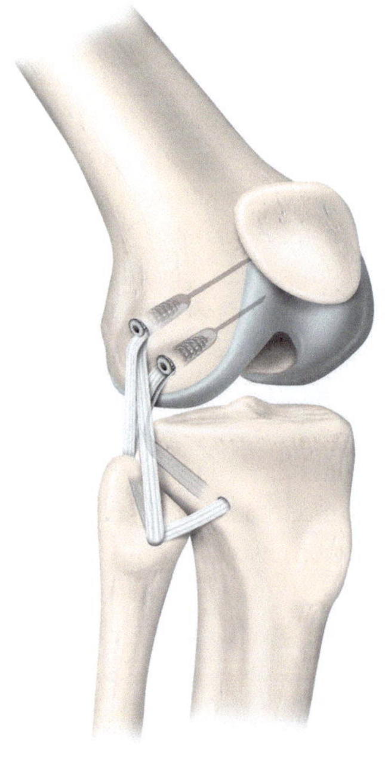

Fig. 21.4 Posterolateral corner reconstruction using two grafts: one to reconstruct the fibular collateral ligament (FCL) and the other to reconstruct the popliteal tendon and the popliteo-fibular ligament. One graft through the tibia and attached to the femur and the other a classic location of LCL/FCL reconstruction between the fibula and the distal femur

chain exercises are usually started around 6–8 weeks, as full weight-bearing is permitted. Return to activity is recommended after 9–12 months and to sports after 12 months, depending on the progress of range of motion and muscle strength, but it often takes longer than 12 months. In some cases, return to sports is not possible after a PLC injury [5, 6, 11, 12].

21.7 Conclusion

PLC injuries comprise fewer than 10% of all knee ligament injuries. There are often difficulties in terms of an exact anatomic diagnosis, and in most cases, several ligaments are involved. The diagnostic evaluation includes a clinical assessment, stress radiographs and MRI. In spite of this, several ligament injuries may be overlooked. In terms of treatment, timing is important. If at all possible, these injuries should be operated on without undue delay, within 2 weeks of the index injury. Grade I and II PLC injuries are commonly treated non-surgically, while there

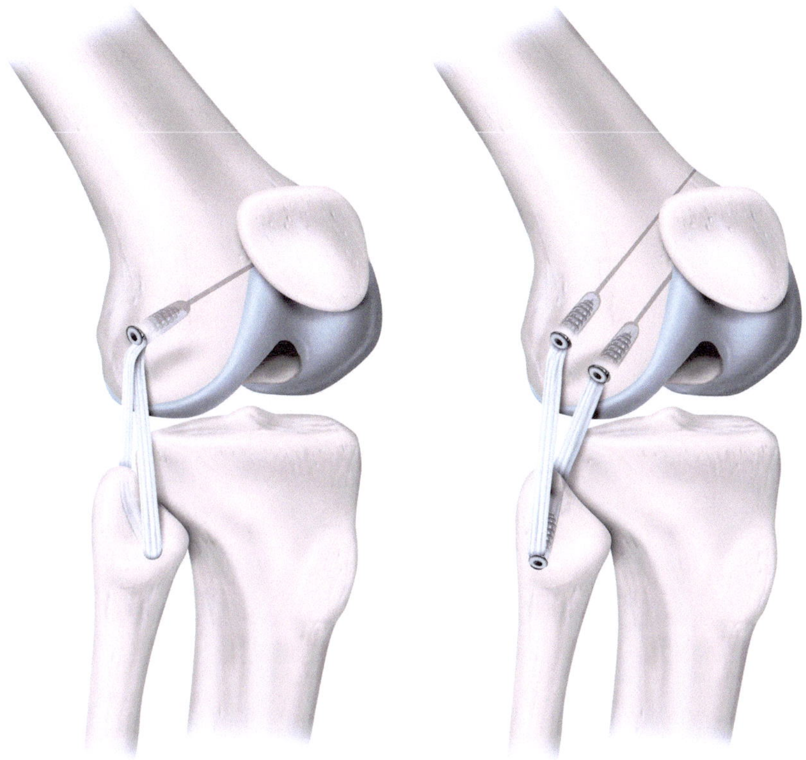

Fig. 21.6 Fibular sling techniques (left), one-femoral tunnel fibular technique and (right) two-femoral tunnel fibular technique. This is the classic and much used technique; however, there are several variations in techniques

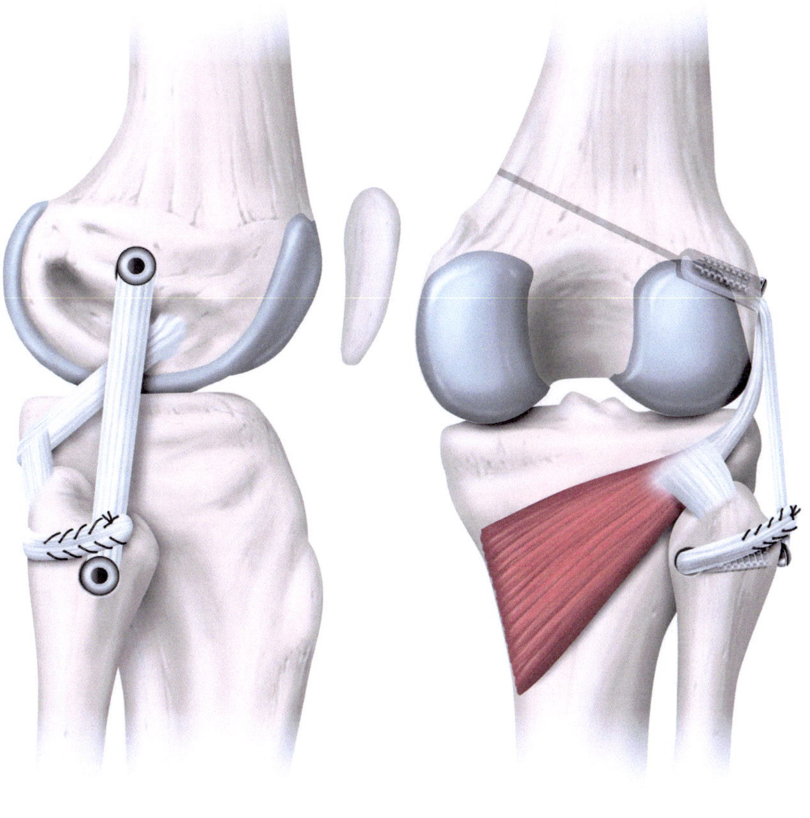

Fig. 21.7 Postero-anterior and lateral views of an isolated lateral (fibular) collateral ligament (LCL/FCL) reconstruction, showing the reconstructed LCL/FCL. A semitendinosus graft is used. Note the location of the fibular fixation

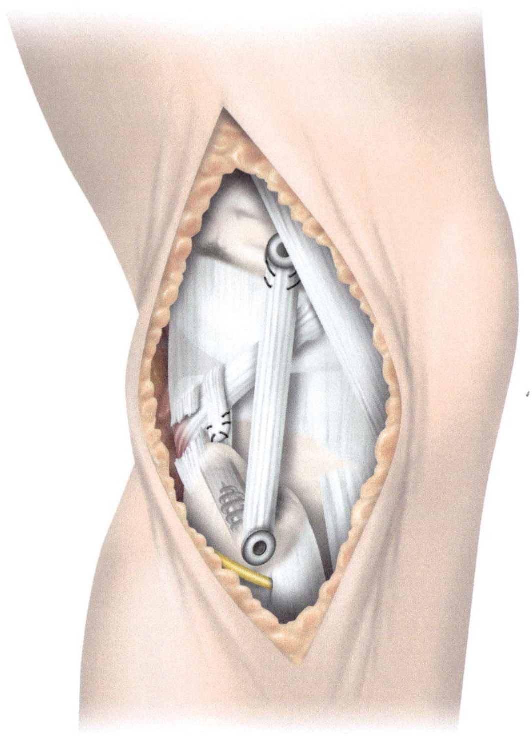

Fig. 21.8 Reconstruction of the LCL/FCL and the popliteo-fibular ligament. Note the proximity of the common peroneal nerve

is consensus that all grade III injuries should be treated surgically. The reconstruction of the involved ligaments is to be preferred to repair alone. It is also important to correct any malalignment of the lower limb, before ligament reconstructions are performed. Moreover, it should be borne in mind that failure to recognise PLC lesions when performing an ACL or PCL reconstruction is an important cause of the failure of these reconstructions.

References

1. Buzzi R, Aglietti P, Vena LM, Giron F. Lateral collateral ligament reconstruction using a semitendinosus graft. Knee Surg Sports Traumatol Arthrosc. 2004;12(1):36–42.
2. Chahla J, Moatshe G, Dean CS, LaPrade RF. Posterolateral corner of the knee: current concepts. Arch Bone Joint Surg. 2016;4(2):97–103.
3. Cinque ME, Geeslin AG, Chahla J, Moatshe G, Pogorzelski J, et al. The heel height test: a novel tool for the detection of combined anterior cruciate ligament and fibular collateral ligament tears. Arthroscopy. 2017;33(12):2177–81.
4. Espregueira M, da Silva MV. Anatomy of the lateral collateral ligament: a cadaver and histological study. Knee Surg Sports Traumatol Arthrosc. 2006;14(3):221–8.
5. Geeslin AG, LaPrade RF. Outcomes of treatment of acute grade-III isolated and combined posterolateral knee injuries: a prospective case series and surgical technique. J Bone Joint Surg Am. 2011;93(18):1672–83.
6. Geeslin AG, Moulton SG, LaPrade RF. A systematic review of the outcomes of posterolateral corner knee injuries, part 1: surgical treatment of acute injuries. Am J Sports Med. 2016;44(5):1336–42.
7. LaPrade RF, Ly TV, Wentorf FA, Engebretsen L. The posterolateral attachments of the knee: a qualitative and quantitative morphologic analysis of the fibular collateral ligament, popliteus tendon, popliteofibular ligament, and lateral gastrocnemius tendon. Am J Sports Med. 2003;31(6):854–60.
8. LaPrade RF, Spiridonov SI, Coobs BR, Ruckert PR, Griffith CJ. Fibular collateral ligament anatomical reconstructions: a prospective outcomes study. Am J Sports Med. 2010;38(10):2005–11.
9. Levy BA, Dajani KA, Morgan JA, Shah JP, Dahm DL, et al. Repair versus reconstruction of the fibular collateral ligament and posterolateral corner in the multiligament-injured knee. Am J Sports Med. 2010;38(4):804–9.
10. Meister BR, Michael SP, Moyer RA, Kelly JD, Schneck CD. Anatomy and kinematics of the lateral collateral ligament of the knee. Am J Sports Med. 2000;28(6):869–78.
11. Moatshe G, Dean CS, Chahla J, Serra Cruz R, LaPrade RF. Anatomic fibular collateral ligament reconstruction. Arthrosc Tech. 2016;5(2):e309–14.
12. Moulton SG, Geeslin AG, LaPrade RF. A systematic review of the outcomes of posterolateral corner knee injuries, part 2: surgical treatment of chronic injuries. Am J Sports Med. 2016;44(6):1616–23.
13. Moulton SG, Matheny LM, James EW, LaPrade RF. Outcomes following anatomic fibular (lateral) collateral ligament reconstruction. Knee Surg Sports Traumatol Arthrosc. 2015;23(10):2960–6.
14. Murphy KP, Helgeson MD, Lehman RA Jr. Surgical treatment of acute lateral collateral ligament and posterolateral corner injuries. Sports Med Arthrosc Rev. 2006;14(1):23–7.
15. Schechinger SJ, Levy BA, Dajani KA, Shah JP, Herrera DA, et al. Achilles tendon allograft reconstruction of the fibular collateral ligament and posterolateral corner. Arthroscopy. 2009;25(3):232–42.
16. Song YB, Watanabe K, Hogan E, D'Antoni AV, Dilandro AC, et al. The fibular collateral ligament of the knee: a detailed review. Clin Anat. 2014;27(5):789–97.

17. Stannard JP, Brown SL, Farris RC, McGwin G Jr, Volgas DA. The posterolateral corner of the knee: repair versus reconstruction. Am J Sports Med. 2005;33(6):881–8.
18. Yuuki A, Muneta T, Ohara T, Sekiya I, Koga H. Associated lateral/medial knee instability and its relevant factors in anterior cruciate ligament-injured knees. J Orthop Sci. 2017;22(2):300–5.

Patellar Instability

22

Seth L. Sherman, Joseph M. Rund, Betina B. Hinckel, and Jack Farr

22.1 Introduction

Patellofemoral instability has a variety of clinical presentations and a multifactorial etiology. Patients with patellofemoral instability have a range of disorders often related to patellar tracking. Maltracking is any deviation from the non-pathologic course of the patellar as it moves from a slightly central lateral position relative to the trochlea at extension to a central position on the trochlea with flexion and is then delivered into the intra-condylar notch during deeper flexion. Subluxation is used to describe an event in which the patella only partially leaves the trochlea. When the patella becomes completely displaced from the trochlea, it is considered a true dislocation. A patient is said to have recurrent patellar dislocations when two or more dislocations have occurred. Patients with abnormal skeletal anatomy are more inclined to experience maltracking and instability. On the other hand, a deviation from normal biomechanics or anatomy may not result in patellofemoral instability (yet, as a subset, these patients may be at risk for pain and/or cartilage wear). Moreover, patellofemoral instability has its place within the spectrum of patellofemoral disorders and can overlap in patients with PF pain, cartilage lesions, or frank arthritis.

Patellar dislocations constitute 2–3% of all knee injuries [1, 2]. The yearly risk of a primary patellar dislocation is 5.8/100,000 [3]. This risk increases in the 10- to 17-year-old age group up to 29 per 100,000 [4]. It was thought that the majority of primary dislocators do not have further instability or persistent dysfunction. However, more recent studies have reported recurrence rates of 15–60% and an annual risk of recurrence of 3.8 per 100,000 [3, 5–8]. Morphologic risk factors, which increase the relative risk of recurrent instability following a dislocation event, are young age with associated open physis, patella alta, large quadriceps vector, and trochlea dysplasia. Usually,

S. L. Sherman
Department of Orthopaedic Surgery, Stanford University Medical Center, Palo Alto, CA, USA
e-mail: shermans@stanford.edu

J. M. Rund
School of Medicine, University of Missouri School of Medicine, Columbia, MO, USA
e-mail: jmrqxc@health.missouri.edu

B. B. Hinckel
Department of Orthopaedic Surgery, William Beaumont Hospital, Royal Oak, MI, USA

Department of Orthopaedic Surgery, Oakland University, William Beaumont School of Medicine, Rochester, MI, USA
e-mail: betinahinckel@me.com

J. Farr (✉)
Department of Orthopedic Surgery, Indiana University School of Medicine, Indianapolis, IN, USA

Knee Preservation and Cartilage Restoration Center of Indiana, OrthoIndy Hospital, Indianapolis, IN, USA
e-mail: jfarr@orthoindy.com

M. Brittberg, K. Slynarski (eds.), *Lower Extremity Joint Preservation*,
https://doi.org/10.1007/978-3-030-57382-9_22

the degree of instability is associated with the presence of an increased number of risk factors and more severe dysplasias [9].

Extensive variability in patient symptoms and pathology of the underlying bony and soft tissue make it difficult to form precise treatment guidelines and recommendations for individual patients. An understanding of the specific patellar abnormalities, the functional ability, and the patient's desired level of activity must be taken into account. Risk stratification through critical identification of contributing anatomic and biomechanical factors is essential to creating an individualized nonoperative or surgical plan for patellofemoral instability.

22.2 History

When assessing for patellofemoral instability, knowledge of demographic information such as age, gender, body mass index, current activity level, goals and expectations for future activity, prior history of injury, and/or surgery is critical. It is important to determine the mechanism of injury from patient history. Sports-related activities account for 61–72% of first-time dislocations [3, 10]. Patellofemoral instability may result from medial direct trauma or more commonly as a noncontact injury, which can be cutting, pivoting, and jumping maneuvers or even activities of daily living in the more unstable patients. Following dislocations, the patella will usually spontaneously reduce in full extension, but will occasionally require manual reduction. If possible, it is helpful to differentiate subluxation from dislocation and number of prior events and to document spontaneous reduction versus requirement for manual reduction with or without sedation. Dislocation and reduction can occur so rapidly that the patient may not realize a dislocation occurred, especially in children. Patients will often report feeling the knee "give out" and "pop" out of place. Soon after the injury, swelling and difficulty weight bearing may occur, except in low-energy dislocators with multiple previous episodes. High-energy dislocation may occur even with "normal anatomy"; thus the high energy required for the patella to exit the trochlea leads to greater injury. As a result, there may be hemarthrosis secondary to ligamentous disruption and chondral/osteochondral injury or fracture. Alongside ACL tear, patella dislocation is a frequent cause of hemarthrosis, particularly in the pediatric population [11]. High index of suspicion for patella instability will allow the clinician to test their hypothesis with careful physical examination and confirmatory imaging studies as indicated.

22.3 Anatomy, Biomechanics, and Risk Factor Stratification

A thorough understanding of the basic anatomy and biomechanics allows the treating physician to identify risk factors for recurrent patellofemoral instability [12]. These risk factors can be divided into problems of the soft tissue stabilizers and/or bony architecture. Soft tissue stabilizers can be further separated into dynamic and static stabilizers. The understanding of those factors allows for a thorough evaluation of each individual patient and forms the basis of personalized treatment recommendations.

22.3.1 Dynamic and Static Soft Tissue Stabilizers

The quadriceps complex, which includes the rectus femoris, vastus lateralis, vastus intermedius, and vastus medialis muscles, is the most important dynamic stabilizer of the patella. Core musculature and hip external rotators are critical secondary dynamic stabilizers of the patellofemoral joint. The vastus medialis and lateralis muscles also connect to the tibia through attachments to the retinaculum. The vastus medialis oblique (VMO) is a part of the vastus medialis, which originates from the lateral intermuscular septum and inserts at an angle of up to 65° on the proximal third of the medial border of the patella [13]. The VMO is the primary dynamic medial restraint to lateral tracking of the patella. If there is atrophy, hypoplasia, or dysfunction of the VMO, there is less opposition to the vastus lateralis, which can contribute to lateral instability [14, 15].

Static soft tissue stabilizers include structures that compose the medial patellar restraints and the lateral patellar restraints. These work together and alongside the dynamic stabilizers to achieve patellofemoral balance and stability. The main medial soft tissue static stabilizers of the patella are the medial patellofemoral (MPFL), patellotibial (MPTL), and patellomeniscal ligaments (MPML). The MPFL is the primary soft tissue restraint to lateral displacement and provides 50–60% restraint in the first 20–30° of flexion [16–19]. The MPFL inserts in the proximal half of the medial patellar border, with some expansion into the quadriceps tendon (medial quadriceps tendon-femoral ligament; MQTFL), and it originates between the adductor tuberosity and medial epicondyle of the femur [9, 20]. For the patella to dislocate, it must laterally displace approximately 50 mm and the MPFL ruptures after elongating to a mean length of 26 mm; therefore, the MPFL must tear with almost every patellar dislocation [18]. The resultant pathological laxity of the MPFL is a frequent contributor to recurrent lateral patellofemoral instability [21, 22]. The MPTL and MPML are secondary soft tissue stabilizers and increasingly contribute to lateral restraint from 26% in extension to 46% at 90° of flexion [23]. The MPML has also been shown to be important in terminal extension, since its isolated lesion leads to subluxation in that knee position [24]. The origins of the MPTL and MPML are both on the distal third of the medial patellar border [25]. The MPTL inserts on the tibia about 10–20 mm distal to the tibial plateau, while the MPML inserts on the anterior horn of the medial meniscus and coronary ligament [9, 25, 26] (Fig. 22.1).

The lateral soft tissue restraints are composed of the interrelated iliotibial band and fibers that run from the iliotibial band to the patella (superficial oblique fibers and deep transverse fibers), the vastus lateralis, the lateral patellofemoral ligament, lateral patellotibial ligament, and the lateral patellomeniscal ligament [12]. The lateral

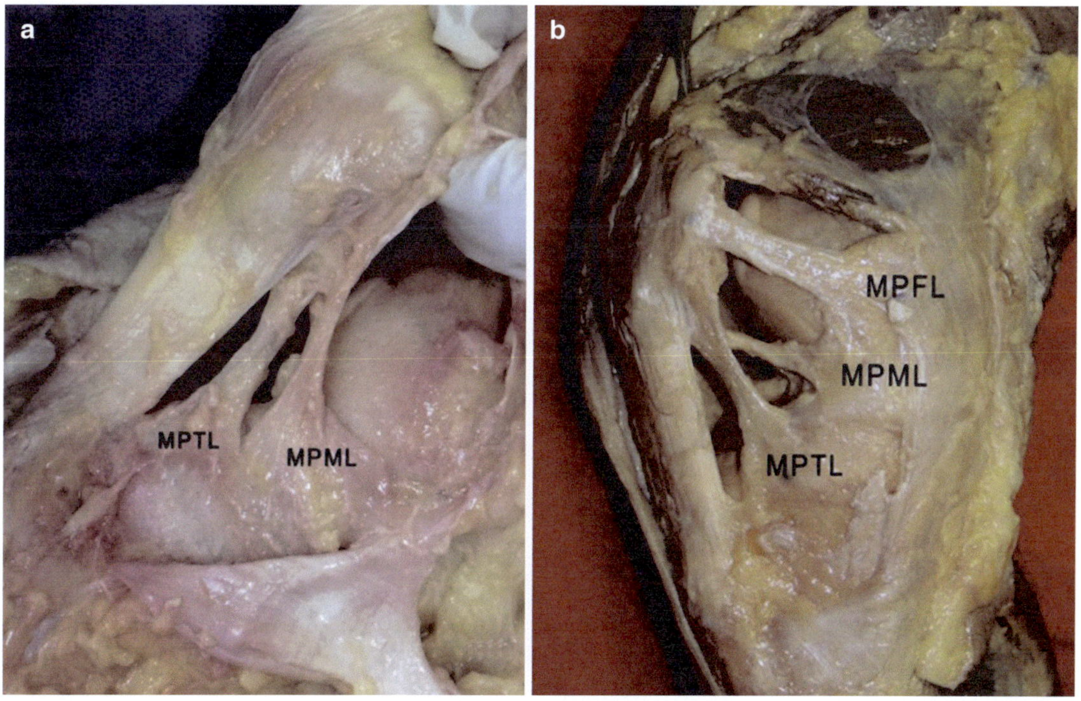

Fig. 22.1 Photograph of two dissected right knees showing (**a**, **b**) the medial patellotibial ligament (MPTL), the medial patellomeniscal ligament (MPML), and the medial patellofemoral ligament (MPFL) (Reprinted from Hinckel et al. [25] with kind permission from Elsevier and the Arthroscopy Association of North America)

retinaculum is an essential secondary stabilizer to lateral translation of the patella. The medial structures are physiologically more compliant than the lateral structures [27]. In low degrees of flexion, the lateral retinaculum contributes 3–13% to the restraint of lateral displacement [16, 28, 29].

Dynamic examination including single-limb squat, step-down, drop vertical jump, and hop tests evaluate for core and hip weakness. Dynamic valgus position during these maneuvers indicates poor neuromuscular coordination and needs to be corrected with rehabilitation to maximize the chance of success of any treatment strategy. Quadriceps musculature can be tested by extending the knee from a flexed position against resistance. Straight leg raise test demonstrates competence of the extensor mechanism along with quadriceps tone and strength. Disorders of the static medial stabilizers are related to insufficiency, while tightness or insufficiency can arise from lateral stabilizers. Of note, the lateral insufficiency is often iatrogenic, resulting in excessive surgical lateral release. Patella mobility is tested by the glide test. With the patient supine at varying degrees of knee flexion, lateral and medial force are applied to the patella. Between one and two quadrants of displacement is considered normal, but should be compared to native laxity and displacement in the opposite limb. A lateral displacement of more than three quadrants with a soft or absent endpoint often indicates medial insufficiency. Medial displacement of one quadrant or less suggests tightness of lateral structures and more than three quadrants is suggestive of lateral soft tissue insufficiency [30]. Apprehension or guarding with lateral displacement suggests symptomatic instability. The patellar tilt test can be conducted to evaluate lateral soft tissue restraints. With the knee fully extended and the quadriceps relaxed, the patella lateral border is lifted. With the patella parallel to the floor, elevation between 0° and 20° is normal. However, a patellar tilt of less than 0° indicates that the lateral retinaculum is tight and greater than 20° means it is loose [31].

Low flexion angle axial radiograph (e.g., Merchant view) can be useful for identifying the position of the patella in relation to the trochlear groove. MRI allows assessment of the soft tissue structures, including the MPFL [32–34]. MRI is 85% sensitive and 70% accurate in detecting injury to the MPFL [35]. Sagittal images are most suitable for the assessment of the MPTL [36]. Patella tilt can be visualized by axial radiographs [37]. On CT or MRI, patellar tilt is measured as the angle between a line coursing through the patellar axis and a line tangential to the posterior condyles. Patellar tilt can indicate the result of a combination of factors [30] including medial restraint insufficiency [38], trochlear dysplasia, lateral quadriceps vector [39], and lateral tightness [30]; an angle greater than 20° is considered abnormal [40, 41].

22.3.2 Q Angle and Lateralized Force Vector

The quadriceps angle (Q angle) is formed between the anterosuperior spine, center of the patella and tibial tuberosity. While the concept is vitally important, precise and reproducible clinical measurement is difficult [42]. It changes during flexion and extension of the knee; smaller in flexion and greatest close to full knee extension due to the external rotation of the tibia on the femur known as the "screw-home mechanism" [43–45]. A normal Q angle in males ranges from 8° to 16° in the supine position and 11–20° in the standing position. Females tend to range from 15° to 19° in supine position and 15–23° in the standing position [46–48]. An abnormal Q angle is one greater than 20° during extension and may lead to increased lateral displacement force and increased patellar contact pressures [12]. Recurrent patellar subluxation or dislocation events might result in falsely low Q angles due to the lateral positioning of the patella. Extension subluxation (subluxation with quadriceps contraction with knee in extension) suggests large increased lateral pull of the quadriceps and insufficiency of the medial stabilizers. Additionally, the offset between the patellar tendon and the trochlea can be used as a measure of the quadriceps vector, acknowledging that it rep-

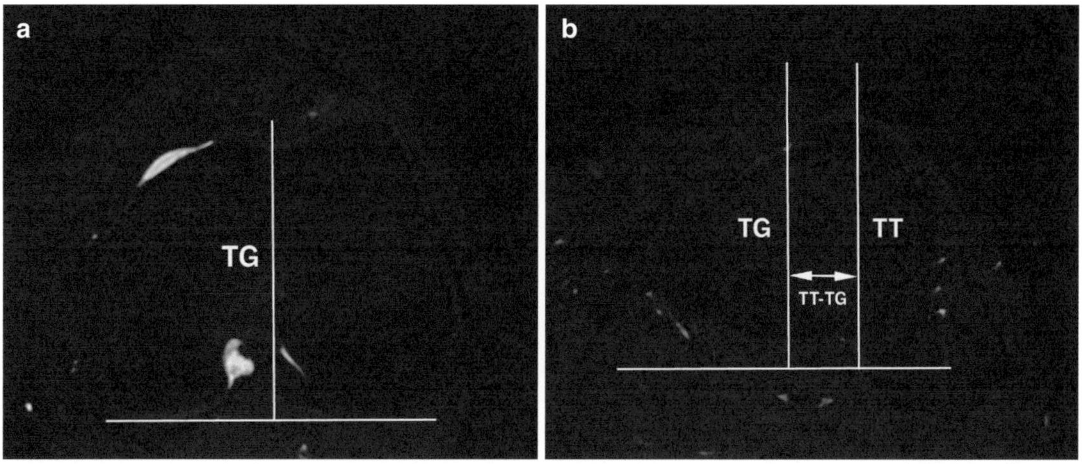

Fig. 22.2 Tibial tuberosity-trochlear groove (TT-TG) measurement with cartilaginous landmarks on magnetic resonance imaging. (**a**) Axial view with the deepest point in the trochlear groove; reference lines are drawn tangent to the medial and lateral posterior condyles. A perpendicular line is drawn at the intersection of the deepest point of the trochlea (line TG). (**b**) Previous lines are transferred to the most cranial axial cut where the patellar tendon fully inserts in the tibial tuberosity; a line perpendicular to the condylar line is drawn at the midpoint of the patellar tendon insertion (line TT). The distance between lines TT and TG is the TT-TG distance

resents only the distal vector of forces, since the relationship between the proximal insertion of quadriceps is not being evaluated. CT or MRI can be used to measure the TT-TG (tibial tuberosity-trochlear groove distance) [49–51] (Fig. 22.2). A TT-TG distance greater than 15–20 mm is associated with patellofemoral instability [41]. In one series, 56% of knees with at least one episode of dislocation had a TT-TG distance of >20 mm [41]. While the TT-TG can be influenced by trochlear dysplasia, knee rotation, and lateral insertion of the patellar tendon, the TT-PCL (tibial tuberosity-posterior cruciate ligament distance) gives an independent measure of the position of the tibial tuberosity in the tibia [52, 53].

22.3.3 Coronal and Axial Alignment

Lower extremity alignment is primarily dictated by the relationship between the femur and tibia. Abnormality in the relationship of these bony structures results in malalignment, which may predispose patients to patellofemoral instability. In most patients, the knee has an anatomical tibiofemoral angle of approximately 5–7° of valgus [54, 55]. With excess valgus alignment, the mechanical pull of the quadriceps muscle changes, which increases the lateral force vector on the patella. Other causes of lateralization of the tibial tuberosity (TT) relative to the center of the patella increase force on the patella and may lead to maltracking. These include femoral and tibial rotation and anatomic foot variations [56]. Increased rotation between the femur (i.e., excessive femoral anteversion) and tibia (i.e., external tibial torsion) results in malalignment of the extensor mechanism as the trochlear groove internally rotates and the patellar tendon insertion externally rotates [56, 57]. Hindfoot valgus and excessive pronation of the foot place a valgus force on the knee, which places a greater lateral force on the patella [58].

These lower extremity abnormalities can be visualized while the patient is standing. Malalignment including valgus alignment, pes planus, hindfoot valgus, and pronation of the foot may be identified. Patients with rotational malalignment can have toe in or toe out posture. With the patient in prone position and their knee flexed to 90°, femoral anteversion can be measured using Craig's test and compared to the opposite limb [59, 60] (Fig. 22.3).

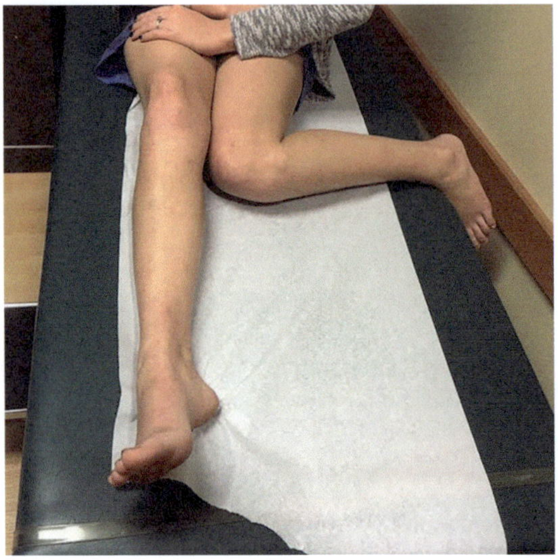

Fig. 22.3 Clinic patient in supine position with range of motion suggestive of femoral anteversion. This is best evaluated during prone examination with the knee flexed to 90°. Femoral anteversion can be measured using Craig's test and compared to the opposite limb

The extremity alignment or mechanical axis view is useful for examining the tibiofemoral alignment (Fig. 22.4). Rotational alignment can be evaluated by CT or MRI [57]. Noyes reported a method for using MRI cuts through the hip, knee, and ankle for measuring femoral anteversion and tibial torsion while avoiding the ionizing radiation of CT [61]. Femoral anteversion is defined as the angle formed between the axis of the femoral neck and distal femur. By measuring the angle of the proximal tibia relative to the distal tibia, the degree of tibial torsion can be assessed. Knee rotation of the femorotibial joint is given by the angles between the distal femur condyles line and the proximal tibia posterior condyles line. Normally, the femoral anteversion is 10–20°, tibial torsion is 25–41°, and the knee rotation angle is 5–9° [41, 57, 62–64].

22.3.4 Patellar Height

Increased height of the patella results in decreased patellofemoral contact with the trochlear groove [65–67] and abnormal concentration of forces at the distal patella. Additionally, a greater degree of knee flexion is required before the patella engages the trochlear groove, contributing to patellofemoral instability and subsequent risk for recurrent patellar dislocation [68, 69].

Clinically, patella alta can be recognized in the seated position by an elongated patella tendon or when the patella faces upward instead of forward in 90° of flexion. Also, mild J-sign can be present. This results from patellar disengagement from the proximal trochlea that occurs through a longer range of motion.

Patellar height is best assessed on a lateral radiograph obtained with the knee flexed to 30°. Various methods of assessing relative patellar height have been described including the Insall-Salvati [70], modified Insall-Salvati [71], Blackburne-Peel [72], Caton-Deschamps [73], and Labelle-Laurin [74] indices. The Caton-Deschamps index is the most widely used method because its value does not vary with knee flexion. In comparison, the Insall-Salvati measurement does not change with tibial tuberosity distalization. Caton-Deschamps allows the surgeon to use the measurement to accurately template and implement the desired amount of correction of patella height as indicated during surgery. The patellatrochlear index quantifies the engagement between the patella and the trochlea and should be evaluated [75, 76] (Fig. 22.5).

22.3.5 Trochlear Dysplasia

Trochlear dysplasia is present in 68.3–99.3% [41, 77–79] of patients with patellofemoral instability. It is also the most significant risk factor for both primary and recurrent patellofemoral instabilities. At 20° of knee flexion, the patella is engaged in the trochlea such that it sufficiently restricts lateral patellar deviation [80]. Trochlear dysplasia is characterized by a loss of the normal concave anatomy and depth of the trochlear groove, which creates a shallow, flat, or convex trochlea.

A key finding in the physical exam indicating the presence of severe trochlea dysplasia is the J-sign [46, 58]. The J-sign refers to the shape of an inverted J of the patella tracking as the knee

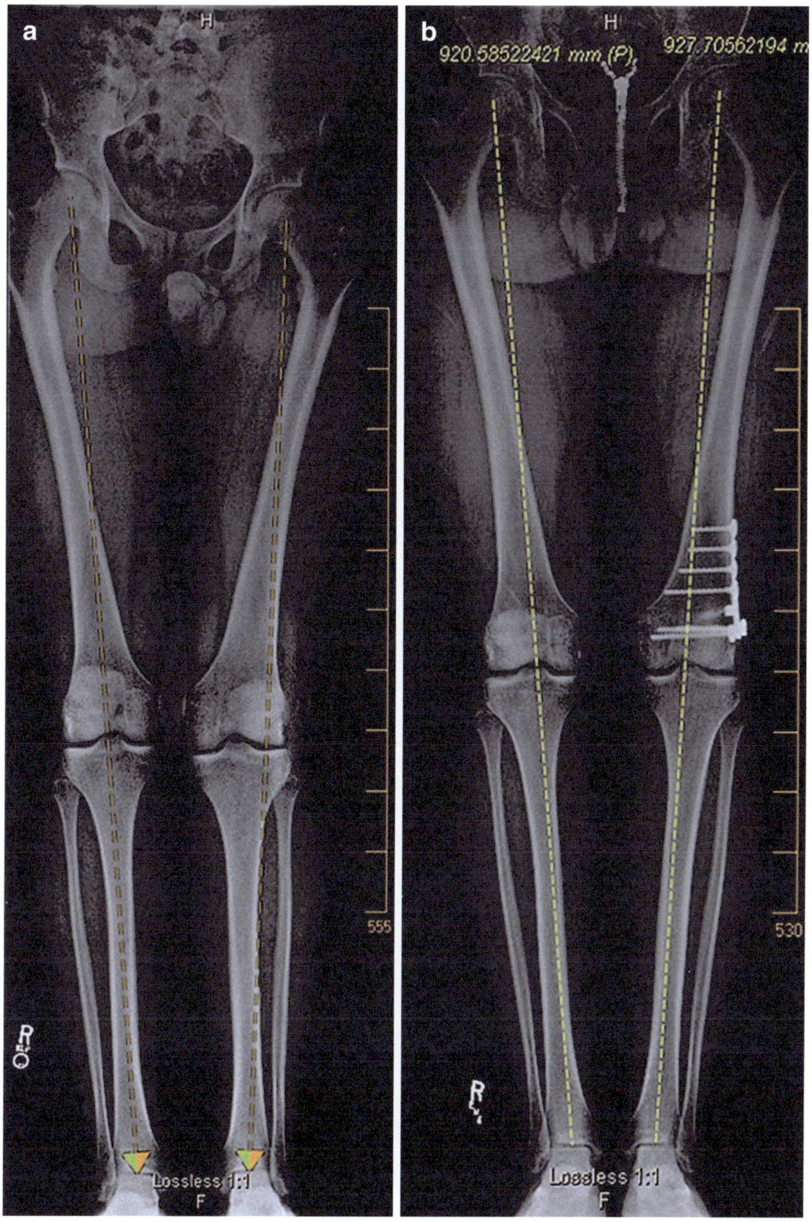

Fig. 22.4 (**a**) Mechanical alignment radiograph demonstrating valgus deformity in the left knee; weight-bearing line is in the lateral tibiofemoral compartment. (**b**) Neutral alignment after a distal femoral osteotomy with open-wedge technique; weight-bearing line is in the center of the knee

extends from a flexed position. As the knee extends from 90° of flexion, the patella moves laterally as it disengages from the proximal trochlea close to full extension (10–20° of flexion). A "clunk" or sudden change in patellar tracking is associated with a trochlear "bump" or "spur."

Trochlear dysplasia is best evaluated on a true lateral radiograph [19, 40, 41, 81]. In a normal knee, the Blumensaat's line continues anteriorly as the trochlear groove line, which should stay posterior to the projection of the trochlear facets. However, when the lines of the lateral trochlear facet, medial trochlear facet, and trochlear groove coincide, it is called the "crossing sign" (Fig. 22.6). The crossing sign indicates that the femoral condyles and trochlear groove are at the same height and that the trochlea is flat [41]. Dejour et al. [41] reported the presence of the crossing sign in 96% of patients with a history of

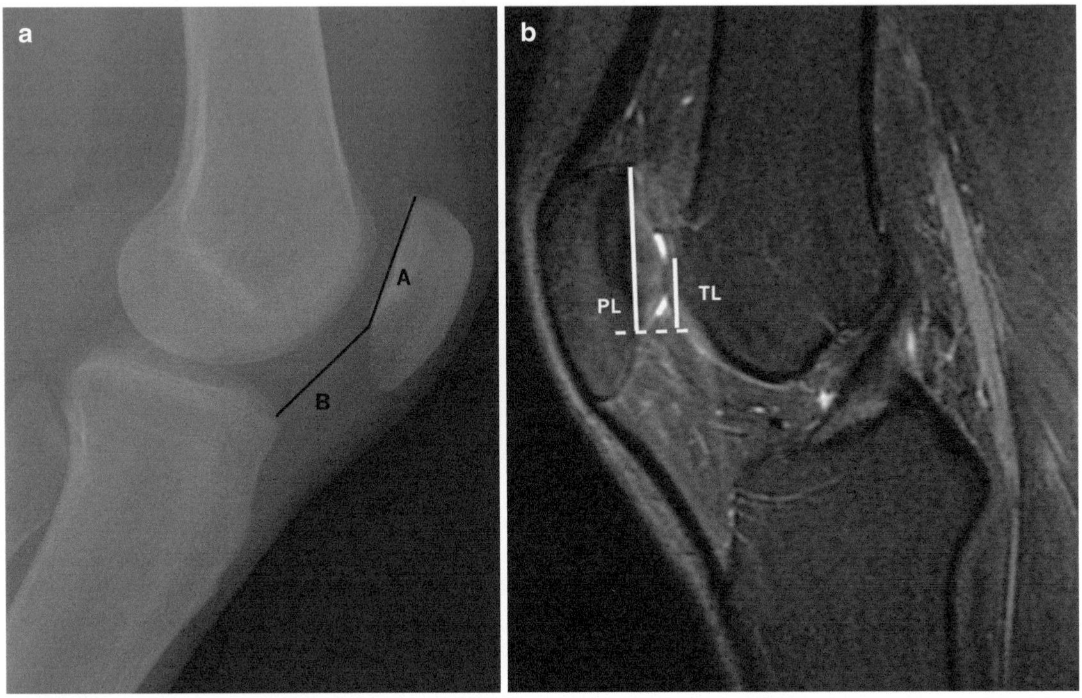

Fig. 22.5 Patellar height measurements. (**a**) Lateral radiograph of a left knee. The Caton-Deschamps Ratio is defined as *B*/*A*, where *B* is the distance between the inferior portion of the patellar cartilage to the antero-proximal tibial plateau and *A* is the patellar cartilage length. (**b**) Sagittal cut of magnetic resonance imaging T2. Patellofemoral engagement ratio is defined as TL/PL, where TL is the distance from the proximal trochlea point to the tangent of the distal patellar cartilage and PL is the length of the patellar cartilage

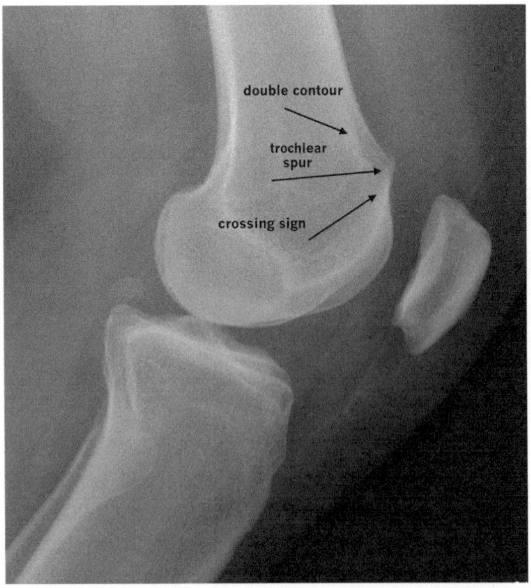

Fig. 22.6 Lateral radiograph of a left knee. Type D trochlear dysplasia: crossing sign, double contour, and trochlear spur are present

a true patellar dislocation compared with 3% in the control group. A trochlear spur or bump is an anterior prominence of the proximal trochlea. The double contour can be seen when the line of the hypoplastic medial condyle is posterior to the lateral trochlear facet line. All of these findings are outlined in the most commonly used classification system established by Dejour [82]. In the Merchant view, the sulcus angle is measured as the angle between two lines originating from highest points of the medial and lateral condyles and converging on the deepest part of the femoral trochlear groove. A value greater than 145° suggests trochlear dysplasia [83]. The cartilaginous bump can be measured in the MRI as the distance between a line paralleling the anterior femoral cortical line and the most anterior cartilaginous point of the trochlea and >8 mm is considered abnormal [84]. A cliff sign in the axial view is also a sign of severe type D trochlear dysplasia.

22.4 Treatment Plan

Treatment of patellofemoral instability is pathology and patient specific. Important knee pathologic details from the history, physical examination, and imaging studies help the clinician make evidence-based treatment recommendations for the pathology within the context of patient-specific requirements. These requirements might include, for example, a patient's tolerance for limited vs extensive surgery, time available to return to school/work, or "career changing" atheletic transitions.

22.4.1 Nonoperative Treatment

Initial management after patellar instability whether first or recurrent is to provide symptomatic relief and to initiate a period or protection and core to floor rehabilitation. Pain is controlled with cryotherapy, analgesic and/or anti-inflammatory medications, rest, compression, and elevation. Knee aspiration may aid in reducing pain in patients with tense hemarthrosis and even more importantly decrease the quadriceps inhibition. There is no consensus on early treatment regarding bracing, so common sense would suggest brace protection. Early range of motion and core/limb exercises are initiated as pain allows. Although immobilization may facilitate ligamentous healing (theoretically in flexion, when the ligament attachments sites are closest—yet practically difficult), it also may lead to muscle atrophy and stiffness that can increase the risk of arthritis [85].

Nonsurgical treatment remains the mainstay of treatment for subluxation patients and for the majority of first-time dislocators without osteochondral fracture or symptomatic loose body [2, 86]. However, recurrence rates ranging from 15% to 60% have been reported following nonsurgical care [3, 5–8, 85]. More recently, risk stratification protocols may help to identify a subset of patients with aberrant underlying anatomy and high risk of recurrent instability that may benefit from discussion about early soft tissue surgical stabilization. That is, for high-risk patients (e.g., a first-time dislocator with a history of recurrent dislocations on the contralateral knee), if a discrete single MPR ligament tear is identified, repair may make sense, and for similar at-risk patients with diffuse MPR injury, MPR reconstruction may make sense when the knee is "ready"—think of the approach to acute ACL tears.

Regarding nonoperative treatment, a comprehensive "core-to-floor" rehabilitation plan should be undertaken to correct any underlying muscular weakness or neuromuscular imbalance. Physical therapy should focus not only on quadriceps strengthening but also on the core and posterior chain musculature including the gluteus, hip external rotators, and hamstrings. The hamstring to quadriceps ratio should be optimized to reduce loads on the knee joint during joint activity. Proprioception and flexibility training can also help to improve symptoms and reduce the risk of recurrent episodes. The use of a compression sleeve or patella stabilization brace may help with proprioception and swelling during the rehabilitation process [65]. Formal referral to a physical therapist allows for a supervised functional progression back to baseline. Similar to ACL prevention programs, the patient needs to be instructed on proper landing from jumps and proper cutting to avoid the functional valgus/internal rotation positioning. Sedentary activities can be resumed in days to weeks, while returning to athletic activities may take weeks to months. Return to sport functional evaluation should be routinely recommended prior to clearance for return to play. This should include clinical examination followed by subjective and objective tests of ROM, strength, and power, ideally performed by an independent evaluator if possible (Table 22.1).

22.4.2 Surgical Treatment

Indications for surgery after a first-time dislocation are evolving. In that setting, traditional indications are irreducible dislocations, large osteochondral or chondral lesions, and/or symptomatic loose bodies. These lesions may be

Table 22.1 Suggested criteria for return to play (RTP) after patellofemoral instability

Criteria for return to play
Complete radiographic healing of the bone if bony surgery is involved
Full range of motion
No knee effusion at rest or with activity
No objective or subjective knee instability
No knee pain
Full core-to-floor strength and endurance
90% or greater limb strength compared to the noninvolved limb
Pass testing of neuromuscular coordination training including dynamic control landing from a jump and cutting activities (no dynamic valgus internal hip rotation)/symmetrical proprioception to noninvolved limb
Complete a sport-specific functional progress evaluation under the direction/observation of a certified athletic trainer or physical therapist
Mental confidence and psychological readiness to return to sport

located along the medial patella, lateral trochlea (less common), or weight-bearing portion of the lateral femoral condyle (more common and typically begin at the level of the notch roof). Large osteochondral or even chondral-only fragments should be repaired if at all possible, often through limited arthrotomy. Osteochondral lesions can be fixed with metallic or bioabsorbable compression screws. "Chondral-only" lesions have healing potential in younger patients and can be fixed with special techniques including transosseous sutures and chondral "darts," or by using knotless suture anchors [87–89] [90]. In this setting, soft tissue stabilization is often recommended concomitantly (i.e., MPFL repair if a focal lesion is noted or reconstruction if the MPR injury is diffuse) to reduce the risk of recurrent instability and to protect the chondral or osteochondral repair.

While somewhat controversial, surgical stabilization may also be considered in first-time dislocators without fracture or loose body who have significant risk factors for recurrent instability. Jaquith et al. [90] found that the significant risk factors for recurrence after nonoperative treatment are trochlear dysplasia, skeletal immaturity, CD ratio >1.45, and a history of contralateral patellar dislocation. With all four factors, patients had a predicted risk of recurrent instability of 88% in their study [91]. Other studies have similarly confirmed risk factors for recurrence (young age, trochlear dysplasia, patella alta) and high recurrence rates in this subset of patients [92]. In addition, limitations to return to previous level of activity can persist after nonoperative treatment even in the absence of further true patellar dislocation [93], which can be perceived as failure of nonoperative treatment.

To date, few studies have compared nonoperative versus operative treatment in patients with first-time patellar dislocations. In most studies, the authors evaluated techniques of MPFL repair that were current at the time, but may differ from modern techniques or procedures other than MPFL reconstruction, and found no major differences in postoperative episodes of instability, activity level or function, and subjective patient outcome measures. However, in a randomized control trial, MPFL reconstruction resulted in higher Kujala outcome scores and lower rates of recurrence when compared to nonoperative treatment [94]. Additional quality studies are needed to determine the potential role of surgical treatment for first-time patellofemoral instability episodes in high-risk patients without loose body or fracture.

Surgery is clearly indicated for recurrent patellofemoral dislocation or for patients who have failed conservative treatment following recurrent subluxation episodes. The goal of surgical intervention is to "individualize, customize, and normalize," a solution tailored to the unique condition that is leading to the recurrent instability events [95]. The proximal MPR (MQTFL and MPFL) are the essential lesions of patellofemoral instability and are always addressed at the time of surgery. Other procedures can be added, as indicated, for soft tissue balance or bony realignment such as medialization and/or distalization.

22.5 Surgical Indications

22.5.1 Soft Tissue Procedures

22.5.1.1 Medial Patellofemoral Restraint Reconstruction (MPRR)

Proximal Restraints: MPFL and/or MQTFL

In the setting of patellofemoral instability, MPR repair/reconstruction is indicated in all patients as it treats the essential lesion common to all patients with lateral patellofemoral instability [96].

Distal Restraint: MPTL

In some circumstances, MPTL reconstruction can be combined with MPFL reconstruction. This may be a useful adjunct in the setting of extension subluxation, flexion instability, skeletal immaturity with associated risk factors (e. g., trochlear dysplasia), and knee hyperextension associated with generalized laxity [97–99].

22.5.1.2 Lateral Retinacular Lengthening (LRL)

Isolated lateral release is not a treatment option for patellofemoral instability. This may worsen the instability and lead to poor results [30]. However, lateral lengthening is a useful adjunct to MPR reconstruction when there is lateral soft tissue tightness and fixed patellar tilt [96]. The main advantage of lateral lengthening over lateral release is to maintain continuity in lateral soft tissue, which contributes to lateral stability, prevents medial instability, and prevents persistent pain from unhealed tissue [16, 100, 101].

22.5.2 Bony Procedures

In general, the following bony procedures are evolving in their indications in the setting of recurrent patellar instability. Proper MPR balance/desired length changes with range of motion without addressing excessive lateral position of the tubercle or excessive patellar alta are difficult [102]. In addition, in knees with associated chondral lesions, tuberosity surgery is often essential in optimizing the load to this damage/repaired area. Thus, tubercle surgery is more commonly performed to correct severe malalignment and to off-load chondral lesions, with or without instability, and in revision instability surgery when soft tissue stabilization has failed. Bony procedures may also be used in the setting of fixed or habitual dislocation and in patients with syndromic causes of severe maltracking with or without instability.

22.5.2.1 Tibial Tuberosity Osteotomy (TTO)

MPR reconstruction should never be used to "pull" the patella medially into the groove. A TTO can be performed to restore normal patella position prior to MPFL reconstruction. This allows the soft tissue repair or reconstruction to act properly as a check rein to lateral patella displacement exclusively [96]. For the treatment of instability, TTO may be important for medialization to correct a large quadriceps vector (i.e., TT-TG >20 mm) and for distalization, to correct patella alta (CD ratio >1.2) [41]. Straight anteriorization unloads the trochlea, and distal poles of the patella, and can be added if there is an associated distal chondral lesion [103].

22.5.2.2 Coronal Plane or Rotational Osteotomy

Femoral osteotomies are indicated to correct excessive valgus alignment, femoral anteversion, or tibial torsion. They are addressed with a distal femoral varus osteotomy, femoral derotation osteotomy, or tibial derotation osteotomy, respectively [104–107].

22.5.2.3 Trochleoplasty

Trochleoplasty indications continue to evolve. They are most commonly used in the setting of maltracking due to severe trochlear dysplasia, that is, patients with a clunk in the J-sign and a spur/bump on imaging exams. They are contraindicated when there is open physes or significant chondrosis/arthritis.

22.6 Surgical Technique

22.6.1 Soft Tissue Procedures

22.6.1.1 Medial Patellofemoral Restraint Reconstruction (MPRR)

Indicated bony procedures and/or lateral lengthening should be performed prior to completing MPR reconstruction.

Proximal Restraints: MPFL and/or MQTFL Reconstruction

There are many different described techniques in the literature. Reconstruction can be performed with autograft (semitendinosus, gracilis, quadriceps, or patellar tendon) or allograft (semitendinosus, gracilis, or other soft tissue grafts) tendon. Fixation can be achieved by maintenance of the attachment, sutures, suspensory fixation, interference screws, or anchors.

Key Points

- Exam under anesthesia confirms lateral patella instability.
- Meticulous dissection to identify layer between retinaculum and capsule to permit free excursion of the graft in an extra-articular location (between layers 2 and 3).
- Patella portion (MPFL) may be placed in the proximal half or proximal third; the quadriceps portion (MQTFL) immediately adjacent to the proximal patellar pole.
- Femoral placement can be confirmed by anatomical landmarks in the saddle region between the medial femoral epicondyle and the adductor tubercle and checked with fluoroscopy identification just anterior to the posterior cortex extension line and between the posterior origin of the medial femoral condyle and the posterior point of the Blumensaat line on a lateral radiograph [108].
- Confirm adequate metric graft behavior (mainly isometric between 20° and 60° of flexion and mild slack in flexion).
- Fix to length, usually between 30° and 45° of flexion (where distance between the attachment points is the longest).
- Confirm adequate patella mobility (one to two quadrants medially and laterally) to avoid overconstraint. Tensioning the graft is avoided as this causes increased pressure on the patellofemoral compartment [109].

Distal Restraint: MPTL Reconstruction

A number of techniques are described for the MPTL reconstruction combined with the MPFL reconstruction [21, 99, 110, 111]. Within these techniques, there are variations in graft choice, harvesting, and fixation [97]. The two most common graft choices are the hamstrings and medial portion of the patellar tendon. The hamstrings can be used as a free graft, or the tibial attachment can be maintained. With the medial patellar tendon, the patellar attachment is preserved, and the distal portion can be detached as soft tissue only or with a bone plug.

Key Points

- Patellar placement in the distal media corner of the patella.
- Tibial placement (anatomical landmarks, 1.5–2 cm below the joint line and 1.5–2 cm medial to the patellar tendon and 20° angle with the patellar tendon; fluoroscopy, medial border of the medial spine and 9–10 mm distal to the joint in the AP view).
- Fixation at 90° of flexion to avoid overtightening in flexion (tension in graft must be similar to the patellar tendon so they can act synergistically). Similar to the MPFL, tensioning the graft should be avoided as this causes increased pressure on the patellofemoral compartment [109].

22.6.1.2 Lateral Retinacular Lengthening (LRL)

As compared to lateral release, lengthening more precisely balances the patellofemoral forces by having more control over the exact amount of tissue that is being lengthened/released. In addi-

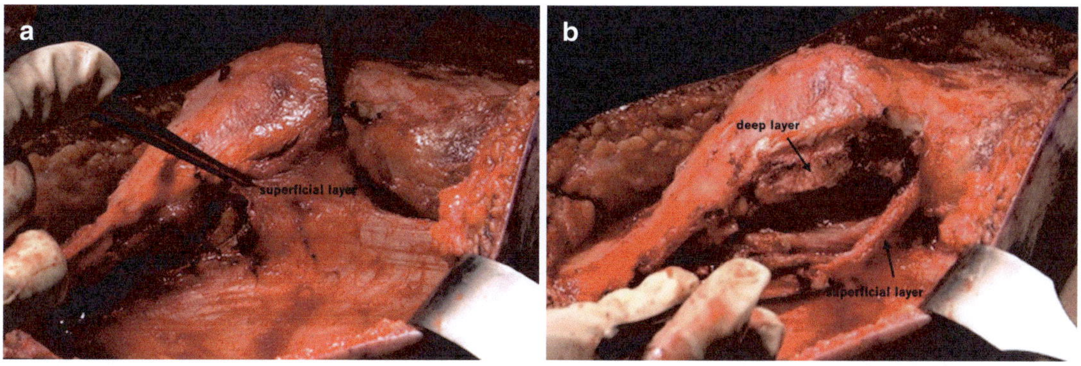

Fig. 22.7 Lateral retinacular lengthening. (**a**) Superficial layer, with oblique fibers coursing from the iliotibial band. (**b**) Superficial layer connected to the iliotibial band is reapproximated with the deep fibers connected to the patella

tion to eliminating the risk of excessive medial patellofemoral translation, it also reduces the risk of surgical hematoma. Conversely, lateral retinacular lengthening requires a larger incision (Fig. 22.7).

Key Points
- Identify the superficial oblique fibers of the lateral reticulum (as they course from the iliotibial band); incise the superficial fibers and dissect them from the deeper fibers (transverse).
- Deeper transverse fibers cut approximately 1.5–2 cm posteriorly.
- Two borders are sutured at 30–60° of flexion with the patella centered on the trochlear groove.

22.6.2 Bony Procedures

22.6.2.1 Tibial Tuberosity Osteotomy (TTO)

Depending on the individual patient and their anatomy, the tibial tubercle can undergo medialization, anteriorization, anteromedialization, or distalization (Fig. 22.8).

Key Points
- Tibial tuberosity and patellar tendon exposure.
- Anterior compartment of the leg is reflected and neurovascular structures protected.
- Plane of posterior cut is defined with the angle planned for desired effect; two distal cuts are performed parallel if distalization is indicated; posterior cut of the osteotomy is performed with an oscillating saw (free hand or use of a guide), cut between the TT and Gerdy's tubercle; proximal cut is made with an osteotome with the patellar tendon retracted.
- TT is lifted carefully and shifted to desired position; avoid overmedialization (the Q angle should not be less than zero in any angle of flexion); provisory fixation is performed; two bicortical screws are placed with compression technique.

22.6.2.2 Trochleoplasty

Many trochleoplasty techniques have been described. In the proximal open "grooveplasty" by Peterson [112], the groove is not deepened, but instead, resection of the proximal dysplastic portion facilitates the entrance in the trochlea and engagement of the patella in the deeper distal groove. In the resection wedge Goutallier technique [113], a wedge is resected from the lateral cortex, and the bump is posteriorized to the level of the anterior cortex. In the V-shaped deepening trochleoplasty by Dejour [114], an osteotomy is performed in a thick osteochondral flap. In the U-shaped deepening trochleoplasty by Bereiter, deepening is through a thinner flap that is molded. Arthroscopic deepening by Blønd [115] is similar to Bereiter [116]. Although there are many different techniques, they all accomplish the goal of establishing a deeper trochlear track for the patella to engage.

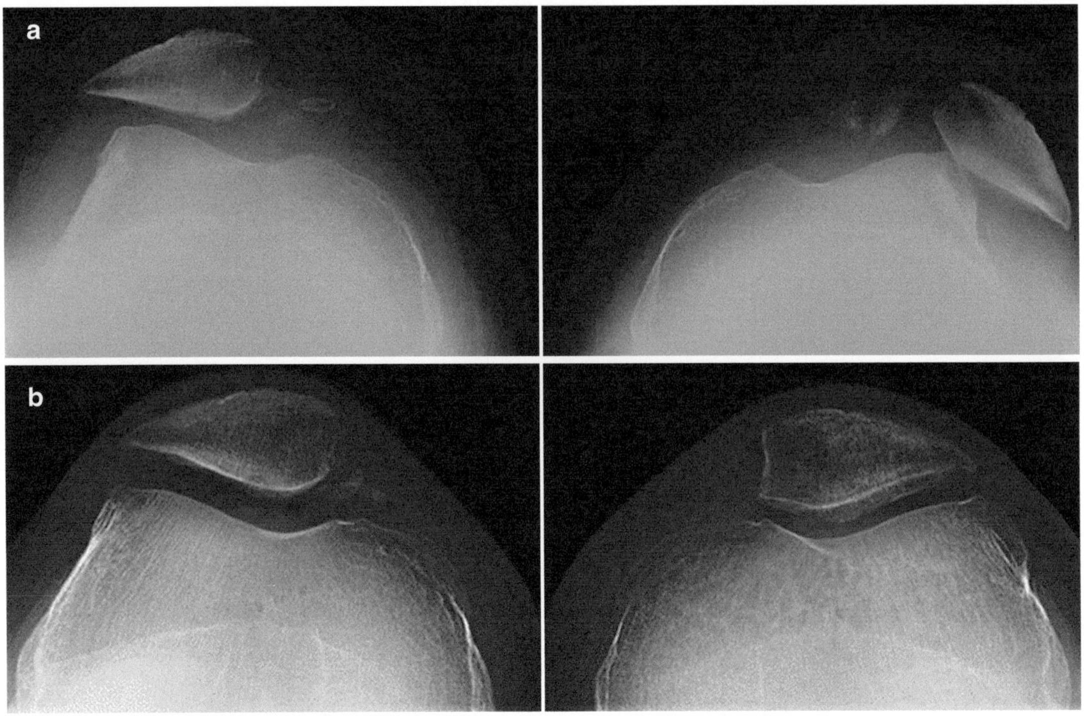

Fig. 22.8 Merchant view radiograph of bilateral knees. (**a**) Dislocated patella in the left knee. (**b**) Patella reduced after soft tissue realignment procedure

22.7 Rehabilitation

22.7.1 Soft Tissue Procedures

Patients are discharged with crutches and allowed to weight bear as tolerated with the brace locked in extension until the nerve block wears off. Gravity-assisted range of motion as tolerated may begin immediately out of the brace, and a continuous passive motion machine may be used per surgeon discretion. Early full range of motion is essential. Patients are instructed to perform isometric quadriceps sets, short arc quadriceps, and ankle pumps. Formal physical therapy is initialized. Adequate quadriceps strength and full range of motion are usually reached by 6–8 weeks. Through this progression of activities, crutches and a hinged brace are discontinued, usually by 6 weeks. Low-impact activities including the bike and elliptical can be used within the first several months, and jogging can be accomplished by 3–4 months. While following a criteria-based progression, return to sport may occur any time after 4–6 months.

22.7.2 Bony Procedures

Patients are discharged home with crutches with limited weight bearing, progressing to full weight bearing by 6–8 weeks, brace locked in extension while weight bearing [117]. Continuous passive motion and/or gravity-assisted range of motion is initiated as tolerated immediately. Isometric quadriceps sets, heel slides, and ankle pumps are performed. When adequate bone healing is demonstrated by x-ray and quadriceps control is achieved, the brace can be unlocked and then discontinued, and patient can progress to therapy [4], usually by 6–8 weeks. Full range of motion should be achieved by 6–12 weeks. Low-impact activities can be initiated within the first 3 months.

Jogging and sport-related drills may be initiated between 4 and 6 months. Following a criteria-based progression, patient can often return to sport by 6–8 months.

22.8 Outcomes and Complications

22.8.1 Soft Tissue Procedures

22.8.1.1 MPRR: Proximal Restraints – MPFL and/or MQTFL Reconstruction

Outcomes

Isolated reconstruction of the MPFL can provide good clinical outcomes and low recurrence rate of less than 10% in primary or revision surgeries [94, 118–126]. Failure with recurrence of dislocation after isolated MPFL reconstruction in children has been associated with severe trochlea dysplasia and rotational deformities with femoral anteversion [127]. The isolated reconstruction of the MPFL in adults has led to a low rate of recurrent dislocations even in the presence of risk factors, although patients with high-grade trochlear dysplasia and increased TT-TG had worse clinical outcomes [121]. However, in addition to small sample sizes and short-term follow-up, population characteristics, risk factors, and the surgical techniques are varied. These variances make it difficult to generalize the outcomes of MPFL reconstruction. When compared to MPFL reconstruction, MPFL repair or medial retinacular reefing has higher rates of recurrent dislocation (9–28%) and lower clinical outcomes in adults.

Complications

In a systematic review, a total of 164 complications occurred in 629 knees (26.1%) [128]. These complications ranged from minor to major events including patellar fracture, failures, clinical instability on postoperative examination, loss of knee flexion, wound complications, and pain. Twenty-six patients returned to the operating room for additional procedures. A total of 12% had objective or subjective instability [128].

22.8.1.2 MPRR: Distal Restraint – MPTL Reconstruction

Outcomes

By providing additional ligamentous support in carefully selected patients, combined reconstruction of the MPTL and MPFL can potentially improve outcomes relative to isolated MPFL reconstructions [21, 110, 111, 133–135]. A recent systematic review concluded that good clinical outcomes were achieved with MPTL reconstruction [97], with low rate of recurrent dislocations similar to recurrent dislocations reported after isolated MPFL reconstruction surgeries [94, 119, 120, 122, 125]. Good and excellent outcomes were achieved in more than 75% of cohorts. In the studies that reported the presence of risk factors or factors associated with worse outcomes, their presence did not seem to negatively affect clinical outcomes [97].

Complications

The most common were wound complications [111, 136–138], quadriceps atrophy [139], and subjective instability complaints [136]. Wound complications happened in patients with habitual dislocations and more extensive surgical procedures [137, 138]. Other concerning complications, such as patella baja and arthritis, which could be associated with the increase in the medial and distal restriction by the MPTL, were very rare [97].

22.8.1.3 Lateral Retinacular Lengthening (LRL)

Outcomes

Two randomized control trials showed that lateral lengthening results in better knee functional outcomes [129, 130] and return to previous athletic activities [130] when compared to lateral release. Lateral lengthening is also the preference of 59% of the surgeons in the International Patellofemoral Study Group [3].

Complications

The complication rates of loss of range of motion, muscle mass, and strength were similar between the lengthening and release procedures [130]. However, lateral release was associated with a higher risk of iatrogenic medial patellar instability [129]. There have not been any reports of medial instability after lateral lengthening. In patients with continued disability after lateral release, the incidence of medial instability ranges from 50% to 72% [100, 131]. Most common symptoms are pain, swelling, and giving way that can be exacerbated by twisting/pivoting [100, 131, 132].

22.8.2 Bony Procedures

22.8.2.1 Tibial Tuberosity Osteotomy (TTO)

Outcomes

In the setting of patellofemoral instability, studies in the past have shown that tibial tubercle osteotomies produce good outcomes in 72.5–78.9% of patients [140–142]. In a systematic review including more than 1000 knees, Saltzman et al. revealed that tibial tubercle osteotomies were most frequently performed for patellofemoral instability when pain was present [143]. Pritsch et al. reported on TTO procedures for patellofemoral instability or maltracking and described 72.5% good or excellent results at 6.2-year follow-up [142]. In this study, patients with preoperative pain and instability experienced inferior outcomes to those with isolated instability. Long-term studies have shown rates of recurrent patellofemoral instability between 8% and 15% [144–147].

However, tibial tubercle osteotomies are not currently used as the sole treatment for patellofemoral instability. Instead, the current debate is over when TTOs should be added to MPFL reconstructions. Studies have shown successful outcomes when TTOs are performed concomitantly with MPFL reconstructions [148–152]. Allen et al. and Mikashima et al. noted excellent postoperative outcomes in Kujala and IKDC scores [148, 149]. Other studies have reported significantly improved patient-reported outcome measures from pre- to post-operation including Kujala, KOOS, Lysholm, Tegner, and VAS pain scores [150–152]. Within these studies, low rates of complications and recurrence of patellofemoral instability were reported. The rate of recurrent instability varied from 0% to 6.7% between studies, which is a lower rate when compared to TTO without MPFL reconstruction. Due to excellent patient-reported outcomes and low rates of complications, studies support the use of TTO with concomitant MPFL reconstruction for patellofemoral instability when indicated.

Complications

A variety of complications have been described with tibial tuberosity osteotomies including delayed wound healing, infections, and skin necrosis over the tuberosity in the Maquet procedure [153–155], tuberosity fractures, proximal tibial fractures, delayed union of the osteotomy, and the need for later hardware removal [156–160]. Compartment syndrome has been reported, and surgeons must remain vigilant for this potentially catastrophic complication [161, 162]. Pulmonary emboli [162] and deep venous thrombosis [158] have also been reported, although the role for chemoprophylaxis remains unclear. Arthrofibrosis which can require arthroscopic lysis of adhesions and/or manipulation under anesthesia [156, 161, 163] can also occur. Early motion [164] is imperative to prevent this complication, and in selected situations, a continuous passive motion machine can be helpful [158]. Because the osteotomy site can serve as a stress riser, a period of restricted weight bearing is critical to avoid proximal tibial fractures [158, 164]. Nonunion at the osteotomy site is rare at 3.7% because of compressive interfragmentary fixation [165, 166].

22.8.2.2 Coronal Plane or Rotational Osteotomy

Outcomes

Distal femoral osteotomies indicated for patellar instability have resulted in improved patient-reported functional outcomes [105, 106, 167–169]. In these studies, concomitant procedures performed alongside femoral osteotomies included MPFL reconstructions [105, 167], lateral release

[106], or both medial reefing and lateral releases [168, 169]. Patient-reported outcomes have commonly included statistical improvements in both Kujala and VAS pain scores. Additionally, these studies presented high patient satisfaction rates which varied from 70% to 100% [105, 167]. Within a cohort of 11 patients, Wilson et al. reported that 90% returned to their desired level of activity [105].

In the setting of combined femoral derotation osteotomies with MPFL reconstructions, Nelitz et al. also reported a significant increase in patient-reported outcomes. These included Kujala, IKDC, and VAS. Additionally, no patient was not satisfied at the last follow-up [170].

Complications

In a systematic review, DFO was found to have an approximately 10% complication rate and a 35–40% reoperation rate [171]. The most common reason cited for reoperation was conversion to arthroplasty in patients with previous arthritis or removal of hardware. Complications, although not commonly experienced, have included decreased range of motion, delayed union, and recurrent subluxation events [105, 106, 167–169]. These papers reported minor complications, but did not report the occurrence of more severe complications, which might include dislocation, infection, compartment syndrome, thrombosis, or nonunion.

In femoral derotation osteotomies, Nelitz et al. also reported no recurrent dislocations, infections, or delayed unions. However, like the DFO papers, two patients experienced decreased range of motion. Full range of motion was eventually achieved following a lengthened rehabilitation program [170].

22.8.2.3 Trochleoplasty

Outcomes

Two systematic reviews compared trochleoplasty with non-trochleoplasty procedures in patients with patellofemoral instability and severe trochlear dysplasia. Song et al. evaluated 329 knees in 17 studies who had a trochleoplasty through a number of techniques (112 knees had MPFL reconstruction associated) and 130 knees in six studies undergoing MPFL reconstruction (28 patients) or other procedures [172]. The most important finding was significant postoperative improvement shown in all included studies regardless of the specific procedures performed. The trochleoplasty group showed improved postoperative patellar stability and less patellofemoral arthritis, but also showed reduced range of motion. Importantly, there were also a significantly greater number of revision cases in the trochleoplasty group [172]. Balcarek et al. provided an analysis of ten studies which included four MPFL studies with 221 knees and six trochleoplasty studies with 186 knees. They found that trochleoplasty in conjunction with other procedures, including MPFL, decreased the rate of dislocation to 2.1% compared to a dislocation rate of 7% in MPFL reconstructions alone [173].

Complications

A recent meta-analysis was conducted on the complications of trochleoplasties in 20 studies. Decreased range of motion has also been found to be a more common complication. Patellofemoral osteoarthritis occurred in 7% of knees in Bereiter and 12% in the Dejour technique. Lastly, 8% of knees in the Berieter technique required further surgery with 20% in the Dejour [174].

22.9 Conclusion

The diagnosis and treatment of patellofemoral instability remains a challenge. Individualized treatment plans based on clinical evaluation and imaging studies can be tailored to improve patient outcome. Despite numerous studies examining the treatment of patellofemoral instability, high-quality outcomes are lacking [174]. Randomized controlled studies, larger sample sizes, and long-term follow-up are needed to better define the role of nonoperative, soft tissue, and/or bony surgical management. Additional biomechanical studies should provide insight regarding the surgical procedures that will best correct patellofemoral instability. Finally, surgical techniques must be standardized to make studies comparable.

References

1. Harilainen A, Myllynen P, Antila H, Seitsalo S. The significance of arthroscopy and examination under anaesthesia in the diagnosis of fresh injury haemarthrosis of the knee joint. Injury. 1988;19(1):21–4. https://doi.org/10.1016/0020-1383(88)90168-4.
2. Stefancin JJ, Parker RD. First-time traumatic patellar dislocation: a systematic review. Clin Orthop Relat Res. 2007;455:93–101. https://doi.org/10.1097/BLO.0b013e31802eb40a.
3. Fithian DC, Paxton EW, Post WR, Panni AS, International Patellofemoral Study Group. Lateral retinacular release: a survey of the International Patellofemoral Study Group. Arthroscopy. 2004;20(5):463–8. https://doi.org/10.1016/j.arthro.2004.03.002.
4. Sherman SL, Erickson BJ, Cvetanovich GL, et al. Tibial tuberosity osteotomy: indications, techniques, and outcomes. Am J Sports Med. 2014;42(8):2006–17. https://doi.org/10.1177/0363546513507423.
5. Camanho GL, Viegas Ade C, Bitar AC, Demange MK, Hernandez AJ. Conservative versus surgical treatment for repair of the medial patellofemoral ligament in acute dislocations of the patella. Arthroscopy. 2009;25(6):620–5. https://doi.org/10.1016/j.arthro.2008.12.005.
6. Hawkins RJ, Bell RH, Anisette G. Acute patellar dislocations. The natural history. Am J Sports Med. 1986;14(2):117–20. https://doi.org/10.1177/036354658601400204.
7. Mäenpää H, Huhtala H, Lehto MU. Recurrence after patellar dislocation. Redislocation in 37/75 patients followed for 6–24 years. Acta Orthop Scand. 1997;68(5):424–6.
8. Palmu S, Kallio PE, Donell ST, Helenius I, Nietosvaara Y. Acute patellar dislocation in children and adolescents: a randomized clinical trial. J Bone Joint Surg Am. 2008;90(3):463–70. https://doi.org/10.2106/JBJS.G.00072.
9. Hinckel BB, Gobbi RG, Kaleka CC, Camanho GL, Arendt EA. Medial patellotibial ligament and medial patellomeniscal ligament: anatomy, imaging, biomechanics, and clinical review. Knee Surg Sports Traumatol Arthrosc. 2018;26(3):685–96. https://doi.org/10.1007/s00167-017-4469-y.
10. Atkin DM, Fithian DC, Marangi KS, Stone ML, Dobson BE, Mendelsohn C. Characteristics of patients with primary acute lateral patellar dislocation and their recovery within the first 6 months of injury. Am J Sports Med. 2000;28(4):472–9. https://doi.org/10.1177/03635465000280040601.
11. Askenberger M, Ekstrom W, Finnbogason T, Janarv PM. Occult intra-articular knee injuries in children with hemarthrosis. Am J Sports Med. 2014;42(7):1600–6. https://doi.org/10.1177/0363546514529639.
12. Sherman SL, Plackis AC, Nuelle CW. Patellofemoral anatomy and biomechanics. Clin Sports Med. 2014;33(3):389–401. https://doi.org/10.1016/j.csm.2014.03.008.
13. Jacobson KE, Flandry FC. Diagnosis of anterior knee pain. Clin Sports Med. 1989;8(2):179–95.
14. Fox TA. Dysplasia of the quadriceps mechanism: hypoplasia of the vastus medialis muscle as related to the hypermobile patella syndrome. Surg Clin North Am. 1975;55(1):199–226.
15. Sakai N, Luo ZP, Rand JA, An KN. The influence of weakness in the vastus medialis oblique muscle on the patellofemoral joint: an in vitro biomechanical study. Clin Biomech (Bristol, Avon). 2000;15(5):335–9. https://doi.org/10.1016/S0268-0033(99)00089-3.
16. Desio SM, Burks RT, Bachus KN. Soft tissue restraints to lateral patellar translation in the human knee. Am J Sports Med. 1998;26(1):59–65. https://doi.org/10.1177/03635465980260012701.
17. Hautamaa PV, Fithian DC, Kaufman KR, Daniel DM, Pohlmeyer AM. Medial soft tissue restraints in lateral patellar instability and repair. Clin Orthop Relat Res. 1998;349:174–82.
18. Mountney J, Senavongse W, Amis AA, Thomas NP. Tensile strength of the medial patellofemoral ligament before and after repair or reconstruction. J Bone Joint Surg Br. 2005;87(1):36–40.
19. Senavongse W, Amis AA. The effects of articular, retinacular, or muscular deficiencies on patellofemoral joint stability: a biomechanical study in vitro. J Bone Joint Surg Br. 2005;87(4):577–82. https://doi.org/10.1302/0301-620X.87B4.14768.
20. Tanaka MJ. Variability in the patellar attachment of the medial patellofemoral ligament. Arthroscopy. 2016;32(8):1667–70. https://doi.org/10.1016/j.arthro.2016.01.046.
21. Ebied AM, El-Kholy W. Reconstruction of the medial patello-femoral and patello-tibial ligaments for treatment of patellar instability. Knee Surg Sports Traumatol Arthrosc. 2012;20(5):926–32. https://doi.org/10.1007/s00167-011-1659-x.
22. Redziniak DE, Diduch DR, Mihalko WM, et al. Patellar instability. J Bone Joint Surg Am. 2009;91(9):2264–75.
23. Philippot R, Boyer B, Testa R, Farizon F, Moyen B. The role of the medial ligamentous structures on patellar tracking during knee flexion. Knee Surg Sports Traumatol Arthrosc. 2012;20(2):331–6. https://doi.org/10.1007/s00167-011-1598-6.
24. Garth WP Jr, Connor GS, Futch L, Belarmino H. Patellar subluxation at terminal knee extension: isolated deficiency of the medial patellomeniscal ligament. J Bone Joint Surg Am. 2011;93(10):954–62. https://doi.org/10.2106/JBJS.H.00103.
25. Hinckel BB, Gobbi RG, Demange MK, et al. Medial patellofemoral ligament, medial patellotibial ligament, and medial patellomeniscal ligament: anatomic, histologic, radiographic, and biomechanical study. Arthroscopy. 2017;33(10):1862–73. https://doi.org/10.1016/j.arthro.2017.04.020.

26. Kaleka CC, Aihara LJ, Rodrigues A, de Medeiros SF, de Oliveira VM, de Paula Leite Cury R. Cadaveric study of the secondary medial patellar restraints: patellotibial and patellomeniscal ligaments. Knee Surg Sports Traumatol Arthrosc. 2017;25(1):144–51. https://doi.org/10.1007/s00167-016-4322-8.
27. Johnson RP. Lateral facet syndrome of the patella. Lateral restraint analysis and use of lateral resection. Clin Orthop Relat Res. 1989;238:148–58.
28. Panagiotopoulos E, Strzelczyk P, Herrmann M, Scuderi G. Cadaveric study on static medial patellar stabilizers: the dynamizing role of the vastus medialis obliquus on medial patellofemoral ligament. Knee Surg Sports Traumatol Arthrosc. 2006;14(1):7–12. https://doi.org/10.1007/s00167-005-0631-z.
29. Conlan T, Garth WP Jr, Lemons JE. Evaluation of the medial soft-tissue restraints of the extensor mechanism of the knee. J Bone Joint Surg Am. 1993;75(5):682–93.
30. Hinckel BB, Arendt EA. Lateral retinaculum lengthening or release. Oper Tech Sports Med. 2015;23(2):100–6. https://doi.org/10.1053/j.otsm.2015.02.012.
31. Smith TO, Clark A, Neda S, et al. The intra- and inter-observer reliability of the physical examination methods used to assess patients with patellofemoral joint instability. Knee. 2012;19(4):404–10. https://doi.org/10.1016/j.knee.2011.06.002.
32. Nomura E, Horiuchi Y, Inoue M. Correlation of MR imaging findings and open exploration of medial patellofemoral ligament injuries in acute patellar dislocations. Knee. 2002;9(2):139–43.
33. Post WR, Teitge R, Amis A. Patellofemoral malalignment: looking beyond the viewbox. Clin Sports Med. 2002;21(3):521–46, x. https://doi.org/10.1016/S0278-5919(02)00011-X.
34. Stäubli HU, Dürrenmatt U, Porcellini B, Rauschning W. Anatomy and surface geometry of the patellofemoral joint in the axial plane. J Bone Joint Surg Br. 1999;81(3):452–8.
35. Sanders TG, Morrison WB, Singleton BA, Miller MD, Cornum KG. Medial patellofemoral ligament injury following acute transient dislocation of the patella: MR findings with surgical correlation in 14 patients. J Comput Assist Tomogr. 2001;25(6):957–62.
36. Thawait SK, Soldatos T, Thawait GK, Cosgarea AJ, Carrino JA, Chhabra A. High resolution magnetic resonance imaging of the patellar retinaculum: normal anatomy, common injury patterns, and pathologies. Skelet Radiol. 2012;41(2):137–48. https://doi.org/10.1007/s00256-011-1291-3.
37. Maldague B, Malghem J. Radiology of patellar instability: contribution of the lateral radiography and the 30-degree axial view with external rotation. Acta Orthop Belg. 1989;55(3):311–29.
38. Arendt EA, Dejour D. Patella instability: building bridges across the ocean a historic review. Knee Surg Sports Traumatol Arthrosc. 2013;21(2):279–93. https://doi.org/10.1007/s00167-012-2274-1.
39. Biyani R, Elias JJ, Saranathan A, et al. Anatomical factors influencing patellar tracking in the unstable patellofemoral joint. Knee Surg Sports Traumatol Arthrosc. 2014;22(10):2334–41. https://doi.org/10.1007/s00167-014-3195-y.
40. Dejour H, Walch G, Neyret P, Adeleine P. Dysplasia of the femoral trochlea. Rev Chir Orthop Reparatrice Appareil Mot. 1990;76(1):45–54.
41. Dejour H, Walch G, Nove-Josserand L, Guier C. Factors of patellar instability: an anatomic radiographic study. Knee Surg Sports Traumatol Arthrosc. 1994;2(1):19–26.
42. Post WR, Fithian DC. Patellofemoral instability: a consensus statement from the AOSSM/PFF Patellofemoral Instability Workshop. Orthop J Sports Med. 2018;6(1):2325967117750352. https://doi.org/10.1177/2325967117750352.
43. Markolf KL, Mensch JS, Amstutz HC. Stiffness and laxity of the knee—the contributions of the supporting structures. A quantitative in vitro study. J Bone Joint Surg Am. 1976;58(5):583–94.
44. Shoemaker SC, Adams D, Daniel DM, Woo SL. Quadriceps/anterior cruciate graft interaction. An in vitro study of joint kinematics and anterior cruciate ligament graft tension. Clin Orthop Relat Res. 1993;294:379–90.
45. Trent PS, Walker PS, Wolf B. Ligament length patterns, strength, and rotational axes of the knee joint. Clin Orthop Relat Res. 1976;117:263–70.
46. Johnson LL, van Dyk GE, Green JR 3rd, et al. Clinical assessment of asymptomatic knees: comparison of men and women. Arthroscopy. 1998;14(4):347–59. https://doi.org/10.1016/S0749-8063(98)70001-5.
47. Sojbjerg JO, Lauritzen J, Hvid I, Boe S. Arthroscopic determination of patellofemoral malalignment. Clin Orthop Relat Res. 1987;215:243–7.
48. Woodland LH, Francis RS. Parameters and comparisons of the quadriceps angle of college-aged men and women in the supine and standing positions. Am J Sports Med. 1992;20(2):208–11. https://doi.org/10.1177/036354659202000220.
49. Hinckel BB, Gobbi RG, Filho EN, et al. Are the osseous and tendinous-cartilaginous tibial tuberosity-trochlear groove distances the same on CT and MRI? Skelet Radiol. 2015;44(8):1085–93. https://doi.org/10.1007/s00256-015-2118-4.
50. Hinckel BB, Gobbi RG, Kihara Filho EN, Demange MK, Pecora JR, Camanho GL. Patellar tendon-trochlear groove angle measurement: a new method for patellofemoral rotational analyses. Orthop J Sports Med. 2015;3(9):2325967115601031. https://doi.org/10.1177/2325967115601031.
51. Hinckel BB, Gobbi RG, Kihara Filho EN, et al. Why are bone and soft tissue measurements of the TT-TG distance on MRI different in patients with patellar instability? Knee Surg Sports Traumatol Arthrosc. 2017;25(10):3053–60. https://doi.org/10.1007/s00167-016-4095-0.
52. Daynes J, Hinckel BB, Farr J. Tibial tuberosity-posterior cruciate ligament distance. J Knee

Surg. 2016;29(6):471–7. https://doi.org/10.1055/s-0035-1564732.
53. Tensho K, Akaoka Y, Shimodaira H, et al. What components comprise the measurement of the tibial tuberosity-trochlear groove distance in a patellar dislocation population? J Bone Joint Surg Am. 2015;97(17):1441–8. https://doi.org/10.2106/JBJS.N.01313.
54. Johnson F, Leitl S, Waugh W. The distribution of load across the knee. A comparison of static and dynamic measurements. J Bone Joint Surg Br. 1980;62(3):346–9.
55. Karachalios T, Sarangi PP, Newman JH. Severe varus and valgus deformities treated by total knee arthroplasty. J Bone Joint Surg Br. 1994;76(6):938–42.
56. Seitlinger G, Moroder P, Scheurecker G, Hofmann S, Grelsamer RP. The contribution of different femur segments to overall femoral torsion. Am J Sports Med. 2016;44(7):1796–800. https://doi.org/10.1177/0363546516639945.
57. Diederichs G, Kohlitz T, Kornaropoulos E, Heller MO, Vollnberg B, Scheffler S. Magnetic resonance imaging analysis of rotational alignment in patients with patellar dislocations. Am J Sports Med. 2013;41(1):51–7. https://doi.org/10.1177/0363546512464691.
58. Post WR. Clinical evaluation of patients with patellofemoral disorders. Arthroscopy. 1999;15(8):841–51. https://doi.org/10.1053/ar.1999.v15.015084.
59. Reider B, Martell JM. Pelvis, hip and thigh. In: The orthopedic physical examination. Philadelphia, PA: WB Saunders; 1999. p. 159–99.
60. Takagi S, Sato T, Watanabe S, et al. Alignment in the transverse plane, but not sagittal or coronal plane, affects the risk of recurrent patella dislocation. Knee Surg Sports Traumatol Arthrosc. 2017; https://doi.org/10.1007/s00167-017-4806-1.
61. Parikh S, Noyes FR. Patellofemoral disorders: role of computed tomography and magnetic resonance imaging in defining abnormal rotational lower limb alignment. Sports Health. 2011;3(2):158–69. https://doi.org/10.1177/1941738111399372.
62. Kuo TY, Skedros JG, Bloebaum RD. Measurement of femoral anteversion by biplane radiography and computed tomography imaging: comparison with an anatomic reference. Investig Radiol. 2003;38(4):221–9. https://doi.org/10.1097/01.RLI.0000059542.90854.EF.
63. Tamari K, Tinley P, Briffa K, Aoyagi K. Ethnic-, gender-, and age-related differences in femorotibial angle, femoral antetorsion, and tibiofibular torsion: cross-sectional study among healthy Japanese and Australian Caucasians. Clin Anat. 2006;19(1):59–67. https://doi.org/10.1002/ca.20170.
64. Schneider B, Laubenberger J, Jemlich S, Groene K, Weber HM, Langer M. Measurement of femoral antetorsion and tibial torsion by magnetic resonance imaging. Br J Radiol. 1997;70(834):575–9. https://doi.org/10.1259/bjr.70.834.9227249.
65. Colvin AC, West RV. Patellar instability. J Bone Joint Surg Am. 2008;90(12):2751–62. https://doi.org/10.2106/JBJS.H.00211.
66. Insall J, Goldberg V, Salvati E. Recurrent dislocation and the high-riding patella. Clin Orthop Relat Res. 1972;88:67–9.
67. Ward SR, Terk MR, Powers CM. Patella alta: association with patellofemoral alignment and changes in contact area during weight-bearing. J Bone Joint Surg Am. 2007;89(8):1749–550. https://doi.org/10.2106/JBJS.F.00508.
68. Aglietti P, Insall JN, Cerulli G. Patellar pain and incongruence. I: measurements of incongruence. Clin Orthop Relat Res. 1983;176:217–24.
69. Simmons E Jr, Cameron JC. Patella alta and recurrent dislocation of the patella. Clin Orthop Relat Res. 1992;274:265–9.
70. Insall J, Salvati E. Patella position in the normal knee joint. Radiology. 1971;101(1):101–4. https://doi.org/10.1148/101.1.101.
71. Grelsamer RP, Meadows S. The modified Insall-Salvati ratio for assessment of patellar height. Clin Orthop Relat Res. 1992;282:170–6.
72. Blackburne JS, Peel TE. A new method of measuring patellar height. J Bone Joint Surg Br. 1977;59(2):241–2.
73. Caton J, Deschamps G, Chambat P, Lerat JL, Dejour H. Patella infera. Apropos of 128 cases. Rev Chir Orthop Reparatrice Appar Mot. 1982;68(5):317–25.
74. Labelle H, Laurin CA. Radiological investigation of normal and abnormal patellae. J Bone Joint Surg Br. 1975;57:530.
75. Biedert RM, Albrecht S. The patellotrochlear index: a new index for assessing patellar height. Knee Surg Sports Traumatol Arthrosc. 2006;14(8):707–12. https://doi.org/10.1007/s00167-005-0015-4.
76. Dejour D, Ferrua P, Ntagiopoulos PG, et al. The introduction of a new MRI index to evaluate sagittal patellofemoral engagement. Orthop Traumatol Surg Res. 2013;99(8 Suppl):S391–8. https://doi.org/10.1016/j.otsr.2013.10.008.
77. Askenberger M, Janarv PM, Finnbogason T, Arendt EA. Morphology and anatomic patellar instability risk factors in first-time traumatic lateral patellar dislocations: a prospective magnetic resonance imaging study in skeletally immature children. Am J Sports Med. 2017;45(1):50–8. https://doi.org/10.1177/0363546516663498.
78. Steensen RN, Bentley JC, Trinh TQ, Backes JR, Wiltfong RE. The prevalence and combined prevalences of anatomic factors associated with recurrent patellar dislocation: a magnetic resonance imaging study. Am J Sports Med. 2015;43(4):921–7. https://doi.org/10.1177/0363546514563904.
79. Tompkins MA, Rohr SR, Agel J, Arendt EA. Anatomic patellar instability risk factors in primary lateral patellar dislocations do not predict injury patterns: an MRI-based study. Knee Surg

Sports Traumatol Arthrosc. 2017;26(3):677–84. https://doi.org/10.1007/s00167-017-4464-3.
80. Albee F. The bone graft wedge in the treatment of habitual dislocation of the patella. Med Rec. 1915;88(7):257–9.
81. Feller JA, Amis AA, Andrish JT, Arendt EA, Erasmus PJ, Powers CM. Surgical biomechanics of the patellofemoral joint. Arthroscopy. 2007;23(5):542–53. https://doi.org/10.1016/j.arthro.2007.03.006.
82. Dejour D, Le Coultre B. Osteotomies in patellofemoral instabilities. Sports Med Arthrosc Rev. 2007;15(1):39–46. https://doi.org/10.1097/JSA.0b013e31803035ae.
83. Malghem J, Maldague B. Depth insufficiency of the proximal trochlear groove on lateral radiographs of the knee: relation to patellar dislocation. Radiology. 1989;170(2):507–10. https://doi.org/10.1148/radiology.170.2.2911676.
84. Pfirrmann CW, Zanetti M, Romero J, Hodler J. Femoral trochlear dysplasia: MR findings. Radiology. 2000;216(3):858–64. https://doi.org/10.1148/radiology.216.3.r00se38858.
85. Mäenpää H, Lehto MU. Patellar dislocation. The long-term results of nonoperative management in 100 patients. Am J Sports Med. 1997;25(2):213–7. https://doi.org/10.1177/036354659702500213.
86. Cosgarea AJ, Browne JA, Kim TK, McFarland EG. Evaluation and management of the unstable patella. Phys Sportsmed. 2002;30(10):33–40. https://doi.org/10.3810/psm.2002.10.492.
87. Fabricant PD, Yen YM, Kramer DE, et al. Fixation of traumatic chondral-only fragments of the knee in pediatric and adolescent athletes: a retrospective multicenter report. Orthop J Sports Med. 2018;6(2):2325967117753140. https://doi.org/10.1177/2325967117753140.
88. Cavalheiro CM, Gobbi RG, Hinckel BB, Demange MK, Pécora JR, Camanho GL. Lesão condral do fêmur tratada com sutura óssea após luxação aguda de patela: um relato de caso. Rev Bras Ortop. 2017; https://doi.org/10.1016/j.rbo.2017.04.003.
89. Hinckel BB, Gomoll AH, Farr J II. Cartilage restoration in the patellofemoral joint. Am J Orthop (Belle Mead NJ). 2017;46(5):217–22.
90. Anderson CN, Magnussen RA, Block JJ, Anderson AF, Spindler KP. Operative fixation of chondral loose bodies in osteochondritis dissecans in the knee: a report of 5 cases. Orthop J Sports Med. 2013;1(2):2325967113496546. https://doi.org/10.1177/2325967113496546.
91. Jaquith BP, Parikh SN. Predictors of recurrent patellar instability in children and adolescents after first-time dislocation. J Pediatr Orthop. 2017;37(7):484–90. https://doi.org/10.1097/BPO.0000000000000674.
92. Christensen TC, Sanders TL, Pareek A, Mohan R, Dahm DL, Krych AJ. Risk factors and time to recurrent ipsilateral and contralateral patellar dislocations. Am J Sports Med. 2017;45(9):2105–10. https://doi.org/10.1177/0363546517704178.
93. Magnussen RA, Verlage M, Stock E, et al. Primary patellar dislocations without surgical stabilization or recurrence: how well are these patients really doing? Knee Surg Sports Traumatol Arthrosc. 2017;25(8):2352–6. https://doi.org/10.1007/s00167-015-3716-3.
94. Bitar AC, Demange MK, D'Elia CO, Camanho GL. Traumatic patellar dislocation: nonoperative treatment compared with MPFL reconstruction using patellar tendon. Am J Sports Med. 2012;40(1):114–22. https://doi.org/10.1177/0363546511423742.
95. Andrish J. The management of recurrent patellar dislocation. Orthop Clin North Am. 2008;39(3):313–27, vi. https://doi.org/10.1016/j.ocl.2008.03.005.
96. Sherman SL, Nuelle CW, Farr J. Issues specific to cartilage restoration in the patellofemoral joint. In: Amendola A, Gomoll AH, editors. AAOS let's discuss joint preservation of the knee. Rosemont, IL: American Academy of Orthopaedic Surgeons; 2015. p. 213–37.
97. Baumann CA, Pratte EL, Sherman SL, Arendt EA, Hinckel BB. Reconstruction of the medial patellotibial ligament results in favorable clinical outcomes: a systematic review. Knee Surg Sports Traumatol Arthrosc. 2018; https://doi.org/10.1007/s00167-018-4833-6.
98. Hinckel BB, Gobbi RG, Bonadio MB, Demange MK, Pécora JR, Camanho GL. Reconstruction of medial patellofemoral ligament using quadriceps tendon combined with reconstruction of medial patellotibial ligament using patellar tendon: initial experience. Rev Bras Ortop. 2016;51(1):75–82. https://doi.org/10.1016/j.rboe.2015.03.012.
99. Hinckel BB, Gobbi RG, Demange MK, Bonadio MB, Pecora JR, Camanho GL. Combined reconstruction of the medial patellofemoral ligament with quadricipital tendon and the medial patellotibial ligament with patellar tendon. Arthrosc Tech. 2016;5(1):e79–84. https://doi.org/10.1016/j.eats.2015.10.004.
100. Hughston JC, Deese M. Medial subluxation of the patella as a complication of lateral retinacular release. Am J Sports Med. 1988;16(4):383–8. https://doi.org/10.1177/036354658801600413.
101. Aglietti P, Pisaneschi A, Buzzi R, Gaudenzi A, Allegra M. Arthroscopic lateral release for patellar pain or instability. Arthroscopy. 1989;5(3):176–83.
102. Redler LH, Meyers KN, Brady JM, Dennis ER, Nguyen JT, Shubin Stein BE. Anisometry of medial patellofemoral ligament reconstruction in the setting of increased tibial tubercle-trochlear groove distance and patella alta. Arthroscopy. 2018;34(2):502–10. https://doi.org/10.1016/j.arthro.2017.08.256.
103. Beck PR, Thomas AL, Farr J, Lewis PB, Cole BJ. Trochlear contact pressures after anteromedialization of the tibial tubercle. Am J Sports Med. 2005;33(11):1710–5. https://doi.org/10.1177/0363546505278300.
104. Franciozi CE, Ambra LF, Albertoni LJ, et al. Increased femoral anteversion influence over surgically treated recurrent patellar instability patients.

Arthroscopy. 2017;33(3):633–40. https://doi.org/10.1016/j.arthro.2016.09.015.
105. Wilson PL, Black SR, Ellis HB, Podeszwa DA. Distal femoral valgus and recurrent traumatic patellar instability: is an isolated varus producing distal femoral osteotomy a treatment option? J Pediatr Orthop. 2018;38(3):e162–e7. https://doi.org/10.1097/BPO.0000000000001128.
106. Swarup I, Elattar O, Rozbruch SR. Patellar instability treated with distal femoral osteotomy. Knee. 2017;24(3):608–14. https://doi.org/10.1016/j.knee.2017.02.004.
107. Hinterwimmer S, Minzlaff P, Saier T, Niemeyer P, Imhoff AB, Feucht MJ. Biplanar supracondylar femoral derotation osteotomy for patellofemoral malalignment: the anterior closed-wedge technique. Knee Surg Sports Traumatol Arthrosc. 2014;22(10):2518–21. https://doi.org/10.1007/s00167-014-2993-6.
108. Schöttle PB, Schmeling A, Rosenstiel N, Weiler A. Radiographic landmarks for femoral tunnel placement in medial patellofemoral ligament reconstruction. Am J Sports Med. 2007;35(5):801–4. https://doi.org/10.1177/0363546506296415.
109. Beck P, Brown NA, Greis PE, Burks RT. Patellofemoral contact pressures and lateral patellar translation after medial patellofemoral ligament reconstruction. Am J Sports Med. 2007;35(9):1557–63. https://doi.org/10.1177/0363546507300872.
110. Sobhy MH, Mahran MA, Kamel EM. Midterm results of combined patellofemoral and patellotibial ligaments reconstruction in recurrent patellar dislocation. Eur J Orthop Surg Traumatol. 2013;23(4):465–70. https://doi.org/10.1007/s00590-012-0999-7.
111. Hinckel BB, Gobbi RG, Bonadio MB, Demange MK, Pecora JR, Camanho GL. Reconstruction of medial patellofemoral ligament using quadriceps tendon combined with reconstruction of medial patellotibial ligament using patellar tendon: initial experience. Rev Bras Ortop. 2016;51(1):75–82. https://doi.org/10.1016/j.rboe.2015.03.012.
112. Peterson L, Karlsson J, Brittberg M. Patellar instability with recurrent dislocation due to patellofemoral dysplasia. Results after surgical treatment. Bull Hosp Jt Dis Orthop Inst. 1988;48(2):130–9.
113. Goutallier D, Raou D, Van Driessche S. Retro-trochlear wedge reduction trochleoplasty for the treatment of painful patella syndrome with protruding trochleae. Technical note and early results. Rev Chir Orthop Reparatrice Appar Mot. 2002;88(7):678–85.
114. Hinckel BB, Arendt EA, Ntagiopoulos PG, Dejour D. Trochleoplasty: historical overview and Dejour technique. Oper Tech Sports Med. 2015;23(2):114–22. https://doi.org/10.1053/j.otsm.2015.02.005.
115. Blønd L, Schöttle PB. The arthroscopic deepening trochleoplasty. Knee Surg Sports Traumatol Arthrosc. 2010;18(4):480–5. https://doi.org/10.1007/s00167-009-0935-5.
116. von Knoch F, Böhm T, Bürgi ML, von Knoch M, Bereiter H. Trochleaplasty for recurrent patellar dislocation in association with trochlear dysplasia. A 4- to 14-year follow-up study. J Bone Joint Surg Br. 2006;88(10):1331–5. https://doi.org/10.1302/0301-620X.88B10.17834.
117. Bellemans J, Cauwenberghs F, Brys P, Victor J, Fabry G. Fracture of the proximal tibia after Fulkerson anteromedial tibial tubercle transfer. A report of four cases. Am J Sports Med. 1998;26(2):300–2. https://doi.org/10.1177/03635465980260022401.
118. Witoński D, Kęska R, Synder M, Sibiński M. An isolated medial patellofemoral ligament reconstruction with patellar tendon autograft. Biomed Res Int. 2013;2013:637678. https://doi.org/10.1155/2013/637678.
119. Ma LF, Wang F, Chen BC, Wang CH, Zhou JW, Wang HY. Medial retinaculum plasty versus medial patellofemoral ligament reconstruction for recurrent patellar instability in adults: a randomized controlled trial. Arthroscopy. 2013;29(5):891–7. https://doi.org/10.1016/j.arthro.2013.01.030.
120. Zhao J, Huangfu X, He Y. The role of medial retinaculum plication versus medial patellofemoral ligament reconstruction in combined procedures for recurrent patellar instability in adults. Am J Sports Med. 2012;40(6):1355–64. https://doi.org/10.1177/0363546512439193.
121. Wagner D, Pfalzer F, Hingelbaum S, Huth J, Mauch F, Bauer G. The influence of risk factors on clinical outcomes following anatomical medial patellofemoral ligament (MPFL) reconstruction using the gracilis tendon. Knee Surg Sports Traumatol Arthrosc. 2013;21(2):318–24. https://doi.org/10.1007/s00167-012-2015-5.
122. Howells NR, Barnett AJ, Ahearn N, Ansari A, Eldridge JD. Medial patellofemoral ligament reconstruction: a prospective outcome assessment of a large single centre series. J Bone Joint Surg Br. 2012;94(9):1202–8. https://doi.org/10.1302/0301-620X.94B9.28738.
123. Ahmad CS, Brown GD, Shubin Stein BE. The docking technique for medial patellofemoral ligament reconstruction: surgical technique and clinical outcome. Am J Sports Med. 2009;37(10):2021–7. https://doi.org/10.1177/0363546509336261.
124. Sillanpää P, Mattila VM, Visuri T, Mäenpää H, Pihlajamäki H. Ligament reconstruction versus distal realignment for patellar dislocation. Clin Orthop Relat Res. 2008;466(6):1475–84. https://doi.org/10.1007/s11999-008-0207-6.
125. Christiansen SE, Jacobsen BW, Lund B, Lind M. Reconstruction of the medial patellofemoral ligament with gracilis tendon autograft in transverse patellar drill holes. Arthroscopy. 2008;24(1):82–7. https://doi.org/10.1016/j.arthro.2007.08.005.
126. Schöttle PB, Fucentese SF, Romero J. Clinical and radiological outcome of medial patellofemoral ligament reconstruction with a semitendinosus autograft for patella instability. Knee Surg Sports Traumatol Arthrosc. 2005;13(7):516–21. https://doi.org/10.1007/s00167-005-0659-0.

127. Nelitz M, Williams RS, Lippacher S, Reichel H, Dornacher D. Analysis of failure and clinical outcome after unsuccessful medial patellofemoral ligament reconstruction in young patients. Int Orthop. 2014;38(11):2265–72. https://doi.org/10.1007/s00264-014-2437-4.
128. Shah JN, Howard JS, Flanigan DC, Brophy RH, Carey JL, Lattermann C. A systematic review of complications and failures associated with medial patellofemoral ligament reconstruction for recurrent patellar dislocation. Am J Sports Med. 2012;40(8):1916–23. https://doi.org/10.1177/0363546512442330.
129. Pagenstert G, Wolf N, Bachmann M, et al. Open lateral patellar retinacular lengthening versus open retinacular release in lateral patellar hypercompression syndrome: a prospective double-blinded comparative study on complications and outcome. Arthroscopy. 2012;28(6):788–97. https://doi.org/10.1016/j.arthro.2011.11.004.
130. O'Neill DB. Open lateral retinacular lengthening compared with arthroscopic release. A prospective, randomized outcome study. J Bone Joint Surg Am. 1997;79(12):1759–69.
131. Shellock FG, Mink JH, Deutsch A, Fox JM, Ferkel RD. Evaluation of patients with persistent symptoms after lateral retinacular release by kinematic magnetic resonance imaging of the patellofemoral joint. Arthroscopy. 1990;6(3):226–34. https://doi.org/10.1016/0749-8063(90)90079-S.
132. Heyworth BE, Carroll KM, Dawson CK, Gill TJ. Open lateral retinacular closure surgery for treatment of anterolateral knee pain and disability after arthroscopic lateral retinacular release. Am J Sports Med. 2012;40(2):376–82. https://doi.org/10.1177/0363546511428600.
133. Brown GD, Ahmad CS. Combined medial patellofemoral ligament and medial patellotibial ligament reconstruction in skeletally immature patients. J Knee Surg. 2008;21(4):328–32.
134. Drez D Jr, Edwards TB, Williams CS. Results of medial patellofemoral ligament reconstruction in the treatment of patellar dislocation. Arthroscopy. 2001;17(3):298–306. https://doi.org/10.1053/jars.2001.21490.
135. Giordano M, Falciglia F, Aulisa AG, Guzzanti V. Patellar dislocation in skeletally immature patients: semitendinosous and gracilis augmentation for combined medial patellofemoral and medial patellotibial ligament reconstruction. Knee Surg Sports Traumatol Arthrosc. 2012;20(8):1594–8. https://doi.org/10.1007/s00167-011-1784-6.
136. Baker RH, Carroll N, Dewar FP, Hall JE. The semitendinosus tenodesis for recurrent dislocation of the patella. J Bone Joint Surg Br. 1972;54(1):103–9.
137. Hall JE, Micheli LJ, McManama GB Jr. Semitendinosus tenodesis for recurrent subluxation or dislocation of the patella. Clin Orthop Relat Res. 1979;144:31–5.
138. Joo SY, Park KB, Kim BR, Park HW, Kim HW. The 'four-in-one' procedure for habitual dislocation of the patella in children: early results in patients with severe generalised ligamentous laxity and aplasia of the trochlear groove. J Bone Joint Surg Br. 2007;89(12):1645–9. https://doi.org/10.1302/0301-620X.89B12.19398.
139. Letts RM, Davidson D, Beaule P. Semitendinosus tenodesis for repair of recurrent dislocation of the patella in children. J Pediatr Orthop. 1999;19(6):742–7.
140. Caton JH, Dejour D. Tibial tubercle osteotomy in patello-femoral instability and in patellar height abnormality. Int Orthop. 2010;34(2):305–9. https://doi.org/10.1007/s00264-009-0929-4.
141. Dantas P, Nunes C, Moreira J, Amaral LB. Anteromedialisation of the tibial tubercle for patellar instability. Int Orthop. 2005;29(6):390–1. https://doi.org/10.1007/s00264-005-0015-5.
142. Pritsch T, Haim A, Arbel R, Snir N, Shasha N, Dekel S. Tailored tibial tubercle transfer for patellofemoral malalignment: analysis of clinical outcomes. Knee Surg Sports Traumatol Arthrosc. 2007;15(8):994–1002. https://doi.org/10.1007/s00167-007-0325-9.
143. Saltzman BM, Rao A, Erickson BJ, et al. A systematic review of 21 tibial tubercle osteotomy studies and more than 1000 knees: indications, clinical outcomes, complications, and reoperations. Am J Orthop (Belle Mead NJ). 2017;46(6):E396–e407.
144. Akgun U, Nuran R, Karahan M. Modified Fulkerson osteotomy in recurrent patellofemoral dislocations. Acta Orthop Traumatol Turc. 2010;44(1):27–35. https://doi.org/10.3944/AOTT.2010.2143.
145. Barber FA, McGarry JE. Elmslie-Trillat procedure for the treatment of recurrent patellar instability. Arthroscopy. 2008;24(1):77–81. https://doi.org/10.1016/j.arthro.2007.07.028.
146. Tecklenburg K, Feller JA, Whitehead TS, Webster KE, Elzarka A. Outcome of surgery for recurrent patellar dislocation based on the distance of the tibial tuberosity to the trochlear groove. J Bone Joint Surg Br. 2010;92(10):1376–80. https://doi.org/10.1302/0301-620X.92B10.24439.
147. Tsuda E, Ishibashi Y, Yamamoto Y, Maeda S. Incidence and radiologic predictor of postoperative patellar instability after Fulkerson procedure of the tibial tuberosity for recurrent patellar dislocation. Knee Surg Sports Traumatol Arthrosc. 2012;20(10):2062–70. https://doi.org/10.1007/s00167-011-1832-2.
148. Allen MM, Krych AJ, Johnson NR, Mohan R, Stuart MJ, Dahm DL. Combined tibial tubercle osteotomy and medial patellofemoral ligament reconstruction for recurrent lateral patellar instability in patients with multiple anatomic risk factors. Arthroscopy. 2018;34(8):2420–6.e3. https://doi.org/10.1016/j.arthro.2018.02.049.
149. Mikashima Y, Kimura M, Kobayashi Y, Asagumo H, Tomatsu T. Medial patellofemoral ligament reconstruction for recurrent patellar instability. Acta Orthop Belg. 2004;70(6):545–50.

150. Mulliez A, Lambrecht D, Verbruggen D, Van Der Straeten C, Verdonk P, Victor J. Clinical outcome in MPFL reconstruction with and without tuberositas transposition. Knee Surg Sports Traumatol Arthrosc. 2017;25(9):2708–14. https://doi.org/10.1007/s00167-015-3654-0.
151. Watanabe T, Muneta T, Ikeda H, Tateishi T, Sekiya I. Visual analog scale assessment after medial patellofemoral ligament reconstruction: with or without tibial tubercle transfer. J Orthop Sci. 2008;13(1):32–8. https://doi.org/10.1007/s00776-007-1196-0.
152. Frings J, Krause M, Wohlmuth P, Akoto R, Frosch KH. Influence of patient-related factors on clinical outcome of tibial tubercle transfer combined with medial patellofemoral ligament reconstruction. Knee. 2018;pii:S0968–0160(18)30609-4. https://doi.org/10.1016/j.knee.2018.07.018.
153. Maquet P. Advancement of the tibial tuberosity. Clin Orthop Relat Res. 1976;115:225–30.
154. Mendes DG, Soudry M, Iusim M. Clinical assessment of Maquet tibial tuberosity advancement. Clin Orthop Relat Res. 1987;222:228–38.
155. Silvello L, Scarponi R, Guazzetti R, Bianchetti M, Fiore AM. Tibial tubercle advancement by the Maquet technique for patellofemoral arthritis or chondromalacia. Ital J Orthop Traumatol. 1987;13(1):37–44.
156. Bessette GC, Hunter RE. The Maquet procedure. A retrospective review. Clin Orthop Relat Res. 1988;232:159–67.
157. Ebinger TP, Boezaart A, Albright JP. Modifications of the Fulkerson osteotomy: a pilot study assessment of a novel technique of dynamic intraoperative determination of the adequacy of tubercle transfer. Iowa Orthop J. 2007;27:61–4.
158. Fulkerson JP, Becker GJ, Meaney JA, Miranda M, Folcik MA. Anteromedial tibial tubercle transfer without bone graft. Am J Sports Med. 1990;18(5):490–6; discussion 496–7. https://doi.org/10.1177/036354659001800508.
159. Klecker RJ, Winalski CS, Aliabadi P, Minas T. The aberrant anterior tibial artery: magnetic resonance appearance, prevalence, and surgical implications. Am J Sports Med. 2008;36(4):720–7. https://doi.org/10.1177/0363546507311595.
160. Shelbourne KD, Porter DA, Rozzi W. Use of a modified Elmslie-Trillat procedure to improve abnormal patellar congruence angle. Am J Sports Med. 1994;22(3):318–23. https://doi.org/10.1177/036354659402200304.
161. Cox JS. Evaluation of the Roux-Elmslie-Trillat procedure for knee extensor realignment. Am J Sports Med. 1982;10(5):303–10. https://doi.org/10.1177/036354658201000509.
162. Wiggins HE. The anterior tibial compartmental syndrome. A complication of the Hauser procedure. Clin Orthop Relat Res. 1975;113:90–4.
163. Fulkerson JP. Anteromedialization of the tibial tuberosity for patellofemoral malalignment. Clin Orthop Relat Res. 1983;177:176–81.
164. Farr J. Tibial tubercle osteotomy. Tech Knee Surg. 2003;2(1):28–42.
165. Farr J, Schepsis A, Cole B, Fulkerson J, Lewis P. Anteromedialization: review and technique. J Knee Surg. 2007;20(2):120–8.
166. Mayer C, Magnussen RA, Servien E, et al. Patellar tendon tenodesis in association with tibial tubercle distalization for the treatment of episodic patellar dislocation with patella alta. Am J Sports Med. 2012;40(2):346–51. https://doi.org/10.1177/0363546511427117.
167. Frings J, Krause M, Akoto R, Wohlmuth P, Frosch KH. Combined distal femoral osteotomy (DFO) in genu valgum leads to reliable patellar stabilization and an improvement in knee function. Knee Surg Sports Traumatol Arthrosc. 2018; https://doi.org/10.1007/s00167-018-5000-9.
168. Nha KW, Ha Y, Oh S, et al. Surgical Treatment with closing-wedge distal femoral osteotomy for recurrent patellar dislocation with genu valgum. Am J Sports Med. 2018;46(7):1632–40. https://doi.org/10.1177/0363546518765479.
169. Chang CB, Shetty GM, Lee JS, Kim YC, Kwon JH, Nha KW. A combined closing wedge distal femoral osteotomy and medial reefing procedure for recurrent patellar dislocation with genu valgum. Yonsei Med J. 2017;58(4):878–83. https://doi.org/10.3349/ymj.2017.58.4.878.
170. Nelitz M, Dreyhaupt J, Williams SR, Dornacher D. Combined supracondylar femoral derotation osteotomy and patellofemoral ligament reconstruction for recurrent patellar dislocation and severe femoral anteversion syndrome: surgical technique and clinical outcome. Int Orthop. 2015;39(12):2355–62. https://doi.org/10.1007/s00264-015-2859-7.
171. Wylie JD, Jones DL, Hartley MK, et al. Distal femoral osteotomy for the valgus knee: medial closing wedge versus lateral opening wedge: a systematic review. Arthroscopy. 2016;32(10):2141–7. https://doi.org/10.1016/j.arthro.2016.04.010.
172. Song GY, Hong L, Zhang H, et al. Trochleoplasty versus nontrochleoplasty procedures in treating patellar instability caused by severe trochlear dysplasia. Arthroscopy. 2014;30(4):523–32. https://doi.org/10.1016/j.arthro.2014.01.011.
173. Balcarek P, Rehn S, Howells NR, et al. Results of medial patellofemoral ligament reconstruction compared with trochleoplasty plus individual extensor apparatus balancing in patellar instability caused by severe trochlear dysplasia: a systematic review and meta-analysis. Knee Surg Sports Traumatol Arthrosc. 2017;25(12):3869–77. https://doi.org/10.1007/s00167-016-4365-x.
174. van Sambeeck JDP, van de Groes SAW, Verdonschot N, Hannink G. Trochleoplasty procedures show complication rates similar to other patellar-stabilizing procedures. Knee Surg Sports Traumatol Arthrosc. 2017;26(9):2841–57. https://doi.org/10.1007/s00167-017-4766-5.

23 Arthroscopic Trochleoplasty

Lars Blond

23.1 Introduction and Basic Science

Trochleoplasty is a well-established procedure for many years; however, the indications for the surgery are still debatable [1, 2]. The trochlea dysplasia classification systems are unreliable and there is a lack of randomized studies using patient-related outcome systems.

The aim of the trochleoplasty procedure is to restore anatomy, when trochlear dysplasia (TD) is present and when patients have symptoms secondary to this type of malalignment. Biomechanics has demonstrated how trochlear dysplasia significantly affects the kinematics of the patellofemoral joint and negatively influences the stabilizing forces on the patella [3, 4].

Trochlear dysplasia has been found to predispose to

- Patellar instability.
- Anterior knee pain.
- Patellofemoral osteoarthritis [5–11].

The first arthroscopic trochleoplasty (AT) was done back in 2008, and today it is a well-accepted procedure that slowly spreads to more and more centers. The general impression for those being used to perform the open trochleoplasty and who starts to perform the arthroscopic version is very positive. Several trochleoplasty techniques have been described, and arthroscopic trochleoplasty (AT) [12–15] is a variant based upon the Bereiter technique, also called the thin flap technique [16]. AT is less invasive and is considered to have the same known advantages of the other techniques based on minimal invasive surgery. Moreover, AT is more precise, and the risk of cartilage flap fracture is significantly reduced. Moreover, open trochleoplasty is associated with the risk of arthrofibrosis, infection, prolonged pain, and scar formation [17], and those complications have not yet been observed by the AT method. After several cadaver experiments, the first in person athroscopic trochleoplasty was done in Denmark in the start of 2008, and soon followed by several other cases. Those experiencies from those first cases was presented at ISAKOS meeting in Osaka, Japan in 2009. Today it is a well-accepted procedure [18]. To perform AT you need to be very experienced with arthroscopic knee surgery and have a good understanding of the underlying biomechanical mechanism of patellar femoral problems. It is recommended to read this chapter closely and to practice on cadaver knees. An important issue is that cadaver knees contain a

L. Blond (✉)
Department of Orthopaedic Surgery, Aleris-Hamlet Hospital, Copenhagen, Denmark

Department of Orthopaedic Surgery, The Zealand University Hospital, Koege, Denmark

Greve Strand, Denmark
e-mail: Lars-blond@dadlnet.dk

M. Brittberg, K. Slynarski (eds.), *Lower Extremity Joint Preservation*,
https://doi.org/10.1007/978-3-030-57382-9_23

V-shaped trochlea and a fragile cartilage, which means that the release of the cartilage flake can be close to impossible. However, in living human knees having trochlea dysplasia the release of the cartilage is more easy since the trochlea is flat. The purpose of the AT procedure is to unload the compressive forces in the PF joint and provide osseous stability by creating a lateral trochlea wall. Ideally the trochlea is approximately 4.5 mm deep and the it should be lateralized to approximate a more normal figure of 50% trochlear symmetry [19]. By lateralizing the groove the TT-TG is also reduced by several millimeters [20].

The AT technique is typically combined with MPFL reconstruction and lateral release or lateral lengthening. This chapter concentrates only on the AT technique.

23.2 Indications

The main indication for AT in combination with MPFL reconstruction is symptomatic patellar instability in patients with severe trochlear dysplasia evaluated by MRI axial scans. In rare cases, the procedure has been found indicated in patients having chronic anterior knee pain and severe trochlear dysplasia. The author's preferred parameters for evaluation of the degree of trochlear dysplasia is the lateral trochlea inclination angle and the trochlear asymmetry [21]. Clinically, patellar instability patients must have a positive reverse dynamic apprehension sign at a minimum of 30° of flexion.

23.3 Contraindications

Contraindication is severe PF osteoarthritis; however in some patients having smaller grade 4 cartilage lesions AT surgery has resulted in good outcomes. Open growth plates are a relative contraindication. If the growing potential is near its end, meaning that the patients are close to the height of the parents and if the girls have had menstruation for more than a year, the procedure can be done.

23.4 Technique

A tourniquet is not needed, and in cases of intraoperative bleeding the arthroscopic pump pressure can be gradually elevated until the bleeding is reduced. One dose of intravenous antibiotics is given pre- and postoperatively. Antithrombotic prophylactic treatment is considered in patients above the age of 40 years or in cases with a history of thrombotic complications.

23.5 Preparation and Portal Placement

Initially a standard knee arthroscopy is done through two standard anterior portals and the knee is inspected for other intraarticular pathologies. The trochlear configuration and cartilage are evaluated to confirm the MRI findings. A superior portal must be created as proximal as possible to reach an optimal view of the trochlea and it is placed just medial to the quadriceps tendon. By insertion of a hypodermic needle the correct placement is identified, and a switching stick is introduced in the same direction into the most proximal part of the suprapatellar pouch followed by introduction of the arthroscope. The author's preferable scope is 45°, but a 30 or 70° scope can be used as well. With the scope introduced in the suprapatellar portal, the position for the lateral suprapatellar portal is localized by the needle technique. Correct placement of this portal is vital. The correct location is parallel to the proximal extent of the flat part of the trochlear groove in both the frontal and transversal planes, in order to give the right working angle for the instruments. A too distal or too posterior placement can be detrimental, since it will not be possible to create the correct lateral wall angulation. A too proximal portal can make it difficult to reach the most distal part of the trochlea. A 8 mm PassPort Button Canula (ArthrexInc. Naples, FL) is useful as a working portal (Fig. 23.1).

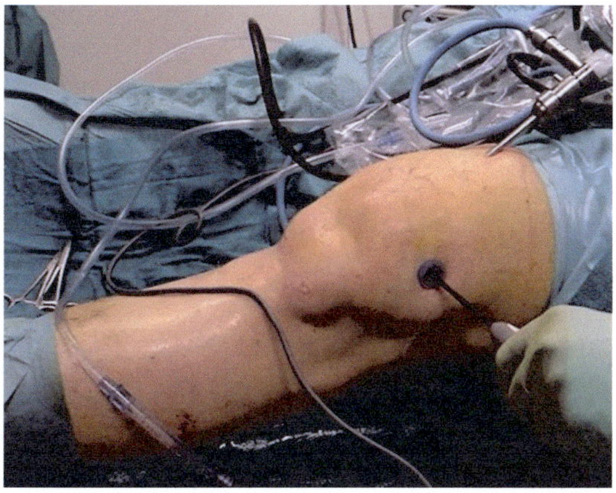

Fig. 23.1 This demostrates the superior suprapatellar portal with the arthroscope introduced and the lateral superopatellar portal with a PassPort canula mounted

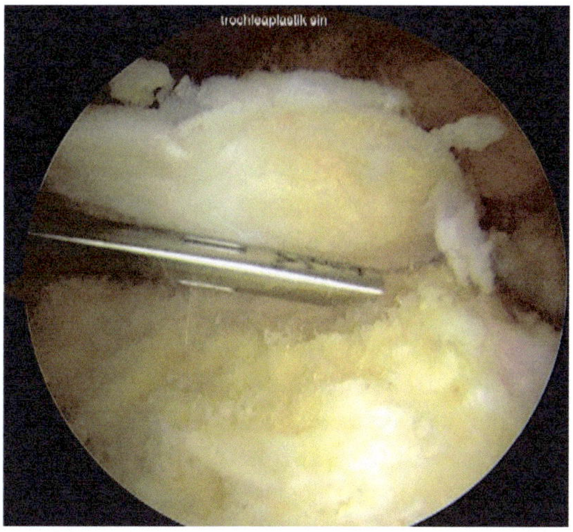

Fig. 23.2 This demonstrates the release of the cartilage flap using a shaverburr

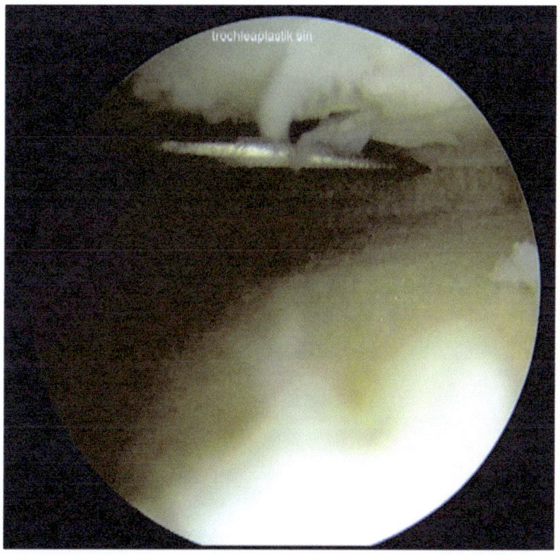

Fig. 23.3 This demonstrates the use of the osteotome to avoid taking away too much bone most lateral

23.6 Creation of the Cartilage Flap

By the use of a 90° radiofrequency device introduced through the lateral suprapatellar portal, the synovium/periosteum is released from the area proximal to the trochlear cartilage.

The release is continued proximal in order to achieve a clear area for the placement of the proximal anchors in the end of the procedure. Once the bone is cleared, a 3 and/or 4 mm round shaver burr without a shield is used to take away bone proximal and posterior to the trochlea cartilage. The release of the cartilage flap is initiated by moving the shaver burr from medial to lateral and vice versa. Slowly, the cartilage is undermined, and the progression of the shaver continues more and more distally beneath the cartilage (Fig. 23.2).

As a supplement to the shaver, both a straight and a curved lambotte osteotome (6 mm × 27 cm) can be helpful. By adding the osteotome, the bone resection at the most lateral part of the trochlea is minimized, helping to achieve a normal lateral trochlear wall and thereby achieving a more anatomic lateral trochlea inclination angle (Fig. 23.3). The cartilage flap separation from bone is continued distally until the shaver meets the curvature of the femoral condyles. Before this point is reached distally, it is recommended to change the 4 mm shaver burr to a smaller 3 mm burr, thereby minimizing the bone resection in the area close to the hinge of the cartilage flap. The release should be continued in the medial and lateral directions, otherwise the hinge of the flap will not become sufficiently elastic.

23.6.1 Formation and Shaping of a Deeper Trochlear Groove

The aim is to achieve the correct trochlear depth and sulcus orientation of the new groove. Therefore the groove needs to be deepened and centralized using shaver burrs. A PowerRasp (Arthrex Inc., Naples FL) can be useful for smoothening the bony surface of the lateral wall of the trochlea. Part of the trochlear dysplasia is the medialized groove, so the amount of lateralization of the new groove should reflect the increased TT-TG measured preoperatively. A trochlea depth of 4.5 mm is sought, taking into account the size of the involved knee. The amount of bone resection for the deepening of the trochlea and for taking away the trochlear bump can be estimated during surgery by looking at the most anterior part of the femur, since the resection proximally should allow for a smooth transition between groove and anterior cortex of the femur. The new groove is therefore trimmed with the shaver burr or PowerRasp according to the preoperative plan, and a good lateral wall is aimed (Fig. 23.4).

The cartilage flap needs to have sufficient elasticity to integrate into the new groove, to get in contact with the underlying bone, and to achieve the correct trochlea shape. The flap elasticity is tested, by pressing the flap into the new

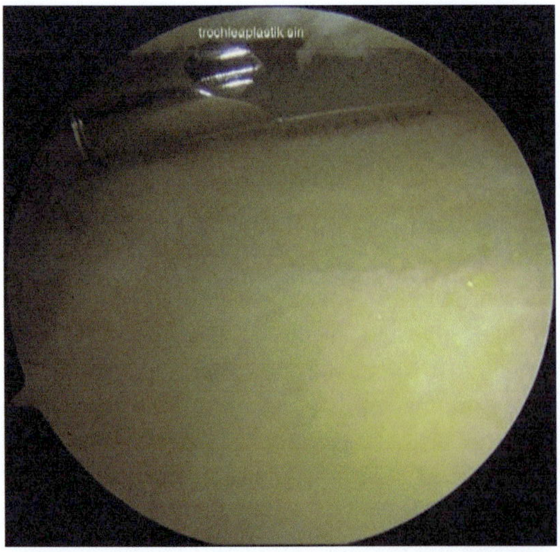

Fig. 23.4 This demonstrates how the PowerRasp can help create a smooth lateral wall of the new trochlea

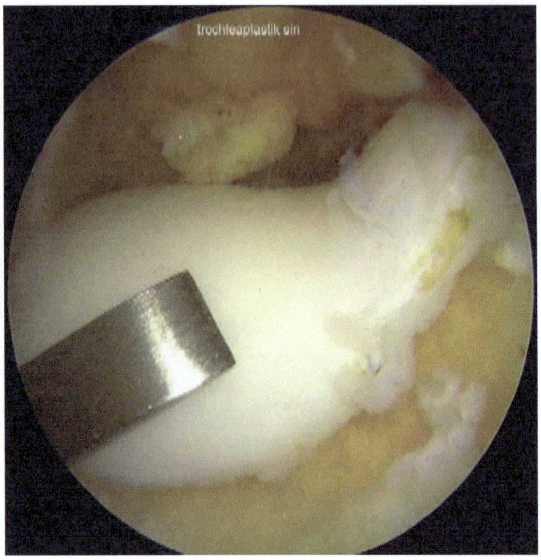

Fig. 23.5 This demonstrates how the elasticity of cartilage flap can be tested using stump instrument

deepened trochlea using a blunt instrument (Fig. 23.5).

In cases where the cartilage flap is too stiff, excessive bone on the rear side of the flap should be gently and gradually removed until the needed elasticity is reached.

23.6.2 Fixation of the Cartilage Flap

The fixation of the cartilage flap is started, with the arthroscope remaining in the superior medial portal, by placing a suture anchor distal to the cartilage hinge through the medial joint line portal. In order to achieve a 90° insertion angle of the anchor, the knee has to be flexed close to 45°. A bone socket for the anchor is initially drilled central in the most distal part of the trochlea, just proximal to the notch and still distally from the cartilage flap. A biocomposite 3.5 mm PushLock anchor (Arthrex Inc., Naples FL) with the eyelet is loaded with a resorbable tape and a suture, so that the end of the tape and sutures are equal in length. The anchor is placed into the bone socket (one tape—Vicryl 3 mm BP-1, V152G, Ethicon and one 1–0 suture Vicryl CT-2 plus, V335 H). Eventually the tapes can be replaced successfully with multiple resorbable sutures. A suture grasper

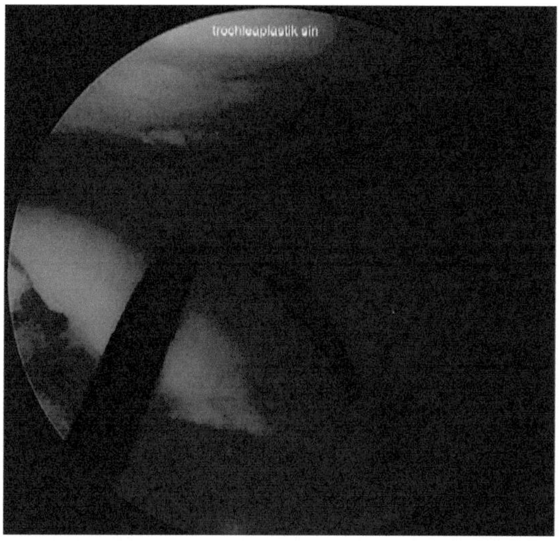

Fig. 23.6 This demonstrates how the cartilage flap in pressed into the new trochlear groove by the tape fixation

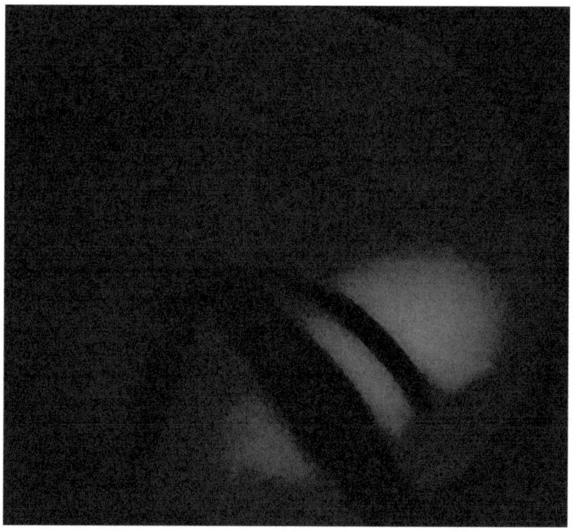

Fig. 23.7 This demonstrates a case with the use of the extra vicryl sutures in order to provide extra fixation compared to Fig. 23.6

is introduced through the superior lateral portal, grasping one of the tape endings and bringing it out through the canula, and loaded into another similar anchor.

On the lateral side, based upon the hardness of the bone, the socket can be prepared using either a taping device or a burr, placed in a spot superior to the cartilage flap and lateral to the center of the groove. The tape is gradually tensioned thereby pressing the cartilage flap into the new groove, and the anchor is inserted into its position. With the anchor positioned, the tape is locked and the excess is cut. Next, the arthroscope is introduced through the superior lateral canula.

The superior medial portal is used for the insertion of the next anchor in a similar way. This should also be placed superior to cartilage flap and medial to the center of the groove. The cartilage flap is now sufficiently stabilized into the new trochlea groove (Fig. 23.6). In about 50% of the cases, there is a gap between the cartilage flap and the new trochlea, and this requires an additional anchor now loaded with the vicryl (Fig. 23.7). Obviously, comorbidities are treated as indicated, such as medial patellofemoral ligament insufficiency with MPFL reconstruction.

When the MPFL reconstruction is done in conjunction to an AT, the following issues have to be taken into consideration. The axis of rotation around the femoral epicondylar axis, as described by Coughlin et al. [22], is affected due to the bone resection caused by the AT. The distance (radius) from the center of rotation (the foot print in the epicondyle) to the resection area in the new groove is shortened. Consequently, both the native MPFL and the MPFL graft are relatively slack in extension.

If this is not taken into account, it can have a detrimental impact on the outcome. The MPFL insertion point needs to be placed in a more distal anisometrical position and should be fixed with the knee in the specific degree of flexion (approx. 70°), where the patella is placed in the unaffected trochlea area, otherwise the graft will become too tight in flexion and consequently leads to flexion problems resulting in over tensioning of the graft and compression of the PF articular cartilage.

23.7 Postoperative Regime

Immediately after the surgery, patients are allowed to do full range of movements and full weight bearing. No brace are prescripted.

Postoperative rehabilitation is detailed in Table 23.1.

Table 23.1 Protocol for Trochleoplasty with MPFL reconstruktion

Day	Goal	Exercise	Physical therapy
0–1	Range of motion (ROM): CPM machine	Ankel pumps	
	RICE: Rest, Compression, Ice 2–3 × day: 30 min. Elevation		
2–3	ROM, focus extension	Heel slides, ankel pumps, seated heel slides	PROM, retrograde massage, Pain control
	Strength	Isometric quadriceps, VMO	Maybe NMES (neuromuscular stimulation 30–40 Hz)
	Gait	FWB (full weight bearing) with two crutches	Gait training; heel-toe AlterG Anti-Gravity: 40–50% WB, 0.5–1 km/h, 4–5 incline. 5–10 min
	RICE: Rest, Compression, Ice 2–3 × day: 30 min. Elevation		
	Electrotherapy		Vascularization 8 Hz and pain relief (Endorfin 5 Hz, or TENS)
	Laser		Level IV laser for pain and swelling
4–7	ROM: focus extension	Heel slides, ankel pumps, seated heel slides	PROM
	Strength	Isometric quad sets, Assisted straight leg raises: FLX, ABD, EXT, Terminal knee extension (TKE), Bridge	NMES (neuromuscular stimulation 30–40 Hz)
	Stretching	Hamstring supine with strap Quad: prone with strap Calf: standing on step, push heel down	
	Gait	Weight bearing exercises	Gait traingn using two crutches AlterG Anti-Gravity: 50% WB, 1–2 km/h, 2–3 incline. 10–15 min
	Stationary bike	High seat, slowly back and forth for ROM, do not force the knee around	
	Manual therapy		Retrograde massage, Scar massage with vitamin-e, Patella mobes Superior-inferior. No Medial-lateral with MPFL reconstuction for 4 weeks
	Prioprioception	Standing on one leg on even surface, if able to stand without knee extension dysfunction then close eyes	
	Electrotherapy		Vascularization 8 Hz and pain relief (Endorfin 5 Hz, or TENS)
	Laser		Level IV laser for pain and swelling

1–4 weeks	ROM: focus extension	Heel slides, ankel pumps, seated heel slides, prone FLX-EXT with strap If problems with getting full knee extension, try low load long duration stretch prone with rubber band 5–10 min daily	PROM
	Strength	Isometric quad sets, Assisted straight leg raises: FLX, ABD, EXT, Terminal knee extension (TKE), Bridge, mini squat, Heel glides on cloth supine	NMES (neuromuscular stimulation 35–40 Hz) AlterG Anti-Gravity: 50% WB, 0 km/h, 0 incline: bilateral heel lifts (progres to eccentric and unilateral), mini squat, single leg stance
	Stretching	Hamstring supine with strap Quad: prone with strap Calf: standing on step, push heel dow	Manual stretching
	Gait	Heel –Toe with 1–2 crutche	Gait training using 1–2 crutches AlterG Anti-Gravity: 50% WB, 2–3 km/h, 2 incline. 15–20 min
	Stationary bike	High seat, slowly back and forth for ROM, try to cycle around back and forth with resistance: 10–15 min	
	Manual therapy		Retrograde massage, Scar massage with vitamin-e, Patella mobes Superior-inferior. No Medial-lateral with MPFL reconstuction for 4 wks. Knee mobilisering: tibia A-P mobes, general mobes for FLX/EXT gr I–II
	Priopriоception	Standing on one leg on even surface, if able to stand without knee extension dysfunction then close eyes	
	Electrotherapy		Vascularization 8 Hz and pain relief (Endorfin 5 Hz, or TENS)
	Laser		Level IV laser for pain and swelling

(continued)

Table 23.1 (continued)

Day	Goal	Exercise	Physical therapy
4–6 weeks	ROM: Full Extension. Fleksion 90–120	Heel slides, seated heel slides, prone heel to buttocks with strap	PROM
	Strength	Isometric quad sets, straight leg raises (SLR): FLX, ABD, EXT, Terminal knee extension (TKE), Bridge, mini squat, Heel glides on cloth supine	NMES (neuromuscular stimulation 50–70 Hz) AlterG Anti-Gravity: 50–80% WB, 0 km/h, 0 incline: bilateral heel lifts (progres to eccentric and unilateral), mini squat, single leg stance
	Stretching	Hamstring supine with strap Quad: prone with strap Calf: standing on step, push heel dow	Manual stretching
	Gait	Gait training without crutche	Gait training without crutches: heel-toe AlterG Anti-Gravity: 50–80% WB, 2–4 km/h, 2–3 incline. 15–20 min
	Stationary bike	High seat, slowly back and forth for ROM, do not force the knee around	
	Manual therapy		Retrograde massage, Scar massage with vitamin-e, Patella mobes Superior-inferior. No Medial-lateral with MPFL reconstuction for 4 weeks
	Priopricoeption	Standing on one leg on even surface, if able to stand without knee extension dysfunction then close eye	Single leg stance in trampoline, ball catch
	Electrotherapy	Vascularization 8 Hz and pain relief (Endorfin 5 Hz, or TENS	
	Laser		Level IV laser for pain and swelling

6–? weeks progression as tolerated	ROM: full extension. Fleksion 135–140	Heel slides, seated heel slides, prone heel to buttocks with strap	PROM
	Strength	Isometric quad sets, SLR: FLX, ABD, EXT (should be able to hold knee in full extension, otherwise cont. Ass), SLR with rubberband, Terminal knee extension (TKE), Bridge with leg lifts, wall squat, Heel glides on cloth supine. Progression: standing slides on cloth, side step without and with rubberband, lunges, squats. Machines: Leg press, squat in smith rack, leg curls Free weights when full AROM and able to hold knee in full extension with SLR	NMES (neuromuscular stimulation 50–70 Hz) AlterG Anti-Gravity: 50–80% WB, 0 km/h, 0 incline: bilateral heel lifts (progres to eccentric and unilateral), mini squat, single leg stance
	Stretching	Hamstring supine with strap Quad: prone with strap Calf: standing on step, push heel down	Manual stretching
	Gait	Gait training without crutches	Gait training without crutches: heel-toe AlterG Anti-Gravity: 50–80% WB, 2–4 km/h, 2–3 incline. 15–20 min
	Stationary bike	Normal cykling on stationary bike, able to bike outside about 3 months after surgery if full AROM and Isometric strength normal compare to opposite leg	
	Manual therapy		Retrograde massage, Scar massage with vitamin-e, Patella mobes Superior-inferior. Medial-lateral gr I–II Knee mobilisering: tibia A-P mobes, general mobes for FLX/EXT gr I–II
	Priopriocеption	Standing on one leg on even surface, if able to stand without knee extension dysfunction then close eyes	Single leg stance in trampoline, ball catch. Mini jog on trampoline
	Electrotherapy		Vascularization 8 Hz and pain relief (Endorfin 5 Hz, or TENS)
	Laser		Level IV laser for pain and swelling

In 2016 physiotherapist Dorte Nielsen, Proalign.dk developed this rehabilitation protocol after having had several years of experience treating a significant number of patients both pre- and postoperatively with physiotherapy in patients undergoing arthroscopic trochleoplasty and MPFL reconstruction, and it remains unchanged since

23.8 Expected Outcomes

The author has conducted the AT procedure in 129 knees in 97 patients (69 women and 28 male) with a median age of 20 (range 12–51). In 116 cases, the surgery has been combined with MPFL reconstructions. For those thirteen cases without MPFL reconstruction, the isolated AT has been done for instability and previous MPFL reconstruction in two case and for severe chronic anterior knee pain in eleven cases. It is a one-day surgery. The results from the first 29 cases of AT in combination with MPFL reconstruction have been published [12], in which significant improvements in Kujala and KOOS scores were observed with 93% satisfied with the outcome and 55% returning to sports. In all cases the preoperative range of movements or more have been achieved. A later smaller case series with similar results has been published as an abstract [23].

23.9 Complications

Two complications (DVT) have occurred. Eight patients have had further surgery. Three patients who had high TT-TG distances above 20 mm developed symptomatic subluxations postoperatively and were subsequently corrected by medialization of the tibial tubercle. Those cases were all operated in the start of the series, and at that phase, due to lack of knowledge, the new trochlear grooves were not lateralized during the trochleoplasty procedure.

Three patients also from the start of the series experienced pronounced postoperative anterior knee pain in flexion. On examination, tightness of the lateral retinaculum was found, indicating lateral hyperpressure syndrome, and they all responded positively to a subsequent lateral release. This finding has resulted in a more liberal use of a subsequent lateral release. Since then there have been no further cases developing symptoms of hyperpressure. One patient who already have had five operation, developed severe anterior knee pain due to degeneration of cartilage in the lateral part of the trochlear. At further examination increased femoral anteversion was recognized. The patients had undergone external rotational distal femoral osteotomy and tibial internal osteotomy elsewhere. This procedure worsened the situation. One patient had redislocated (by report) and undergone a revision trochleoplasty elsewhere.

23.10 Discussion

The author has performed AT in 129 knees in the past eleven years, with no cases of arthrofibrosis or infections; however, complications as mentioned above have occurred. Since the original paper was published in 2010, the procedure has undergone minor changes in addition to above-mentioned technique. The superior lateral canula has been omitted, based on the fact that it was not necessary, and the PowerRasp 4.0 mm × 13 cm AR-8400PR (Arthrex Inc., Naples FL) has lately been introduced for smoothening of the new trochlear groove, but this is not mandatory. The fixation method for the cartilage flap, with the use of absorbable tapes in combination with suture anchors, has now been adopted by several open trochleoplasty surgeons. In the primary study, a median VAS pain score of 3 was observed 24 h postoperatively, and this equalized the level of pain scores from MPFL reconstructions alone. Based on these findings and later observations, we have experienced that the combined AT and MPFL procedure is unproblematic and can be carried out as a 1-day surgery.

In a follow-up study of a consecutive series of 29 knees in patients troubled by patella instability and treated by combined AT and MPFL reconstruction, significantly improved median knee scores for all measured parameters with no redislocations were found [12]. These results have later been confirmed in a second follow-up study including 18 more knees [23]. Within the first 0 - 30 degrees of flexion, the patella has not engaged the trochlea and therefore the trochlea cannot provide stability in those first degrees of flexion. To solve that lack of stability, a concomitan MPFL reconstruction are more frequently added as a supplement to a trochleoplasty as i evident in four recent series [15, 24–27].

A significant relationship between trochlea cartilage lesions and trochlea dysplasia has been documented [8, 28, 29]. Neumann et al. observed, in a 50-month follow-up of 46 patients after trochleoplasty, that in a subgroup of 26 patients with radiographic degenerative changes or intraoperative findings of chondromalacia, there were comparable subjective postoperative improvements in this group, compared to the patients without chondral changes [30]. Based on these results the author has found it reasonable to include patients with more degenerative cartilage changes in the trochlea as an indication for AT and the results until now have been positive.

23.11 Conclusion

This is a description of AT, a technique that has been slightly optimized since the original paper. The technique has been found to be a reproducible and safe technique with limited serious complications. Based upon personal communications, other centers have implemented the technique achieving similar results. Clinically, AT has been found to give significant improvements in postoperative Kujala and KOOS scores and also provide stable patellae with no reported cases of arthrofibrosis.

Acknowledgements Thanks to physiotherapist Dorte Nielsen, Proalign.dk for providing the rehabilitation protocol.

References

1. Van SJDP, Van De GSAW, Verdonschot N, Hannink G. Trochleoplasty procedures show complication rates similar to other patellar-stabilizing procedures. Knee Surg Sports Traumatol Arthrosc. 2018;26(9):2841–57. https://doi.org/10.1007/s00167-017-4766-5.
2. Longo UG, Vincenzo C, Mannering N, Ciuffreda M, Salvatore G, Berton A, et al. Trochleoplasty techniques provide good clinical results in patients with trochlear dysplasia. Knee Surg Sports Traumatol Arthrosc. 2018;26(9):2640–58. https://doi.org/10.1007/s00167-017-4584-9.
3. Van Haver A, De Roo K, De Beule M, Labey L, De Baets P, Dejour D, et al. The effect of trochlear dysplasia on patellofemoral biomechanics: a cadaveric study with simulated trochlear deformities. Am J Sports Med. 2015;43(6):1354–61. https://doi.org/10.1177/0363546515572143.
4. Amis AA, Oguz C, Bull AMJ, Senavongse W, Dejour D. The effect of trochleoplasty on patellar stability and kinematics: a biomechanical study in vitro. J Bone Joint Surg Br. 2008;90(7):864–9. https://doi.org/10.1302/0301-620X.90B7.20447.
5. Tuna BK, Semiz-Oysu A, Pekar B, Bukte Y, Hayirlioglu A. The association of patellofemoral joint morphology with chondromalacia patella: a quantitative MRI analysis. Clin Imaging. 2014;38(4):495–8.
6. Duran S, Cavusoglu M, Kocadal O, Sakman B. Association between trochlear morphology and chondromalacia patella: an MRI study. Clin Imaging. 2017;41:7–10.
7. Keser S, Savranlar A, Bayar A, Ege A, Turhan E. Is there a relationship between anterior knee pain and femoral trochlear dysplasia? Assessment of lateral trochlear inclination by magnetic resonance imaging. Knee Surg Sports Traumatol Arthrosc. 2008;16(10):911–5. https://doi.org/10.1007/s00167-008-0571-5.
8. Stefanik JJ, Roemer FW, Zumwalt AC, Zhu Y, Gross KD, Lynch JA, et al. Association between measures of trochlear morphology and structural features of patellofemoral joint osteoarthritis on MRI: the MOST study. J Orthop Res. 2012;30(1):1–8. https://doi.org/10.1002/jor.21486.
9. Kalichman L, Zhang Y, Niu J, Goggins J, Gale D, Felson DT, et al. The association between patellar alignment and patellofemoral joint osteoarthritis features-an MRI study. Rheumatology (Oxford). 2007;46(8):1303–8.
10. Askenberger M, Janarv P-M, Finnbogason T, Arendt EA. Morphology and anatomic patellar instability risk factors in first-time traumatic lateral patellar dislocations. Am J Sports Med. 2017;45(1):50–8. https://doi.org/10.1177/0363546516663498.
11. Lewallen LW, McIntosh AL, Dahm DL. Predictors of recurrent instability after acute patellofemoral dislocation in pediatric and adolescent patients. Am J Sports Med. 2013;41(3):575–81. https://doi.org/10.1177/0363546512472873.
12. Blønd L, Haugegaard M. Combined arthroscopic deepening trochleoplasty and reconstruction of the medial patellofemoral ligament for patients with recurrent patella dislocation and trochlear dysplasia. Knee Surg Sports Traumatol Arthrosc. 2014;22(10):2484–90. https://doi.org/10.1007/s00167-013-2422-2.
13. Blønd L. Arthroscopic deepening trochleoplasty: the technique. Oper Tech Sports Med. 2015;23(2):136–42.
14. Blønd L, Schöttle PB. The arthroscopic deepening trochleoplasty. Knee Surg Sports Traumatol Arthrosc. 2010;18(4):480–5. https://doi.org/10.1007/s00167-009-0935-5.

15. Blønd L. Arthroscopic deepening trochleoplasty for chronic anterior knee pain after previous failed conservative and arthroscopic treatment. Report of two cases. Int J Surg Case Rep. 2017;40:63–8.
16. Bereiter H, Gautier E. Die trochleaplastik als chirurgische therapie der reziderenden patellaluxation bei trochleadysplasie. Arthroskopie. 1994;7:281–6.
17. Song G-Y, Hong L, Zhang H, Zhang J, Li X, Li Y, et al. Trochleoplasty versus nontrochleoplasty procedures in treating patellar instability caused by severe trochlear dysplasia. Arthroscopy. 2014;30(4):523–32. https://doi.org/10.1016/j.arthro.2014.01.011.
18. Balcarek P, Rehn S, Howells NR, Eldridge JD, Kita K, Dejour D, et al. Results of medial patellofemoral ligament reconstruction compared with trochleoplasty plus individual extensor apparatus balancing in patellar instability caused by severe trochlear dysplasia: a systematic review and meta-analysis. Knee Surg Sports Traumatol Arthrosc. 2017;25(12):3869–77. https://doi.org/10.1007/s00167-016-4365-x.
19. Ridley TJ, Hincke BB, Kruckeberg BM, Agel J, Arendt EA. Anatomical patella instability risk factors on MRI show sensitivity without specificity in patients with patellofemoral instability: a systematic review. J ISAKOS. 2016;1(3):141–52.
20. Fucentese SF, Schottle PB, Pfirrmann CW, Romero J. CT changes after trochleoplasty for symptomatic trochlear dysplasia. Knee Surg Sports Traumatol Arthrosc. 2007;15(2):168–74.
21. Paiva M, Blønd L, Hölmich P, Steensen RN, Diederichs G, Feller JA, et al. Quality assessment of radiological measurements of trochlear dysplasia; a literature review. Knee Surg Sport Traumatol Arthrosc. 2017;26(3):1–10.
22. Coughlin KM, Incavo SJ, Churchill DL, Beynnon BD. Tibial axis and patellar position relative to the femoral epicondylar axis during squatting. J Arthroplasty. 2003;18(8):1048–55.
23. Blønd L. Arthroscopic trochleoplasty belongs to the future. In: The 1st annual world congress of orthopaedics, Xian, China; 2014. p. 131.
24. Von Engelhardt L, Weskamp P, Lahner M, Spahn G, Jerosch J. Deepening trochleoplasty combined with balanced medial patellofemoral ligament reconstruction for an adequate graft tensioning. World J Orthop. 2017;8(2):935–45.
25. Nelitz M, Dreyhaupt J, Lippacher S. Combined trochleoplasty and medial patellofemoral ligament reconstruction for recurrent patellar dislocations in severe trochlear dysplasia: a minimum 2-year follow-up study. Am J Sports Med. 2013;41(5):1005–12. https://doi.org/10.1177/0363546513478579.
26. Ntagiopoulos PG, Byn P, Dejour D. Midterm results of comprehensive surgical reconstruction including sulcus-deepening trochleoplasty in recurrent patellar dislocations with high-grade trochlear dysplasia. Am J Sports Med. 2013;41(5):998–1004. https://doi.org/10.1177/0363546513482302.
27. Banke IJ, Kohn LM, Meidinger G, Otto A, Hensler D, Beitzel K, et al. Combined trochleoplasty and MPFL reconstruction for treatment of chronic patellofemoral instability: a prospective minimum 2-year follow-up study. Knee Surg Sports Traumatol Arthrosc. 2014;22(11):2591–8.
28. Mehl J, Feucht MJ, Bode G, Dovi-Akue D, Südkamp NP, Niemeyer P. Association between patellar cartilage defects and patellofemoral geometry: a matched-pair MRI comparison of patients with and without isolated patellar cartilage defects. Knee Surg Sports Traumatol Arthrosc. 2016;24(3):838–46. https://doi.org/10.1007/s00167-014-3385-7.
29. Teichtahl AJ, Hanna F, Wluka AE, Urquhart DM, Wang Y, English DR, et al. A flatter proximal trochlear groove is associated with patella cartilage loss. Med Sci Sports Exerc. 2012;44(3):496–500. https://doi.org/10.1249/MSS.0b013e31822fb9a6.
30. Neumann MV, Stalder M, Schuster a J. Reconstructive surgery for patellofemoral joint incongruency. Knee Surg Sports Traumatol Arthrosc. 2016;24(3):873–8.

Open Trochleoplasty

24

Philip B. Schoettle, Armin Keshmiri,
and Florian Schimanski

24.1 Introduction and Basic Science

24.1.1 Trochlear Dysplasia and Trochleoplasty

One of the most common causes of patellofemoral dysfunction is (habitual) patellar dislocation or subluxation. The importance of trochlear dysplasia and its treatment are discussed below.

24.1.2 Factors of Patellofemoral Stability

Throughout the complete cycle of the leg's motion, various factors complexly interact to grant the patellofemoral joint stability [1].

These are the three main factors:

1. Static factors (bone-morphology): The trochlea, patella, and their congruence [2–5]. In the assessment of congruence, the morphology of the trochlea is of crucial importance [6]. It forms the guide channel, into which the patella engages and glides [7]. Another static / bony factor is the orientation between the femur and tibia. Both, a rotational malalignment as well as a valgus deformity increase the Q-angle and lead to an increased force vector of the quadriceps muscles laterally and thus to an increased dislocation tendency of the patella.
2. Passive factors (passive stabilizers): The medial patellofemoral ligament (MPFL) [8–11], and also the entire patellofemoral ligamentous apparatus and the retinacula. The MPFL is a passive medial stabilizer that counteracts the lateral force vector and prevents dislocation of the patella. Especially when close to full extension, before the patella plunges into the trochlear groove and experiences bony guidance, the MPFL is of particular importance [10, 12–15].
3. Active factors (active stabilizers): Here, the femoral quadriceps muscle, especially the oblique part, should be emphasized. Between 60° and 90° flexion, the quadriceps muscle's direction vector is pointed posterior, pulling the patella into the trochlear groove and counteracting patellofemoral instability [16–18].

Of all the factors mentioned, the bony shape of the trochlea has the greatest influence on the patellofemoral stability. Trochlear dysplasia results in a "function follows form" situation that leads to instability and, in most cases, dislocation.

P. B. Schoettle (✉) · A. Keshmiri · F. Schimanski
Knee and Health Institute, Munich, Germany
e-mail: info@prof-schoettle.de

M. Brittberg, K. Slynarski (eds.), *Lower Extremity Joint Preservation*,
https://doi.org/10.1007/978-3-030-57382-9_24

24.1.3 "Pathologic" Anatomy of Trochlear Dysplasia

The differentiation between a dysplastic trochlea and an isolated dysplasia or flattening of the lateral femoral condyle is important. A dysplastic trochlea is defined as a hypoplastic medial femoral condyle associated with a relatively hyperplastic lateral trochlea facet. The resulting silhouette is similar to a breaking wave. The trochlea is therefore shifted medially and flat or even convex. Radiologically, the medial displacement of the trochlea can be determined by an increased tibia–tubercle/trochlea–grove distance [19–21], an increased patellar shift and a patella alta. The consequence is an increased Q-angle and increased susceptibility to dislocation events. This pathoanatomical exploration is of crucial importance, since almost all nontraumatic patellofemoral instabilities are caused by trochlear dysplasia.

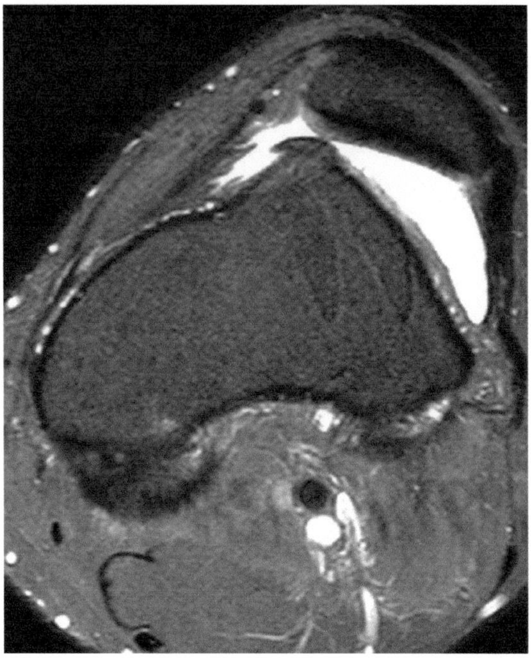

Fig. 24.1 Trochlear bump in trochlear dysplasia

24.1.4 Pathomechanism of Patella Dislocation in Trochlear Dysplasia

About 85% of all habitual patellar dislocations are due to trochlear dysplasia [22]. Most patellar dislocations occur in between 0° and 40° active extension. In those angles, the missing trochlear groove is equivalent to a missing lateral barrier; the lateral facet of the trochlea, which counteracts the laterally directed force vector of the quadriceps femoral muscle, is too shallow, thus subluxation or dislocation of the patella is the consequence. The more distal this dysplasia reaches, the greater is the resulting instability in the patellofemoral joint. The posteriorly directed force vector, increasing with higher degrees of flexion, loses its stabilizing effect and only leads to an increase in patellofemoral pressure and the corresponding clinical symptoms. If a severe trochlear dysplasia exists with an additional "bump" (Fig. 24.1), it is particularly difficult for the patella to glide into the trochlea. Additional to the missing groove, the patella has to overcome another obstacle. Since trochlear dysplasia is a congenital pathology, the patella is lateralized from childhood on, which results in an persistent increased risk of dislocation [2, 22].

The cause of patellofemoral instability is multifactorial, but with strong genetic association.

Trochlear dysplasia is an inherited anatomical deformity which explains the familiar accumulation of habitual patellar dislocations [23]. It is subdivided-according to D. Dejour-into four types, found as a "mix type" in almost all patients [24] with an increasing risk of patellar dislocation [25].

A radiological examination has shown that the patellar form is not affected by an existing trochlear dysplasia [26]. This explains the patellar tilt due to the lack of congruence between the trochlea and patella. The convex patella lies on the convexity of the trochlea like an egg balancing on another egg (Fig. 24.2). The increased punctate peak pressure leads to instability and additionally premature cartilage damage.

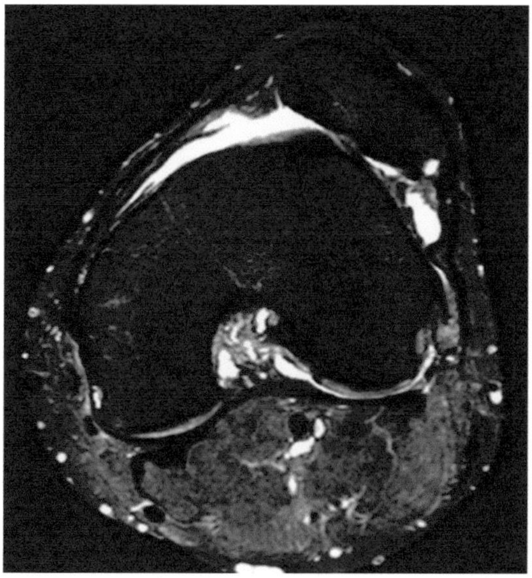

Fig. 24.2 Anatomy of trochlear dysplasia and a normal shaped trochlea. The two convex surfaces of the patella and the dysplastic trochlea do not fit together. Thus, the patella is dancing on the trochlea like trying to balance an egg on another

24.1.5 Surgical Indication for a Trochleoplasty

Not every trochlear dysplasia needs to be treated through surgery. However, this should be considered as a primary intervention if necessary. The indication is based on the clinical assessment and MRI results [26–28]. A positive apprehension test and a positive J-sign of more than 30° are clinically indicative of the existing patellofemoral instability. If a trochlear "bump" is confirmed by magnetic resonance imaging and a convex trochlea morphology, a trochleoplasty is indicated. Arthrotic changes and advanced patellofemoral cartilage damage are contraindications.

24.1.6 Target of Trochleoplasty

The aim of trochlea surgery is to lateralize and deepen the trochlear groove to minimize the Q-angle and to create a lateral trochlear facet as a static barrier to balance out the laterally directed force vector. The sole increase of the lateral trochlea facet would merely increase the patellofemoral contact pressure [2, 27]. This cannot reduce the laterally directed vector.

24.1.7 Surgical Technique

24.1.7.1 The Surgical Procedure

The knee is bent to 45° and the lateral retinaculum is prepared via a lateral parapatellar approach. By sharply separating the two layers of the lateral retinaculum longitudinally (Fig. 24.3a) a lateral retinacular elongation [27] is performed. Following this, the lateral joint capsule is opened and the patella is retracted medially in order to clearly present the complete trochlea. The proximodistal expression of the trochlear dysplasia determines how distally the cartilage must be lifted to model the subchondral bone. With a scalpel, the periosteum is cut at the lateral periostal chondral boarder, separated from the synovium, and lifted by elevator. The proximal cartilage is lifted with a straight chisel, the distal part with a curved one (Fig. 24.3b, c). After this, 1–3 mm of the subchondral bone remains on the cartilage. The cartilage is carefully chiseled off the lateral femoral condyle from proximal to distal direction until 5 mm of a cartilage flap is mobile. This can be done either with a chisel or with a milling cutter (Fig. 24.3d). After that the bone sticking to the cartilage is thinned so far that the cartilage can be modulated. This leaves enough subchondral bone to secure healing, while leaving the lifted cartilage lamella flexible.

Now, the new trochlear groove is formed: using a curved chisel, the proximal portion is slightly lateralized (Fig. 24.3e). If present, the trochlear bump is ablated and the trochlear groove is placed below the level of the distal femoral diaphysis. The formation of the bony trochlear groove is now finished with the aid of the rongeur, a sharp spoon and/or a milling cutter (Fig. 24.3f).

The osteochondral lamella is then incorporated into the newly formed bone bed using a blunt or a

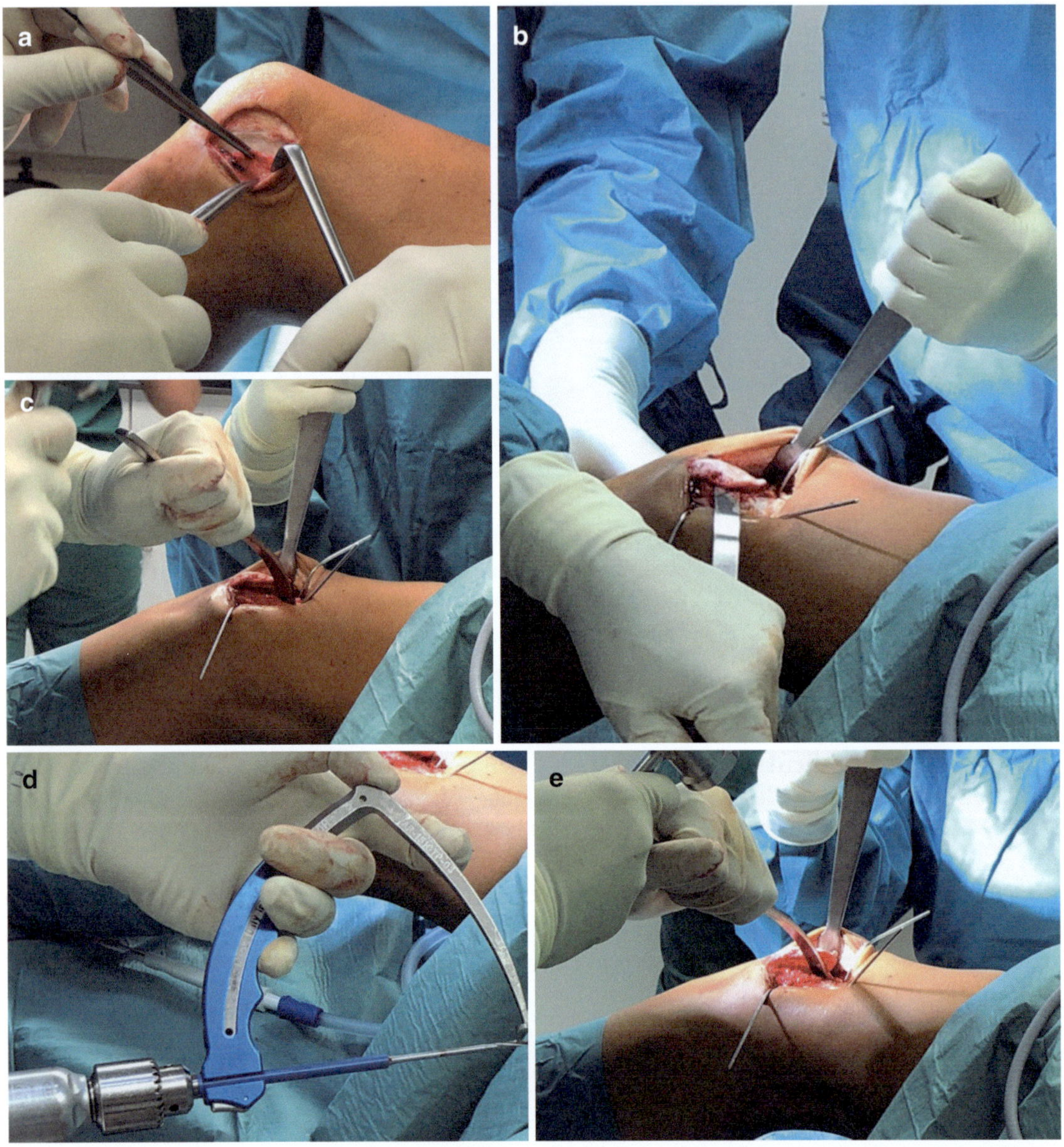

Fig. 24.3 **a–g** Trochlear plastic surgery steps. (**a**) A lateral retinacular elongation is performed by sharply separating the two layers of the lateral retinaculum longitudinally. (**b**) The proximal cartilage is lifted with the help of a straight chisel. (**c**) The proxolateral cartilage is lifted with a curved chisel. (**d**) The cartilage lamella is loosened towards distally over the entire medio-lateral extent using a specially designed tiller beginning with the 5 mm and finalising with a 5 mm distance switch. (**e**) Forming the new trochlear groove. With a straight chisel, the proximal portion is slightly lateralized. (**f**) Forming the bony trochlear groove with the aid of a high-speed milling machine. (**g**) Two 3 mm Vicryl tapes (Ethicon Products, Norderstedt, Germany) are threaded into a 3.5 mm Pushlock anchor (Arthrex GmbH, Freiham, Germany) and centrally fixed at the distal end of the new trochlear groove. (**h**) Also using Pushlock anchors, the three free ends are fixed in a "star shape" technique proximally, centrally, medially and laterally off bone-cartilage border in order to press the cartilage lamella onto the bone and promote healing. (**i**) The initially prepared lateral expansion plastic is now closed in appropriate tension

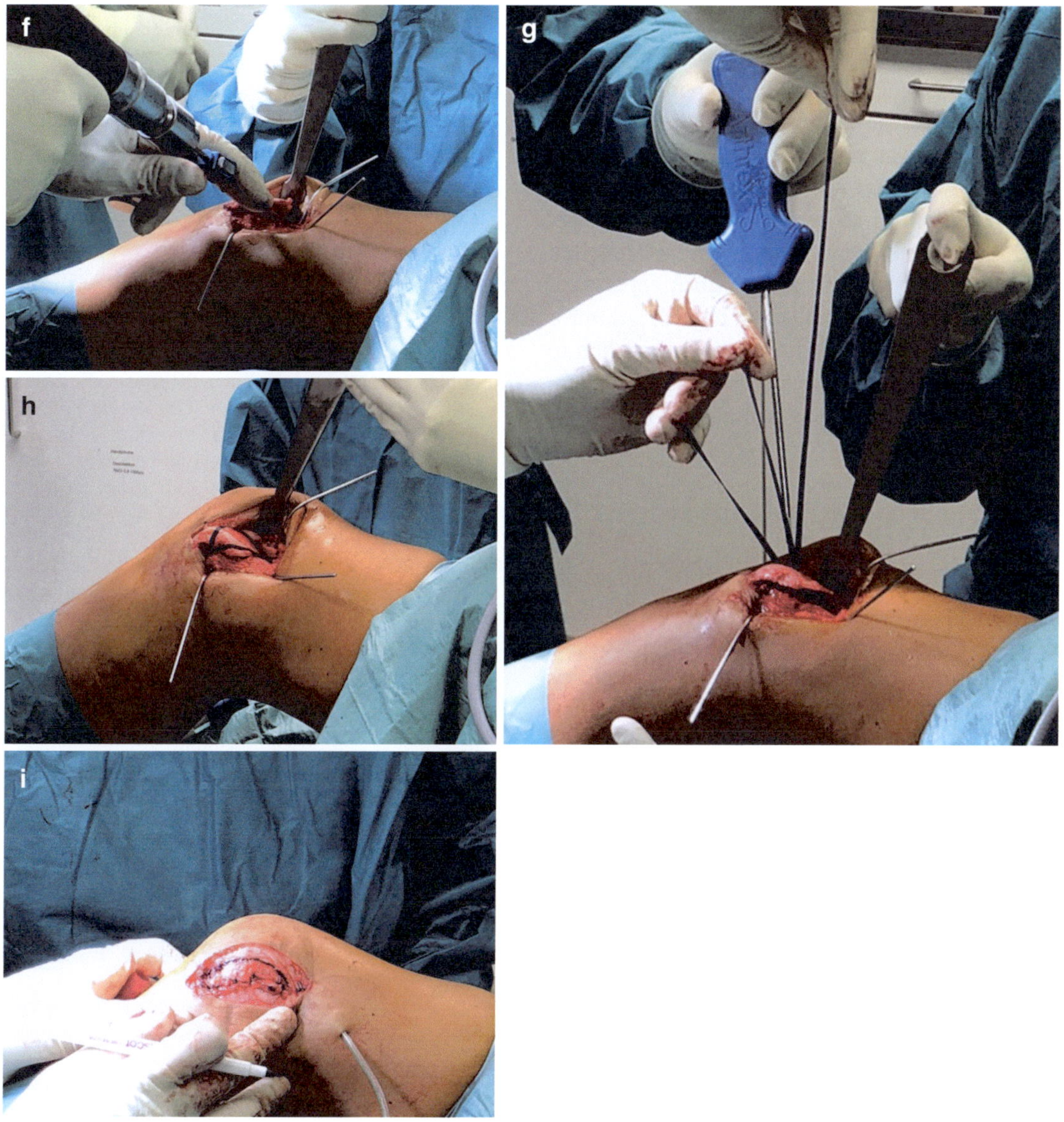

Fig. 24.3 (continued)

rounded impactor. Once the cartilage is well molded onto the boney groove, the fixation is carried out. To do so, two 3 mm Vicryl tapes (Ethicon Products, Norderstedt, Germany) are threaded into a 3.5 mm pushlock anchor (Arthrex GmbH, Freiham, Germany) and centrally fixed at the distal end of the new trochlear groove (Fig. 24.3g). The three free ends are then fixed with pushlock anchors in a "star shape" technique proximally, centrally, medially, and laterally off bone–cartilage border in order to press the cartilage lamella onto the bone and promote healing (Fig. 24.3h). After fixation, the edges of the cartilage lamella are sealed with fibrin glue to avoid postoperative bleeding from the bone. Before the lateral retinaculum is closed in 70° flexion, an intraarticular redon-drainage is inserted. If lateral enlargement is necessary, the initially prepared lateral expansion plastic can be closed accordingly in 70° of knee flexion (Fig. 24.3i).

24.1.7.2 The Role of the MPFL

As already mentioned, the MPFL has an important function for patellofemoral stability. Especially in close-to-the-point flexion, since the patella is not yet immersed into the stabilizing trochlear groove [29]. It is also shown that in more than 90% of all patellar dislocation events, the MPFL is either ruptured or at least deficient [12, 30]. So when performing a trochleoplasty, it is advisable to closely examine the indication for an additionally required MPFL reconstruction to ensure patellofemoral stability during the entire range of motion of the knee joint [31, 32].

24.2 Postoperative Management

For the rest of his or her hospitalization, the patient should be exercised ideally in a CPM machine four times 20 min a day, without limitation of the degree of freedom on a CPM splint. Inpatient discharge should not be performed before reaching a minimum of 60° flexion to prevent the occurrence of postoperative scarring. During the first 2 weeks after operation, it is important to pay attention to only weight the leg with 20 kg or less. Afterwards the pain-adapted increase up to the full load can take place. Only after a total of 6 weeks the gradual return to everyday activities is advisable. Sportive activities should not be started before 3 months after surgery.

References

1. Meidinger G, Schöttle P. Pathogenese und Diagnostik der patellofemoralen Arthrose. Arthroskopie. 2010;23(3):201–7.
2. Dejour H, Walch G, Neyret P, Adeleine P. Dysplasia of the femoral trochlea. Rev Chir Orthop Reparatrice Appar Mot. 1989;76(1):45–54.
3. Malghem J, Maldague B. Depth insufficiency of the proximal trochlear groove on lateral radiographs of the knee: relation to patellar dislocation. Radiology. 1989;170(2):507–10.
4. Merchant AC, Mercer RL, Jacobson RH, Cool CR. Roentgenographic analysis of patellofemoral congruence. J Bone Joint Surg. 1974;56(7):1391–6.
5. Senavongse W, Amis A. The effects of articular, retinacular, or muscular deficiencies on patellofemoral joint stability. A biomechanical study in vitro. J Bone Joint Surg Br. 2005;87(4):577–82.
6. Shih Y-F, Bull AM, Amis AA. The cartilaginous and osseous geometry of the femoral trochlear groove. Knee Surg Sports Traumatol Arthrosc. 2004;12(4):300–6.
7. Heegaard J, Leyvraz P, Curnier A, Rakotomanana L, Huiskes R. The biomechanics of the human patella during passive knee flexion. J Biomech. 1995;28(11):1265–79.
8. Fithian DC, Meier SW. The case for advancement and repairof the medial patellofemoral ligament in patients with recurrent patellar instability. Oper Tech Sports Med. 1999;7(2):81–9.
9. Fithian DC, Mishra DK, Balen PF, Stone ML, Daniel DM. Instrumented measurement of patellar mobility. Am J Sports Med. 1995;23(5):607–15.
10. Hautamaa PV, Fithian DC, Kaufman KR, Daniel DM, Pohlmeyer AM. Medial soft tissue restraints in lateral patellar instability and repair. Clin Orthop. 1998;349:174–82.
11. Teitge RA, Faerber W, Des Madryl P, Matelic TM. Stress radiographs of the patellofemoral joint. J Bone Joint Surg Am. 1996;78(2):193–203.
12. Burks RT, Desio SM, Bachus KN, Tyson L, Springer K. Biomechanical evaluation of lateral patellar dislocations. Am J Knee Surg. 1997;11(1):24–31.
13. Conlan T, Garth WP, Lemons JE. Evaluation of the medial soft-tissue restraints of the extensor mechanism of the knee. J Bone Joint Surg Am. 1993;75(5):682–93.
14. Desio SM, Burks RT, Bachus KN. Soft tissue restraints to lateral patellar translation in the human knee. Am J Sports Med. 1998;26(1):59–65.
15. Sandmeier RH, Burks RT, Bachus KN, Billings A. The effect of reconstruction of the medial patellofemoral ligament on patellar tracking. Am J Sports Med. 2000;28(3):345–9.
16. Ahmed A, Duncan N. Correlation of patellar tracking pattern with trochlear and retropatellar surface topographies. J Biomech Eng. 2000;122(6):652–60.
17. Farahmand F, Tahmasbi M, Amis A. Lateral force–displacement behaviour of the human patella and its variation with knee flexion—a biomechanical study in vitro. J Biomech. 1998;31(12):1147–52.
18. Heegaard J, Leyvraz P-F, Van Kampen A, Rakotomanana L, Rubin PJ, Blankevoort L. Influence of soft structures on patellar three-dimensional tracking. Clin Orthop Relat Res. 1994;299:235–43.
19. Goutallier D, Bernageau J, Lecudonnec B. The measurement of the tibial tuberosity. Patella groove distanced technique and results. Rev Chir Orthop Reparatrice Appar Mot. 1977;64(5):423–8.
20. Beaconsfield T, Pintore E, Maffulli N, Petri GJ. Radiological measurements in patellofemoral disorders: a review. Clin Orthop Relat Res. 1994;308:18–28.

21. Schoettle PB, Zanetti M, Seifert B, Pfirrmann CW, Fucentese SF, Romero J. The tibial tuberosity–trochlear groove distance; a comparative study between CT and MRI scanning. Knee. 2006;13(1):26–31.
22. Dejour H, Walch G, Nove-Josserand L, Guier C. Factors of patellar instability: an anatomic radiographic study. Knee Surg Sports Traumatol Arthrosc. 1994;2(1):19–26.
23. Tardieu C, Dupont J. The origin of femoral trochlear dysplasia: comparative anatomy, evolution, and growth of the patellofemoral joint. Rev Chir Orthop Reparatrice Appar Mot. 2001;87(4):373–83.
24. Tscholl PM, Wanivenhaus F, Fucentese SF. Conventional radiographs and magnetic resonance imaging for the analysis of trochlear dysplasia: the influence of selected levels on magnetic resonance imaging. Am J Sports Med. 2017;45(5):1059–65. https://doi.org/10.1177/0363546516685054. Epub 2017 Feb 8. PMID: 28177645
25. Dejour D, Reynaud P, Lecoultre B. Douleurs et instabilité rotulienne. Essai de classification. Méd Hyg. 1998;56(2217):1466–71.
26. Fucentese SF, von Roll A, Koch PP, Epari DR, Fuchs B, Schottle PB. The patella morphology in trochlear dysplasia—a comparative MRI study. Knee. 2006;13(2):145–50.
27. Trochleoplasty MY. Restoration of the intercondylar groove in subluxations and dislocations of the patella. Rev Chir Orthop Reparatrice Appar Mot. 1977;64(1):3–17.
28. Salzmann GM, Weber TS, Spang JT, Imhoff AB, Schöttle PB. Comparison of native axial radiographs with axial MR imaging for determination of the trochlear morphology in patients with trochlear dysplasia. Arch Orthop Trauma Surg. 2010;130(3):335–40.
29. Senavongse W, Farahmand F, Jones J, Andersen H. Quantitative measurement of patellofemoral joint stability: force-displacement behavior of the human patella in vitro. J Orthop Res. 2003;21(5):780.
30. Kang HJ, Wang F, Chen BC, Zhang YZ, Ma L. Nonsurgical treatment for acute patellar dislocation with special emphasis on the MPFL injury patterns. Knee Surg Sports Traumatol Arthrosc. 2013;21(2):325–31.
31. Banke IJ, Kohn LM, Meidinger G, Otto A, Hensler D, Beitzel K, et al. Combined trochleoplasty and MPFL reconstruction for treatment of chronic patellofemoral instability: a prospective minimum 2-year follow-up study. Knee Surg Sports Traumatol Arthrosc. 2014;22(11):2591–8.
32. Schoettle P, Werner C, Romero J. Reconstruction of the medial patellofemoral ligament for painful patellar subluxation in distal torsional malalignment: a case report. Arch Orthop Trauma Surg. 2005;125(9):644–8.

Patellofemoral Osteotomies

25

Jacek Walawski and Florian Dirisamer

25.1 Introduction

Form follows function. Does the function follow the form? Essentially the concept of osteotomy means change of the shape, the load and the relation in the joint. We do change the environment and the forces' directions as well as the congruency of joint surfaces. Once we think about the patellofemoral joint we must admit that nothing is certain and definite considering the normal shape and position in the patellofemoral joint (PFJ). Neither anatomical nor biomechanical factors are described by a single value as "normal" value. There is nothing like the universal, correct patella and trochlea shape and position. Malposition and dysplasia are common but on the other hand, a vast number of individuals present abnormal alignment or shape but without having any symptoms. Others report severe complaints having virtually no anatomical abnormalities.

J. Walawski (✉)
Department of Biomechanics and Computer Science, Faculty of Physical Education and Sport, Józef Piłsudski University of Physical Education, Biała Podlaska, Poland

Poland Orthopedic Department, ŻagielMed Hospital, Lublin, Poland

F. Dirisamer
Orthopädie & Sportchirurgie Dr. Dirisamer | Dr. Patsch, Linz, Austria

Klinik Diakonissen Linz, Linz, Austria
e-mail: florian.dirisamer@orthopaedie-linz.com

The shape of the patella reflects the shape of the trochlea; long axis alignment directs forces and creates vectors. The extensor mechanism drives the patella, anatomical and functional rotation of tibia and femur alters the patella and trochlea relation during arc of motion. The extension and flexion moves patella in and out of the groove. All those ingredients collaborate to transmit the load through 140° of ROM. However, even if we have a definite bony shaped PF joint, it is influenced by numerous functional factors. Actually we rather should talk about relation or relative position of the moving elements. Teitge [1] stated that in the PFJ "geometry of the skeleton is ultimately the determinant of the direction of the load on the PFJ". If we admit that point of view, there must be a limit for soft tissue repair. Osteotomies in PFJ improve or just change the bony alignment.

The PFJ is a very specific joint, since it carries a load that exceeds 3–7 × body weight. Additionally this is a relatively flat joint that holds the inherited risk of instability. A combination of abnormal load transfer and low-profile congruency may lead to instability or/and cartilage wear.

There are three important issues that should be mentioned about PF joint preservation and osteotomies.

- The PFI was initially treated with only bony procedures. About 20 years ago "soft tissue" started to play the dominant role and osteotomy left the first row of the stage. Now the pendulum swings

M. Brittberg, K. Slynarski (eds.), *Lower Extremity Joint Preservation*,
https://doi.org/10.1007/978-3-030-57382-9_25

back. The bone becomes more important and joint reshaping is desired. That turn holds a potential "band wagon" effect, meaning that we actually might miss the whole joint as the target.

- Many orthopaedic surgeons dealing with patellar problems are arthroscopy-educated and experienced. That fact inevitably delivers an attitude that one should use minimal invasive techniques, which the arthroscopy in fact is but osteotomy is not. Psychological, social, legal and medical evidence drives to the conclusion that we are to make interventions not bigger and not more than necessary and not less than needed. Furthermore, more extensive procedures hold greater chance for complications (greater procedure – greater complications). That known fact expressed by Arendt is the base of current PF surgery and should be remembered [2]. Thus the bony procedures, especially extensive ones, are of some potential fear. However, there is a limit where soft tissue steps back facing the bone [3].

The interest in joint preservation surgery rapidly grows as we face younger patients with severely degenerative knees. Facing this situation means that we should try everything to buy these patients time to delay arthroplasty. The metal elements we "glue" to the bone covered by impaired cartilage are reluctant to stick long enough to satisfy the patient and please the surgeon. Because of such factors, we should fight longer for preserving bone stock and cartilage cover than to dispose it.

25.2 Indications

Osteotomies have been indicated to play a role in PF instability, pain and osteoarthritis. Episodic patellar dislocation (EPD) is the most common clinical presentation of patellar instability. Patients with EPD are the main target when the tibial tubercle osteotomy (TTO) is addressed.

We divide those patients (EPD) into two groups.

The majority of them are mild to moderate dysplastic from the anatomical point of view and might be successfully addressed with TTO and soft tissue arrangements.

The second group is far lower in number along with even far more difficult PFJ geometry and muscle imbalance. These patients are much more demanding and difficult to diagnose and treat, and derotational and angular bony changes are often required. One should keep in mind that we must use and equibalance the spectrum of possible treatment options from minimal interventions to extended corrections. Indications for osteotomies in PFJ disorders are presented (Table 25.1).

25.2.1 Diagnostic Parameters

It is true that we do not know how the ideal PFJ should look like. It is due to the fact that some, as we call them, healthy individuals do have dysplastic PFJ. However, we know how to approximate to ideal geometry and the relation of the PFJ parts. Parameters describe PFJ in range. Ideal geometry would be one with every single parameter just "in the middle" value. So, we have to correct to mean values—it is enough to be in the desired range. That is what we call approximate to the ideal geometry. Approximate means—one does not have to

Table 25.1 Indications for osteotomies in patellofemoral joint

Indication	Treatment
TTTG >20 mm and TTPCL >24 mm	TT medialization
Patella alta (CD ratio > 1.2 (1.4[a]))	TT distalization
Patella baja	TT proximalization
Tibial external rotation >45°	Tibial derotation osteotomy
Femoral internal rotation >25°	Femoral derotation osteotomy
Femoral valgus >5°	Femoral varization osteotomy

TTTG tibial tuberosity–trochlear groove distance, *TTPCL* tibial tuberosity—posterior cruciate ligament distance
[a]Bartsch et al. [4]

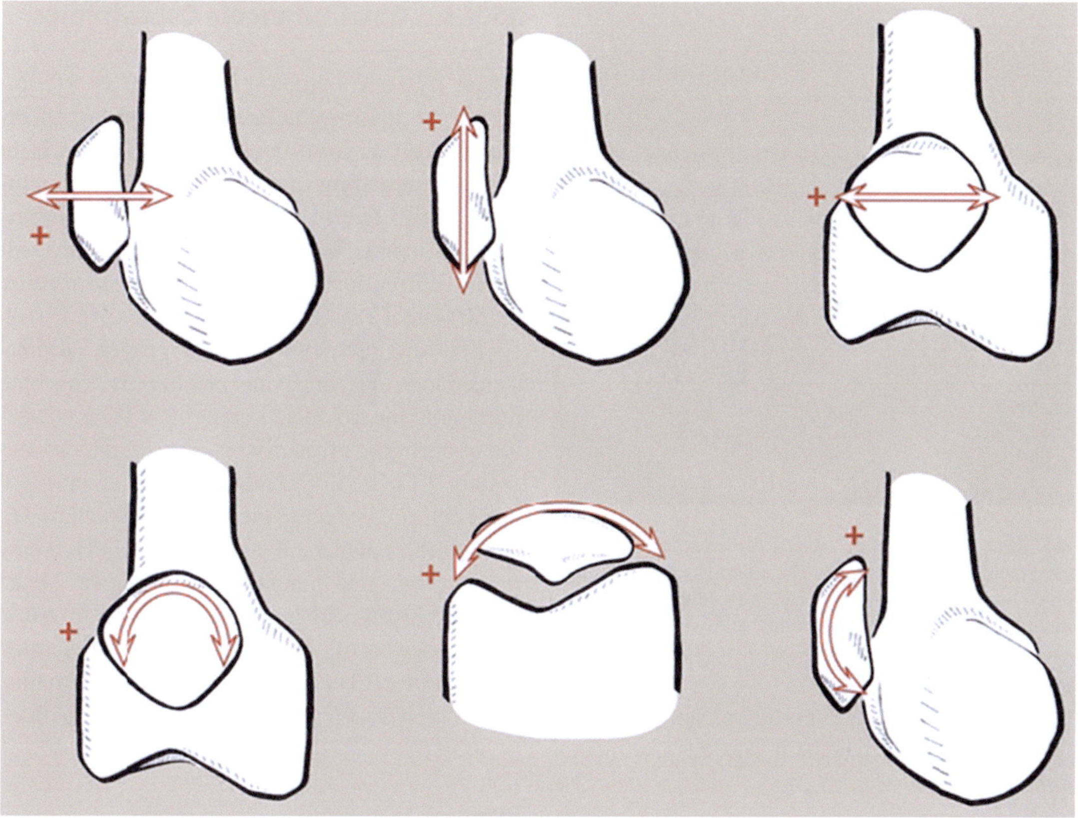

Fig. 25.1 Three-dimensional relation of PFJ

be ideal—just be in the range. Do not force too far—just approximate.

We can speak about a three-dimensional bony model (Fig. 25.1). It is described by limited and counted number of parameters at least for the everyday surgical practice. Most common parameters in the authors' opinion in use are as follows:

- Patellar height (distal-proximal) Caton-Deschamp [5], Bernageau [6].
- Patellar tracking (TTTG, TTPCL) Goutallier, Bernageau [6], Seitlinger [7].
- Patellar shape in relation to the trochlea [Dejour classification] [8].
- Tibia and femur rotational indexes.
- Lateral patellofemoral length (LPL) Nicolaas [9].
- Frontal alignment of the lower limb (mLDFA and mMPTA).

The patellofemoral system must be corrected according to those parameters within the known, desired range. We have to measure and count them before surgery. This allows for efficient planning and choice of the selected bony procedure accordingly. Since the indexes describe bony abnormalities, it is clear that none of the above can be changed with acceptable and durable soft tissue technique. At a certain threshold, the soft tissue correction will fail as opposed to the bone border [10]. If the PFJ relations leave the accepted "normal range parameters area we must discuss and presumably implement osteotomy.

Tibial tubercle osteotomy (TTO) alone does not correct the co-working trochlear shape. A majority of the techniques generally correct just one factor leaving co-working partners unchanged. Actually it might from some point change joint congruency and lead to overload and

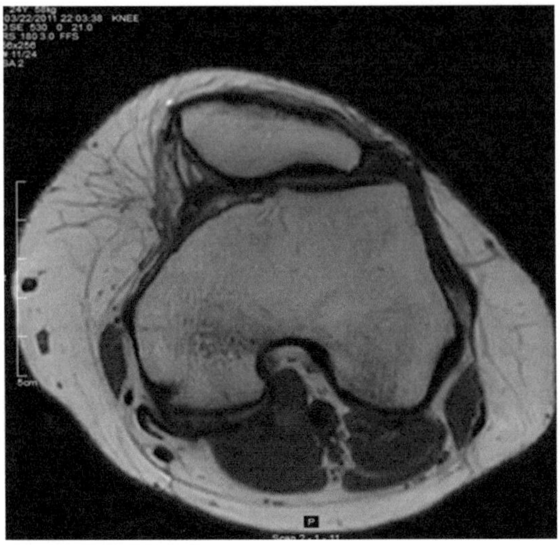

Fig. 25.2 Incongruence caused by over-medialization and extensive lateral release. The effect is somehow magnified by the MRI coil. In clinical presentation patient has true medial luxation of the patella)

OA. Subsequently, we should be cautious not to overcorrect. Overcorrection can be detrimental and irreversible (Fig. 25.2).

25.3 Techniques

PF osteotomies are directed to correct bony malalignment in the selected areas. While those start from hip and end on tibia a variety is offered. Lyon Group (H. Dejour) suggested the very French title "menu a la carte" to cover all the demands by the tailored surgeries. That approach requires that the long axis alignment, PF relations, shape of trochlea and patella must all be addressed according to the measurements (parameters).

All calculations must be done before surgery. Once we correct numeric values the surgery must be emphasized in numeric values. Simply speaking, if one individual is presented with abnormal Caton-Deschamps (CD) index of 1.5 (e.g. ratio of the patellar tendon length of 35 mm and joint surface of the patella length 23 mm) and normal TTTG distance (10 mm) *n* only TT distalization is indicated. Calculation is simple. The patella must be lowered at least 7 mm to reach the CD index 1.2 (28 mm: 23 mm = 1.2).

25.3.1 Tibial Tubercule Osteotomies

Tibial tubercle osteotomies (TTO) is a common treatment option to modify patellar tracking as well as joint contact forces. This is to achieve unloading or alter existing load conditions in PFJ and/or correct alignment in multiple dimensions. PF instability may require soft tissue corrections as concomitant procedure along with TTO.

TTO are probably the best proven surgical procedures to change the patellar tracking and relation to the trochlea. In fact the TTO are capable of changing primarily patellar height and secondary TTTG/TTPCL relation (medialization of the patella). The techniques also have potential to change the patellar tilt and rotation [11]. Many procedures and modifications have been described—all primarily relocate distal insertion of the extensor mechanism. The indication threshold for TTO in patellar height abnormality, tracking on trochlea and instability is well defined [4, 12–15].

Surgical Technique

TTO might be performed either by medial approach facilitating the gracillis tendon harvest or by lateral approach allowing for better exposure of tibial tubercule. Direct medial approach keeps advantages and disadvantages of the former two. Introduction of mechanical saw brings accuracy and good shape of the cut part, but saw speed brings potential risk of bone overheating and delayed/non-union (Fig. 25.3). A sharp chisel is essential and helpful. Two bicortical cannulated screws are advocated in most techniques; however, the three or four screws is a valuable fixation option (Fig. 25.4). Special care must be taken not to break the osteotomized part of the tibia since solid fixation is crucial.

There are generally two possible technical options: wedge TT osteotomy as described by Roux and modified by Elmslie and Trillat [16, 17] and complete detachment described by Caton and Dejour [8].

Hauser osteotomy (TT moved medially and posterior) and Maquet osteotomy (anterioriza-

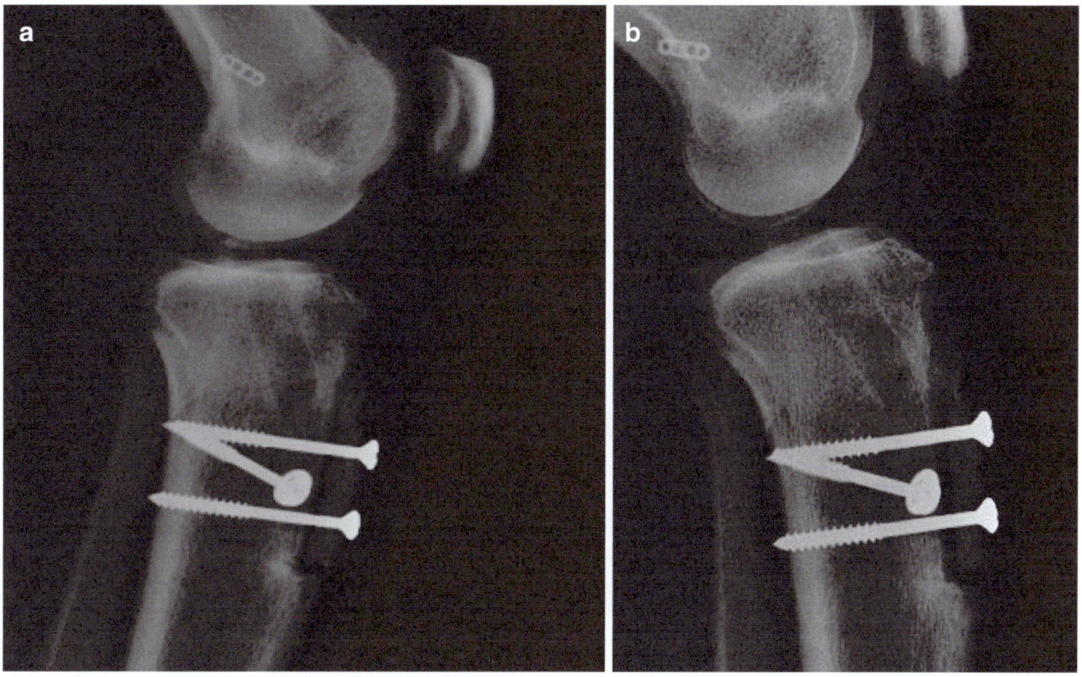

Fig. 25.3 (**a**, **b**). Delayed union after ultra-fast minisaw use. Additional, oblique screw serves for ACL graft fixation. (**a**) Six weeks postop. (**b**) Twelve weeks postop. Delayed union. Patient was revised and grafted

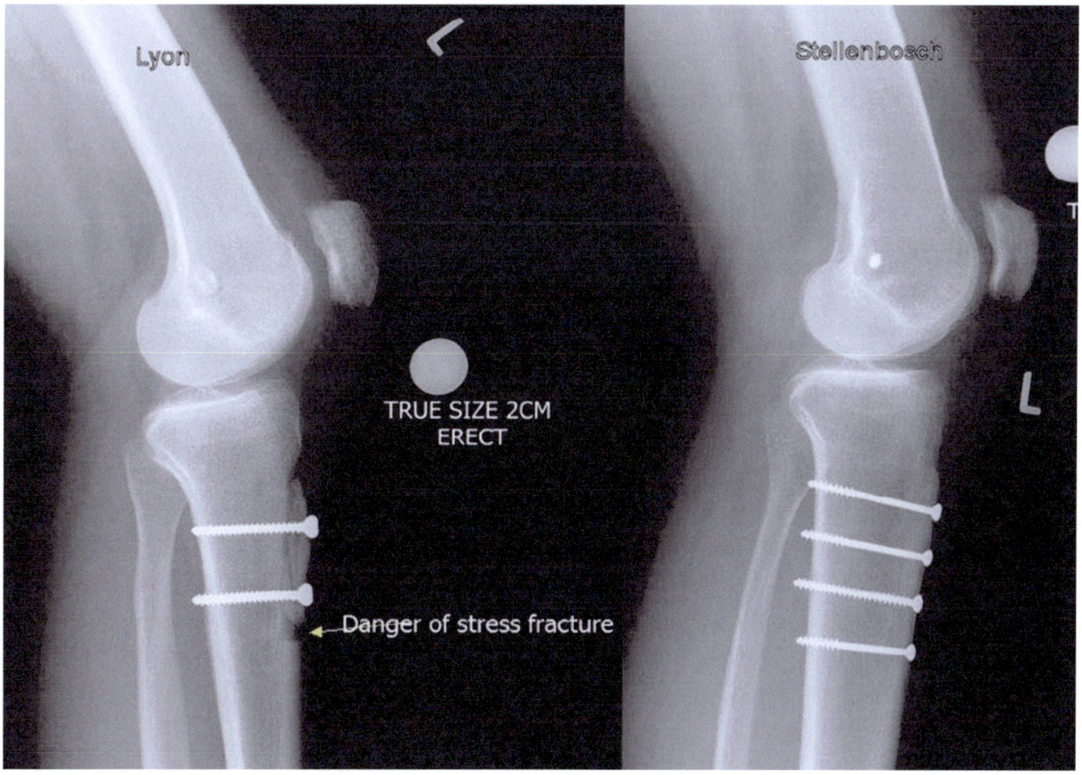

Fig. 25.4 Four screws fixation vs. two screws (courtesy of Dr. "Spike" Erasmus)

tion) were abandoned in the 1990s. Hauser TTO caused residual pain in over 50% of patients; presumably due to posterior displacement of TT and Maquet TTO, which caused many complications and frequent extension lag [18].

25.3.1.1 Distalization (Lyon Procedure)

This method is used to correct CD index over 1.2 in patients who have a patella alta without significant change in TTTG index. Some authors define that point to 1.4 [4]. The most common amount of distalization is around 7 mm [19]. Expected amount is assessed before procedure (Figs. 25.5 and 25.6). It is suggested that osteotomy is performed with a biplanar "L"-shaped cut (Figs. 25.7 and 25.8). Even if it is a straight distalization, an approximately 3 mm functional medialization effect occurs due to the tibial rotation during knee flexion. This is a reverse effect of screw home mechanism. Distalization itself does not change the length of

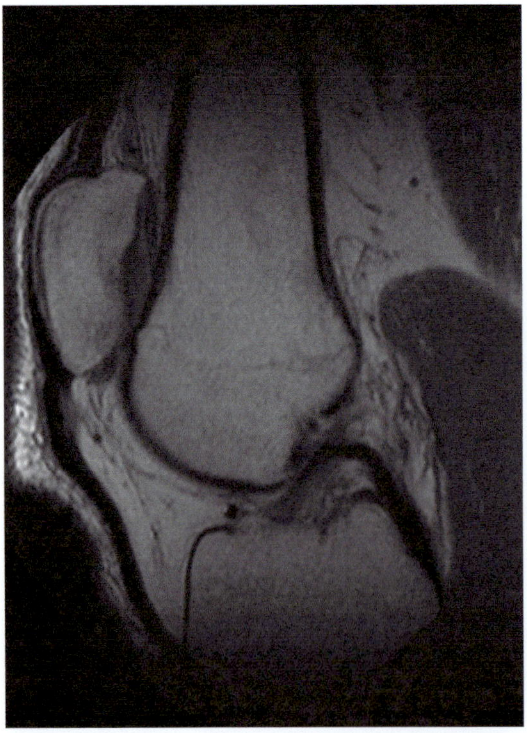

Fig. 25.5 Preoperative CD index app >1, 6 (note "waving" ligament patella – with knee flexed measured CD would be probably much closer to 2)

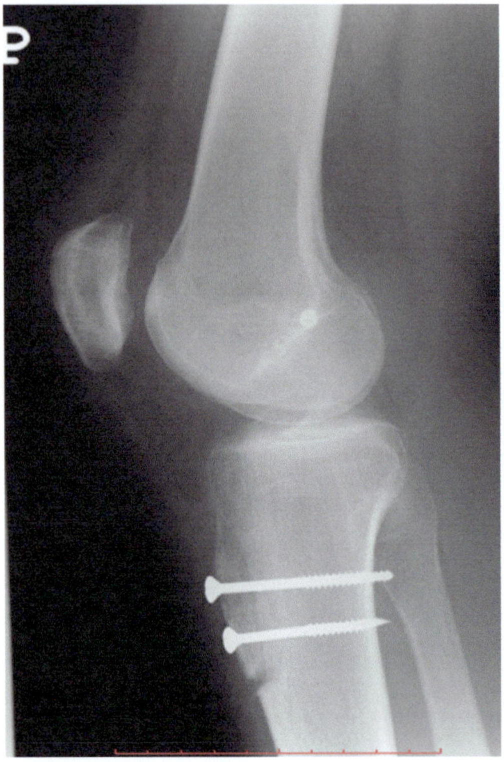

Fig. 25.6 Post-op x-ray. CD = 1, 1

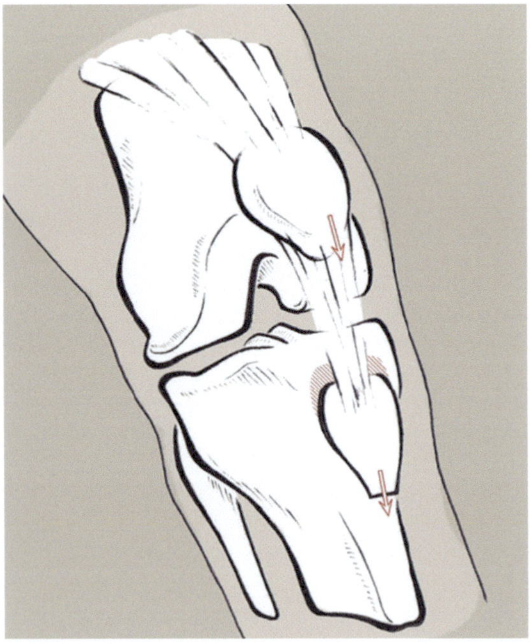

Fig. 25.7 TTO distalization modified Lyon" technique

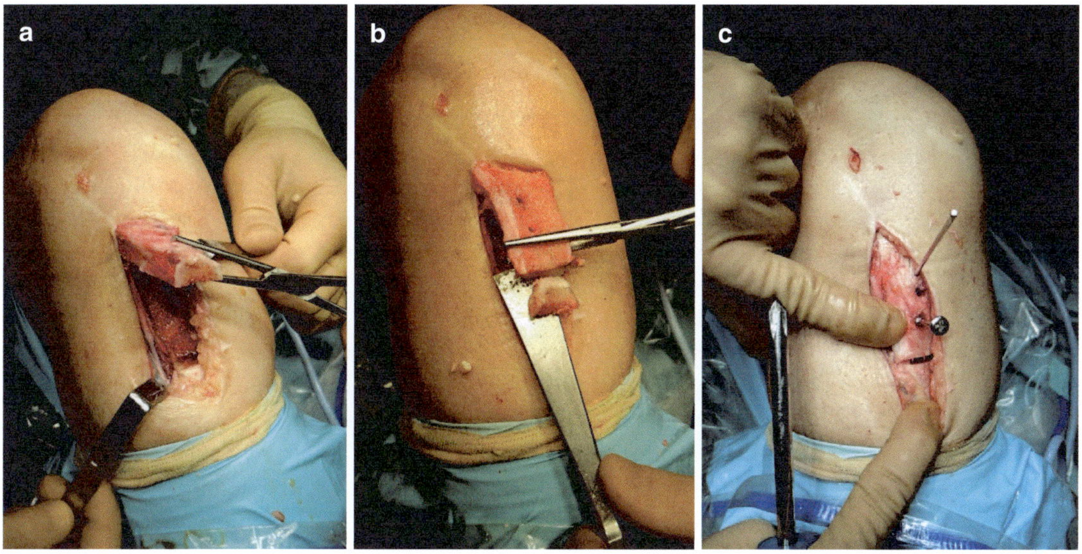

Fig. 25.8 Distalization in revision case of failed medialization. Intraoperative views. (**a**) Biplanar "L"-shaped piece of tibial tubercle. (**b**) Resection of distal part, (**c**) lowering and fixation

patellar tendon but it changes the relative length of the "tibial" part. If the patellar tendon is longer than 52 mm, a tenodesis is to be considered since biomechanical tests demonstrate kinematic changes in the PFJ [19, 20].

Historically there have been a lot of concerns regarding patella distalization in terms of increasing the patellofemoral pressure. New biomechanical studies could clearly demonstrate that this is vice versa in patella alta. In a preexisting patella alta, the patellofemoral pressure can be lowered to normal by distalization of the TTO; however, in normal patella height this manoeuvre has to be avoided [21].

25.3.1.2 Proximalization

Proximalization is a much less common indication (Fig. 25.9). It corrects patella baja despite the origin of the abnormality. It should be options if CD index is lower than 0.8. It is to some extent a disputable indication in patients with anterior knee pain if the CD ratio is around 0.8 and no other anatomical pathology is present. TTO ssurgery when the Caton–Deschamp's index is over 0.6 (between 0.6 and 0.8) gives unsatisfactory results [22].

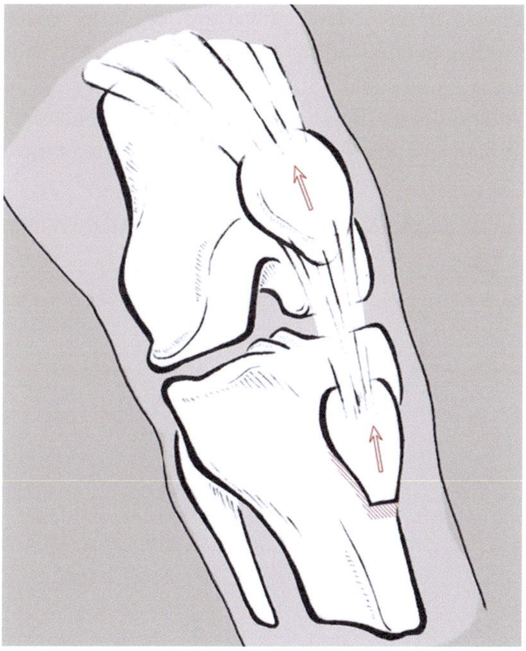

Fig. 25.9 Proximalization of the TT

It is indicated as adjunctive procedure facilitating the access to the knee joint during prosthetic revision surgery if the flexion of less than

60° is present. TTO allows for extensor mechanism release and facilitates flexion. It should be remembered that if the patellar tendon is shorter than 2,5 cm, than lengthening of the tendon is to be considered as well [23].

25.3.1.3 Medialization-Distalization (Elmslie-Trillat Technique, ET)

This is a very well described technique (Fig. 25.10) [17]. It is indicated for patellar instability without significant patella alta. This fact is expressed by high TTTG index and normal or near-normal CD index. A high TTTG is not always due to a lateralized TT, but sometimes due to femoral abnormality (valgus, internal rotation).

The use of TTPCL makes it clear that we face a tibial problem. In the authors' opinion, first measure TTTG—if increased measures TTPCL—if increased go for medialization (if not check femur). The procedure contains distal wedge medialization osteotomy. Precisely it is more a rotational TT osteotomy and the centre of rotation is the tibial wedge. Medialization safety limit is about 8-9 mm, as some bone contact must remain. So if medialization is required inevitably some distalization occurs as a result of downward moving of the TT and subsequent folding of the patellar tendon. It is understood as the correction tool for increased TTPCL distance and mild patella alta. Expected lowering of the patella might be 5-6 mm maximum. There are still some doubts about which modification of TTTG index is to be used and what is the threshold for medialization [7, 15, 24].

Special care must be taken not to cut too small TT piece—potentially risk of non-union and/or fracture. It should be at least 5 cm long and 1.5 cm wide. Careful periosteal and soft tissue treatment/reconstruction and TTO site cover are mandatory.

25.3.1.4 Anteromedialization (Fulkerson) [18]

It was introduced in 1983 as an alternative to Maquet anteriorization aiming to combine effect of release of the stress forces in PFJ by anterior and medial TT reorientation (Fig. 25.11). The original technique's main target is anteromedialization of the tibial tubercle. It was

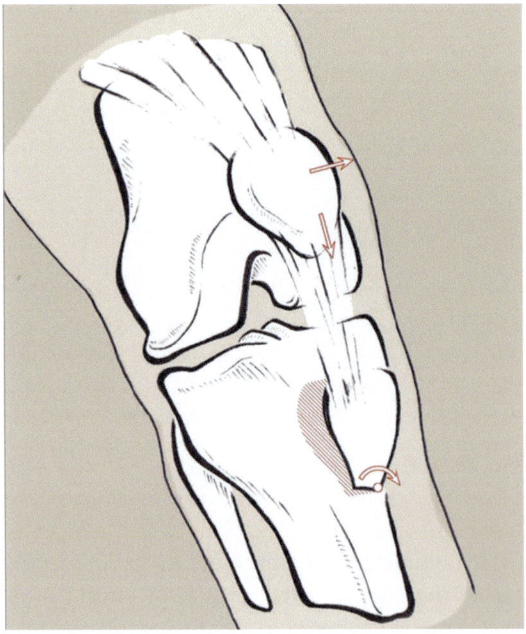

Fig. 25.10 ET technique and patellar tendon folding due to medialization/rotation

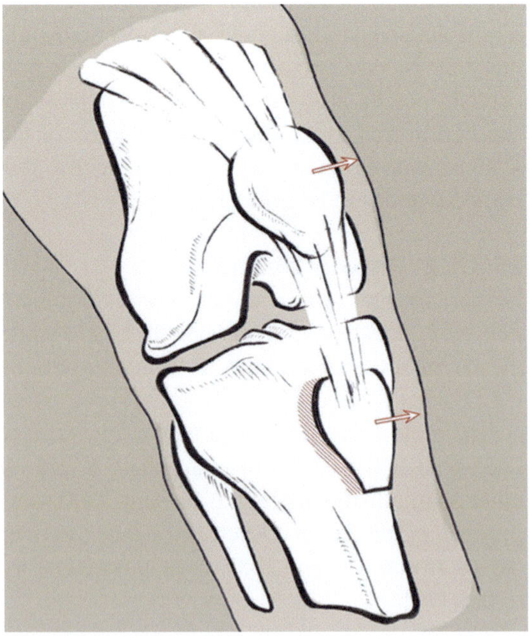

Fig. 25.11 Anteromedialization acc. Fulkerson

designed for patients with PF instability and chondral lesions (lateral facet) and patients with anterior knee pain. It corrects TT lateralization and diminishes load forces in PFJ [18]. Fulkerson TTO assumes a relatively large bone block cut detached completely from the tibia. It is well described and has many modifications and might be used for distalization as well [25]. The technique assures a very good healing contact. However, severe complications are described including tibia fracture and neurovascular damage (deep peroneal nerve and anterior tibial artery). Its main advantage—anterior movement of TT—is somehow disputable if needed at all having the alternative of the proximalization. Kinematic changes and expected unloading of PFJ might play only a theoretical role, while the technique itself requires a rather extensive open approach and holds a risk of potentially serious complications. It is far more popular in the US than in Europe.

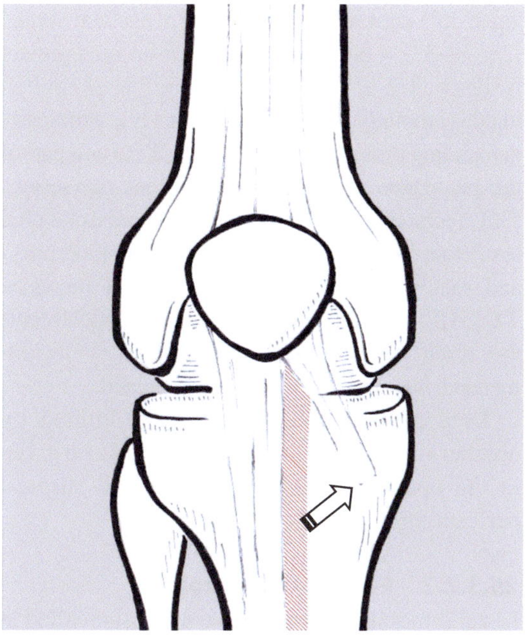

Fig. 25.12 Medial transfer of the LP

25.3.1.5 Partial Medialization [MPTL Reconstruction acc. Zaffagnini]

Another concept has been presented by Zaffagnini et al. [11] with a partial TT osteotomy that uses the medial transfer of the medial 1/3 of TT (Fig. 25.12). Thus it is expected to recreate opposing, medializing forces restraint to the laterally directed force vector of rectus femoris. This relatively delicate and distinctive procedure according the authors is indicated in mild cases of patellar subluxation [11]. Interestingly it is suggested that it may additionally change patellar tilt resulting in unloading effect of the lateral facet of patella.

25.3.2 Rotational and Frontal Malalignment

Rotational malalignment is typically expressed by excessive external rotation of the tibia or/and excessive internal rotation of the femur. Actually, the above-described TTO medialization in the form of Elmslie-Trillat serves as solution for mild symptoms of external tibial rotation. During this procedure, TT is transferred medially and that results in a relative reduction of external tibial rotation. However, if the rotational disarrangements exceed the value of 30–40° ET is incapable to correct it.

No clear and defined limits of normal values exist in literature for this kind of malalignment. What is more complicated—there is a substantial difference between the various proposed CT rotational measurement results [26]. Frontal plane deviations are firmly bonded to rotational deviations. It is proven that if changing the former, the latter changes along and the final result might be unintentional and not desired. That is explained by the fact that proximal derotational femoral osteotomy done on average level (20–30° amount of angular correction) creates the varus femoral deviation in frontal plane [27].

25.3.2.1 Tibial Derotational Osteotomies

Excessive external tibial torsion is an extra-articular deformity that may be a predisposing factor of PF instability and lateral overload. This is a relatively uncommon condition and might be associated with excessive femoral anteversion. Generally it resolves with growth [28, 29]. The threshold for derotational osteotomy is stated between over 30° or 45° (normal value 20°) depending on population, age and source [28, 30–32]. Correction requires distal realignment by derotation, as TTO alone is incapable of correcting this amount of displacement. This is a technically demanding procedure, including the TTO as a part of the procedure. Reported complications are serious [30]. Technically it can be done in the proximal tibia (osteotomy level proximal to the tibial tuberosity) and usually fixed with staples on tibia and screws on TT [31]. In open growth plate children/adolescents the distal tibia derogation osteotomy is recommended, but even less frequently indicated.

Data presented in literature are limited by number of adult patients and care must be given in the operative inclusion criteria and surgical performing.

25.3.2.2 Femoral Osteotomies

Distal femoral osteotomies are well established in the treatment of lateral OA and are capable of controlling the varus–valgus frontal plane. Excessive internal torsion of the femur is a predisposing factor for PF instability and overload. Derotation osteotomies have been proven to address this issue [31, 32]. The modification—supracondylar biplanar femoral osteotomy—has been developed to assure higher stability and better bone-to-bone contact and control femoral rotation [29, 33, 34]. This modification is capable to correct in one stage malalignment in frontal plane along with derotation. The same features are also described for oblique single planar DFO [35].

However, there is no true threshold value for pathological internal femoral torsion reported in the literature [35, 37] It is recommended to consider derotation if the femoral antetorsion is greater than 25–30° [29]. It is important to know which technique is used for measuring the femoral rotation as different techniques lead to different values. Therefore it is recommended to use the same technique for every single measurement [38].

For the indication of varization osteotomies in patellofemoral problems there is even less evidence in literature. However, experts recommend varization DFO in femoral valgus deformities greater than 5°.

In patients with open growth plates and patellofemoral instability combined with malalignment of the lower limb, temporary epiphyseodesis is a minimal invasive and easy procedure to eliminate a risk factor for instability and further on pain in the PFJ. The procedure is very effective and can help avoid the later eventually necessary osteotomy for these patients. To our knowledge there is no evidence for rotational corrections using epiphyseodesis so far.

From a biomechanical point of view both varization and external derotation unload the lateral patellofemoral joint and reduce the lateralizing forces. Therefore it can be considered for patella instability situations as well as in the degenerative PFJ.

25.3.3 Patella Osteotomies (Patelloplasty)

In the recent years we focus on trochlear dysplasia as an anatomical cause of PF instability or pain and eventually the OA predisposing factor. We tend to forget that the term "patellofemoral dysplasia" describes the malformation of both the corresponding joint parts—femoral trochlea and the patella.

Surgical correction of the femoral part (trochleoplasty) inevitably drives to incongruence if the dysplastic patella remains. A surgical technique adapting the dysplastic patella to the reshaped trochlea potentially would be beneficial [33]. Historically, several techniques were proposed to correct the patella shape, probably as many as the number of trochleoplasty techniques. Up to date three main patelloplasty techniques are available.

- Saragaglia [49] described a medial facet patelloplasty technique performed by resection of the medial and distal patellar bulge with the cartilage cover.
- Morscher [39] developed a procedure that involves anterior closing or opening wedge sagittal osteotomy depending on the patella shape.
- Choufani proposed lateral closing wedge osteotomy preserving the cartilage layer [40].

The only series of Morscher open-wedge type technique was described with reported good

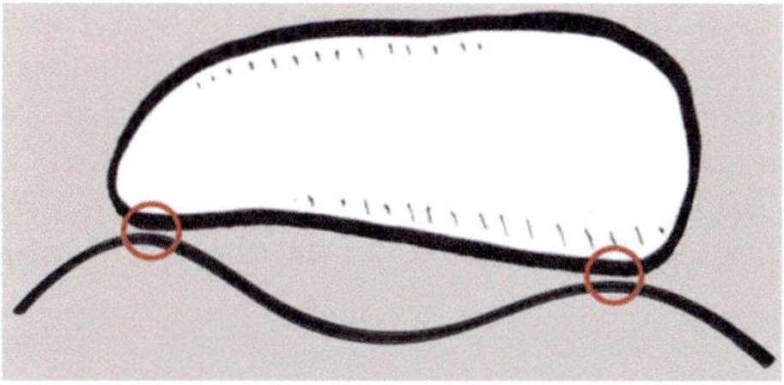

Fig. 25.13 Bridging patella

long-term follow-up by Pecina [41]. According to the author the crucial aspect of planning this type of osteotomy is Wiberg's angle. The patella and the sulcus angle should be approximately equal. Otherwise the so-called bridging of the patella will be created (Fig. 25.13).

The patella osteotomy approach is more or less historic. The techniques were mainly used in dysplastic patellofemoral joints, where the trochlea geometry was pathologic as well and was not addressed. We found only two articles by Koch [33] and Badhe [34] describing concomitant procedures of trochleoplasty and patella osteotomy. Both are case series.

In summary patella-osteotomies may be an option in severe dysplastic situations with a size and shape mismatch of patella and trochlea where both have to be addressed. The potential risk of non-union, cartilage damage or fracture has to be considered very carefully when indicating this unique procedure.

Exceptional care must be taken since the above described techniques are presented on limited number of patients. Dejour and Coultre criticized the overall results of patelloplasty in their literature review [42].

25.3.3.1 Partial Facetectomy

A typical change in the process of degenerative joint disease is the formation of osteophytes. In many arthritic PFJs large such develop on the lateral facet of the patella making it wider and causing mechanical irritation. Many describe it as the raven's beak.

By resecting the most lateral part of the lateral patella facet (usually about 10 mm), a kind of lateral release effect in combination with solving the problem of mechanical irritation can be achieved [43, 52]. If necessary, it can be combined with a lengthening of the lateral retinaculum—but resecting the osteophytes (= resecting the hypomochlion) leads to untensioning of the retinaculum itself. It is done via a small parapatellar lateral approach. If necessary lateral trochlea osteophytes can be removed as well.

The arthroscopic technique has been described with good clinical results [44].

There are satisfactory mid/long-term results available, reporting a realistic delay of arthroplasty in 50–66% after 10 years [45, 46].

25.4 Fractures, OA and Patellectomy

Fractures of the patella once occur are still a challenge to manage. It is known since 40 years that the step in the articular cartilage of more than 1 mm increases risk of patellar osteoarthritis [47]. ORIF with meticulous cartilage surface reconstruction is as mandatory as difficult to achieve. In cases of failure and early onset of OA, patellectomy was found as potentially beneficial. However, following patellectomy, a 30% increase in torque is needed to hold the leg in full extension [48] and the procedure itself compromises results of subsequent TKA. Overall results of this procedure are detrimental. This desperate step is no longer advocated and should be restricted to very unique indications (tumors) [49, 50].

25.5 HTO for the OA and PFJ

25.5.1 Technical Note

Change in patellar height is the undesired phenomenon after open wedge HTO. The hinge effect results in lowering patella in open-wedge and altering in closed-wedge tibial osteotomies [36, 37]. The incidence of patella infera after HTO was reported to be as high as 89% [37]. Lowering the patella overloads the PF leading to OA and compromises the clinical effect of HTO and is correlated with poorer functional outcome [38].

Patella baja also leads to challenging total knee arthroplasty in the future. Exposure of the knee joint would be difficult, especially the eversion of the patella. This increases the risk of patella tendon avulsion. On top of that, the major drawback is the change in the biomechanics of the patellofemoral joint, which may lead to patellofemoral osteoarthritis.

A new technique for TTO during HTO was developed by Gaasbeck, Ihle [36, 51–53]. It is described as descending HTO [54]. This might be advocated if the osteotomy correction angle is over 10°.

25.6 Rehabilitation

Rehabilitation protocols are dedicated to assure fastest possible joint function recovery [55]. However, there is no universal agreement on how this should be addressed [56]. Despite very fast improvement in surgical techniques, the practical approach is generally based on Fithian's statement that it is similar to ACL patients [57].

Authors support the opinion that we used to be too conservative and "stay on safe side" far too far. That attitude results in delayed and often disregarded final functional results. We must keep in mind that "stable" patella or corrected malalignment is not the end of the story. If the operated PFJ is not regaining full and unrestricted function, it remains disabled. Functional overload on the contralateral side leads to overuse and ultimately to OA. Further investigation is required if the surgical improvement is to be followed by adequate rehabilitation.

References

1. Teitge RA. Osteotomy in the treatment of patellofemoral instability. Tech Knee Surg. 2006;5(1):2–18.
2. Arendt EA, Fithian DC, Cohen E. Current concepts of lateral patella dislocation. Clin Sports Med. 2002;21(3):499–519. Review
3. Stephen JM, Dodds AL, Lumpaopong P, Kader D, Williams A, Amis AA. The ability of medial patellofemoral ligament reconstruction to correct patellar kinematics and contact mechanics in the presence of a lateralized tibial tubercle. Am J Sports Med. 2015;43:2198–207.
4. Bartsch A), Lubberts B, Mumme M, Egloff C, Pagenstert G. Does patella alta lead to worse clinical outcome in patients who undergo isolated medial patellofemoral ligament reconstruction? A systematic review. Arch Orthop Trauma Surg 2018 138(11):1563-1573.
5. Caton J. Méthode de mesure de la hauteur de la rotule. Acta Orthop Belg. 1989;55:385–6.
6. Bernageau J, Goutallier D. Examen radiologique de l'articulation fémoro-patellaire. In: L'actualité rhumatologique de Seze et Coll. Paris: Expansion Scientifique Française; 1984. p. 105–10.
7. Seitlinger G, Scheurecker G, Högler R, Labey L, Innocenti B, Hofmann S. Tibial tubercle-posterior cruciate ligament distance: a new measurement to define the position of the tibial tubercle in patients with patellar dislocation. Am J Sports Med. 2012;40(5):1119–25.
8. Caton J, Deschamp G, Chambat P, Lerat JL, Dejour H. Les rotules basses (Patellae inferae) – A propos de 128 observations. Rev Chir Orthop. 1982;68:317–25.
9. Nicolaas L, Tigchelaar S, Koëter S. Patellofemoral evaluation with magnetic resonance imaging in 51 knees of asymptomatic subjects. Knee Surg Sports Traumatol Arthrosc. 2011;19(10):1735–9.
10. Redler LH, Meyers KN, Brady JM, Dennis ER, Nguyen JT, Shubin Stein BE. Anisometry of Medial Patellofemoral Ligament Reconstruction in the Setting of Increased Tibial Tubercle-Trochlear Groove Distance and Patella Alta. Arthroscopy. 2018;34(2):502–10.
11. Zaffagnini S, Dejour D, Arendt E. Patellofemoral pain, instability and arthritis. Berlin: Springer; 2010.
12. Simmons E Jr, Cameron JC. Patella alta and recurrent dislocation of the patella. Clin Orthop Relat Res. 1992;274:265–9. PubMed PMID: 1729011.
13. Dejour H, Walch G, Nove-Josserand L, Guier C. Factors of patellar instability: an anatomic radiographic study. Knee Surg Sports Traumatol Arthrosc. 1994;2(1):19–26.
14. Monk AP, Doll HA, Gibbons CL, Ostlere S, Beard DJ, Gill HS, Murray DW. The patho-anatomy of patellofemoral subluxation. J Bone Joint Surg Br. 2011;93(10):1341–7.
15. Colvin AC, West RV. Patellar instability. J Bone Joint Surg Am. 2008;90:2751–62.
16. Trillat A, Dejour H, Couette A. Diagnostic et traitement des subluxations récidivantes de la rotule. Rev Chir Orthop. 1964;50:813–24.
17. Cox JS. An evaluation of the Elmslie Trillat procedure for management of patellar dislocation and subluxation. A preliminary report. Am J Sports Med. 1976;4:72–7.
18. Fulkerson JP. Anteromedialization of the tibial tuberosity for patellofemoral malalignment. Clin Orthop. 1983;177:176-181.
19. Servien E, Lustig S, Neyret P. Bony surgery distal realignment for episodic patellar dislocations. In: Zaffagnini S, et al., editors. Patellofemoral pain, instability and arthritis. Berlin: Springer; 2010.

20. Mayer C, Magnussen RA, Servien E, Demey G, Jacobi M, Neyret P, Lustig S. Patellar tendon tenodesis in association with tibial tubercle distalization for the treatment of episodic patellar dislocation with patella alta. Am J Sports Med. 2012;40(2):346–51.
21. Luyckx T, Didden K, Vandenneucker H, Labey L, Innocenti B, Bellemans J. Is there a biomechanical explanation for anterior knee pain in patients with patella alta? Influence of patellar height on patellofemoral contact force, contact area and contact pressure. J Bone Joint Surg Br. 2009;91(3):344–50.
22. Caton JH, Dejour D. Tibial tubercle osteotomy in patello-femoral instability and in patellar height abnormality. Int Orthop. 2010;34(2):305–9.
23. Dejour D, Levigne C, Dejour H. Postoperative low patella. Treatment by lengthening of the patellar tendon. Rev Chir Orthop Reparatrice Appar Mot. 1995;81(4):286–95. French.
24. Matsushita T, Kuroda R, Oka S, Matsumoto T, Takayama K, Kurosaka M. Clinical outcomes of medial patellofemoral ligament reconstruction in patients with an increased tibial tuberosity-trochlear groove distance. Knee Surg Sports Traumatol Arthrosc. 2014;22(10):2438–44.
25. Ridley TJ, Baer M, Macalena JA. Revisiting Fulkerson's original technique for tibial tubercle transfer: easing technical demand and improving versatility. Arthrosc Tech. 2017;6(4):e1211–4.
26. Kaiser P, Attal R, Kammerer M, Thauerer M, Hamberger L, Mayr R, Schmoelz W. Significant differences in femoral torsion values depending on the CT measurement technique. Arch Orthop Trauma Surg. 2016;136(9):1259–64.
27. Nelitz M, Wehner T, Steiner M, Dürselen L, Lippacher S. The effects of femoral external derotational osteotomy on frontal plane alignment. Knee Surg Sports Traumatol Arthrosc. 2014;22(11):2740–6.
28. Cameron JC, Saha S. External tibial torsion: an underrecognized cause of recurrent patellar dislocation. Clin Orthop Relat Res. 1996;328:177–84.
29. Turner MS, Smillie IS. The effect of tibial torsion of the pathology of the knee. J Bone Joint Surg Br. 1981;63:396–8.
30. Drexler M, Dwyer T, Dolkart O, Goldstein Y, Steinberg EL, Chakravertty R, Cameron JC. Tibial rotational osteotomy and distal tuberosity transfer for patella subluxation secondary to excessive external tibial torsion: surgical technique and clinical outcome. Knee Surg Sports Traumatol Arthrosc. 2014;22(11):2682–9.
31. Fouilleron N, Marchetti E, Autissier G, Gougeon F, Migaud H, Girard J. Proximal tibial derotation osteotomy for torsional tibial deformities generating patello-femoral disorders. Orthop Traumatol Surg Res. 2010;96(7):785–92.
32. Staheli LT. Torsion—treatment indications. Clin Orthop Relat Res. 1989;247:61–6.
33. Koch PP, Fuchs B, Meyer DC, Fucentese SF. Closing wedge patellar osteotomy in combination with trochleoplasty. Acta Orthop Belg. 2011;77(1):116–21.
34. Badhe NP, Forster W. Patellar osteotomy and Albee's procedure for dysplastic patellar instability. Eur J Orthop Surg Traumatol. 2003;13:43–7.
35. Scuderi GR, Windsor RE, Insall JN. Observations on patellar height after proximal tibial osteotomy. J Bone Joint Surg Am. 1989;71:245–8.
36. Bin SI, Kim HJ, Ahn HS, Rim DS, Lee DH. Changes in patellar height after opening wedge and closing wedge high tibial osteotomy: a meta-analysis. Arthroscopy. 2016;32:2393–400.
37. El-Azab H, Glabgly P, Paul J, Imhoff AB, Hinterwimmer S. Patellar height and posterior tibial slope after open- and closed-wedge high tibial osteotomy: a radiological study on 100 patients. Am J Sports Med. 2010;38:323–9.
38. Izadpanah K, Weitzel E, Vicari M, Hennig J, Weigel M, Sudkamp NP, Niemeyer P. Influence of knee flexion angle and weight bearing on the Tibial Tuberosity-Trochlear Groove (TTTG) distance for evaluation of patellofemoral alignment. Knee Surg Sports Traumatol Arthrosc. 2013;22(11):2655–61.
39. Morscher E. Osteotomy of the patella in chondromalacia. Preliminary report. Arch Orthop Trauma Surg. 1978;92(2–3):139–47.
40. Choufani C, Barbier O, Versier G. Patellar lateral closing-wedge osteotomy in habitual patellar dislocation with severe dysplasia. Orthop Traumatol Surg Res. 2015;101(7):879–82.
41. Pećina M, Ivković A, Hudetz D, Smoljanović T, Janković S. Sagittal osteotomy of the patella after Morscher. Int Orthop. 2010;34(2):297–303.
42. Dejour D, Le Coultre B. Osteotomies in patellofemoral instabilities. Sports Med Arthrosc. 2007;15(1):39–46.
43. van Jonbergen HP, Poolman RW, van Kampen A. Isolatedpatellofemoral osteoarthritis. Acta Orthop. 2010;81:199–205.
44. Ferrari MB, Sanchez G, Chahla J, Moatshe G, LaPrade RF. Arthroscopic Patellar Lateral Facetectomy. Arthrosc Tech. 2017;6(2):e357–62.
45. López-Franco M, Murciano-Antón MA, Fernández-Aceñero MJ, De Lucas-Villarru- bia JC, López-Martín N, Gómez-Barrena E. Evaluation of a minimally aggressive method of patellofemoral osteoarthritis treatment at 10 years minimum follow-up. Knee. 2013;20:476–81.
46. Wetzels T, Bellemans J. Patellofemoral osteoarthritis treated by partial lateral facetectomy: results at long-term follow up. Knee. 2012;19:411–5.
47. Boström A. Longitudinal fractures of the patella. Reconstr Surg Traumatol. 1974;14(0):136–46.
48. Maquet P. Mechanics and osteoarthritis of the patellofemoral joint. Clin Orthop Relat Res. 1979;70:144.
49. Gwinner C, Märdian S, Schwabe P, Schaser KD, Krapohl BD, Jung TM. Current concepts review: frac-

tures of the patella. GMS Interdiscip Plast Reconstr Surg DGPW. 2016;5:Doc01.
50. Müller EJ, Wick M, Muhr G. Patellektomie nach Traumabeeinflusst der Zeitpunkt das Ergebnis [Patellectomy after trauma: is there a correlation between the timing and the clinical outcome]. Unfallchirurg. 2003;106(12):1016–9.
51. El Amrani MH, Lévy B, Scharycki S, Asselineau A. Patellar height relevance in opening-wedge high tibial osteotomy. Orthop Traumatol Surg Res. 2010;96:37–43.
52. Gaasbeek RD, Sonneveld H, van Heerwaarden RJ, Jacobs WC, Wymenga AB. Distal tuberosity osteotomy in open wedge high tibial osteotomy can prevent patella infera: a new technique. Knee. 2004;11(6):457–61.
53. Ihle C, Ahrend M, Grünwald L, Ateschrang A, Stöckle U, Schröter S. No change in patellar height following open wedge high tibial osteotomy using a novel femur-referenced measurement method. Knee. 2017;24(5):1118–28.
54. Krause M, Drenck TC, Korthaus A, Preiss A, Frosch KH, Akoto R. Patella height is not altered by descending medial open-wedge high tibial osteotomy (HTO) compared to ascending HTO. Knee Surg Sports Traumatol Arthrosc. 2018;26(6):1859–66.
55. McGee TG, Cosgarea AJ, McLaughlin K, Tanaka M, Johnson K. Rehabilitation After Medial Patellofemoral Ligament Reconstruction. Sports Med Arthrosc Rev. 2017;25(2):105–13.
56. Lightsey HM, Wright ML, Trofa DP, Popkin CA, Ahmad CS, Redler LH. Rehabilitation variability following medial patellofemoral ligament reconstruction. Phys Sportsmed. 2018;46(4):441–8.
57. Fithian DC, Powers CM, Khan N. Rehabilitation of the knee after medial patellofemoral ligament reconstruction. Clin Sports Med. 2010;29(2):283–90.

26 Unloading Osteotomies Around the Knee

Ronald J. van Heerwaarden

26.1 Introduction

In the past decades an evolution of osteotomies around the knee has taken place [1], which is still evolving and holds a dominant position in joint preservation [2].

New techniques for medial opening wedge high tibial osteotomy (HTO) and medial closing wedge distal femur osteotomy (DFO), and specifically designed fixation plates based on locking-compression-plate (LCP) concepts, providing superior initial stability, are now available [3, 4]. These factors have led to a trend back towards osteotomy around the knee. In this chapter the current knowledge on osteotomies around the knee is presented in relation to joint preservation. The focus is on the treatment of varus and valgus osteoarthritis of the knee and more specifically on indications and goals of osteotomies, procedures and techniques, expected outcomes, and possible joint restoration as well as ability to return to work and sports after osteotomies around the knee.

R. J. van Heerwaarden (✉)
Centre for Deformity Correction & Joint Preserving Surgery, Mill, The Netherlands

International Knee & Joint Centre, Abu Dhabi, UAE

London Knee Osteotomy Centre, London, UK
e-mail: r.vanheerwaarden@viasana.nl

26.2 Indication and Goals of Osteotomies

The main indication for HTO is the correction of varus malalignment in medial unicompartmental osteoarthritis of the knee, and the main aim for DFO is the correction of valgus malalignment in lateral unicompartmental osteoarthritis. In HTO, the aim is to unload the medial compartment by slightly overcorrecting into valgus, in order to reduce pain, stop or slow the degenerative process and delay joint replacement [3]. For similar reasons, a DFO's aim is to unload the lateral compartment correcting to neutral or slight varus leg alignment [4]. These effects of unloading also apply to the offloading of localized osteochondral defects [5] and therefore promote the healing of these defects irrespective of the regenerative treatment chosen. Besides unloading, the aim of an osteotomy may also be to neutralize, i.e., correction to neutral mechanical axis, or normalize, i.e., correction to normal bone shape or symmetric leg alignment. HTOs are also performed to replace or assist the function of insufficient ligaments, and HTOs and DFOs can correct patellar maltracking caused by rotational malalignment or valgus malalignment (Table 26.1). Objective criteria for patient selection are not defined to a full extent, and recent research on HTOs questions some of the old dogmas in patient selection as results in a large patient cohort were found to be good to excellent (Oxford knee scores >37) in

M. Brittberg, K. Slynarski (eds.), *Lower Extremity Joint Preservation*,
https://doi.org/10.1007/978-3-030-57382-9_26

Table 26.1 Indications for high tibial osteotomy (HTO) and distal femoral osteotomy (DFO) related to pathology

Indication	High tibial osteotomy	Distal femoral osteotomy
Cartilage pathology		
– Osteochondral lesions	Unloading HTO	Unloading DFO
– Osteochondritis dissecans	Unloading HTO	Unloading DFO
– Osteonecrosis	Unloading HTO	Unloading DFO
– Osteoarthritis	Unloading HTO	Unloading DFO
Meniscus pathology		
– Post (subtotal) meniscectomy	Unloading HTO	Unloading DFO
– With meniscal transplant	Neutralizing HTO	Neutralizing DFO
Ligament pathology		
– ACL/PCL	Normalizing (S) HTO	
– MCL/LCL	Ligament tensioning HTO	
– Posterolateral corner	Biplanar (F + S) HTO	
Deformity		
– Congenital	Normalizing HTO	Normalizing
– Developmental	Normalizing HTO	Normalizing
– Posttraumatic	Normalizing HTO	Normalizing
– Iatrogenic (post-surgery)	Normalizing/unloading HTO	Normalizing/unloading
Patella maltracking	Rotational HTO	Normalizing DFO Rotational DFO

ACL anterior cruciate ligament, *PCL* posterior cruciate ligament, *MCL* medial collateral ligament, *LCL* lateral collateral ligament, *S* sagittal plane, *F* frontal plane

patients with grade 4 osteoarthritis, age >60 years, and BMI > 30 [6].

Besides proper patient selection criteria, the achievement of the optimal amount of correction is key for the success of osteotomies around the knee [7]. Both under- and overcorrection lead to failure of the osteotomy and poor results [8]. Systematic deformity analysis helps to recognize the magnitude, level, plane, and direction of the deformity [9]. Once the nature of the deformity is understood, the correctional goal has to be defined [10]. Finally, a careful and precise planning will help achieve the desired correction [11].

26.3 Procedure and Techniques

Since the introduction of HTO, the surgical technique has evolved. Recently, the open-wedge technique (OW-HTO) has become more popular, since it provides some potential benefits including less risk of intraoperative damage of the peroneal nerve, less soft tissue damage, and the ability of continuously variable correction. Concerning the surgical technique, a biplanar, intraligamentous OW-HTO has been recommended (Fig. 26.1). Using this technique, a large proximal bone fragment is made available, the osteotomy is performed in well healing metaphysial bone, and rotational stability is provided by the biplanar tuberosity osteotomy [3]. In most HTOs the tibial tuberosity remains attached to the distal fragment. In patients that need large corrections (>12 mm) and those with preexisting patella baja, the biplanar technique can also be modified in terms that the osteotomy of the tuberosity is performed distally [3, 12]. Bone healing has been proven superior in biplanar HTOs compared to single planar osteotomies [13]. Concerning collateral ligaments, a controlled release of the medial collateral ligament is essential in order to achieve unloading of the medial compartment [14]. For OW-HTO, specific implants are needed in order to stabilize the osteotomy and enable a functional rehabilitation including early full weight bearing [15, 16].

The preferred surgical technique of the DFO has evolved to a biplanar medial closing wedge technique (Fig. 26.2). In this technique a medially based wedge is removed using incomplete sawcuts ending at a hinge point within the lateral cortex from the posterior three-fourth of the bone. After that, a third sawcut is made proximally in the anterior one-fourth of the bone parallel to the posterior femur cortex. After wedge removal, closure of the wedge fixation is

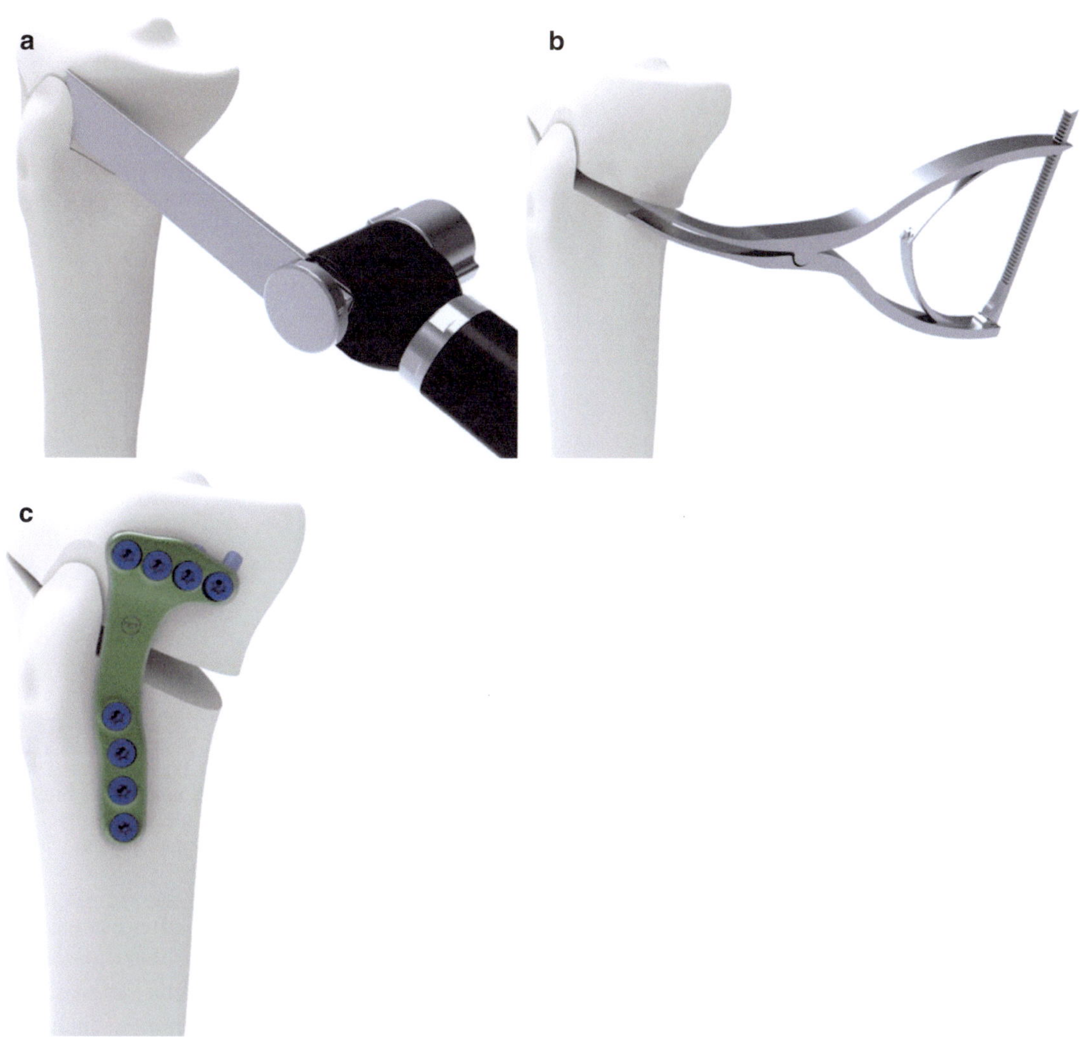

Fig. 26.1 Surgical technique for a biplane opening-wedge HTO fixated with an internal fixator plate. (**a**) The biplanar tuberosity osteotomy cut is made after the transverse osteotomy cut. (**b**) Wedge opening with a bone spreader. (**c**) Configuration after Activmotion™ NewclipTechnics™ plate fixation

performed with an internal fixator implant [4]. Biomechanical testing has shown that the biplanar DFO with internal fixator plate fixation shows superior fixation strength compared to previously performed single-plane DFOs and lateral opening wedge DFO techniques [17, 18]. With this technique the bone healing potential is increased compared to single-plane osteotomies [19], and due to decreased time for partial weight bearing, rehabilitation time after DFO is already reduced until 4–6 weeks after surgery [4, 16].

26.4 Expected Outcomes and Possible Joint Restoration

Outcomes reported for HTO and DFO differ according to the osteotomy technique used, follow-up time, and outcome measures used [6, 7, 20–27]. The location and amount of the preoperative bone deformity as well as the orientation of the knee joint line after the correction have been identified as prognostic factors important for the

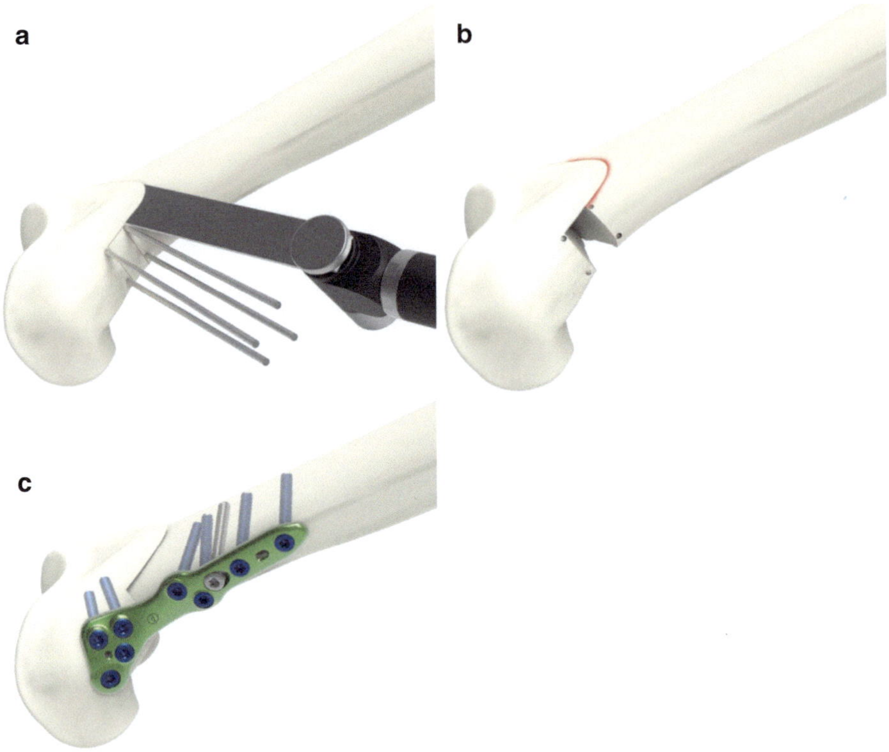

Fig. 26.2 Surgical technique for a biplane medial closing-wedge DFO fixated with an internal fixator plate. (**a**) The biplanar osteotomy cut is made after the transverse osteotomy cuts. (**b**) Wedge removed after biplanar osteotomy. (**c**) Configuration after closure and Activmotion™ NewclipTechnics™ plate fixation

outcome of osteotomies around the knee. Bonnin and Chambat [28] looked at tibial deformities and measured the tibial bone varus angle (TBVA). They found that HTO was more or less curative in patients with an abnormal TBVA (>5°). The osteotomy corrected the congenital deformity in these patients and normalized the obliquity of the joint line while it was palliative in patients with a normal TBVA (<5°). If patients are selected for osteotomy based on the TBVA, a successful result is obtained in >90% at 10 years' follow-up [21, 28] Babis et al. [29] also looked at the obliquity of the joint line as a prognostic factor. In a series of patients with large varus deformities, double osteotomies, i.e., combining a distal femoral with a proximal tibial osteotomy, preserved normal obliquity of the joint line. In 24 patients this resulted in a 96% survival rate at a mean follow-up of 82.7 months. They concluded that preservation of obliquity of the joint line within narrow boundaries of 0° knee joint line orientation (SD 4) was the key to success.

Evidence of joint restoration after osteotomies around the knee in humans has been described using different evaluation methods. Arthroscopic evaluation of cartilage regeneration including biopsies proved fibrocartilage tissue restoration in a direct method of evaluation [30, 31, 32, 33]. Indirect methods providing joint restoration evidence in the subchondral bone as well as cartilage tissues include bone scans [34], dGEMRIC-MRIs [35, 36], and knee images digital analyses showing increase of joint space width [37].

26.5 Return to Work and Sports

Return to work (RTW) and return to sports (RTS) recently have been given more attention. For HTO and for DFO, large cohort studies have now become available, which help to manage patient expectations for these procedures [38, 39, 40].

Out of the author's cohort of HTOs performed between 2012 and 2015, eligible patients treated with HTOs for medial and lateral osteoarthritis were retrospectively followed-up at mean 3.7 years [41, 42]. Out of a cohort of 294 patients, 256 participating in sports preoperatively, it was found that 210 patients (82%) returned to sports postoperatively. RTS in 75% of patients was within 6 months. A shift to participation in lower-impact activities was observed and the median Tegner score decreased from 5.0 presymptomatically to 4.0 at follow-up. The mean Lysholm score at follow-up was 68 (SD ± 22) and no significant differences were found between varus or valgus osteoarthritis. The strongest prognostic factor for RTS was continued sports participation in the year prior to surgery.

A larger cohort of patients was available to study return to work (RTW) after HTO: 349 patients could be included, of whom preoperatively 299 patients worked, and 284 (95%) could RTW. Of these patients, 90% returned within 6 months. Patients reported significant postoperative improvements in performing knee-demanding activities. Being the family's breadwinner was the strongest predictor of RTW, and in contrast, preoperative sick leave was associated with lower RTW [42].

Hoorntje et al. also studied the DFO population of the author's practice between 2012 and 2015 and found that at 3.4 years' follow-up 126 patients were eligible for evaluation of RTW and RTS [43]. Out of 84 patients participating in sports preoperatively, 65 patients (77%) returned to sport postoperatively. Forty-six patients (71%) returned to sports within 6 months. Postoperative participation in high-impact sports was possible, though less frequent, compared to preoperative participation. The median presymptomatic Tegner activity score [4.0 (range 0–10)] was significantly higher ($p < 0.01$) than the reported Tegner score at follow-up [3.0 (range 0–10)]. The mean Lysholm score at follow-up was 68 (±22). For RTW after DFO, results were similar to HTOs: out of 80 patients working preoperatively, 73 (91%) returned to work postoperatively, of whom 59 patients (77%) returned within 6 months.

26.6 Conclusion

Osteotomies around the knee behold a dominant position in joint preservation because of predictable good mid- and long-term results. Indications are increasing and goals of corrections are defined more accurately because of improved planning and osteotomy techniques and fixation methods. Prognostic factors for better outcomes are available and proven cases of joint restoration after osteotomies around the knee are increasing. Eight out of ten athletes return to sports after HTO and after DFO, and 95% and 90% of workers return to work after HTO and DFO, respectively.

References

1. Seil R, van Heerwaarden R, Lobenhoffer P, Kohn D. The rapid evolution of knee osteotomies. Knee Surg Sports Traumatol Arthrosc. 2013;21:1–2.
2. van Heerwaarden RJ, Hirschmann MT. Knee joint preservation: a call for daily practice revival of realignment surgery and osteotomies around the knee. Knee Surg Sports Traumatol Arthrosc. 2017;25:3655–6.
3. Brinkman J-M, Lobenhoffer P, Agneskirchner JD, Staubli AE, Wymenga AB, van Heerwaarden RJ. Aspects of current management: osteotomies around the knee – patient selection, stability of fixation and bone healing in high tibial osteotomies. J Bone Joint Surg Br. 2008;90(12):1548–57.
4. van Heerwaarden RJ, Brinkman JM, Pronk Y. Correction of femoral valgus deformity. J Knee Surg. 2017;30(8):746–55.
5. Mina C, Garrett WE, Garrett J, Pietrobon R, Glisson R, Higgins L. High tibial osteotomy for unloading osteochondral defects in the medial compartment of the knee. AJSM. 2008;36:949–55.
6. Floerkemeier S, Staubli AE, Schroeter S, Goldhahn S, Lobenhoffer P. Outcome after high tibial open-wedge osteotomy: a retrospective evaluation of 533 patients. Knee Surg Sports Traumatol Arthrosc. 2012;21:1–2.
7. Ivarsson I, Myrnerts R, Gillquist J. High tibial osteotomy for medial osteoarthritis of the knee: a 5 to 7 and 11 year follow-up. J Bone Joint Surg (Br). 1990;72:238–44.
8. Tjornstrand B, Egund N, Hagstedst B, Lindstrand A. Tibial osteotomy in medial gonarthrosis: the importance of over-correction of varus deformity. Arch Orthop Trauma Surg. 1981;99:83–9.
9. Hofmann S, Pietsch M, van Heerwaarden R. Biomechanische Grundlagen und Planung

bei Umstellungsosteotomien am Kniegelenk. Orthopädische Praxis. 2007;43(3):109–15.
10. van Heerwaarden RJ, Mast JW, Paccola CAJ. Diagnostics and planning of deformity correction: formation of a surgical plan. In: Marti RK, van Heerwaarden RJ, editors. Osteotomies for posttraumatic deformities. Stuttgart: Georg Thieme Verlag; 2008. p. 33–55.
11. Schröter S, Ihle C, Mueller J, Lobenhoffer P, Stöckle U, van Heerwaarden R. Digital planning of high tibial osteotomy. Interrater reliability by using two different software. Knee Surg Sports Traumatol Arthrosc. 2013;21:189–96.
12. Gaasbeek RDA, Sonneveld H, van Heerwaarden RJ, Jacobs WCH, Wymenga AB. Distal tuberosity osteotomy in open wedge high tibial osteotomy can prevent patella infera: a new technique. Knee. 2004;11:457–61.
13. Pape D, Dueck K, Haag M, Lorbach O, Seil R, Madry H. Wedge volume and osteotomy surface depend on surgical technique for high tibial osteotomy. Knee Surg Sports Traumatol Arthrosc. 2013;21(1):127–33.
14. Agneskirchner JD, Hurschler C, Wrann CD, Lobenhoffer P. The effects of valgus medial opening wedge high tibial osteotomy on articular cartilage pressure of the knee: a biomechanical study. Arthroscopy. 2007;23:852–61.
15. Brinkman JM, Luites JW, Wymenga AB, van Heerwaarden RJ. Early full weight bearing is safe in open-wedge high tibial osteotomy. Acta Orthop. 2010;81(2):193–8. https://doi.org/10.3109/17453671003619003.
16. Takeuchi R, Martijn C, van Heerwaarden R, Seil R. Rehabilitation nach kniegelenknaher osteotomie. In: Lobenhoffer P, van Heerwaarden R, Agneskirchner JD, editors. Kniegelenknahe osteotomien indikation, planung, operationstechnik mit plattenfixateuren. Stuttgart: Georg Thieme Verlag; 2014. p. 150–8.
17. Brinkman J-M, Hurschler C, Agneskirchner JD, Freiling D, van Heerwaarden RJ. Axial and torsional stability of supracondylar femur osteotomies: a biomechanical investigation of five different plate and osteotomy configurations. Knee Surg Sports Traumatol Arthrosc. 2011;19:579–87.
18. Brinkman J-M, Hurschler C, Agneskirchner JD, Freiling D, van Heerwaarden RJ. Axial and torsional stability of an improved single plane and a new biplane osteotomy technique for supracondylar femur osteotomies. Knee Surg Sports Traumatol Arthrosc. 2011;19:1090–8.
19. van Heerwaarden R, Najfeld M, Brinkman M, Seil R, Madry H, Pape D. Wedge volume and osteotomy surface depend on surgical technique for distal femoral osteotomy. Knee Surg Sports Traumatol Arthrosc. 2013;21:206–12.
20. Flecher X, Parratte S, Aubaniac JM, Argenson JN. A 12–28-year followup study of closing wedge high tibial osteotomy. Clin Orthop Relat Res. 2006;452:91–6.
21. Jenny JY, Tavan A, Jenny G, Kehr P. Long-term survival rate of tibial osteotomies for valgus gonarthrosis. Rev Chir Orthop Reparatrice Appar Mot. 1998;84:350–7.
22. Akizuki S, Shibakawa A, Takizawa T, Yamazaki I, Horiuchi H. The long-term outcome of high tibial osteotomy: a ten- to 20-year follow-up. J Bone Joint Surg Br. 2008;90(5):592–6. https://doi.org/10.1302/0301-620X.90B5.20386.
23. Aglietti P, Buzzi R, Vena LM, Baldini A, Mondaini A. High tibial valgus osteotomy for medial gonarthrosis: a 10- to 21-year study. J Knee Surg. 2003;16(1):21–6.
24. Saithna A, Kundra R, Modi CS, Getgood A, Spalding T. Distal femoral varus osteotomy for lateral compartment osteoarthritis in the valgus knee. A systematic review of the literature. Open Orthop J. 2012;6:313–9.
25. Haviv B, Bronak S, Thein R, Thein R. The results of corrective osteotomy for valgus arthritic knees. Knee Surg Sports Traumatol Arthrosc. 2013;21(01):49–56.
26. Chahla J, Mitchell JJ, Liechti DJ, et al. Opening- and closing-wedge distal femoral osteotomy: a systematic review of outcomes for isolated lateral compartment osteoarthritis. Orthop J Sports Med. 2016;4(06):2325967116649901.
27. Wylie JD, Jones DL, Hartley MK, et al. Distal femoral osteotomy for the valgus knee: medial closing wedge versus lateral opening wedge: a systematic review. Arthroscopy. 2016;32(10):2141–7.
28. Bonnin M, Chambat P. Current status of valgus angle, tibial head closing wedge osteotomy in medial gonarthrosis. Orthopade. 2004;33:135–42.
29. Babis GC, An KN, Chao EY, Rand JA, Sim FH. Double level osteotomy of the knee: a method to retain joint-line obliquity. J Bone Joint Surg Am. 2002;84-A:1380–8.
30. Fujisawa Y, Masuhara K, Shiomi S. The effect of high tibial osteotomy on osteoarthritis of the knee. An arthroscopic study of 54 knee joints. Orthop Clin North Am. 1979;10:585–608.
31. Koshino T, Wada S, Ara Y, Saito T. Regeneration of degenerated articular cartilage after high tibial valgus osteotomy for medial compartmental osteoarthritis of the knee. Knee. 2003;10:229–36.
32. Wakabayashi S, Akizuki S, Takizawa T, Yasukawa Y. A comparison of the healing potential of fibrillated cartilage versus eburnated bone in osteoarthritic knees after high tibial osteotomy: an arthroscopic study with 1-year follow-up. Arthroscopy. 2002;18:272–8.
33. Jung WH, Takeuchi R, Chun CW, Lee JS, Ha JH, Kim JH, Jeong JH. Second-look arthroscopic assessment of cartilage regeneration after medial opening-wedge high tibial osteotomy. Arthroscopy. 2014;30:72–9.
34. Kröner AH, Berger CE, Kluger R, Oberhauser G, Bock P, Engel A. Influence of high tibial osteotomy on bone marrow edema in the knee. Clin Orthop Relat Res. 2007;454:155–62.
35. Besselink NJ, Vincken KL, Bartels LW, van Heerwaarden RJ, Concepcion AN, Marijnissen ACA, Spruijt S, Custers RJH, van der Woude JAD, Wiegant K, Welsing PMJ, Mastbergen SC, Lafeber FPJG. Cartilage quality (dGEMRIC Index) follow-

ing knee joint distraction or high tibial osteotomy. Cartilage. 2018;1:1–13.

36. d'Entremont AG, McCormack RG, Agbanlog K, Horlick SG, Stone TB, Manzary MM, Wilson DR. Cartilage health in high tibial osteotomy using dGEMRIC: relationships with joint kinematics. Knee. 2015;22(3):156–62.
37. van der Woude JA, Wiegant K, van Heerwaarden RJ, Spruijt S, van Roermund PM, Custers RJ, Mastbergen SC, Lafeber FP. Knee joint distraction compared with high tibial osteotomy: a randomized controlled trial. Knee Surg Sports Traumatol Arthrosc. 2017;25(3):876–86.
38. Ekhtiari S, Haldane CE, De Sa D, Simunovic N, Musahl V, Ayeni OR. Return to work and sport following high tibial osteotomy: a systematic review. J Bone Joint Surg Am. 2016;98(18):1568–77. https://doi.org/10.2106/JBJS.16.00036.
39. Faschingbauer M, Nelitz M, Urlaub S, Reichel H, Dornacher D. Return to work and sporting activities after high tibial osteotomy. Int Orthop. 2015;39(8):1527–34. https://doi.org/10.1007/s00264-015-2701-2.
40. Hoorntje A, Witjes S, Kuijer PPFM, et al. High rates of return to sports activities and work after osteotomies around the knee: a systematic review and meta-analysis. Sports Med. 2017;47(11):1–26. https://doi.org/10.1007/s40279-017-0726-y.
41. Hoorntje A, Kuijer PPFM, van Ginneken BT, Koenraadt KLM, van Geenen RCI, Kerkhoffs GMMJ, van Heerwaarden RJ. Prognostic factors for return to sport after high tibial osteotomy: a directed acyclic graph approach. Am J Sports Med. 2019;47(8):1854–62. https://doi.org/10.1177/0363546519849476.
42. Hoorntje A, Kuijer PPFM, van Ginneken BT, van Geenen RCI, Kerkhoffs GMMJ, van Heerwaarden RJ. Predictors of return to work after high tibial osteotomy. The importance of being a breadwinner. Orthop J Sports Med. 2019;7(12):232596711989005. https://doi.org/10.1177/2325967119890056.
43. Hoorntje A, van Ginneken BT, Kuijer PPFM, van Geenen RCI, Kerkhoffs GMMJ, van Heerwaarden RJ. Eight respectively nine out of ten patients return to sport and work after distal femoral osteotomy. Knee Surg Sports Traumatol Arthrosc. 2019;27(7):2345–53. https://doi.org/10.1007/s00167-018-5206-x.

27 Joint Preservation by Articular Joint Unloading

Konrad Slynarski

Therapeutic joint unloading is recommended for a number of knee disorders. Very often, knees may be unloaded as part of postoperative rehabilitation protocols after surgical procedures, such as microfracture, osteochondral allografts, autologous chondrocyte implantation, repair for osteonecrosis, and others. Joint unloading may also be indicated as a primary treatment for bone marrow edema, osteochondral defects, meniscal defects, cartilage defects, and, most commonly, osteoarthritis.

Osteoarthritis (OA) is one of the most common forms of musculoskeletal disease worldwide [1]. The World Health Organization (WHO) estimates that 10% of the world's population over 60 years old suffers from symptomatic OA [2].

OA is a progressive, irreversible disease for which there is no cure. Treatment usually consists of symptom managing, with an expectation of improving the patient's functional abilities. Pharmacological interventions, consisting largely of analgesics and anti-inflammatory agents or supplements such as glucosamine and chondroitin sulfates are available, but their effect is temporary and limited. More invasive, intra-articular injections of corticosteroid, hyaluronic acid (HA), platelet-rich plasma are commonly used [3–5]. Innovative injection therapies such as bone marrow—or adipose—derived mesenchymal stem cells gain lots of attention and emerge as new option for nonsurgical treatment of OA symptoms, but there is certainly a need for further evaluation of their clinical application in randomized high-quality studies [6–8]. For patients who do not respond favorably to these conservative treatment options, surgical interventions might be recommended, including arthroscopy and osteotomies in some patients [9] and replacement of the knee joint as a last resort. The risk of future revision surgery is a major concern for especially young patients suffering from knee OA, who will likely outlive a prosthesis. Just as the number of younger arthritics is increasing rapidly, the incidence of arthroplasty procedures is increasing disproportionately quickly in this younger patient population with knee OA. Younger patients are more likely to experience failure of the prosthesis and, subsequently, require a revision surgery [10–13]. In a study of 88,000 patients in California, Meehan et al. [14] found that patients with TKA < 50 years old experienced a 2-year revision rate of 9% due to infection and aseptic loosening, a rate nearly four times that of patients >65 years old. Furthermore, multiple recent studies have reported dissatisfaction rates near 30% in arthroplasty patients <55 years old, with the authors recommending that patients younger than 55 years be informed about the increased risk of dissatisfaction [12, 15].

K. Slynarski (✉)
Słynarski Knee Clinic, Warsaw, Poland
e-mail: konrad@slynarski.pl

M. Brittberg, K. Slynarski (eds.), *Lower Extremity Joint Preservation*,
https://doi.org/10.1007/978-3-030-57382-9_27

Current medical treatments for knee osteoarthritis are not always suitable for some people, and as a result, these people often live with severe pain and have significant difficulty conducting their normal day-to-day activities [16]. Many such patients fall into what has been called the "treatment gap." This gap exists for the younger patient with symptomatic knee OA who is unresponsive to conservative care yet refuses to undergo or is not an appropriate candidate for more invasive surgical procedures.

We are able to successfully treat severe OA changes with prosthetic joint replacements especially in older patients' population, but younger population and patients with mild to moderate disease need more attention, as their goal is to preserve as much of their pre-injury activity and functional level as possible, without pain. This population is reluctant to undergo surgeries of the knee that involve bone cutting [17].

Pathology in the young adult and early OA population is a challenging condition [18]. In most cases the natural disease history begins with trauma to the knee, with OA changes occurring 3.86 times more frequently after initial joint trauma [19]. Initial trauma acts in two different ways [20]. First, a molecular reaction begins when tissue (such as meniscus, cartilage, ligaments) is subjected trauma. This reaction initiates osteoarthritic changes in the joint that lead to a degenerative cascade toward full spectrum of OA. The second, and most obvious, situation is that traumatized tissue cannot sustain its proper mechanical function (e.g. an injured meniscus loses its ability to function as a shock absorber).

Emerging evidence suggests that treatments for early knee OA should incorporate unloading the knee joint since any potential therapeutic benefit of regenerative therapies will likely be weakened by excessive mechanical stress at the knee joint [21, 22]. Until recently, unloading treatments for knee pathology included only external knee braces, wedged shoe insoles, and, high tibial osteotomy. Knee unloader braces provide an opportunity to reduce pain and regain normal activity status. Lee PY et al. analyzed 63 patients with medial knee osteoarthritis with up to 8 years of follow-up, demonstrating good clinical scores and a cost-effective result compared to unicompartmental knee arthroplasty [23]. Unfortunately, patients demonstrate poor long-term compliance, as the brace must be worn for long periods, may be uncomfortable, and may invite social stigma. Unloader brace relieve pain with compliant use, but it can cause severe skin abrasion or deep vein thrombosis when used often, and thus knee braces are not a practical long-term solution [24].

The only predictable surgical procedure capable of lastingly unloading the joint was osteotomy. Osteotomy around the knee (distal femoral osteotomy—DFO, or high tibial osteotomy—HTO) is a surgical procedure in which a wedge of bone is removed from the bone or the bone is cut and bent by certain millimeters. The angle of the bone is adjusted to effectively shift the load from the damaged compartment to the intact compartment of the knee. Patients with OA that has been primarily caused by limb malalignment have been shown to benefit from an osteotomy to provide pain relief.

In 1958, Jackson was one of the first to describe a modern unloading procedure for medial compartment osteoarthritis [25]. Coventry's closing-wedge osteotomy was one of the first procedures popularized worldwide to attempt osteotomy as a treatment for OA [26–28]. More recently, osteotomies are gaining renewed interest because of significant advances of the surgical techniques and materials, resulting in much shorter recovery period, improved rate of return to sport after such surgery [29, 30], but also due to lack of other treatment options for active, young patents with osteoarthritis and limb malalignment. While this procedure does accomplish the goal of transferring the load of weight-bearing forces from arthritic portions to healthier locations of a joint, it requires bone resection or healing of bone gap, a relatively long recovery period accompanied with extensive physical therapy and is only recommended in highly motivated and healthy patients. It is also important to mention, that osteotomy is indicated only when the values of proximal or distal epiphyseal measurements of the femoral or tibial bone are incorrect, and not every single compartment knee degeneration is correlated with malalignment. In such situation osteotomy should not be performed as it would result in iatrogenic deformity, compromising the results of such osteotomy and results of future conversion of knee osteotomy to arthroplasty.

Approaches to dealing with OA that attempt to reduce the medial compartment loads have been shown to be clinically effective. Additionally, published literature describing the importance of joint unloading in other indications is expanding [31–33]. Unloading the medial compartment of a painful knee when medically indicated can decrease pain and even increase the radiographic joint space [34]. There is further evidence in the clinical literature that a reduction in knee adduction movement (which is a direct indicator of loads on the knee joint) results in a relief of pain and improvement in function [35].

Although there is substantial scientific evidence to support the need for altering joint loading, there is still a need for a less invasive treatment option to fill the "treatment gap" between noninvasive treatment and joint-altering surgery such as HTO or joint replacement that is effective and durable. The fundamental need is to decrease the loads on the knee joint which is key to addressing the underlying disease mechanism and has been shown to result in pain relief and improvement in function. If this could be accomplished without having to replace the joint or shift the entire load to another portion of the joint, this would be a much more preferable path for the patient. Furthermore, delaying the need for arthroplasty will reduce the need for future revision surgery, which is expensive and associated with higher risk of complications.

To address the need to unload the medial compartment, a load absorber has been developed to reduce the load acting on the medial compartment of the knee without transferring this overload to the lateral compartment.

The KineSpring Knee Implant System absorbs a maximum load of 13 kg (29 lb) during full knee extension and reduces chronic medial compartment loading without imparting additional forces on the lateral compartment [36]. This magnitude of unloading is comparable to the magnitude of knee adduction moment reduction that has been shown to improve function and alleviate knee pain in OA patients [37, 38]. The KineSpring has been evaluated in three, single-arm, prospective, multicenter studies (OASYS, ACTRN12608000451303; OAKS, ACTRN12609001068257; COAST, ISRCTN63048529) [39–41]. Results from these investigations support the safety and effectiveness of the KineSpring to treat the symptoms of medial knee OA. Amongst 100 patients enrolled across three studies, 18 subjects with KineSpring Knee Implants have completed 36-month follow-up, 36 have completed 24-month follow-up, and 62 have exceeded 12 months. The number of subjects with implants reporting >20% improvement in WOMAC pain and function scores compared to baseline are 94.4% (17/18) at 36 months, 83.3% (30/36) at 24 months and 70.9% (44/62) at 12 months.

Comparing these improvements to historical data available in the HTO literature suggests that the KineSpring System offers comparable OA symptom relief [42].

Clinical experience with the KineSpring System has also demonstrated the safety of the device. There were no unanticipated events reported. Device removals were uncomplicated and did not require immediate conversion to arthroplasty. Following early OASYS first in human experience (n = 30), 70 subjects have been studied. The rate of removals in these 70 subjects is 18.6% (13/70). HTO secondary procedure rates are similar, ranging from 8.7% to 48.9% [43–47]. Based on both clinical occurrence and significance, complications associated with the KineSpring System and high tibial osteotomy are comparable. An interesting study by Kloos et al. compared the impact of different HTO techniques and implantation of KineSpring absorber on patellofemoral contact forces. HTO with a proximal biplanar osteotomy of the tuberositas tibia significantly increased patellofemoral pressure conditions depending on the correction angle. In contrast a distally directed biplanar osteotomy diminished these effects while implantation of an extracapsular, extra-articular absorber had no influence on the patellofemoral compartment at all [48]. Unloading implant may modify knee OA disease progression by increasing joint space width and improving subchondral bone trabecular integrity, thereby reducing pain and improving joint function. In the study by Miller et al., nine patients with unilateral medial knee OA resistant to nonsurgical therapy were treated with the KineSpring System and followed for 2 years [49]. WOMAC scores, on average, improved by 92% for pain, 91% for function, and 79% for stiffness over the 2-year follow-up period. Joint space width in the medial compartment of the treated knee significantly increased from 0.9 mm at baseline to 3.1 mm at 2 years; joint space width in the medial compartment of the untreated knee was unchanged. Fractal signatures of the vertically oriented trabeculae in the medial compartment decreased by 2.8% in the treated knee and increased by 2.1% in the untreated knee over 2 years. No statistically significant fractal signature changes were observed in the horizontally oriented trabeculae in the medial compartment or in the horizontal or vertical trabeculae of the lateral compartment in the treated knee.

The Phantom Knee System (Moximed, Hayward, CA, USA) is a next generation of KineSpring System but has a lower profile and modified surgical technique, designed to reduce load by approximately 11 kg (25 lb). The device consists of titanium alloy femoral and tibial bases, and a polycarbonate urethane (PCU) absorber that reduces the load transferred through the affected medial compartment of the knee joint. The absorber consists of central PCU body that provides compressive load absorption and an articulating ball and socket joint at each end that allows the device to accommodate the natural motions of the knee (Fig. 27.1). Load absorption occurs at low knee flexion angles, such as during the stance phase of gait, while the device is passive at higher knee flexion angles. The absorber is implanted in the subcutaneous tissue of the medial extra-capsular space and remains extra-articular. The compressible load absorber spans the joint, positioned superficial to the medial collateral ligament and isolated from the articular surfaces of the knee. The device is designed to be implanted through a single, relatively small incision without resection of bone, muscle, or ligaments, and without violation of the joint capsule.

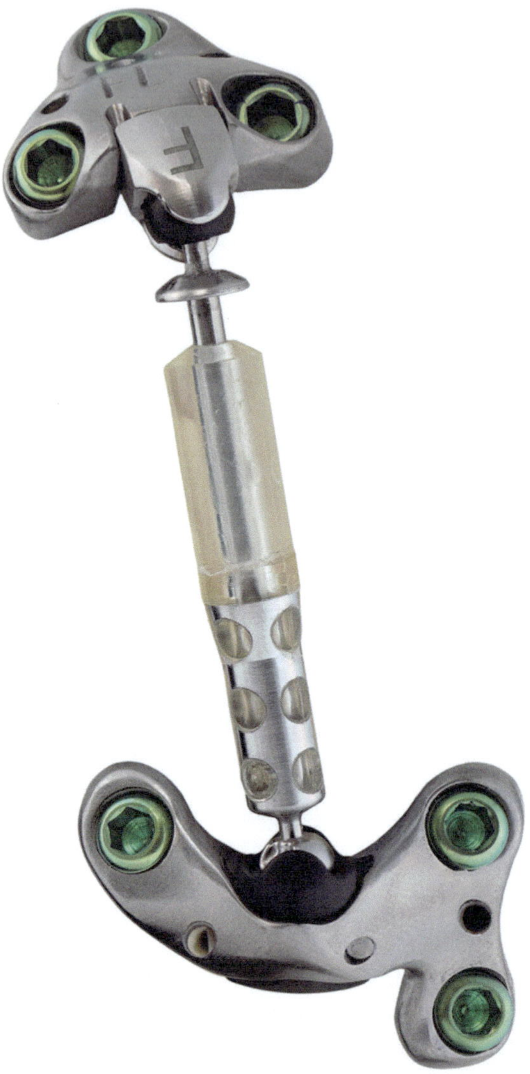

Fig. 27.1 Knee absorber

It is important to note that minimally invasive device implantation without joint invasion provides a surgical procedure that is essentially reversible. The device can be removed without disruption to the joint and surrounding tissues. Notably, the implantation of the device does not interfere with any of the bone used for future joint replacement, if necessary.

In the feasibility study of Phantom unloader, 26 patients with mean age at the time of surgery of 51 ± 1.7 years were treated and evaluated (PHANTOM High Flex Trial) [50]. Importantly, the inclusion criteria targeted a younger patient population for whom arthroplasty is not the ideal treatment. All concomitant procedures, including arthroscopy, were prohibited in this study, so the outcomes can be attributed to the joint unloading provided by the implant. This patient cohort demonstrated statistically significant improvements across a number of disease-specific outcome measures over 12 months. Impressive responder rates of 96.2% and 92.3% of patients demonstrating a clinically significant ≥20% improvement in KOOS pain and WOMAC pain scores, respectively, at 12 months indicate that the treatment is well targeted toward the difficult-to-treat young arthritic population. Average KOOS pain scores significantly improved from 44.2 ± 2.1 at baseline to 78.9 ± 3.7 points at 12 months. Western Ontario and McMaster Universities Osteoarthritis Index pain, stiffness, and function subscales all significantly improved over 12 months. The KSS knee scores improved from 61.9 ± 3.0 at baseline to 94.6 ± 1.6 at 12 months, and KSS function scores improved from 73.4 ± 2.8 at baseline to 98.1 ± 1.1 at 12 months. Nine patients (34.6%) experienced at least one adverse event (AE) during the 12-month follow-up period. A total of 14 events were reported, and none of them resulted in study discontinuation. Of the 14 events, three were classified as serious AEs and occurred in three patients (11.5%). One patient (3.8%) had his implant removed due to ongoing knee pain and decreased ROM at 12 months. This patient was a professional triathlonist; unfortunately, his treatment expectations were not met. Importantly, the explant procedure consisted of implant removal and cartilage debridement only, without conversion to any subsequent implant. During removal surgery, the proper function of the device was confirmed.

The two years follow-up of a same study, all had a clinically meaningful improvement in pain and 96% had a clinically meaningful improvement function [51]. WOMAC pain and function subscales all improved over the 2 years relative to baseline (Figs. 27.2 and 27.3). Pain scores improved from 53.5 ± 8.6 at baseline to

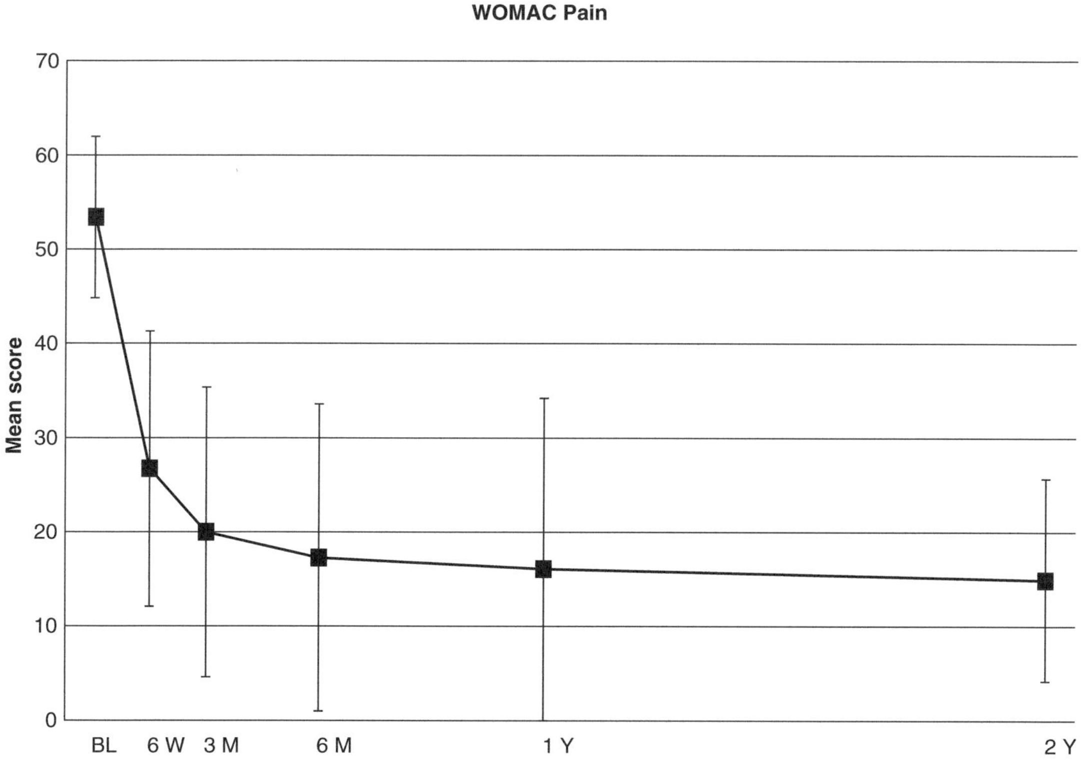

Fig. 27.2 Mean (±SD) WOMAC pain scores from baseline to 2 years. Lower scores indicate improvement. *BL* baseline, *M* months, *W* weeks, *Y* years. WOMAC indicates Western Ontario and McMaster. Universities Osteoarthritis Index

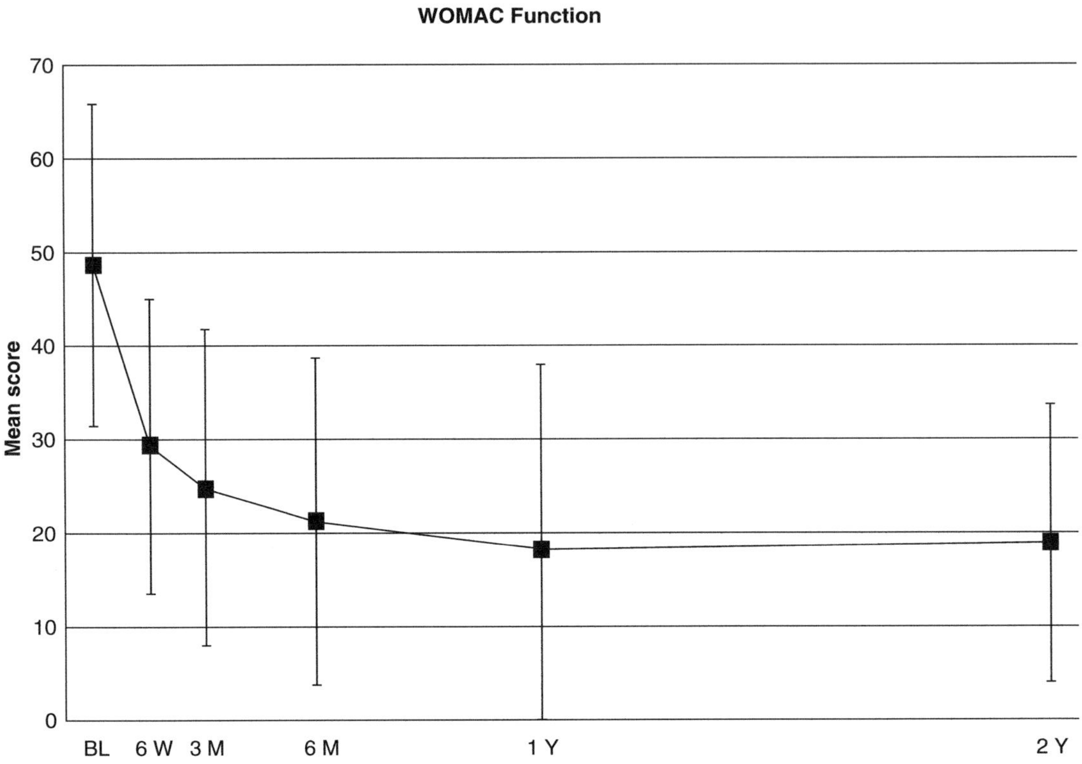

Fig. 27.3 Mean (±SD) WOMAC function scores from baseline to 2 years. Lower scores indicate improvement. *BL* baseline, *M* months, *W* weeks, *Y* years. WOMAC indicates Western Ontario and McMaster. Universities Osteoarthritis Index

15.0 ± 10.8, and function scores improved from 48.4 ± 17.2 at baseline to 18.8 ± 14.8. Range of motion values initially decreased from baseline (133.5 ± 8.7) to 6 weeks (119.7 ± 14.1) but returned to normal at the 6-month visit, and this ROM was maintained over the 2 years (Fig. 27.4).

In addition, the subjects reported a rapid return to preoperative activity levels within a mean of 23 days, which compares favorably to a prior report that patients were unable to work for a median of 87 days after an HTO procedure [52]. These results indicate that the treatment is well-targeted toward the difficult-to-treat young arthritic population. A strength of this study was the strict eligibility criteria and rigorous protocol, which ensured that the sample included the targeted patient population and treatment effects could only be attributed to the investigation device. These results also confirmed that the findings seen at 1 year were sustained to 2 years. A limitation of this trial was its limited sample size. There was also no comparator to evaluate how the unloader performs against one of the many knee OA treatments.

Finally, it is worth mentioning the similar attempts to develop implantable devices designed to unload the knee joint. Shenoy et al. conducted a study focused on unloading of the medial compartment of the knee. Authors assumed that changing the lever arm of forces acting on the knee can change load distribution in knee compartments. They introduced a device which displaces the iliotibial band from lateral femoral condyle and changes the effective moment arm to displace load distribution toward the lateral compartment, similar to an HTO [53]. Preclinical cadaver results are promising and load distribution changes from the medial compartment to the lateral compartment range between 34% and

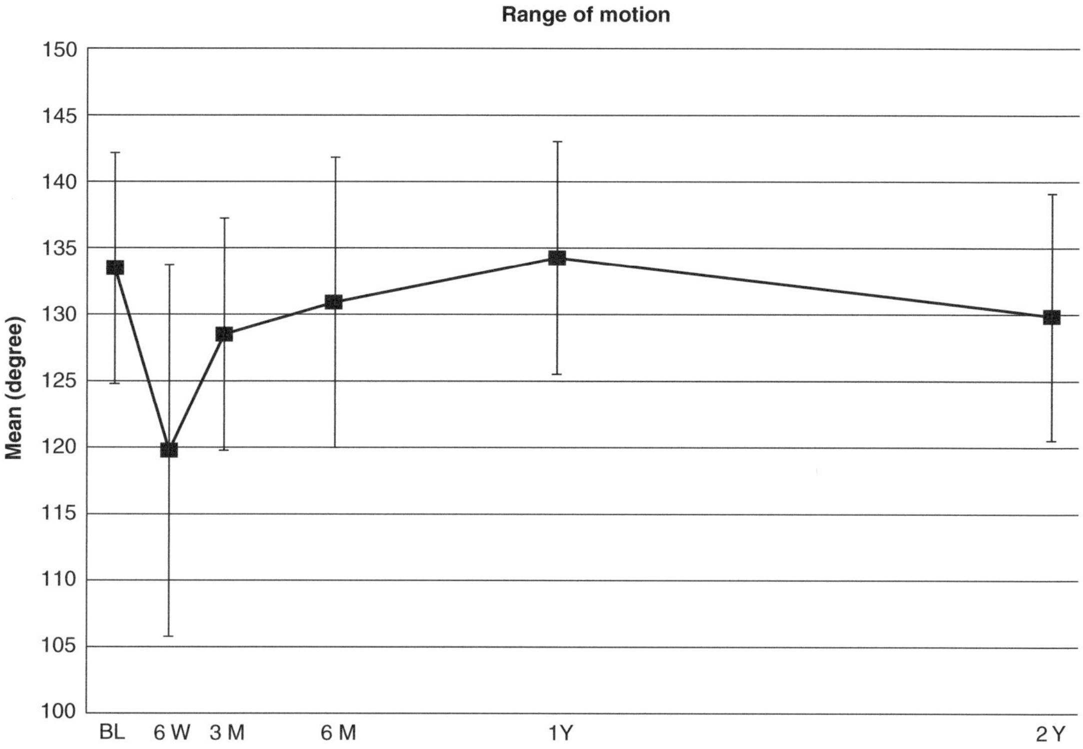

Fig. 27.4 Mean (±SD) range of motion values (in degrees) from baseline to 2 years. *BL* baseline, *M* months, *W* weeks, *Y* years

65%. This was obtained by lateral displacement of illiotibial band between 15 and 20 millimeters. One concern would be illiotibial band syndrome, which can be a serious problem in an osteoarthritic patient even without implantation of such a device, and further investigation is necessary.

The clinically meaningful improvements in pain and function, clean safety profile, and rapid return to preoperative activity level suggest that the implantable unloaders may serve as a potential bridge therapy for patients with medial knee OA who hope to delay arthroplasty.

References

1. Wieland HA, Michaelis M, Kirschbaum BJ, Rudolphi KA. Osteoarthritis—an untreatable disease? Nat Rev Drug Discov. 2005;4(4):331–44.
2. Das SK, Farooqi A. Osteoarthritis. Best Pract Res Clin Rheumatol. 2008;22(4):657–75.
3. Jüni P, Hari R, Rutjes AW, et al. Intra-articular corticosteroid for knee osteoarthritis. Cochrane Database Syst Rev. 2015;10:CD005328. https://doi.org/10.1002/14651858.CD005328.pub3.
4. Bellamy N, Campbell J, Robinson V, Gee T, Bourne R, Wells G. Viscosupplementation for the treatment of osteoarthritis of the knee. Cochrane Database Syst Rev. 2006;2:CD005321. https://doi.org/10.1002/14651858.CD005321.pub2.
5. Dong Y, Zhang B, Yang Q, Zhu J, Sun X. The effects of platelet-rich plasma injection in knee and hip osteoarthritis: a meta-analysis of randomized controlled trials. Clin Rheumatol. 2020; https://doi.org/10.1007/s10067-020-05185-2.
6. Maheshwer B, Polce EM, Paul K, et al. Regenerative potential of mesenchymal stem cells for the treatment of knee osteoarthritis and chondral defects: a systematic review and meta-analysis. Arthroscopy. 2020;2020:S0749-8063(20)30456-4. https://doi.org/10.1016/j.arthro.2020.05.037.
7. Migliorini F, Rath B, Colarossi G, et al. Improved outcomes after mesenchymal stem cells injections for knee osteoarthritis: results at 12-months follow-up: a systematic review of the literature. Arch Orthop Trauma Surg. 2019; https://doi.org/10.1007/s00402-019-03267-8.
8. Anz AW, Hubbard R, Rendos NK, Everts PA, Andrews JR, Hackel JG. Bone marrow aspirate concentrate is equivalent to platelet-rich plasma

for the treatment of knee osteoarthritis at 1 year: a prospective, randomized trial. Orthop J Sports Med. 2020;8(2):2325967119900958. https://doi.org/10.1177/2325967119900958.
9. Floerkemeier S, Staubli AE, Schroeter S, Goldhahn S, Lobenhoffer P. Outcome after high tibial open-wedge osteotomy: a retrospective evaluation of 533 patients. Knee Surg Sports Traumatol Arthrosc. 2013;21(1):170–80. https://doi.org/10.1007/s00167-012-2087-2.
10. W-Dahl A, Robertsson O, Lidgren L. Surgery for knee osteoarthritis in younger patients. Acta Orthop. 2010;81:161–4.
11. Kurtz SM, Lau E, Ong K, Zhao K, Kelly M, Bozic KJ. Future young patient demand for primary and revision joint replacement: national projections from 2010 to 2030. Clin Orthop Relat Res. 2009;467:2606–12.
12. Scott CE, Oliver WM, MacDonald D, Wade FA, Moran M, Breusch SJ. Predicting dissatisfaction following total knee arthroplasty in patients under 55 years of age. Bone Joint J. 2016;98:1625–34.
13. Stambough JB, Clohisy JC, Barrack RL, Nunley RM, Keeney JA. Increased risk of failure following revision total knee replacement in patients aged 55 years and younger. Bone Joint J. 2014;96:1657–62.
14. Meehan JP, Danielsen B, Kim SH, Jamali AA, White RH. Younger age is associated with a higher risk of early periprosthetic joint infection and aseptic mechanical failure after total knee arthroplasty. J Bone Joint Surg Am. 2014;96:529–35.
15. Parvizi J, Nunley RM, Berend KR, et al. High level of residual symptoms in young patients after total knee arthroplasty. Clin Orthop Relat Res. 2014;472:133–7.
16. New trial to bring hope for people with knee osteoarthritis. Arthritis Research UK; 2013 . http://www.arthritisresearchuk.org/news/press-releases/2013/september/new-trial-to-bring-hope-for-people-with-knee-osteoarthritis.aspx.
17. Moorman T, Kirwan T, Share J, Vannabouathong C. Patient preferences regarding surgical interventions for knee osteoarthritis. Clin Med Insights. 2017;10:1–12.
18. Luyten FP, Bierma-Zeinstra S, Dell'Accio F, Kraus VB, Nakata K, Sekiya I, Arden NK, Lohmander LS. Toward classification criteria for early osteoarthritis of the knee. Semin Arthritis Rheum. 2017;pii:S0049-0172(17)30098-7. https://doi.org/10.1016/j.semarthrit.2017.08.006.
19. Blagojevic M, Jinks C, Jeffery A, Jordan KP. Risk factors for onset of osteoarthritis of the knee in older adults: a systematic review and meta-analysis. Osteoarthr Cartil. 2010;18:24–33.
20. Cattano NM, Barbe MF, Massicotte VS, Sitler MR, Balasubramanian E, Tierney R, Driban JB. Joint trauma initiates knee osteoarthritis through biochemical and biomechanical processes and interactions. OA Musculoskelet Med. 2013;1:3–8.
21. Gomoll AH, Angele P, Condello V, et al. Load distribution in early osteoarthritis. Knee Surg Sports Traumatol Arthrosc. 2016;24(6):1815–25. https://doi.org/10.1007/s00167-016-4123-0.
22. Arendt EA, Miller LE, Block JE. Early knee osteoarthritis management should first address mechanical joint overload. Orthop Rev (Pavia). 2014;6(1):5188. https://doi.org/10.4081/or.2014.5188.
23. Lee PY, Winfield TG, Harris SR, Storey E, Chandratreya A. Unloading knee brace is a cost-effective method to bridge and delay surgery in unicompartmental knee arthritis. BMJ Open Sport Exerc Med. 2017;2(1):e000195. https://doi.org/10.1136/bmjsem-2016-000195. eCollection 2016.
24. Hurwitz DE, et al. Knee pain and joint loading in subjects with osteoarthritis of the knee. J Orthop Res. 2000;18(4):572–9.
25. Jackson JP, Waugh W. Tibial osteotomy for osteoarthritis of the knee. Proc R Soc Med. 1960;53(10):888.
26. Coventry MB. Osteotomy of the upper portion of the tibia for degenerative arthritis of the knee. A preliminary report. J Bone Joint Surg Am. 1965;47:984–90.
27. Coventry MB. Upper tibial osteotomy. Clin Orthop Relat Res. 1984;182:46–52.
28. Coventry MB, Ilstrup DM, Wallrichs SL. Proximal tibial osteotomy. A critical long-term study of eighty-seven cases. J Bone Joint Surg Am. 1993;75(2):196–201.
29. Seil R, van Heerwaarden R, Lobenhoffer P, Kohn D. The rapid evolution of knee osteotomies. Knee Surg Sports Traumatol Arthrosc. 2013;21(1):1–2. https://doi.org/10.1007/s00167-012-2175-3.
30. Hoorntje A, van Ginneken BT, Kuijer PPFM, et al. Eight respectively nine out of ten patients return to sport and work after distal femoral osteotomy. Knee Surg Sports Traumatol Arthrosc. 2019;27(7):2345–53. https://doi.org/10.1007/s00167-018-5206-x.
31. Arnold MP, Hirschmann MT, Verdonk PC. See the whole picture: knee preserving therapy needs more than surface repair. Knee Surg Sports Traumatol Arthrosc. 2012;20(2):195–6.
32. Becker R, Kopf S, Karlsson J. Loading conditions of the knee: what does it mean? Knee Surg Sports Traumatol Arthrosc. 2013;21(12):2659–60.
33. Stiebel M, Miller LE, Block JE. Post-traumatic knee osteoarthritis in the young patient: therapeutic dilemmas and emerging technologies. Open Access J Sports Med. 2014;5:73–9.
34. Andriacchi TP, et al. Methods for evaluating the progression of osteoarthritis. J Rehabil Res Dev. 2000;37(2):163–70.
35. Hunt MA, et al. Associations among knee adduction moment, frontal plane ground reaction force, and lever arm during walking in patients with knee osteoarthritis. J Biomech. 2006;39(12):2213–20.
36. Clifford A, O'Connell M, Gabriel S, Miller LE, Block JE. The KineSpring load absorber implant: rationale, design and biomechanical characterization. J Med Eng Technol. 2011;35:65–71.
37. Zhao D, Banks SA, Mitchell KH, D'Lima DD, Colwell CW Jr, Fregly BJ. Correlation between the knee

adduction torque and medial contact force for a variety of gait patterns. J Orthop Res. 2007;25(6):789–97.
38. Clifford AG, Gabriel SM, O'Connell M, Lowe D, Miller LE, Block JE. The KineSpring® Knee Implant System: an implantable joint-unloading prosthesis for treatment of medial knee osteoarthritis. Med Devices (Auckl). 2013;6:69–76. https://doi.org/10.2147/MDER.S44385.
39. Moximed, Inc. Safety and feasibility of a load bypass knee support system (LBKSS) for the treatment of osteoarthritis. Camperdown, NSW: The Australian New Zealand Clinical Trials Registry; 2008. anzctr.org.au. https://www.anzctr.org.au/Trial/Registration/TrialReview.aspx?id=82977. ANZCTR Trial ID: ACTRN12608000451303. Accessed 7 Mar 2013.
40. Moximed, Inc. A multi-center, open-label, interventional study of patients with medial compartment knee osteoarthritis (OA) treated with the KineSpring® System. Camperdown, NSW: The Australian New Zealand Clinical Trials Registry; 2009. https://www.anzctr.org.au/ Trial/Registration/TrialReview.aspx?id = 320854. ANZCTR Trial ID: ACTRN12609001068257. Accessed March 7, 2013.
41. Moximed, Inc. The treatment of medial compartmental knee osteoarthritis (OA) symptoms with the KineSpringTM Unicompartmental Knee Arthroplasty (UKA) System. In: [website on the Internet]. London: Current Controlled Trials Ltd, 2009. http://www.controlled-trials.com/ISRCTN63048529. ISRCTN identifier: ISRCTN63048529. Accessed 7 Mar 2013.
42. Amendola A, Panarella L. High tibial osteotomy for the treatment of unicompartmental arthritis of the knee. Orthop Clin North Am. 2005;36(4):497–504.
43. Birmingham TB, et al. Medial opening wedge high tibial osteotomy: a prospective cohort study of gait, radiographic, and patient-reported outcomes. Arthritis Rheum. 2009;61(5):648–57.
44. Brouwer RW, et al. Osteotomy for medial compartment arthritis of the knee using a closing wedge or an opening wedge controlled by a Puddu plate. A one-year randomised, controlled study. J Bone Joint Surg Br. 2006;88(11):1454–9.
45. Gaasbeek RD, et al. Correction accuracy and collateral laxity in open versus closed wedge high tibial osteotomy. A one-year randomised controlled study. Int Orthop. 2009;34(2):201–7.
46. Niemeyer P, et al. Open-wedge osteotomy using an internal plate fixator in patients with medial-compartment gonarthritis and varus malalignment: 3-year results with regard to preoperative arthroscopic and radiographic findings. Arthroscopy. 2010;26(12):1607–16.
47. Takeuchi R, et al. Medial opening wedge high tibial osteotomy with early full weight bearing. Arthroscopy. 2009;25(1):46–53.
48. Kloos F, Becher C, Fleischer B, et al. High tibial osteotomy increases patellofemoral pressure if adverted proximal, while open-wedge HTO with distal biplanar osteotomy discharges the patellofemoral joint: different open-wedge high tibial osteotomies compared to an extra-articular unloading device. Knee Surg Sports Traumatol Arthrosc. 2019;27(7):2334–44. https://doi.org/10.1007/s00167-018-5194-x.
49. Miller LE, Sode M, Fuerst T, Block JE. Joint unloading implant modifies subchondral bone trabecular structure in medial knee osteoarthritis: 2-year outcomes of a pilot study using fractal signature analysis. Clin Interv Aging. 2015;10:351–7. https://doi.org/10.2147/CIA.S76982.
50. Slynarski K, Walawski J, Smigielski R, van der Merwe W. Feasibility of the Atlas Unicompartmental Knee System load absorber in improving pain relief and function in patients needing unloading of the medial compartment of the knee: 1-year follow-up of a Prospective, Multicenter, Single-Arm Pilot Study (PHANTOM High Flex Trial). Clin Med Insights Arthritis Musculoskelet Disord. 2017;10:1179544117733446. https://doi.org/10.1177/1179544117733446.
51. Slynarski K, Walawski J, Smigielski R, van der Merwe W. Two-Year Results of the PHANTOM High Flex Trial: A Single-Arm Study on the Atlas Unicompartmental Knee System Load Absorber in Patients With Medial Compartment Osteoarthritis of the Knee. Clin Med Insights Arthritis Musculoskelet Disord. 2019;12:1179544119877170. https://doi.org/10.1177/1179544119877170.
52. Schroter S, Mueller J, van Heerwaarden R, Lobenhoffer P, Stockle U, Albrecht D. Return to work and clinical outcome after open wedge HTO. Knee Surg Sports Traumatol Arthrosc. 2013;21:213–9.
53. Vivek N, Shenoy MS, Hanson S, Gifford BS III, John T, Kao MD. A novel implant system for unloading the medial compartment of the knee by lateral displacement of the iliotibial band. Orthop J Sports Med. 2017;5(3):2325967117693614.

Overload Assessment and Prevention in Knee Joint Malalignment Using Gait Analysis

28

Martyna Jarocka and Tomasz Sacewicz

28.1 Introduction

Disorders in the lower limbs and the resulting dysfunctions of the musculoskeletal system constitute an important problem for physiotherapists and physicians. Also, the contemporary attitude of the patient, who is often impatient, accustomed to the technique of quick forms of action, forces, in a sense, to create new ways of diagnosing, monitoring, and evaluating the treatment [1, 2]. Not only from the perspective of the attending physician but also from the perspective of the therapist and the patient himself, it is significant to receive an answer to the question concerning the right moment for the return to work or a safe physical activity [3]. Therefore, methods and measurement tools are sought that will allow to precisely specify this time [4].

One of the common methods is to conduct manual tests as well as radiological assessment. In the physiotherapeutic assessment, among others, the following tests are applied:

- Functional fitness assessment tests.
- Kinesiotherapeutic measurements.
- Visual assessment of the patient.

However, the question arises whether the standard patient assessment tools allow us to functionally evaluate the patient during his/her natural, basic activity—which is gait?

Within the range of the lower limb there are numerous mechanoreceptors in the form of Ruffini bodies, Paccini bodies, and Golgi's tendon organs [5, 6].

Injuries in the range of soft tissues on the basis of acute condition or overloading or a breach of joint integrity due to surgical intervention, may affect the maintenance of patient's body balance [7, 8].

Postoperative disturbances or lack of feedback transmitted to the central nervous system by mechanoreceptors located within the joints are, however, subtle. Direct tracking of these disorders is practically impossible; therefore, indirect methods of their detection are applied in the form of static and dynamic stability tests of the patient's posture on dynamographic platforms [9, 10].

The basic function of the lower limb is gait. This movement, which is performed automatically for almost the entire human life, is an everyday life activity that stimulates the basic motoric features of a human being. Disturbances of gait functions limit the ability to move independently, and may over time lead to physical, psychologi-

M. Jarocka (✉)
Department of Rehabilitation, Faculty of Physical Education and Health in Biała Podlaska, Jozef Pilsudski University of Physical Education in Warsaw, Biała Podlaska, Poland

T. Sacewicz
Department of Natural Sciences, Faculty of Physical Education and Health in Biała Podlaska, Jozef Pilsudski University of Physical Eductaion in Warsaw, Biała Podlaska, Poland
e-mail: tomasz.sacewicz@awf-bp.edu.pl

M. Brittberg, K. Slynarski (eds.), *Lower Extremity Joint Preservation*,
https://doi.org/10.1007/978-3-030-57382-9_28

cal, and social degradation of the patients [11]. Such a dysfunction of one of the elements of the locomotor system leads to an increase in the energy expenditure of the others, as well as the fact that this activity becomes mechanically less effective. In correct physiological walking, all biomechanical conditions are met optimally, with moderate energy expenditure. In the variants of pathological gait locomotion needs can be satisfied thanks to the compensation of the locomotor system in space or with the use of orthopedic equipment. Compensation and the maintenance of energy expenditure on the optimal level provoke the organism to activate the so-called substitute movements. Within the lower limbs, the largest energy expenditure is visible while limiting flexion movements in the knee joints. The body compensates for this movement by increasing the pelvis torsion range around the longitudinal axis of the body, which, as a result, leads to the patient's step lengthening. The following lack of knee and foot synchronization movements makes correct walking impossible. Basmajian and DeLuca [12] emphasize that the most significant criterion for natural gait assessment is economical functioning of the locomotor system, since every deviation from the norm leads to increase in energy expenditure by working muscles. Defining the gait functions, its abnormalities/anomalies/deficiencies, identifying areas and ranges of dysfunctions, and their classification is the main goal of gait analysis, enabling further actions to be taken in order to improve it.

28.2 Gait Analysis

Gait analysis has existed for at least 100 years [13], but only recently, with the development of technology, it is becoming one of the main directions in the field of therapeutic, medical, sports, and robotics sciences. Before modern technologies were invented, it was conducted visually and its interpretation was based solely on the observer's clinical experience. Modern technologies have contributed to the development of various tools and devices that ensure accurate and effective measurement of the walking profile with reliable information for researchers. Diagnostic methods, which are applied today, are based on modern solutions, thanks to which a three-dimensional, simultaneous analysis of kinetic and kinematic parameters of motion is possible. In recent years, many publications have been devoted to the problem of various registration techniques and methods of locomotion parameters analysis. A different approach to the registered and analyzed parameters can be observed. Clinicians focus on the analysis of parameters easy to visualize by an assessment/evaluation such as:

- Step length.
- Walking/stride frequency.
- Joint angles.

However, in contrast, neurologists prefer the analysis of the bioelectrical activity of the muscle's nervous system (EMG), and biomechanics evaluates the reaction forces of the ground, moments of strength, etc.

There are two methods of gait assessment applied in the conducted research: qualitative and quantitative. The qualitative method is most frequently used/applied in clinical conditions. Its basis is observation and comparison of properties or behavior of a certain test object with known/familiar patterns. Unquestionably its advantage is the fact that it does not require any equipment and hence it is cheap. However, due to the fact that it is a subjective method, it is overburdened with great mistakes. The imperfection/the limitations of such an examination is/are related to the low time resolution of the investigating eye, with low repetitiveness and comparability of results.

Quantitative gait assessment method is becoming more frequently applied in clinical practice and is increasingly becoming a supplement to medical research. It is based on a numerical analysis of the results obtained during measurements and provides an objective description of kinematics and motion dynamics. It is a useful tool in clinics for functional assessment, diagnosis, planning of therapeutic and rehabilitation interventions as well as assessment of results. Obtained kinematic and kinetic data make it possible to describe the locomotion of the musculoskeletal system in a 2D (two-dimensional) or 3D (three-dimensional) environment [14]. The application/use of reverse dynamic analysis, carried out with the use of musculoskeletal models and experimental data, allows noninvasive assessment of muscle strength as well as external and internal loads during walking [15].

In addition to many indisputable advantages, the biomechanical laboratory gait evaluation has also many disadvantages. First of all, despite the speed of measurement performance, the analysis of the results requires a relatively long time. Research is usually performed by biomechanists or engineers, so the results of analyses may not be fully understood, e.g. for clinicians. The cost of measuring equipment is added to these drawbacks.

In the gait analysis, various devices and measurement systems are used/applied, such as optical, accelerometric, electromagnetic, acoustic systems, platforms for measuring forces, dynamometers, pressure sensors, electromyography, goniometric measurement systems, and medical MRI imaging techniques. In order to obtain the most reliable results, hybrid methods using several measurement techniques are often applied [16, 17].

28.2.1 Optical and Optoelectronic Systems

Measurement systems using cameras in motion analysis are considered to be most valuable due to the quantity and quality of information provided. The most frequently used are sets of cameras recording the position of markers placed on strictly determined anatomical points of the examined subject. They allow, while using special software, to measure the trajectory of selected segments of the human body in space and related parameters such as speed, acceleration, and angles in the joints. We can distinguish two groups of systems depending on the type of markers. The first one is related to active markers (light emitting) and here we can list such systems as, for example, Optotrak, Selspot, and CODA. The second group are systems that use passive markers, passive (reflecting light), e.g. APAS, Vicon (Figs. 28.1 and 28.2), BTS, and Qualisys.

The advantage of these systems is their noninvasiveness (markers are glued on the patient's skin), precision and fast calibration ensuring the accuracy and repetitiveness of tests and the possibility to use them in various work spaces. An important advantage is also the fact that they are compatible with other systems such as EMG,

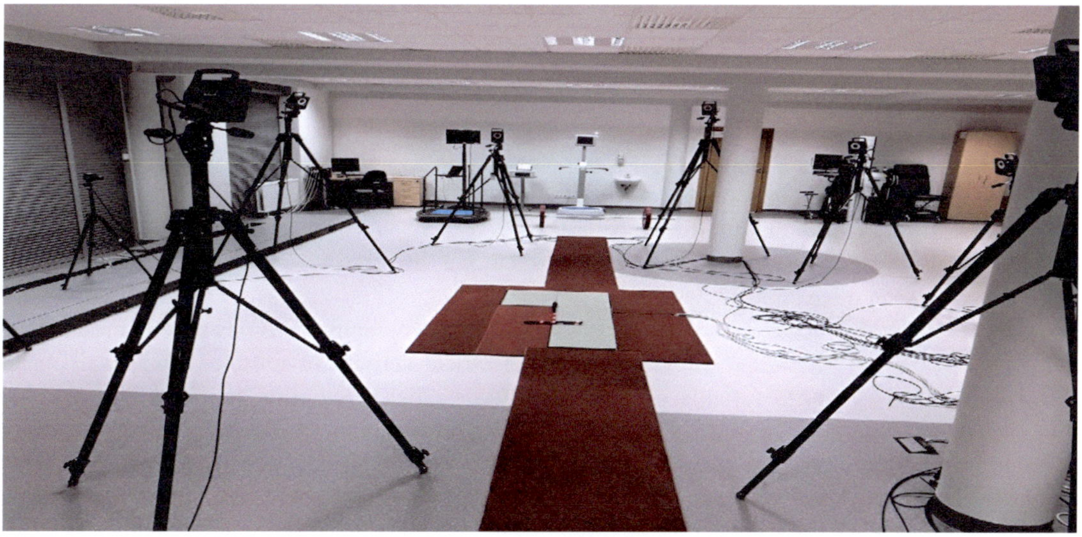

Fig. 28.1 Vicon System in Regional Center for Research and Development in Biała Podlaska (With permission from Rector Josef Pilsudski University of Physical Education in Warsaw, Branch in Biała Podlaska)

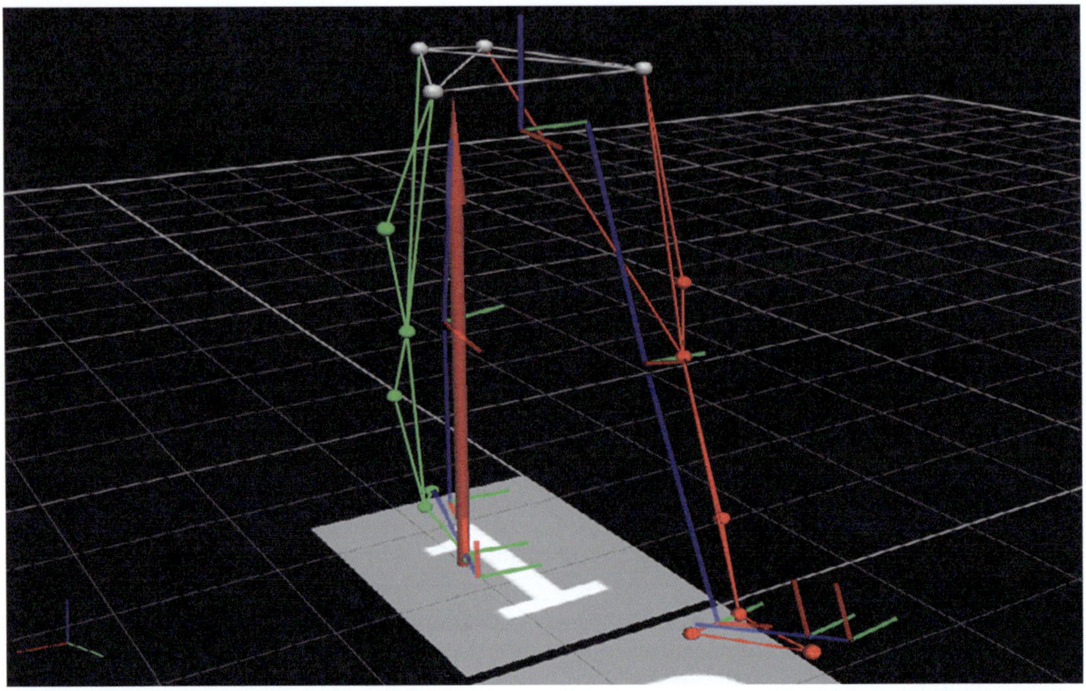

Fig. 28.2 Visualization of the course of a patient's gait examination assessment on Vicon System. Ground reaction

dynamometric platforms, etc. Additionally, while recording the walk/gait with the use of cameras we have the possibility to analyze certain body positions in the desired position and show the patient his way of moving.

The main problem in the research where these systems are applied is to determine the anthropometric parameters of the examined subject and to compensate for soft tissue in relation to the bones underneath.

In the long term/in time perspective, it is possible that imaging of bones and joints in three dimensions (using MRI or fluoroscopy) will replace marker-based systems and eliminate problems occurring there.

28.2.2 Inertial Systems

Inertial systems, thanks to built-in accelerometers (accelerometers) and gyroscopes provide information referring to accelerations, the orientation of the analysed segment in 3D space (in the case of triaxial sensors), as well as the position of joints during gait analysis. Rapid technological progression and the use/application of inertial sensors built into the phones opens new possibilities in gait analysis and traffic monitoring.

The advantage of accelerometers is that they are small and light, and the procedure for their use itself is uncomplicated and the results are reproducible/repetitive.

The basic disadvantages include disturbances resulting from the movement of soft tissues and the influence of the environment in which they work on the correctness of the obtained results (magnetism).

28.2.3 Electromyography

Electromyography (EMG) is used to measure the electrical activity of muscles while walking or during other locomotion activities [18]. We distinguish two types of electromyography: surface EMG (sEMG) using electrodes applied on the skin and intramuscular EMG (iEMG) requiring the insertion of electrodes into the muscles of the examined subject. EMG tests provide information on the extent to which the muscle is active in particular phases of movement. In the case of walking, the head of the thigh quadriceps muscle, the biceps muscle, the gluteus maximus, the tibia front, the gastrocnemius, and the soleus muscle are examined most frequently.

Electromyography does not help to distinguish between primary gait abnormalities and secondary abnormalities. It should be used in conjunction with data informing about the values of moments of forces causing movement in the joint. Kinematic and kinetic parameters allow determining how the muscle tone changes depending on the direction and value of the forces acting and what is the involvement of different muscles in the individual phases of gait.

28.2.4 Systems for the Substrate Reaction Measurement

To measure the dynamics of motion, namely forces and moments of forces, platforms and measuring paths are used, as well as insoles for footwear. These devices are equipped with resistive, piezoelectric, tensometric, and other sensors. They enable registration of dynamic parameters and pressure exerted by the foot on the ground. An example of such devices may be the platforms of Kistler (piezoelectric), AMTI (tensometric), Noraxon or Biodex treadmills (Fig. 28.3), MediLogic insoles used to evaluate load distribution.

Platforms are most frequently used to determine the ground reaction forces during a gait. As a rule, they enable the measurement of three components of ground reaction forces (Fx, Fy, and Fz) and determination of the resultant force vector (value, point of application and inclination angle of this force).

Which gait parameters can we examine?

- Temporal parameters: gait speed, time of stance and swing phase, time of double support, time of step.
- Spatial parameters: stride and step length, step width.
- Joint kinetic parameters (moments): hip/knee/ankle flexion, extension, adduction, abduction, rotation internal, rotation external moments.
- Joint kinematic parameters (movement).

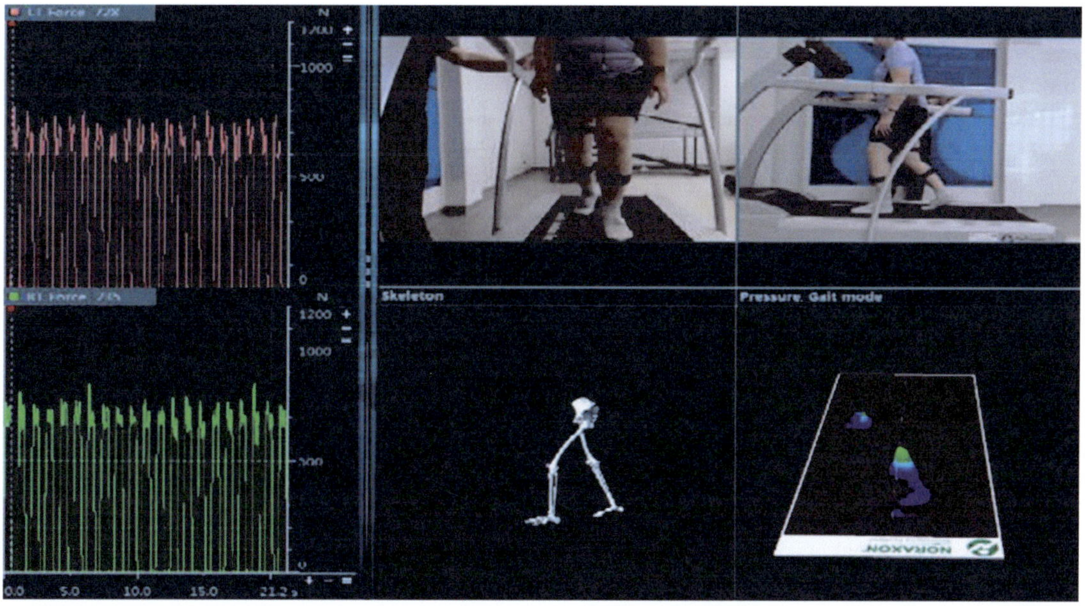

Fig. 28.3 Visualization of the course of a patient's gait examination assessment after osteotomy on a Noraxon device coupled with accelerometers. Regional Center for Research and Development in Biała Podlaska project cofinanced by the European Union under the European Development Fund of the Regional Operational Program Development of Eastern Poland 2007–2013 (With permission from Rector Jozef Pilsudski University of Physical Education in Warsaw, Branch in Biala Podlaska)

28.2.5 Medical Imaging Technique

Biomechanical human modeling is not possible without parameters such as: segment length, segment mass, center of gravity, axis of motion, segment density, and moment of inertia [19]. Medical imaging technique, computer tomography (CT) scans; magnetic resonance imaging (MRI), x-rays, etc. are becoming more frequently being used to facilitate the anthropometric measurement of the examined subjects. They are used to model the geometric structure of the body.

28.2.6 Application of Gait Analysis

The disorders of the lower limbs axis lead to the change in human body biomechanics. Looking at it from another angle, the disorders of the body's biomechanics lead to the changes within the range of the patient's walking. In these two examples it can be concluded that it is extremely reasonable to monitor the changes concerning the patient's walking as the basic form of everyday activity during the whole treatment process. According to Sanguex [20] the measurement of gait kinematic variability provides relevant clinical information under certain conditions which influence/affect neuro-motor control.

Biomechanical gait analysis allows observing the tendency of functional disturbances provoking overloads which may affect the occurrence of osteoarthritis (OA) and lead to the change in limb axis [21]. Stergiou and others [22] claim that plasticity in the joint coordination may reflect the adaptive ability of a motion control system. Interestingly, they also concluded that low walking speed is more difficult for neuromuscular control since it requires increased energy expenditure to maintain certain dynamic balance—it can be suggested that low gait speed is a greater physical effort, a challenge for people who are motorical efficient. Gait analysis is the method used to evaluate in different target groups [23]. The sensitivity of this method allows to apply to the assessment of changes in the locomotor system both in people with degenerative disease [24] and after stroke, sprain of the ankle joint [25], reconstruction of the anterior cruciate ligament [26], patellofemoral ligament reconstruction [27] or with infantile cerebral palsy [28].

According to Resende [29] this method is used in order to assess people with limb symmetry. He showed that limb asymmetry affects the entire kinetic chain of patients with osteoarthritis during gait, increasing the sagittal plane load on the knee joint. A difference in the length of the limbs which is greater than 1 cm increases the treatment of osteoarthritis of the knee in the shorter limb. Further research on gait carried out by the same author [30] shows that increased one-sided foot pronation in osteoarthritis of the knee causes mechanical changes in the lower limbs and torso, which may overload the joint, lower back, resulting in increased knee restraint, stem rotation and tilting the torso. The author concludes that people, who suffer from degenerative disease, should undergo gait analysis in order to assess the work of the foot and provide the basis for proper orthopedic equipment in the form of shoe inserts. Also Beckett [31] states that gait monitoring allow observing the existing relationship between biomechanical disorders within the feet, ankles and knee joint pathology.

Taking into consideration the aforementioned information it is known that structural and functional disorders within the knee joint are very often the resultant of numerous components. Therefore, biomechanical changes within the hip joint lead to:

- Incorrect walk pattern.
- Disordered muscle tension.
- Assymetry position of pelvic girdle.
- Contracture of hip flexors—rectus femoris.
- Increased compression on patella.
- Incorrect sartorius tension.
- Inreased hip joint rotation.
- Lack of correct limb axis.

However, within the foot and ankle joint they can lead to: Foot injuries (bones fractures) changes lead to:

- Reduced longitudinal arch of foot.
- Disordered tibialis anterior tension.
- Pain in the front of the knee.
- Disordered support function of great toe.

Osteotomy, which is a surgical intervention, changes the axis of the joint and leads to the restoration of the proper distribution of forces acting on the growth cartilage. According to Lind and others [32] *osteotomies* are dedicated for/characteristic for young people who lead an active lifestyle with developed or developing osteoarthritis of the knee joint limited to the medial or lateral compartment of the knee joint. Depending on the disturbance of the mechanical axis (genu valgum or knee varus/ bow leg), properly selected tibial or femoral bone osteotomy can be used to correct the mechanical axis in order to relieve the overload in the medial compartment. Gait analysis during the correction of the axis allows to check whether the performed correction affects the improvement of the walking pattern and thus to eliminate the mechanism of overloading the joint in the future. It allows checking whether the desired components of the lower limb locomotor system work properly. Osteoarthritis (OA) for sure disturbs normal walking, especially in periods when pain occurs. Patient with osteoarthritis who has pain starts to use strategies which can decrease joint loading that is way the gait pattern starts to be disturbed. The literature shows a relationship between the degree of knee deformity and the forces acting on the knee. A malalignment of the knee influences the forces and moments acting on the knee during walking. In patients with medial knee OA and a varus alignment, an increased knee adduction moment is typically observed.

According to literature:

- Their walking speed is slower, they make less steps per minute, step and stride length is shorter, single-leg stance time is shorter.
- Degree of maximum knee flexion in stance is reduced, knee extension, hip flexion, and ankle extension are also reduced.
- Stance phase is longer (especially the double-leg stance time is longer), stride time and step time is longer.
- Knee adduction moment and knee flexion moment during stance phase are increased changed (in knee with valgus alignment a decreased knee adduction moment is observed but in varus alignment an increased knee adduction moment is observed).

To put it in detail: there is a decrease in:

- Walking speed (m/s).
- Cadence (steps/min).
- Stride length (m).
- Step length (m).
- Single-leg stance time (s).
- Knee flexion/extension (°).
- Hip flexion (°).
- Ankle extension (°).

However, there is increase in:

- Stance phase (s, %).
- Double support (s).
- Stride time (s).
- Step time (s).
- Knee flexion moment during stance phase.

Some researchers claim that after osteotomy, walking does not change from a clinical perspective—it still deviates from the normal pattern. The only difference is that the patient does not feel pain, he/she is generally more fit, the quality of the life improves and he/she achieves improvement in the results of KOOS, WOMAC, Lysholm [33].

The majority of authors, however, present results which prove that the pattern of gait changes both in case of the osteotomy of valgus as well as varus [32, 34–37].

According to literature:

- Walking speed and step and stride length increase.
- Stance phase time is shorter (especially double support time is shorter), stride and step time is shorter, and knee adduction moment and lateral thrust are decreased.
- Interestingly, the adduction moments in the nonoperated knee increase postoperatively.

- Loading forces and knee ligament balance and reduce progression of OA or the risk of OA.
- Postoperatively, the patients showed kinetics and kinematics of gait similar to that of a healthy control group.
- Knee adduction moment and knee flexion moment during stance phase is changed (in knee with valgus alignment an increased knee adduction moment is observed but in varus alignment a decreased knee adduction moment is observed).

To put it in detail there is increase in:

- Walking speed.
- Stride/step length.
- Adduction moment in the nonoperated knee.

However, there is decrease in:

- Stance phase time.
- Double support time.
- Stride and step time.

Analyzing literature, a question arises: why it is worth combining gait analysis with analysis of changes in the strength of lower limb muscles in malalignment patients? Firstly, the knee joint should be considered as a functional unit of the neuromuscular system, which consists of motor bones, cartilage, ligaments, bags, and muscles. The precise, controlled movement is based on the optimal operation of each component of these devices. If any component is dysfunctional, the joint will be dysfunctional. Hurley et al. [38] have already shown in their studies that motor dysfunction—mainly muscle function—is the cause of OA pathogenesis. According to Øiestad et al. [39], Winters [40], muscle strength affects the quality of walking and the lack of a proper level contributes to the formation of OA. Secondly, as Lind et al. [32] writes, patients who are dedicated to osteotomy are relatively young and physically active. It is a group of patients struggling with symptoms of OA but who want to maintain their current level of fitness [41]. According to Coudeyre [42] isokinetic muscle strengthening (IMS) has a significant impact on the pain and disability and functioning of patients with OA. Thirdly, the muscles that are responsible for movement in the knee joint are relatively easily examined. A common/widespread device applied to measure muscle strength/strength generated by muscles is an isokinetic dynamometer (Medical System PRO-4, produced by Biodex (USA)). Isokinetic studies have been listed among objective tests to assess the possibility of return to preinjury activity, consistent with the guidelines of *Evidence-Based Practice* (EBP) [43].

28.2.7 At What Stages of Rehabilitation Should the Gait Assessment Be Used?

The answer is simple at very stage. Among the people who train, it is reasonable to use gait analysis in order to detect early occurring disorders, which will give rise to the modification of training, elements of physio prophylaxis and orthopedic equipment in the form of, for example, insoles for footwear [23]. According to Nguyen et al. [44, 45], it is reasonable to clearly define the appropriate physical effort that can be used in patients with already appearing OA (Fig. 28.4). According to the author, gait analysis is one of the tools used to properly select and monitor the course of the exercise. The gait parameter, which is very often used to observe overloads on a given limb—the maximum reaction of the ground allows to precisely determining what the value of the overload is. Our own research shows that patients with lower limb disorders present overloads of 2–7 kg on one limb. The inclusion of running elements in such a situation would significantly deepen the given dysfunction.

The analysis of the literature shows that the patient's gait should also be examined at the time of him/her being qualified for osteotomy, namely preoperative surgery [46–49]. The results of these studies form the grounds for postoperative prognosis and provide a reference point for later patient's evaluation results [50]. Our own research shows that it is reasonable to apply these results as part of the patient's qualification for surgery. The communication grounds in the rela-

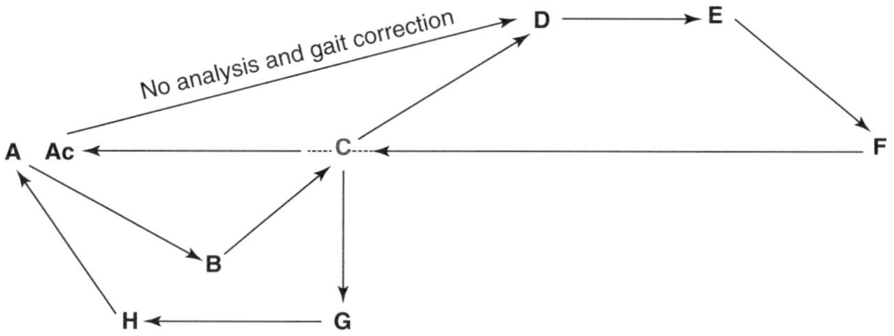

Fig. 28.4 A graph of possible variants of the process leading to or preventing osteotomy. A graph of possible variants of the process leading to or preventing osteotomy. A—sports activity, B—injury/overload, C—gait disorder, D—adding up overload, E—malalignment, F—OA (osteoarthrosis), Ac—sports activity with a coexisting gait disorder, G—gait analysis, H—physiotherapy

tionship between patient–physiotherapist–doctor are significant at each of the stages of the treatment. It seems important to get a clear relationship already at the initial stage of the treatment. Lack of a proper level of agreement at the preoperational stage significantly determines the further course of the process. The lack of the patient's awareness concerning the need to get involved in the preoperative rehabilitation process leads to the lack of growth of the required biomechanical parameters, e.g. muscle strength or the improvement of dynamic stability, and thus impedes the patient's proper preparation for further treatment. The research conducted on our own indicates that the application of selected biomechanical parameters to assess the degree of motoric preparation of the patient to the surgery greatly affects the course of postoperative treatment. In addition, this research constitutes the basis for postponing the date of surgery in case there is lack of the minimal progress of the required parameters registered.

The results of other authors' research show that kinetic disorders of the operated knee joint [51], 49 and the knee extensor strength deficit [49] occur a year or more after surgery [52–54]. That is why it is reasonable to monitor patients undergoing osteotomy even up to 1 year [55–57].

Qualification of patients for surgical intervention involves a medical interview, physical examination, and performing imaging examinations. Imaging examinations constitute a really important element while planning surgical intervention. In the pictures of whole limbs, the angle of the axis correction is determined. However, this has its drawbacks. The measurement of the mechanical axis is performed on the X-ray in a static position. Therefore, the degree of deformation during gait is not measured, when the complaints are usually the greatest and does not take into consideration the individual characteristics of the patient regarding the way of walking. Currently, solutions are being sought through the application of biomechanical studies. Performed before and after osteotomy, they can be used to develop the best possible model on which measurements of the mechanical axis will be made before and after surgical intervention, and comparing the therapeutic effectiveness of osteotomy planned on the basis of static and dynamic study. It is reasonable to take action in order to create a mathematical modeling method among patients undergoing osteotomy.

References

1. Myers CA, Hawkins D. Alterations to movement mechnics can greatly reduce anterior cruciate ligament loading without reducing performance. J Biomech. 2010;43:2657–64.
2. Risberg MA, Holm I, Myklebust G, Engebretsen L. Neuromuscular training versus strength training during first 6 months after anterior cruciate ligament reconstruction: a randomized clinical trial. Phys Ther. 2007;87(6):737–50.

3. Murphy DF, Connolly DA, Beynnon BD. Risk factors for lower extremity injury:a review of the literature. Br J Sports Med. 2003;37:13–29.
4. Neeter C, Gustavsson A, Thomee P, Augustsson J, Thomee R, Karlsson J. Development of a strength test battery for evaluating leg muscle power after anterior cruciate liagament injury and reconstruction. Knee Surg Sports Traumatol Arthreosc. 2006;14:571–80.
5. Fridén T, Roberts D, Ageberg E, Waldén M, Zätterström R. Review of knee proprioception and the relation to extremity function after an anterior cruciate ligament rupture. J Orthop Sports Phys Ther. 2001;31:567–76.
6. Solomonow M, Krogsgaard M. Sensorimotor control of knee stability. A review. Scand J Med Sci Sports. 2001;11:64–80.
7. Rudolph KS, Axe MJ, Buchanan TS, Scholz JP, Snyder-Mackler L. Dynamic stability in the anterior cruciate ligament deficient knee. Knee Surg Sports Traumatol Arthrosc. 2001;9:62–71.
8. Wilken JM, Rodriguez KM, Brawner M, Darter BJ. Reliability and minimal detectible change values for gait kinematics and kinetics in healthy adults. Gait Posture. 2012;35(2):301–7. https://doi.org/10.1016/j.gaitpost.2011.09.105.
9. Bonfirm TR, Paccola CA, Barela JA. Proprioreceptive and behavior impairments in individuals with anterior cruciate ligament reconstructed knees. Arch Phys Med Rehabil. 2003;84:1217–23.
10. Chmielewski TL, Wilk KE, Snyder-Mackler L. Changes in weight-bearing following anterior cruciate ligament reconstruction of the ACL: relationship to quadriceps strength and function. Gait Posture. 2002;16:87–95.
11. Palazzo C, Nguyen C, Lefevre-Colau MM, Poiraudeau S, Rannou F. Risk factors and burden of osteoarthritis. Ann Phys Rehabil Med. 2016;59:134–8.
12. Basmajian JV, Deluca C. Muscles alive: their functions revealed by electromyography. Philadelphia, PA: Lippincott Williams i Wilkins; 1985.
13. Baker R. The history of gait analysis before the advent of modern computers. Gait Posture. 2007;6(3):331–42.
14. Rueterbories J, Spaich EG, Larsen B, Andersen OK. Methods for gait event detectionand analysis in ambulatory systems, improvement in gait pattern after knee arthroplasty followed by proprioceptive neuromuscular facilitation physiotherapy. Med Eng Phys. 2010;32:545–52.
15. Dziewiecki K, Mazur Z, Blajer W. Uwagi o sposobach obróbki danych kinematycznych dla zadań symulacji dynamicznej odwrotnej układów biomechanicznych. Aktualne Problemy Biomechaniki. 2011;5:89–94.
16. McPherson AL, Berry JD, Bates NA, Hewett TE. validity of athletic task performance measures collected with a single-camera motion analysis system as compared to standard clinical measurements. Int J Sports Phys Ther. 2017;12(4):527.
17. Niknam H, Esteki A, Salavati M, Kahrizi S. Reliability of zebris motion analysis system in healthy athletes and athletes with anterior cruciate ligament reconstruction. Asian J Sports Med. 2017;8(1):e42040. https://doi.org/10.5812/asjsm.42040.
18. Davis RB, Ounpuu S, Tyburski D, Gage JR. A gait analysis data collection and reduction technique. Hum Mov Sci. 1991;10(5):575–87.
19. Moreno AS. Optics in gait analysis anthropometry, Proceedings of the SPIE, 8th Iberoamerican optics meeting 11th Latin American meeting on optics, lasers, applications, 18 Nov, vol. 8785, Session VII; 2013. pp. 1–8.
20. Sangeux M, Passmore EH, Graham K, Tirosh O. The gait standard deviation, a single measure of kinematic variability. Gait Posture. 2016;46:194–200.
21. Hewett TE, Torg JS, Boden BP. Video analysis of trunk and knee motion during non-contact anterior cruciate ligament injury in female athletes: lateral trunk and knee abduction motion are combined components of the injury mechanism. Br J Sports Med. 2009;43(6):417–22.
22. Stergiou N, Moraiti C, Giakas G, Ristanis S, Georgoulis AD. The effect of the walking speed on the stability of the anterior cruciate ligament deficient knee. Clin Biomech (Bristol, Avon). 2004;19(9):957–63. https://doi.org/10.1016/j.clinbiomech.2004.06.008.
23. Howell DR, Osternig LR, LI-shan CH. Return to activity after concussion affects dual-task gait balance control recovery. J Am Coll Sports Med. 2014;2014:673–80.
24. Jaczewska-Bogacka J, Stolarczyk A. Clinical and experimental biomedicine. New York, NY: Springer; 2018. https://doi.org/10.1007/5584_2018_187.
25. Doherty C, Bleakley CM, Hertel J, Caulfield B, Ryan J, Delahunt E. Laboratory measures of postural control during the star excursion balance test after acute first-time lateral ankle sprain. J Athl Train. 2015;50(6):651–64.
26. Kaur M, Ribeiro DC, Theis J-C, Webster KE, Sole G. Movement patterns of the knee during gait following ACL reconstruction: a systematic review and meta-analysis. Sports Med. 2016. https://www.researchgate.net/publication/295920315.
27. Asaeda M, Deie M, Fujita N, Shimada N, Orita N, Iwaki D, Kono Y, Ch T, Ochi M. Knee biomechanics during walking in recurrent lateral patellar dislocation are normalized by 1 year after medial patellofemoral ligament reconstruction. Knee Surg Sports Traumatol Arthrosc. 2016; https://doi.org/10.1007/200167-016-4040-2.
28. Gage J. The role of gait analysis in the treatment of cerebral palsy. J Pediatr Orthop. 1994;14:701–2.
29. Resende RA, Kirkwood RN, Deluzio KJ, Morton AM, Fonseca ST. Mild leg length discrepancy affects lower limbs, pelvis and trunk biomechanics of individualswith knee osteoarthritis during gait. Clin Biomech. 2016;38:1–7. https://doi.org/10.1016/j.clinbiomech.2016.08.001.
30. Resende RA, Kirkwood RN, Deluzio KJ, Hassan Sérgio EA, Fonseca T. Ipsilateral and contralateral foot pronation affect lower limb and trunk biome-

chanics of individuals with knee osteoarthritis during gait. Clin Biomech. 2016;34:30–7.
31. Beckett ME, Massie DL, Bowers KD, Stoll DA. Incidence of hyperpronation in the ACL injured knee: a clinical perspective. J Athl Train. 1992;27(1):58–6,62.
32. Lind M, McClelland J, Wittwer JE, Feller WTSJA, Webster KE. Gait analysis of walking before and after medial opening wedge high tibial osteotomy. Knee Surg Sports Traumatol Arthrosc. 2013;21(1):74–81.
33. Morin V, Pailhé R, Duval BR, Mader R, Cognault J, Rouchy R-C, Saragaglia D. Gait analysis following medial opening-wedge high tibial osteotomy. Knee Surg Sports Traumatol Arthrosc. 2018;26(6):1838–44.
34. Birmingham TB, Giffin JR, Chesworth BM. Medial opening wedge high tibia osteotomy: a prospective cohort study of gait, radiographic, and patient-reported outcomes. Arthritis Rheum. 2009;61(5):648–57.
35. Collins B, Getgood A, Abdulaziz Z, Alomar, Robert Giffin J, Willits K, Fowler PJ, Birmingham TB, Robert BT, Litchfield RB. A case series of lateral opening wedge high tibial osteotomy for valgus malalignment. Knee Surg Traumatol Arthrosc. 2013;21(1): 152–60.
36. Lee SH, Lee O-S, Teo SH, Lee YS. Change in gait after high tibial osteotomy: a systematic review and meta-analysis. Gait Posture. 2017;57:57–68.
37. Egmond V, Stolwijk N, van Heerwaarden R, Keijsers A v KNLW. Gait analysis before and after corrective osteotomy in patients with knee osteoarthritis and a valgus deformity. Knee Surg Sports Traumatol Arthrosc. 2017;25(9):2904–13.
38. Hurley MV. The role of muscle weakness in the pathogenesis of osteoarthritis. Rheum Dis Clin N Am. 1999;25(2):1.
39. Øiestad BE, Juhl CB, Eitzen I, Thorlund JB. Knee extensor muscle weakness is a risk factor for development of knee osteoarthritis. A systematic review and meta-analysis. Osteoarthr Cartil. 2015;23(2):171–7.
40. Winters JD, Rudolph KS. Quadriceps rate of force development affects gait and function in people with knee osteoarthritis. Eur J Appl Physiol. 2014;114(2):273–84.
41. Backstein D, Morag G, Samer H, Safir O, Gross A. Long-term follow-up of distal femoral varus osteotomy of the knee. J Arthroplast. 2007;22(4 Suppl):2–6.
42. Coudeyre E, Jegu AG, Giustanini M, Marrel JP, Pereira PEB. Isokinetic muscle strengthening for knee osteoarthritis: a systematic review of randomized controlled trials with meta-analysis. Ann Phys Rehabil Med. 2016;59:207–15.
43. van Grinsven S, Singel REH, Holla CJM, van Loon CJM. Evidence-based rehabilitation following anterior cruciate ligament reconstruction. Knee Surg Sports Traumatol Arthrosc. 2010;18:1128–44.
44. Nguyen C, Lefevre-Colau MM, Poiraudeau S, Rannou F. Evidence and recommendations for use of intra-articular injections for knee osteoarthritis. Ann Phys Rehabil Med. 2016;59:184–9.
45. Nguyen C, Lefevre-Colau MM, Poiraudeau S, Rannou F. Rehabilitation (exercise and strength training) and osteoarthritis: a critical narrative review. Ann Phys Rehabil Med. 2016;59:190–5.
46. Eitzen I, Holm I, Risberg MA. Preoperative quadriceps strngth is a significant predictor sof knee function two years after anterior cruciate ligament reconstruction. Br J Sports Med. 2009;43(5):371–6.
47. Hartigan E, Zeni J Jr, Di Stasi S, Axe MJ, Synder-Mackler L. Preoperative predictors for npncopeers to pass return to sports criteria after ACL reconstruction. J Appl Biomech. 2012;28:366–73.
48. Keays SL, Bullock-Saxon JE, Newcombe P, Keays AC. The relationship between knee strength and functional stability before and after anterior cruciate ligament reconstruction. J Orthop Res. 2003;21:231–7.
49. Scanlan SF, Favre J, Andriacchi TP. The relationship between peak knee extension at heel-strike of walking and the location of thickest femorial cartilage in ACL reconstructwd and healthy contralateral knees. J Biomech. 2013;46:849–54.
50. Lewek M, Rudolph K, Axe M, Synder-Mackler L. The effect of insufficient quadriceps strength an gait after anterior cruciate ligament reconstruction. Clin Biomech. 2002;17:56–63.
51. Konishi Y, Oda T, Tsukazaki S, Kinugasa R, Hirose N, Fukubayashi T. Relationship between quadriceps femoris muscle volume and muscle torque after anterior cruciate ligament rupture. Knee Surg Sports Traumatol Arthrosc. 2011;19:641–5.
52. Deneweth JM, Bey MJ, McLean SG, Lock TR, Kolovich PA, Tashman S. Tibiofemorial joint kinematics of the anterior cruciate ligament-reconstructed knee during a single-legged hop landing. Am J Sports Med. 2010;38:1820–8.
53. Lee KM, Chang CB, Park MS, Kang SB, Kim TK, Chung CY. Changes of knee joint and ankle joint orientations after high tibial osteotomy. Osteoarthr Cartil. 2015;23:232–8.
54. Rower BD, Di Stasi SL, Synder-Mackler L. Quadriceps strength and wright acceptance strategies continue to improve two years after anterior cruciate ligament reconstruction. J Biomech. 2001;44:p. 1948–53.
55. Salomon L, Russel V, Musgrove T, Pieczewski L, Refshauge K. Incidence and risk factors for graft rupture and contrlateral rupture after anterior cruciate ligament recnostruction. Arthroscopy. 2005;21(8):p. 948–57.
56. Damiano DL, Norman T, Stanley CJ, Park H-S. Comparison of elliptical training, stationary cycling, treadmill walking and overground walking. Gait Posture. 2011;34:260–4.
57. Williams GN, Chmielewski T, Rudolph K. Dynamic knee stability: current theory and implications for clinicians and scientists. J Orthop Sports Phys Ther. 2001;31:546–66.

Return to Sports After Knee Surgery for Intraarticular Pathology

29

Konstantinos Epameinontidis and Emmanuel Papacostas

29.1 Introduction

Successful return to sports (RTS) is put on different contexts by different people. For a professional athlete, it may well be the return to unrestricted training and match play, while for a coach, successful return is marked when the athlete returns to his pre-injury performance levels. For the members of the medical team a successful return to sports may be perceived as the absence of re-injury following an athlete's return to training and match play. For an active individual, the ability to perform his recreational sporting activity without symptoms may be all that he/she wants. Setting realistic goals and expectations must be a major priority for everyone involved in the management of patients requiring salvage procedures. Advancements on surgical and rehabilitation techniques continue to remove limitations from treatment options, but the patient/athlete needs to be aware of the possible activity restrictions, or the prolonged rehabilitation required to achieve the desired outcome. This way, an informed decision can be made by all stakeholders involved in a shared decision-making process, which will ensure the best possible outcome. In this chapter, we review the latest findings from the literature regarding return to sport rates following various surgical procedures.

According to Ardern et al. [1], the minimum information needed to define RTS in a way that is acceptable by all stakeholders is the type of sport and the desired level of participation the athlete wants to return to. They also identified that RTS is a continuum that begins with return to participation, followed by return to sport (competition) and, finally, by return to the highest possible level of performance in each individual case. The type of surgery, patient's age and contextual factors will have an impact on which stage of the continuum the patient will be able to return to.

29.2 Return to Sports After ACL Reconstruction Procedures

Surgical reconstruction of the ACL (ACL-R) is a very common procedure in active populations. Although early studies provided high percentages of RTS rates in their cohorts, Ardern et al. [2] have provided evidence that only 55% of of athletes returned to competitive sports. A recent systematic review and meta-analysis reported that, on average, 83% of elite athletes from soccer, American football, rugby and basketball

K. Epameinontidis
Rehabilitation Department, Aspetar Orthopedic & Sports Medicine Hospital, Doha, Qatar
e-mail: Konstantinos.epamino@aspetar.com

E. Papacostas (✉)
Sports Orthopaedic Surgeon, The MIS Orthopaedic Center, Thessaloniki, Greece

M. Brittberg, K. Slynarski (eds.), *Lower Extremity Joint Preservation*,
https://doi.org/10.1007/978-3-030-57382-9_29

returned to their sport. The time frame of RTS was between 6 and 13 months [3].

Many factors seem to have an effect on the time and the level of return to sporting activities. RTS rates drop significantly following revision ACL-R compared to primary ACL-R [4, 5]. The incidence of cartilage and meniscal pathology is higher during revision ACL-R compared to primary ACL-R [6]. In addition, medial meniscal pathology and severe cartilage lesions observed during revision ACL-R result in lower RTS rates at pre-injury level in a study with a mean follow-up of 4.6 years [7]. Patient's self-perceived level of function is one of the most important factors affecting RTS outcomes. Werner et al. [8] demonstrated that although there was no significant difference in objective outcome measures between ACL-R patients who returned to sport and patients who did not, subjective measurements in the non-return group were inferior to the RTS group. This indicates that objective testing alone is not adequate to deem someone ready to return to sporting activity. Self-perceived level of function and psychological readiness must be acknowledged by all stakeholders and accounted for in the decision-making process for RTS [8, 9].

29.3 Return to Sport After Osteotomies Around the Knee

High-tibial osteotomy and distal femoral osteotomy are surgical procedures aiming at correcting lower limb joint alignment and assist in the unloading of compromised, or surgically reconstructed knee joint compartments. Osteotomies are typically reserved for young, active individuals who wish to continue to participate in sporting activities and an active lifestyle in general, or for patients for whom arthroplasty is currently not an option [10].

The overall rate of return to sports (RTS) for patients undergoing osteotomy at the knee is quite high. In a recent systematic review and meta-analysis, Hoorntje et al. [11] reported overall RTS rates ranging from 66% to >100%, with >100% indicating that more patients participated in sports post-operatively compared to pre-operative levels of participation. However, the authors also pointed out that RTS rate varied significantly between studies depending on the definition of RTS. If pre-surgery levels of sports participation were used as a reference, RTS rate reached 111% in studies that provided data for pooling. In the studies that used sports participation at a pre-symptomatic status as a reference for comparison, RTS dropped at 85%. This difference can be attributed to the fact that pre-surgery levels of sporting activity are expected to be much lower due to symptoms, compared to sporting activity levels before symptoms start. Only five out of these 16 studies presented a low risk of bias, and the RTS rate in these studies was 82%. In another systematic review by Ekhtiari et al. [12] 19 studies were included and assessed for methodological quality. Overall, 87.2% of patients returned to sport, with 78.6% returning at the same level or greater post-operatively. However, the quality of the included studies was relatively poor, with only one prospective study identified by the reviewers. Overall, patients with osteotomy seem to maintain their number of sports played and the number of sessions per week, while slightly reducing the duration of the session [11]. Patient-reported outcome measures (PROMs) appear to improve significantly in the medium and long term (2–10 years) [13–15], while short-term results (around 1 year) do not seem to change substantially [16].

Despite the high RTS rates reported, several factors that influence the outcome of osteotomy are equivocal. Bonnin et al. [17] concluded that patient motivation is a significant factor in achieving RTS, and Nagel et al. [18] identified the pre-surgery level of sporting activity as the decisive factor in RTS process. However, Saragaglia et al. [15] reported that the RTS rates in their cohort were not affected by patient motivation, or level of sports participation. In addition, type of osteotomy performed (open-wedge vs. closing-wedge, single vs. double osteotomy), pre- and post-surgery knee angle values, age, sex and pre-operative BMI did not seem to affect the RTS rate [15]. However, BMI values >27.5 have been associated with worse outcomes after osteotomy

[19]. Patients and clinicians should be aware that higher BMI values may affect the desired outcome, especially if RTS in high-impact sports is the goal.

Returning to competitive sports is in many cases the desired outcome. While some studies report very low RTS rates at an elite level [12, 17], other studies have demonstrated successful return to competitive high-impact sports [20], although the number of participants in these studies was very low. In general, patients receiving osteotomy are encouraged to participate in sporting activities, albeit at a low-impact level in order to prolong the survival of the procedure. However, the decision to return to competitive high-impact sports should not be ruled-out in advance. An individualised decision-making approach should be used, taking into account the primary indication for performing the osteotomy, the age and motivation of the patient and the complete healing of the osteotomy [11].

29.4 Return to Sport After Meniscal Repair, or Transplantation

The importance of meniscal contribution in maintaining knee joint homeostasis cannot be overstated. That is why surgeons try to maintain as much meniscal tissue as possible by repairing, or even replacing the menisci with appropriately selected allografts. By preserving an acceptable level of meniscal function, the patient can return to his pre-injury levels of activity, whether this is recreational sports, or athletic competitions.

29.4.1 Meniscal Repair

Eberbach et al. [21] reported that 90% of mixed-level athletes returned to sport at the pre-injury level, while 86% of professional athletes returned to the same level of sporting activity as before the injury. In another study on 29 competitive footballers, isolated meniscal repair allowed 92% of athletes to return to pre-injury levels, but if the repair was combined with ACL reconstruction the RTS rate dropped at 86.6% [22]. In the same study, at 6 years follow-up, the RTS rate dropped significantly (isolated repair; 21.4%, combined repair and ACL reconstruction; 33.3%), but this decrease could be attributed to factors unrelated to the surgery, such as the mean age of the cohort at the time of surgery (27 years) and the small sample size. Logan et al. [23] reported that 81% of athletes returned to sports. With respect to paediatric patient population, the results are somewhat equivalent, with RTS rate reaching 88.9% [24]. The results on most studies show that meniscal repairs with concomitant procedures seem to delay RTS compared to isolated repairs [25]. Overall, meniscal repair procedures seem to allow full return to sports, regardless of the level of participation.

29.4.2 Meniscal Allograft Transplantation (MAT)

Patients with minimal viable meniscal tissue remaining, and symptoms arising at the joint line are often candidates for MAT. The procedure offers substantial pain relief and improved quality of life [26, 27] and early reports in the literature supported the return, or initiation of low-impact activities. However, high-impact sports and activities were not frequently recommended due to potential threat on graft longevity and survival [28]. In recent years, a trend towards using MAT in a younger, more active population (including professional athletes in high-demand sports) has been identified. Alentorn-Geli et al. [29] reported on 15 competitive football players with a history of isolated meniscectomies and a follow-up of 2–5 years. Twelve out of 15 players returned to competition (85.7%) and the existence of a cartilage lesion did not seem to affect the outcome measures, although sample size is small. Chalmers et al. [30] in their case series concluded that 77% of 14 mixed-level athletes (high school, semi-professional and professional athletes) returned to their previous level of activity, with 70% stating that they returned to their desired level of activity. In another study, 12 male professional soccer players were evaluated with a maximum follow-up of 36 months. Ninety-two percentage of returned to competition, with median Tegner score improving (from 8 to 10) and IKDC, WOMAC and VAS also improving at 36 months. Seventy-five percentage of players still played professional soccer at 36 months after surgery [31]. In an older age group, Zaffagnini et al. [32] retrospectively reviewed 89 patients undergoing MAT, with a mean follow-up of 4.2 years. Seventy-four percentage returned to sport at an average of 8.6 months, but only 49% of athletes returned to the same level. Tegner scores were improved, but never reached pre-injury levels for this cohort. Age at the time of surgery seemed to negatively affect KOOS and Tegner scores.

Although MAT is considered a salvage procedure, and despite the fact that meniscal allografts are unable to fully restore the biomechanical properties of the native meniscus, the evidence suggests that MAT can substantially improve the quality of life of patients and allow return to at least low-impact sporting activity at any age. Moreover, recent reports in the literature do not exclude the use of MAT in an appropriately selected patient population of high-level athletes, with the intent to return to strenuous sporting activity. However, professional athletes should be appropriately informed about the possible deterioration of their knee status in the long term.

29.5 Return to Sports After Patellofemoral Stabilisation Procedures

Patellofemoral instability is a significant challenge for young and active populations. The lack of universally accepted criteria to return to sports and prior performance has not helped in the development of high-quality studies related to patellar stabilisation with the use of MPFL reconstruction [33]. Fisher et al. [34] reviewed the literature and identified only two studies that reported RTS data. The mean rate of RTS was 77.3% and the time frame to return to sports was between 3 and 6 months. A recent systematic review reported that 84.1% of patients returned to sports, but did not define at what level of participation [35]. In retrospective case series, the RTS rates reported are high. Nelitz et al. [36] in a cohort of paediatric patients reported a RTS rate of 84% at pre-injury levels of participation. Ambrozic and Novak [37] also identified 88.5% RTS rate, but only 69.6% of their patient cohort returned to pre-injury level of sporting activities. Lippacher et al. [38] reported that 100% of their patients returned to some form of sporting activity, but only 53% return to prior level of performance. Data related to RTS following patellar stabilisation using concomitant procedures like MPFL reconstruction combined with lateral release, or tibial tubercle transfer, or other procedures, are sparse in the literature. Some studies report very good outcomes regarding return to activities, but they do not define the level of those activities [39, 40].

29.6 Return to Sports After Cartilage Repair Procedures

One of the most exciting tasks in orthopaedics and rehabilitation specialties is to achieve the goal of returning to sports after a surgical procedure for a knee cartilage defect(s). Various techniques have been developed and extensively tested during the last 2–3 decades for the treatment of knee cartilage defects. The range is from palliative to restoring to regenerating methods, from bone marrow stimulation to autologous chondrocyte implantation or osteochondral transfer (auto- or allograft).

A very important parameter, which is not investigated extensively, is the difference between returning to activity and sports or performance [1], although several papers present results for returning to sports after cartilage surgery either prospectively or retrospectively [41–47] or in meta-analyses [48–50].

Bias can be elicited by the heterogeneity of the population in terms of age and sport involvement, age and concomitant procedures [50]. Overall 76% return to sports rate in medium-term follow-up has been presented in 2549 patients [50] ranging from 58% for Mfxs to 93% for

OATS, well in line with a previous publication by Mithoefer et al. [48] with 73% RTS in 1363 patients.

29.6.1 RTP After Debridement

Many surgeons consider simple arthroscopic debridement the first line of treatment in cartilage defects, as this offers symptoms relief and faster return to activities, without burning any bridges. It is reserved for low demanding patients and for high-level athletes as well [51–56], but this approach is not included in published treatment protocols as there is still lack of sound evidence. Faster and high rate of return in the pre-injury level (2.7 months and 100% respectively) were observed, though without long follow-up (1.6 years) [57].

29.6.2 RTP After Bone Marrow Stimulation

Mithoefer and Steadman [58] reported 95% RTS rate in 21 professional soccer players at same level in mean time of 8 months. Meanwhile, in their systematic review for 611 patients the RTS rate was calculated at 67% (±6%), 67% returning at the same level, in 8 (±1) months and continued playing for 2–5 years at 51% (±9%). Other reviews showed RTS rate from 66% (±6%) [48] to 75% [59] and up to 82% when combined with ACL reconstruction [60]. In the most recently published meta-analysis of return to sports after cartilage surgery, Krych et al. found 58% RTS rate in 858 patients out of 19 studies [50], with the results deteriorating from 2 to 5 years.

29.6.3 RTP After Osteochondral Transfer

Patients treated with autologous osteochondral transfer and mosaicplasty managed to have good and excellent results in 89% of cases and returned to sports at same level in 67% according to Panics et al. [61] in a long follow-up cohort in professional soccer players. Similar results were published by Gudas et al. [45] and Marcacci [62] (93% and 73% respectively). Campbell et al. in their systematic review presented 89% and 88% RTS after OAT and OCA, respectively [59]. Krych et al. in their meta-analysis [50] presented 93% RTS after OAT in 300 patients in level 1, 3 and 4 studies.

In the same publication, good results are also yielded by osteochondral allograft transplantation, with 88% RTS, while the most recent paper presented 80% return to play and at the same level, as well, in Elite basketball players [63].

29.6.4 RTP After Autologous Chondrocyte Implantation

Autologous chondrocyte implantation is considered to be the golden standard technique in the treatment of large cartilage defects, having the major drawback of prolonged time to full recovery. Several studies support the mid- and long-term durability of the result after ACI compared to other procedures, especially microfractures. Return to sport after ACI is not only feasible but also in high percentage ranging from 33% [64] to 86% [41]. Krych et al. in their recent meta-analysis presented 83% RTS in approximately 1360 patients out of level 1–4 studies [50], while previous systematic review published by Mithoefer et al. showed 67% return rates for 362 patients [48]. Patients submitted to autologous chondrocyte implantation seem to sustain long-term durability of the result and high rate of return to sport. Both the above-mentioned parameters lead to the conclusion that ACI needs to be considered as first line treatment for KNEE PRESERVATION and RESTORATION of function when all joint pathology is addressed and homeostasis is established.

In summary, return to play following salvage procedures in the knee is possible; however, further high-quality research is needed in order to provide more accurate information on objective and subjective evaluation of RTS rates. In addition, it is important to establish universal consensus on outcome measures utilised in studies of various conditions and to agree on specific criteria for progression to return to sport and, in some cases, return to prior performance.

References

1. Ardern CL, et al. 2016 Consensus statement on return to sport from the First World Congress in Sports Physical Therapy, Bern. Br J Sports Med. 2016;50(14):853–64.
2. Ardern CL, et al. Fifty-five per cent return to competitive sport following anterior cruciate ligament reconstruction surgery: an updated systematic review and meta-analysis including aspects of physical functioning and contextual factors. Br J Sports Med. 2014;48(21):1543–52.
3. Lai CCH, et al. Eighty-three per cent of elite athletes return to preinjury sport after anterior cruciate ligament reconstruction: a systematic review with meta-analysis of return to sport rates, graft rupture rates and performance outcomes. Br J Sports Med. 2018;52(2):128–38.
4. Anand BS, et al. Return-to-sport outcomes after revision anterior cruciate ligament reconstruction surgery. Am J Sports Med. 2016;44(3):580–4.
5. Grassi A, et al. After revision anterior cruciate ligament reconstruction, who returns to sport? A systematic review and meta-analysis. Br J Sports Med. 2015;49(20):1295–304.
6. Wright RW, et al. Outcome of revision anterior cruciate ligament reconstruction: a systematic review. J Bone Joint Surg Am. 2012;94(6):531–6.
7. Webster KE, et al. Medial meniscal and chondral pathology at the time of revision anterior cruciate ligament reconstruction results in inferior mid-term patient-reported outcomes. Knee Surg Sports Traumatol Arthrosc. 2018;26(4):1059–64.
8. Werner JL, et al. Decision to return to sport participation after anterior cruciate ligament reconstruction, part II: self-reported and functional performance outcomes. J Athl Train. 2018;53(5):464–74.
9. Ardern CL, et al. Return to the preinjury level of competitive sport after anterior cruciate ligament reconstruction surgery: two-thirds of patients have not returned by 12 months after surgery. Am J Sports Med. 2011;39(3):538–43.
10. Brinkman JM, et al. Osteotomies around the knee: patient selection, stability of fixation and bone healing in high tibial osteotomies. J Bone Joint Surg Br. 2008;90(12):1548–57.
11. Hoorntje A, et al. High rates of return to sports activities and work after osteotomies around the knee: a systematic review and meta-analysis. Sports Med. 2017;47(11):2219–44.
12. Ekhtiari S, et al. Return to work and sport following high tibial osteotomy: a systematic review. J Bone Joint Surg Am. 2016;98(18):1568–77.
13. Voleti PB, et al. Successful return to sport following distal femoral varus osteotomy. Cartilage. 2017;10(1):19–25.
14. Salzmann GM, et al. Sporting activity after high tibial osteotomy for the treatment of medial compartment knee osteoarthritis. Am J Sports Med. 2009;37(2):312–8.
15. Saragaglia D, et al. Return to sports after valgus osteotomy of the knee joint in patients with medial unicompartmental osteoarthritis. Int Orthop. 2014;38(10):2109–14.
16. Bastard C, et al. Return to sports and quality of life after high tibial osteotomy in patients under 60 years of age. Orthop Traumatol Surg Res. 2017;103(8):1189–91.
17. Bonnin MP, et al. Can patients really participate in sport after high tibial osteotomy? Knee Surg Sports Traumatol Arthrosc. 2013;21(1):64–73.
18. Nagel A, Insall JN, Scuderi GR. Proximal tibial osteotomy. A subjective outcome study. J Bone Joint Surg Am. 1996;78(9):1353–8.
19. Akizuki S, et al. The long-term outcome of high tibial osteotomy: a ten- to 20-year follow-up. J Bone Joint Surg Br. 2008;90(5):592–6.
20. Warme BA, Aalderink K, Amendola A. Is there a role for high tibial osteotomies in the athlete? Sports Health. 2011;3(1):59–69.
21. Eberbach H, et al. Sport-specific outcomes after isolated meniscal repair: a systematic review. Knee Surg Sports Traumatol Arthrosc. 2018;26(3):762–71.
22. Alvarez-Diaz P, et al. Return to play after all-inside meniscal repair in competitive football players: a minimum 5-year follow-up. Knee Surg Sports Traumatol Arthrosc. 2016;24(6):1997–2001.
23. Logan M, et al. Meniscal repair in the elite athlete: results of 45 repairs with a minimum 5-year follow-up. Am J Sports Med. 2009;37(6):1131–4.
24. Vanderhave KL, et al. Meniscus tears in the young athlete: results of arthroscopic repair. J Pediatr Orthop. 2011;31(5):496–500.
25. Lee YS, Lee OS, Lee SH. Return to sports after athletes undergo meniscal surgery: a systematic review. Clin J Sport Med. 2019;29(1):29–36.
26. Elattar M, et al. Twenty-six years of meniscal allograft transplantation: is it still experimental? A meta-analysis of 44 trials. Knee Surg Sports Traumatol Arthrosc. 2011;19(2):147–57.
27. Stone KR, et al. Meniscus transplantation in an active population with moderate to severe cartilage damage. Knee Surg Sports Traumatol Arthrosc. 2015;23(1):251–7.
28. Noyes FR, Barber-Westin SD, Rankin M. Meniscal transplantation in symptomatic patients less than fifty years old. J Bone Joint Surg Am. 2004;86-A(7):1392–404.

29. Alentorn-Geli E, et al. Arthroscopic meniscal transplants in soccer players: outcomes at 2- to 5-year follow-up. Clin J Sport Med. 2010;20(5):340–3.
30. Chalmers PN, et al. Return to high-level sport after meniscal allograft transplantation. Arthroscopy. 2013;29(3):539–44.
31. Marcacci M, et al. Arthroscopic meniscus allograft transplantation in male professional soccer players: a 36-month follow-up study. Am J Sports Med. 2014;42(2):382–8.
32. Zaffagnini S, et al. Is sport activity possible after arthroscopic meniscal allograft transplantation? Midterm results in active patients. Am J Sports Med. 2016;44(3):625–32.
33. Sherman SL, et al. Return to play after patellar stabilization. Curr Rev Musculoskelet Med. 2018;11(2):280–4.
34. Fisher B, et al. Medial patellofemoral ligament reconstruction for recurrent patellar dislocation: a systematic review including rehabilitation and return-to-sports efficacy. Arthroscopy. 2010;26(10):1384–94.
35. Schneider DK, et al. Outcomes after isolated medial patellofemoral ligament reconstruction for the treatment of recurrent lateral patellar dislocations: a systematic review and meta-analysis. Am J Sports Med. 2016;44(11):2993–3005.
36. Nelitz M, Dreyhaupt J, Williams SRM. Anatomic reconstruction of the medial patellofemoral ligament in children and adolescents using a pedicled quadriceps tendon graft shows favourable results at a minimum of 2-year follow-up. Knee Surg Sports Traumatol Arthrosc. 2018;26(4):1210–5.
37. Ambrozic B, Novak S. The influence of medial patellofemoral ligament reconstruction on clinical results and sports activity level. Phys Sportsmed. 2016;44(2):133–40.
38. Lippacher S, et al. Reconstruction of the medial patellofemoral ligament: clinical outcomes and return to sports. Am J Sports Med. 2014;42(7):1661–8.
39. Tjoumakaris FP, Forsythe B, Bradley JP. Patellofemoral instability in athletes: treatment via modified Fulkerson osteotomy and lateral release. Am J Sports Med. 2010;38(5):992–9.
40. Ntagiopoulos PG, Byn P, Dejour D. Midterm results of comprehensive surgical reconstruction including sulcus-deepening trochleoplasty in recurrent patellar dislocations with high-grade trochlear dysplasia. Am J Sports Med. 2013;41(5):998–1004.
41. Kon E, et al. Articular cartilage treatment in high-level male soccer players: a prospective comparative study of arthroscopic second-generation autologous chondrocyte implantation versus microfracture. Am J Sports Med. 2011;39(12):2549–57.
42. Steadman JR, et al. The microfracture technique in the treatment of full-thickness chondral lesions of the knee in National Football League players. J Knee Surg. 2003;16(2):83–6.
43. Gobbi A, Nunag P, Malinowski K. Treatment of full thickness chondral lesions of the knee with microfracture in a group of athletes. Knee Surg Sports Traumatol Arthrosc. 2005;13(3):213–21.
44. Gudas R, et al. A prospective randomized clinical study of mosaic osteochondral autologous transplantation versus microfracture for the treatment of osteochondral defects in the knee joint in young athletes. Arthroscopy. 2005;21(9):1066–75.
45. Gudas R, et al. Osteochondral autologous transplantation versus microfracture for the treatment of articular cartilage defects in the knee joint in athletes. Knee Surg Sports Traumatol Arthrosc. 2006;14(9):834–42.
46. Kon E, et al. Arthroscopic second-generation autologous chondrocyte implantation compared with microfracture for chondral lesions of the knee: prospective nonrandomized study at 5 years. Am J Sports Med. 2009;37(1):33–41.
47. Mithoefer K, et al. High-impact athletics after knee articular cartilage repair: a prospective evaluation of the microfracture technique. Am J Sports Med. 2006;34(9):1413–8.
48. Mithoefer K, et al. Return to sports participation after articular cartilage repair in the knee: scientific evidence. Am J Sports Med. 2009;37(Suppl 1):167S–76S.
49. Steinwachs MR, Engebretsen L, Brophy RH. Scientific evidence base for cartilage injury and repair in the athlete. Cartilage. 2012;3(1 Suppl):11S–7S.
50. Krych AJ, et al. Return to sport after the surgical management of articular cartilage lesions in the knee: a meta-analysis. Knee Surg Sports Traumatol Arthrosc. 2017;25(10):3186–96.
51. Baumgaertner MR, et al. Arthroscopic debridement of the arthritic knee. Clin Orthop Relat Res. 1990;253:197–202.
52. Fond J, et al. Arthroscopic debridement for the treatment of osteoarthritis of the knee: 2- and 5-year results. Arthroscopy. 2002;18(8):829–34.
53. Spahn G, Hofmann GO, Klinger HM. The effects of arthroscopic joint debridement in the knee osteoarthritis: results of a meta-analysis. Knee Surg Sports Traumatol Arthrosc. 2013;21(7):1553–61.
54. McCormick F, et al. Trends in the surgical treatment of articular cartilage lesions in the United States: an analysis of a large private-payer database over a period of 8 years. Arthroscopy. 2014;30(2):222–6.
55. Solheim E, et al. Symptoms and function in patients with articular cartilage lesions in 1,000 knee arthroscopies. Knee Surg Sports Traumatol Arthrosc. 2016;24(5):1610–6.
56. Oliver-Welsh L, et al. Deciding how best to treat cartilage defects. Orthopedics. 2016;39(6):343–50.
57. Levy AS, et al. Chondral delamination of the knee in soccer players. Am J Sports Med. 1996;24(5):634–9.
58. Mithoefer K, Steadman RJ. Microfracture in football (soccer) players: a case series of professional athletes and systematic review. Cartilage. 2012;3(1 Suppl):18S–24S.
59. Campbell AB, et al. Return to sport after articular cartilage repair in athletes' knees: a systematic review. Arthroscopy. 2016;32(4):651–68 e1.

60. Gudas R, et al. Comparison of osteochondral autologous transplantation, microfracture, or debridement techniques in articular cartilage lesions associated with anterior cruciate ligament injury: a prospective study with a 3-year follow-up. Arthroscopy. 2013;29(1):89–97.
61. Panics G, et al. Osteochondral autograft and mosaicplasty in the football (soccer) athlete. Cartilage. 2012;3(1 Suppl):25S–30S.
62. Marcacci M, et al. Multiple osteochondral arthroscopic grafting (mosaicplasty) for cartilage defects of the knee: prospective study results at 2-year follow-up. Arthroscopy. 2005;21(4):462–70.
63. Balazs GC, et al. Return to play among elite basketball players after osteochondral allograft transplantation of full-thickness cartilage lesions. Orthop J Sports Med. 2018;6(7):2325967118786941.
64. Mithofer K, et al. Articular cartilage repair in soccer players with autologous chondrocyte transplantation: functional outcome and return to competition. Am J Sports Med. 2005;33(11):1639–46.

Part III

Ankle

Ankle Joint Cartilage Pathology and Repair

30

Yoshiharu Shimozono, Ashraf M. Fansa, and John G. Kennedy

30.1 Introduction

Articular cartilage is a highly specialized connective tissue that serves to lubricate joint surfaces and distribute loads across the joint. Articular cartilage injury is a significant cause of pain and dysfunction that may eventually lead to posttraumatic arthritis. Management of these injuries is complicated by the complex architecture and poor vascularity of this tissue. As technology has improved over the years, the field of articular cartilage restoration has evolved rapidly and more options have become available to treat these injuries. However, a clear gold standard in management is yet to emerge, and treatment of osteochondral lesions remains challenging. Current concepts of surgical treatments, outcomes, and the potential use of biological augmentation for the management of cartilage injuries of the ankle are reviewed in this chapter.

30.1.1 Pathology

Osteochondral lesions of the talus (OLT) are a common ankle pathology and have been shown to occur in over 65% of patients presenting with chronic ankle sprains and 75% of ankle fractures [1, 2]. OLT are often associated with athletes but can also present in the general population. The widely accepted hypothesis is that articular cartilage damage leads to subchondral bone exposure to high intra-articular hydrostatic pressures during ambulation. Prolonged exposure may in turn lead to the development of subchondral bone sclerosis, osteolysis, and eventually cysts and large defects. This weakened subchondral bone is less likely to support the overlying cartilage, leading to more cartilage damage and collapse. Since cartilage is aneural, pain is most probably propagated by the repetitive high fluid pressures within the joint which irritate the highly innervated subchondral bone [3].

The most common locations for OLT are thought to be the central-medial and the central-lateral aspects of the talar dome [4]. Lateral lesions are mostly associated with trauma and are usually shallow and oval in shape [3]. In contrast, medial lesions are less frequently associated with acute trauma, and are usually deep and cup-shaped, indicating a mechanism of torsional impaction and axial loading [3]. Even though significant interest has gathered over the last several years regarding treatment of OLT, its pathogenesis is still not fully understood. While the pathology is widely accepted to be a sequela of trauma, nontraumatic etiologies such as metabolic and endocrine abnormalities as well as congenital factors have also been suggested [5]. Interestingly,

Y. Shimozono · A. M. Fansa · J. G. Kennedy (✉)
Department of Foot and Ankle, Hospital for Special Surgery, New York, NY, USA
e-mail: fansaa@hss.edu; kennedyj@hss.edu

M. Brittberg, K. Slynarski (eds.), *Lower Extremity Joint Preservation*,
https://doi.org/10.1007/978-3-030-57382-9_30

a significantly higher incidence of OLT has been reported in siblings, suggesting a hereditary component may be contributing [6]. In fact, a missense mutation in the Aggrecan C-type Lectin domain on chromosome 15, responsible for dominant familial osteochondral lesions, was lately identified [7]. Only 10% of patients overall have been found to have a contralateral OLT [8].

Symptomatic OLT often require surgical intervention. Both reparative and replacement surgeries currently used in the treatment of OLT will be discussed as an evidence-based evaluation.

30.2 Treatments

30.2.1 Bone Marrow Stimulation (BMS): Microfracture/Drilling

Microfracture is a reparative technique, where the subchondral bone in the defect is perforated using microfracture awls or drills to release mesenchymal stem cells and growth factors from the bone marrow. This in turn leads to the formation of fibrous cartilage repair tissue. It is traditionally indicated for lesions smaller than 150 mm^2 in area or 15 mm in diameter [9, 10]. However, a recent systematic review demonstrated that microfracture may be optimal for lesions smaller than 100 mm^2 in area and/or 10 mm in diameter [11]. This procedure is low-cost, technically straightforward, and minimally invasive. There are, however, several disadvantages, including the quality of fibrocartilage repair tissue which is inherently inferior to native hyaline cartilage, damage to the subchondral bone, and deterioration of the fibrocartilage grout over time [12].

Microfracture is typically performed arthroscopically through anteromedial and anterolateral portals. The defect is prepared prior by debriding the degenerated cartilage using a ring curette or shaver, and then the layer of calcified cartilage should be carefully removed. Vertical shoulders of stable cartilage should be created [13]. Microfracture is then performed by penetrating the subchondral bone using microfracture awls with various tip angles. The awl providing the most perpendicular angle to the OLT should be chosen. Microfracture holes should be placed 3–4 mm apart to minimize damage to the subchondral bone. An awl of 1 mm or less should be used [14]. After the holes have been created, the tourniquet may be released and arthroscopic inflow turned off to assess for bleeding and fat droplet extrusion. Biological adjuncts, such as platelet rich plasma (PRP) or concentrated bone marrow aspirates (CBMA), which may have the potential to improve the quality of the fibrocartilage repair tissue, may be injected intra-articularly (Fig. 30.1).

Several systematic reviews have demonstrated favorable short- to mid-term outcomes following BMS, with typically >85% of patients reporting good to excellent clinical outcomes [15, 16]. A recent systematic review reports 86.8% of patients returning to previous level of sports at a mean duration of 4.5 months [17].

Despite successful outcomes following BMS for OLT in the short- and mid-term, there is some concern over deterioration of the fibrocartilage repair tissue over time, which may potentially affect the clinical outcomes in the long term [18, 19]. Ferkel et al. reported deterioration of clinical outcome scores in up to 35% of patients within 5 years following BMS [18]. Lee et al. found that only 30% of patients had lesion integration on second look arthroscopy at 12 months post BMS

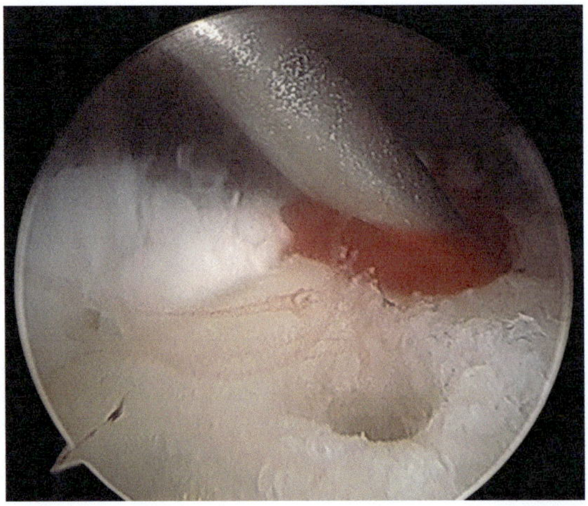

Fig. 30.1 CBMA injection applied into the defect following microfracture

[20]. Furthermore, van Bergen et al. reported that 33% of patients showed progression of ankle arthritis by one grade on plain radiographs at a mean follow-up of 141 months [21].

Mechanically, regenerated fibrocartilage has been shown to be inferior to hyaline cartilage and thus deteriorates over time [22]. Recent studies have increasingly focused on the subchondral bone, which provides the foundation for the overlying articular cartilage [23]. Seow et al. found in a systematic review that subchondral bone was not likely to be restored once damaged by BMS procedures [19]. Similarly, Shimozono et al. recently reported that subchondral bone was not restored following microfracture of OLT and that there was a clear development of subchondral cysts. Furthermore, subchondral bone damage at mid-term follow-up was associated with poorer clinical outcomes [12]. Therefore, techniques minimizing damage to the subchondral bone may be beneficial to the longevity of the reparative cartilage. This has been underscored by a recent translational animal model where the use of small-diameter awls offered improved articular cartilage repair on histological examination compared to large-diameter awls which created greater subchondral bone trauma [24].

30.2.2 Cartilage Allograft Augmentation

In an attempt to improve quality of the cartilage regenerate, particulated juvenile cartilage allograft (PCA) (DeNovo NT; Zimmer Biomet, Inc) and micronized cartilage allograft (MCA) (BioCartilage; Arthrex, Inc) are currently being used in clinical practice for microfracture augmentation. PCA is theoretically advantageous as an adjunct to microfracture, as the high metabolic activity level and differential gene expression may have the potential to produce more hyaline cartilage than adult chondrocytes. However, no animal studies investigating the histological or structural behavior of PCA implantation in osteochondral defects have been published to date. Karnovsky et al. performed a retrospective comparative study assessing the results of patients treated with microfracture and PCA versus those treated with microfracture alone [25]. At a mean follow-up of 30 months the authors found that both groups still showed fibrocartilaginous growth that did not appear normal on MRI. Furthermore, there was no difference in functional outcomes between the two groups at final follow-up. Therefore, the role of PCA remains to be determined, and further long-term high-level studies are warranted.

MCA contains allogeneic extracellular matrix including type II collagen, proteoglycans, and cartilaginous growth factors. MCA is theoretically advantageous as an adjunct to microfracture, by inciting the migration of stem cells to the defect site. They are thought to induce chondrogenesis by acting as a tissue network facilitator promoting cellular interaction. In an equine model with up to 13 months follow-up, Fortier et al. reported that MCA mixed with PRP improved the quality of cartilage repair tissue compared to microfracture alone [26]. In clinical studies, Ahmad et al. reported a case series of 30 patients with an average lesion size of 1.1 cm^2. At a mean follow-up of 20.2 months, the mean Foot and Ankle Ability Measure (FAAM) improved from 51 preoperatively to 89 out of 100 postoperatively, and the mean visual analog scale (VAS) for pain decreased from 8.1 preoperatively to 1.7 postoperatively [27]. However, the literature is void of studies comparing microfracture plus MCA application to microfracture alone. In addition, a recent systematic review revealed that the available studies were of limited data in both PCA and MCA [28]. Therefore, long-term high-level studies are warranted to justify its current widespread use.

30.2.3 Autologous Osteochondral Transplantation

Autologous osteochondral transplantation (AOT) is a replacement technique. The procedure is performed by transferring a cylindrical osteochondral graft, typically harvested from a non-weightbearing portion of the ipsilateral knee, into the appropriately prepared defect site on the talus. It is typically indicated for larger (>10 mm or 10 mm^2), highly cystic lesions that failed previous microfracture [11, 29]. AOT offers the advantage of replacing lesions with viable hyaline cartilage and subchondral bone without the need for a two-stage procedure. Lesion containment, the need for two or more graft plugs, previous BMS, and body mass index may be considered prognostic factors when performing an AOT [30–33]. AOT has several potential disadvantages, including donor site morbidity, the possible need for an osteotomy to access the talar dome, and differences in cartilage biology between the recipient and donor tissues [34].

The OLT can be accessed through a medial or lateral osteotomy depending on the location of the lesion. For medial lesions, a medial malleolar osteotomy may be utilized to adequately reach the lesion. A Chevron-osteotomy is preferred for this approach as it provides appropriate alignment, stability, a large surface area for healing and greater visualization [34]. For lateral lesions, an anterolateral tibial osteotomy may be utilized [35]. Anterior lesions are usually sufficiently exposed through a simple anterior ankle arthrotomy without an osteotomy.

After the lesion is visualized, a trephine is utilized to remove the damaged cartilage and underlying subchondral bone. Multiple donor sites are available for graft harvesting. Our preferred technique is to harvest from the non-weightbearing portion of the ipsilateral lateral femoral condyle as it is technically undemanding to access and the topography closely matches that of the talar dome. Larger lesions may require two grafts, which should be “nested” next to each other to reduce area of fibrocartilage formation [34]. Prior to graft placement, biological adjuncts such as PRP or CBMA are added. Those may improve cartilage repair, reduce cyst formation, and improve subchondral bone incorporation [34, 36]. The final graft position should be as flush as possible with the surrounding native articular surface (Figs. 30.2 and 30.3).

Multiple studies have reported promising outcomes following AOT for OLT. A recent systematic review by Shimozono et al. reported that 87% of patients had good to excellent outcomes at mid-term follow-up [33]. In an athletic population, Fraser et al. found that 90% of professional athletes and 87% of recreational athletes were able to fully return to preinjury activity levels at a mean follow-up of 24 months [37]. However, in a study by Paul et al., patients engaged in

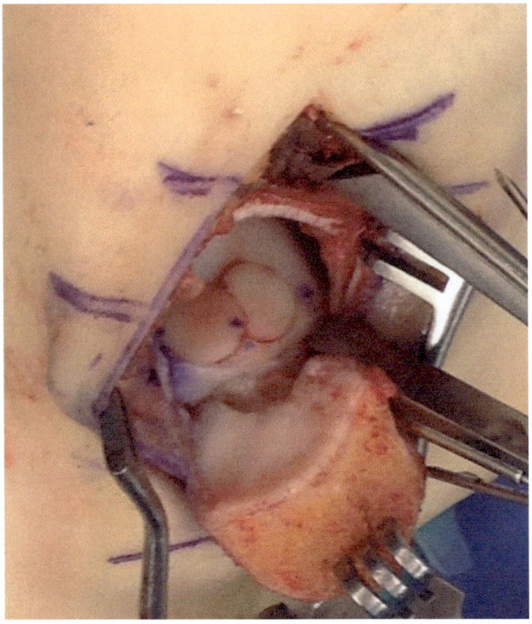

Fig. 30.2 Double osteochondral autograft transplantation into a prepared recipient site

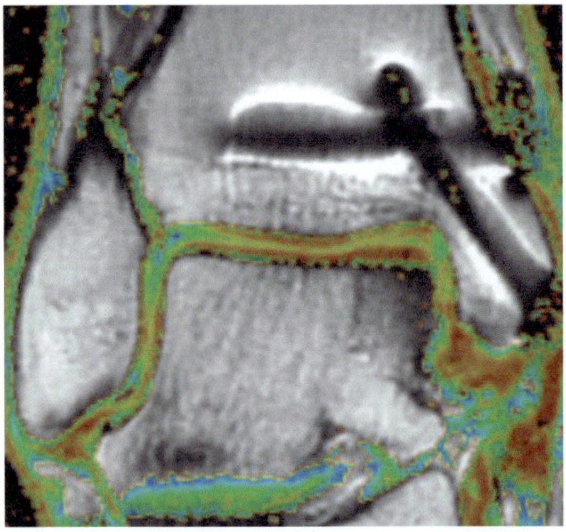

Fig. 30.3 Coronal T2 mapping image showing normal stratification of the interface between the graft and the adjacent native articular cartilage

high-impact and contact sports required partial modification of sporting activities and a reduction in participation [38]. There is still a lack of evidence regarding the long-term outcomes following AOT for OLT.

The most common complication with AOT is donor site morbidity [33]. Yoon et al. found that 9% patients had early donor site morbidity, all of which had resolved at 2 years [39]. Fraser et al. found a 5% donor site morbidity rate at a mean 41.8 months follow-up [40].

Another potential concern is the tibial osteotomy. However, Lamb et al. demonstrated that when utilizing a Chevron-type osteotomy with three screw fixation, 94% of patients were asymptomatic at the osteotomy site with satisfactory healing on T2 mapping MRI [41]. Postoperative cysts have been shown to occur in up to 65% of patients following AOT prompting some concern. Savage-Elliott et al., however, reported that the clinical impact of cyst formation was not found to be significant at a mean follow-up of 15 months [42]. Gül et al. also reported that subchondral cyst formation did not appear to affect clinical outcomes following AOT [43]. Shimozono et al. found that only 1% of patients undergoing AOT were considered a clinical failure at mean follow-up of 5 years, indicating that AOT may have promise for long-term survival [33].

30.2.4 Osteochondral Allograft Transplantation

Osteochondral allograft transplantation is a similar replacement procedure in which an articular cartilage and bone graft are obtained from a cadaveric donor. There are two types of osteochondral allograft:

- Bulk types.
- Cylindrical plug types.

Bulk allograft is generally considered a salvage procedure when previous surgeries have failed but can also be performed as a first line procedure for larger lesions. Cylindrical plug transplantation has similar indications to AOT but is usually preferred over AOT in the presence of knee osteoarthritis, a history of knee infection, and in patients concerned with donor site morbidity in the knee. There are several disadvantages to allograft, including:

- Potential higher failure rate.
- Increased cost.
- Disease transmission.
- Differences in immunology/cartilage biology between the host and cadaveric tissues [44, 45].

Studies have found mixed clinical outcomes following osteochondral allograft transplantation for OLT. The results of osteochondral allograft transplantation differ whether it is a bulk or cylindrical plug allograft. Bulk allograft recipients may experience poorer long-term outcomes due to the larger lesion size being treated, but often these are salvage procedures and the short- to medium-term clinical benefit may be worthwhile for the patient. In a systematic review of 91 OLTs treated with bulk allograft, VanTienderen et al. report average AOFAS and pain VAS score improvements from 48 to 80 and 7.1–2.7, respectively, at a mean follow-up of 45 months [45]. Raikin et al. found in 15 patients treated with bulk allograft at a mean of 54 months that the mean VAS score improved from 8.5 to 3.3 and the mean AOFAS score improved from 38 to 83, with 11 patients reporting good/excellent results [46]. However, two patients required conversion to arthrodesis. On plain radiographs, some evidence of collapse or graft resorption were found in 67% of patients. El-Rashidy et al. showed utilizing cylindrical plug allografts for the treatment of OLT significantly improved clinical outcomes at a mean follow-up of 3 years, although there was a 10.4% failure rate over this time period [47]. Ahmad et al. found similar clinical outcomes following cylindrical plug allograft and autograft implantation for OLT at 35.2 months [48]. In contrast, Shimozono et al. found significantly poorer clinical and MRI outcomes in cylindrical allograft than autograft [49]. The rate of chondral wear on MRI was higher with allograft than with autograft, and allograft-treated patients had a significantly higher rate of clinical failure (25%).

30.2.5 Autologous Chondrocyte Implantation

ACI is a cell-based, two-stage procedure in which healthy articular cartilage is harvested, the chondrocytes isolated from the harvest are cultured and then implanted into the defect site at a later date [50]. ACI aims to regenerate damaged cartilage with hyaline-like tissue and is indicated in larger lesions or revision procedures following a failed primary procedure. However, the disadvantages of ACI include the need for two surgical procedures, increased cost and potential morbidity and decreased graft durability [51].

In the first step of the procedure, chondrocytes are harvested from the ankle, the osteochondral fragment itself or the ipsilateral knee [52]. The cells are then cultured and expanded for 2–3 weeks. After the process of cell culturing is complete, the patient returns for a second procedure to implant the cultured chondrocytes, either arthroscopically or via an open procedure. The recipient site is first prepared by debridement of the OLT and any associated cysts. In larger subchondral cystic defects, a "sandwich" technique can be employed where autologous bone graft obtained from the proximal or distal tibia, iliac crest, or calcaneus is packed into the defect, followed by placement of two periosteal patches typically taken from the proximal or distal tibia. The periosteal patch is typically 1–2 mm larger than the defect to account for shrinkage. The first periosteal patch is sewn over the bone graft with the cambium side up then sealed with fibrin glue. The other patch is sewn over this with the cambium side down and again sealed with fibrin glue.

In a recent systematic review, Niemeyer et al. evaluated the effectiveness of ACI for OLT treatment and reported a clinical success rate of 89.9% in 213 patients [53]. Battaglia et al. evaluated 20 patients following ACI at a mean follow-up of 5 years and found that the mean AOFAS score improved from 59 preoperatively to 84 postoperatively [54]. On MRI T2 mapping, the authors found that all patients demonstrated values consistent with normal hyaline cartilage. Giannini et al. reported clinical and MRI findings at 10-years follow-up following ACI treatment for OLT [51]. This study included ten OLT patients with a mean lesion size of 3.1 cm^2. At the final follow-up timepoint the AOFAS scores improved from 37.9 preoperatively to 92.7 postoperatively. MRI scans demonstrated well-modeled restoration of the articular surface.

30.2.6 Scaffold-Based Therapies

30.2.6.1 Matrix-Induced Autologous Chondrocyte Implantation (MACI)

MACI is a third-generation version of ACI also involving a two-step procedure, where a biodegradable polymer scaffold embedded with chondrocytes is utilized. The scaffold typically contains type I/III collagen, hyaluronan, and polyglycolic/polylactic acid [55]. The traditional ACI procedure had some concerns with harvesting and suturing of the periosteum, delamination of the graft, and periosteal hypertrophy [56]. However, MACI avoids issues related to periosteal graft harvest and does not require fixation with sutures as it is a self-adherent scaffold.

Aurich et al. reported on the results of 19 patients treated with MACI, and observed improvement of the AOFAS score from 58.6 to 80.4 at a final follow-up of 24 months [57]. In the athletic population, 81% of patients returned to sports after MACI, of which 56% returned to preinjury level. Similarly, Magnan et al. showed improvement in the mean AOFAS score from 36.9 to 83.9 in 36 patients, with 18 returning to sports within 2 months [58]. Giannini et al. evaluated 46 ankles with a mean follow-up of 87.2 months [59]. The authors reported a mean AOFAS score of 92 at final follow-up. Among the 29 patients who participated in sports, 20 returned to preinjury sporting levels, three resumed the same sport but at a lower level, two shifted to a noncontact sport, and four patients gave up sports. Four professional soccer players who were included in the study were all able to resume their previous levels of activity.

30.2.6.2 Autologous Matrix-Induced Chondrogenesis (AMIC)

AMIC is a one-step scaffold-based procedure in which BMS is performed on the OLT followed by placement of a porcine collagen I/III matrix over the defect. The supporting theory is that porcine collagen matrix supports the growth of cartilage following microfracture.

The literature on AMIC is limited to a few small case series, but the results seem promising. Wiewiorski et al. investigated the outcomes of 23 patients at a mean follow-up duration of 23 months. At that final timepoint mean AOFAS scores had improved from 60.3 to 90.0 and MOCART scores had a mean of 62.6 [60]. The authors also observed a significant difference in T1 relaxation times between the repair tissue and reference cartilage, suggesting a lower glycosaminoglycan (GAG) content in AMIC-supported repair tissue. In a recent case series by Valderrabano et al., the mean AOFAS score improved from 60 to 89 in 26 patients who underwent AMIC [61]. The authors reported that 35% of patients had complete filling of the defect and 84% of patients had normal or near-normal signal intensity of the repair tissue compared with the adjacent native cartilage on MRI. They also assessed the athletic population within their study group and observed that 45% of patients participating in sports before surgery had returned to their previous level of activity at final follow-up.

30.2.6.3 Bone Marrow-Derived Cell Transplantation (BMDCT)

Bone marrow-derived cell transplantation (BMDCT) is a one-step procedure involving the implantation of a concentrated bone marrow aspirate (CBMA) impregnated scaffold material into an OLT. BMDCT is theoretically beneficial as the mesenchymal stem cells and growth factors in CBMA support the scaffold in chondrogenesis, to develop hyaline-like cartilage at the defect site.

Several clinical studies have shown improvement in clinical outcomes when utilizing this procedure. Vannini et al. reported on 140 athletes treated with BMDCT at a mean follow-up of 48 months, and found the overall mean AOFAS score to improve from 58.7 to 90.9 [62]. The authors also showed that 72.8% of athletes were able to return to preinjury level of sports. Buda et al. compared the clinical outcomes of two groups of patients who underwent either ACI or BMDCT for OLT [63]. There was no significant difference in clinical outcomes at 48 months follow-up, but the rate of return to sports was slightly higher in the BMDCT group. However, this difference did not achieve statistical significance. The results suggest that BMDCT may be a viable alternative to ACI, with the advantage of being a single-stage procedure.

30.2.7 Biologic-Based Therapies

30.2.7.1 Platelet-Rich Plasma (PRP)

PRP is an autologous blood product that contains at least twice the concentration of platelets above the baseline value, or $>1.1 \times 10^6$ platelets/μl. PRP contains an increased number of growth factors and bioactive cytokines, including transforming growth factor, vascular endothelial growth factor, fibroblast growth factor, and platelet-derived growth factor [64].

The current basic science evidence suggests that PRP has positive effects on the cartilage repair process. Smyth et al. performed a systematic review and found that 18 of 21 (85.7%) basic science studies reported positive effects of PRP on cartilage repair, thus establishing a proof of concept [65]. Additionally, Smyth et al. found that the application of PRP at the time of AOT improved the integration of the osteochondral graft at the cartilage interface and decreased graft degeneration in a rabbit model [66]. In clinical investigations, several comparative studies have examined the use of PRP for OLT. In a randomized prospective control trial, Guney et al. found that the group receiving BMS with PRP for OLT had better functional outcomes than the group receiving BMS alone [67]. Görmeli et al. compared the effects of hyaluronic acid (HA) and PRP injections after BMS for OLT in a prospective randomized clinical trial. They found that PRP injections provided significantly better clinical outcomes than HA or saline injections at a mean follow-up duration of 15.3 months [68]. These results suggest that the use of PRP combined with the operative treatment for OLT may improve clinical and functional outcomes.

30.2.7.2 Concentrated Bone Marrow Aspirate (CBMA)

CBMA has been used to deliver mesenchymal stem cells (MSCs) to damaged cartilage to augment cartilage repair. It is produced at the time of surgery by centrifugation of bone marrow aspirate, typically harvested from the iliac crest. CBMA contains a similar growth factor and cytokine profile compared to PRP, with the addition of interleukin 1 receptor antagonist protein in CBMA, which is a potent anti-inflammatory agent [69].

The use of CBMA as an adjunct for the treatment for OLT has been investigated in both in vivo models and clinical studies. Fortier et al. have shown that CBMA improved both histological and radiological outcomes in the repair tissue of cartilage defects in an equine microfracture model, compared to a control without CBMA [70]. Similar results were reported in a goat model when using BMS combined with CBMA and HA [71]. Clinically, Hannon et al. found that patients who underwent BMS with CBMA for OLT had better border repair tissue integration with less evidence of fissuring and fibrillation on MRI compared to BMS alone [72]. Kennedy et al. reported significant improvement of clinical outcomes in 72 patients who underwent AOT with CBMA at a mean duration of 28 months follow-up [34]. Furthermore, the authors demonstrated restoration of the talar dome radius of curvature as well as similar color stratification of the graft relative to the native cartilage on MRI T2 mapping. Overall, the currently available body of evidence suggests that CBMA when used as an adjunct in the treatment for OLT has the potential to improve cartilage repair.

30.3 Summary

The surgical management of OLT remains controversial. Based on the currently available clinical evidence, both reparative and replacement procedures have a role in the surgical treatment of OLT and demonstrate good clinical outcomes. Biological adjuncts and scaffolds have been garnering a lot of attention lately and do provide promising clinical results. However, further high-level studies are required to develop standardized clinical guidelines for the treatment of OLT.

References

1. Hintermann B, Boss A, Schäfer D. Arthroscopic findings in patients with chronic ankle instability. Am J Sports Med. 2002;30:402–9.
2. Hintermann B, Regazzoni P, Lampert C, Stutz G, Gächter A. Arthroscopic findings in acute fractures of the ankle. J Bone Joint Surg Br. 2000;82(3):345–51.
3. van Dijk CN, Reilingh ML, Zengerink M, van Bergen CJ. Osteochondral defects in the ankle: why painful? Knee Surg Sports Traumatol Arthrosc. 2010;18(5):570–80.
4. Elias I, Zoga AC, Morrison WB, Besser MP, Schweitzer ME, Raikin SM. Osteochondral lesions of the talus: localization and morphologic data from 424 patients using a novel anatomical grid scheme. Foot Ankle Int. 2007;28(2):154–61.
5. Hannon CP, Smyth NA, Murawski CD, Savage-Elliott I, Deyer TW, Calder JD, Kennedy JG. Osteochondral lesions of the talus: aspects of current management. Bone Joint J. 2014;96-B(2):164–71.
6. Stougaard J. Familial occurrence of osteochondritis dissecans. J Bone Joint Surg Br. 1964;46:542–3.
7. Stattin EL, Wiklund F, Lindblom K, Onnerfjord P, Jonsson BA, Tegner Y, Sasaki T, Struglics A, Lohmander S, Dahl N, Heinegård D, Aspberg A. A missense mutation in the aggrecan C-type lectin domain disrupts extracellular matrix interactions and causes dominant familial osteochondritis dissecans. Am J Hum Genet. 2010;86(2):126–37.
8. Hermanson E, Ferkel RD. Bilateral osteochondral lesions of the talus. Foot Ankle Int. 2009;30(8):723–7.
9. Chuckpaiwong B, Berkson EM, Theodore GH. Microfracture for osteochondral lesions of the ankle: outcome analysis and outcome predictors of 105 cases. Arthroscopy. 2008;24(1):106–12.
10. Choi WJ, Park KK, Kim BS, Lee JW. Osteochondral lesion of the talus: is there a critical defect size for poor outcome? Am J Sports Med. 2009;37(10):1974–80.
11. Ramponi L, Yasui Y, Murawski CD, Ferkel RD, DiGiovanni CW, Kerkhoffs GMMJ, Calder JDF, Takao M, Vannini F, Choi WJ, Lee JW, Stone J, Kennedy JG. Lesion size is a predictor of clinical outcomes after bone marrow stimulation for Osteochondral lesions of the talus: a systematic review. Am J Sports Med. 2016;45(7):1698–705.
12. Shimozono Y, Coale M, Yasui Y, O'Halloran A, Deyer TW, Kennedy JG. Subchondral bone degradation after microfracture for osteochondral lesions of the talus: an MRI analysis. Am J Sports Med. 2018;46(3):642–8.

13. Takao M, Uchio Y, Kakimaru H, Kumahashi N, Ochi M. Arthroscopic drilling with debridement of remaining cartilage for osteochondral lesions of the talar dome in unstable ankles. Am J Sports Med. 2004;32(2):332–6.
14. Gianakos AL, Yasui Y, Fraser EJ, Ross KA, Prado MP, Fortier LA, Kennedy JG. The effect of different bone marrow stimulation techniques on human talar subchondral bone: a micro-computed tomography evaluation. Arthroscopy. 2016;32(10):2110–7.
15. Dahmen J, Lambers KTA, Reilingh ML, van Bergen CJA, Stufkens SAS, Kerkhoffs GMMJ. No superior treatment for primary osteochondral defects of the talus. Knee Surg Sports Traumatol Arthrosc. 2018;26(7):2142–57.
16. Zengerink M, Struijs PA, Tol JL, van Dijk CN. Treatment of osteochondral lesions of the talus: a systematic review. Knee Surg Sports Traumatol Arthrosc. 2010;18(2):238–46.
17. Hurley ET, Shimozono Y, McGoldrick NP, Myerson CL, Yasui Y, Kennedy JG. High reported rate of return to play following bone marrow stimulation for osteochondral lesions of the talus. Knee Surg Sports Traumatol Arthrosc. 2018;27:2721. https://doi.org/10.1007/s00167-018-4913-7.
18. Ferkel RD, Zanotti RM, Komenda GA, Sgaglione NA, Cheng MS, Applegate GR, Dopirak RM. Arthroscopic treatment of chronic osteochondral lesions of the talus: long-term results. Am J Sports Med. 2008;36(9):1750–62.
19. Seow D, Yasui Y, Hutchinson ID, Hurley ET, Shimozono Y, Kennedy JG. The subchondral bone is affected by bone marrow stimulation: a systematic review of preclinical animal studies. Cartilage. 2017;1:1947603517711220.
20. Lee KB, Bai LB, Yoon TR, Jung ST, Seon JK. Second-look arthroscopic findings and clinical outcomes after microfracture for osteochondral lesions of the talus. Am J Sports Med. 2009;37(Suppl 1):63S–70S.
21. van Bergen CJ, Kox LS, Maas M, Sierevelt IN, Kerkhoffs GM, van Dijk CN. Arthroscopic treatment of osteochondral defects of the talus outcomes at eight to twenty years of follow-up. J Bone Joint Surg Am. 2013;95(6):519–25.
22. Nehrer S, Spector M, Minas T. Histologic analysis of tissue after failed cartilage repair procedures. Clin Orthop Relat Res. 1999;365:149–62.
23. Pugh JW, Radin EL, Rose RM. Quantitative studies of human subchondral cancellous bone. Its relationship to the state of its overlying cartilage. J Bone Joint Surg Am. 1974;56(2):313–21.
24. Orth P, Meyer HL, Goebel L, Eldracher M, Ong MF, Cucchiarini M, Madry H. Improved repair of chondral and osteochondral defects in the ovine trochlea compared with the medial condyle. J Orthop Res. 2013;31(11):1772–9.
25. Karnovsky SC, DeSandis B, Haleem AM, Sofka CM, O'Malley M, Drakos MC. Comparison of juvenile allogenous articular cartilage and bone marrow aspirate concentrate versus microfracture with and without bone marrow aspirate concentrate in arthroscopic treatment of talar osteochondral lesions. Foot Ankle Int. 2018;39(4):393–405.
26. Fortier LA, Chapman HS, Pownder SL, Roller BL, Cross JA, Cook JL, Cole BJ. BioCartilage improves cartilage repair compared with microfracture alone in an equine model of full-thickness cartilage loss. Am J Sports Med. 2016;44(9):2366–74.
27. Ahmad J, Maltenfort M. Arthroscopic treatment of osteochondral lesions of the talus with allograft cartilage matrix. Foot Ankle Int. 2017;38(8):855–62.
28. Seow D, Yasui Y, Hurley ET, Ross AW, Murawski CD, Shimozono Y, Kennedy JG. Extracellular matrix cartilage allograft and particulate cartilage allograft for osteochondral lesions of the knee and ankle joints: a systematic review. Am J Sports Med. 2018;46(7):1758–66.
29. Scranton PE Jr, Frey CC, Feder KS. Outcome of osteochondral autograft transplantation for type-V cystic osteochondral lesions of the talus. J Bone Joint Surg Br. 2006;88(5):614–9.
30. Kim YS, Park EH, Kim YC, Koh YG, Lee JW. Factors associated with the clinical outcomes of the osteochondral autograft transfer system in osteochondral lesions of the talus: second-look arthroscopic evaluation. Am J Sports Med. 2012;40(12):2709–19.
31. Paul J, Sagstetter A, Kriner M, Imhoff AB, Spang J, Hinterwimmer S. Donor-site morbidity after osteochondral autologous transplantation for lesions of the talus. J Bone Joint Surg Am. 2009;91(7):1683–8.
32. Ross AW, Murawski CD, Frase EJ, Ross KA, Do HT, Deyer TW, Kennedy JG. Autologous osteochondral transplantation for osteochondral lesions of the talus: does previous bone marrow stimulation negatively affect clinical outcome? Arthroscopy. 2016;32(7):1377–83.
33. Shimozono Y, Hurley ET, Myerson CL, Kennedy JG. Good clinical and functional outcomes at mid-term following autologous osteochondral transplantation for osteochondral lesions of the talus. Knee Surg Sports Tramatol Arthrosc. 2018;26:3055. https://doi.org/10.1007/s00167-018-4917-3.
34. Kennedy JG, Murawski CD. The treatment of osteochondral lesions of the talus with autologous osteochondral transplantation and bone marrow aspirate concentrate: surgical technique. Cartilage. 2011;2(4):327–36.
35. Gianakos AL, Hannon CP, Ross KA, Newman H, Egan CJ, Deyer TW, Kennedy JG. Anterolateral tibial osteotomy for accessing osteochondral lesions of the talus in autologous osteochondral transplantation: functional and t2 MRI analysis. Foot Ankle Int. 2015;36(5):531–8.
36. Shimozono Y, Hurley ET, Yasui Y, Paugh RA, Deyer TW, Kennedy JG. Concentrated bone marrow aspirate may decrease postoperative cyst occurrence rate in autologous osteochondral transplantation for osteochondral lesions of the talus. Arthroscopy. 2018;35(1):99–105.
37. Fraser EJ, Harris MC, Prado MP, Kennedy JG. Autologous osteochondral transplantation for

osteochondral lesions of the talus in an athletic population. Knee Surg Sports Traumatol Arthrosc. 2016;24(4):1272–9.
38. Paul J, Sagstetter M, Lämmle L, Spang J, El-Azab H, Imhoff AB, Hinterwimmer S. Sports activity after osteochondral transplantation of the talus. Am J Sports Med. 2012;40(4):870–4.
39. Yoon HS, Park YJ, Lee M, Choi WJ, Lee JW. Osteochondral autologous transplantation is superior to repeat arthroscopy for the treatment of osteochondral lesions of the talus after failed primary arthroscopic treatment. Am J Sports Med. 2014;42(8):1896–903.
40. Fraser EJ, Savage-Elliott I, Yasui Y, Ackermann J, Watson G, Ross KA, Deyer T, Kennedy JG. Clinical and MRI donor site outcomes following autologous osteochondral transplantation for talar osteochondral lesions. Foot Ankle Int. 2016;37(9):968–76.
41. Lamb J, Murawski CD, Deyer TW, Kennedy JG. Chevron-type medial malleolar osteotomy: a functional, radiographic and quantitative T2-mapping MRI analysis. Knee Surg Sports Traumatol Arthrosc. 2013;21(6):1283–8.
42. Savage-Elliott I, Smyth NA, Deyer TW, Murawski CD, Ross KA, Hannon CP, Do HT, Kennedy JG. Magnetic resonance imaging evidence of postoperative cyst formation does not appear to affect clinical outcomes after autologous osteochondral transplantation of the talus. Arthroscopy. 2016;32(9):1846–54.
43. Gül M, Çetinkaya E, Aykut ÜS, Özkul B, Saygılı MS, Akman YE, Kabukcuoglu YS. Effect of the presence of subchondral cysts on treatment results of autologous osteochondral graft transfer in osteochondral lesions of the talus. J Foot Ankle Surg. 2016;55(5):1003–6.
44. Neri S, Vannini F, Desando G, Grigolo B, Ruffilli A, Buda R, Facchini A, Giannini S. Ankle bipolar fresh osteochondral allograft survivorship and integration: transplanted tissue genetic typing and phenotypic characteristics. J Bone Joint Surg Am. 2013;95(20):1852–60.
45. van Tienderen RJ, Dunn JC, Kuznezov N, Orr JD. Osteochondral allograft transfer for treatment of osteochondral lesions of the talus: a systematic review. Arthroscopy. 2017;33(1):217–22.
46. Raikin SM. Fresh osteochondral allografts for large-volume cystic osteochondral defects of the talus. J Bone Joint Surg Am. 2009;91(12):2818–26.
47. El-Rashidy H, Villacis D, Omar I, Kelikian AS. Fresh osteochondral allograft for the treatment of cartilage defects of the talus: a retrospective review. J Bone Joint Surg Am. 2011;93(17):1634–40.
48. Ahmad J, Jones K. Comparison of osteochondral autografts and allografts for treatment of recurrent or large talar osteochondral lesions. Foot Ankle Int. 2016;37(1):40–50.
49. Shimozono Y, Hurley ET, Nguyen JT, Deyer TW, Kennedy JG. Allograft compared with autograft in osteochondral transplantation for the treatment of osteochondral lesions of the talus. J Bone Joint Surg. 2018;100(21):1838–44.
50. Brittberg M, Lindahl A, Nilsson A, Ohlsson C, Isaksson O, Peterson L. Treatment of deep cartilage defects in the knee with autologous chondrocyte transplantation. N Engl J Med. 1994;331(14):889–95.
51. Giannini S, Battaglia M, Buda R, Cavallo M, Ruffilli A, Vannini F. Surgical treatment of osteochondral lesions of the talus by open-field autologous chondrocyte implantation: a 10-year follow-up clinical and magnetic resonance imaging T2-mapping evaluation. Am J Sports Med. 2009;37(Suppl 1):112S–8S.
52. Candrian C, Miot C, Wolf F, Bonacina E, Dickinson S, Wirz D, Jakob M, Valderrabano V, Barbero A, Martin I. Are ankle chondrocytes from damaged fragments a suitable cell source for cartilage repair? Osteoarthr Cartil. 2010;18(8):1067–76.
53. Niemeyer P, Salzmann G, Schmal H, Mayr H, Südkamp NP. Autologous chondrocyte implantation for the treatment of chondral and osteochondral defects of the talus: a meta-analysis of available evidence. Knee Surg Sports Traumatol Arthrosc. 2012;20(9):1696–703.
54. Battaglia M, Vannini F, Buda R, Cavallo M, Ruffilli A, Monti C, Galletti S, Giannini S. Arthroscopic autologous chondrocyte implantation in osteochondral lesions of the talus: mid-term T2-mapping MRI evaluation. Knee Surg Sports Traumatol Arthrosc. 2011;19(8):1376–84.
55. Giza E, Sullivan M, Ocel D, Lundeen G, Mitchell ME, Veris L, Walton J. Matrix-induced autologous chondrocyte implantation of talus articular defects. Foot Ankle Int. 2010;31(9):747–53.
56. Nehrer S, Domayer SE, Hirschfeld C, Stelzeneder D, Trattnig S, Dorotka R. Matrix-associated and autologous chondrocyte transplantation in the ankle: clinical and MRI follow-up after 2 to 11 years. Cartilage. 2011;2(1):81–91.
57. Aurich M, Bedi HS, Smith PJ, Rolauffs B, Mückley T, Clayton J, Blackney M. Arthroscopic treatment of osteochondral lesions of the ankle with matrix-associated chondrocyte implantation: early clinical and magnetic resonance imaging results. Am J Sports Med. 2011;39(2):311–9.
58. Magnan B, Samaila E, Bondi M, Vecchini E, Micheloni GM, Bartolozzi P. Three-dimensional matrix-induced autologous chondrocytes implantation for osteochondral lesions of the talus: midterm results. Adv Orthop. 2012;2012:942174.
59. Giannini S, Buda R, Ruffilli A, Cavallo M, Pagliazzi G, Bulzamini MC, Desando G, Luciani D, Vannini F. Arthroscopic autologous chondrocyte implantation in the ankle joint. Knee Surg Sports Traumatol Arthrosc. 2014;22(6):1311–9.
60. Wiewiorski M, Miska M, Kretzschmar M, Studler U, Bieri O, Valderrabano V. Delayed gadolinium-enhanced MRI of cartilage of the ankle joint: results after autologous matrix-induced chondrogenesis (AMIC)-aided reconstruction of osteochondral lesions of the talus. Clin Radiol. 2013;68(10):1031–8.
61. Valderrabano V, Miska M, Leumann A, Wiewiorski M. Reconstruction of osteochondral lesions of the

talus with autologous spongiosa grafts and autologous matrix-induced chondrogenesis. Am J Sports Med. 2013;41(3):519–27.
62. Vannini F, Cavallo M, Ramponi L, Castagnini F, Massimi S, Giannini S, Buda R. Return to sports after bone marrow-derived cell transplantation for osteochondral lesions of the talus. Cartilage. 2017;8(1):80–7.
63. Buda R, Vannini F, Castagnini F, Cavallo M, Ruffilli A, Ramponi L, Pagliazzi G, Giannini S. Regenerative treatment in osteochondral lesions of the talus: autologous chondrocyte implantation versus one-step bone marrow derived cells transplantation. Int Orthop. 2015;39(5):893–900.
64. Baksh N, Hannon CP, Murawski CD, Smyth NA, Kennedy JG. Platelet-rich plasma in tendon models: a systematic review of basic science literature. Arthroscopy. 2013;29(3):596–607.
65. Smyth NA, Murawski CD, Fortier LA, Cole BJ, Kennedy JG. Platelet-rich plasma in the pathologic processes of cartilage: review of basic science evidence. Arthroscopy. 2013;29(8):1399–409.
66. Smyth NA, Haleem AM, Murawski CD, Do HT, Deland JT, Kennedy JG. The effect of platelet-rich plasma on autologous osteochondral transplantation an in vivo rabbit mode. J Bone Joint Surg Am. 2013;95(24):2185–93.
67. Guney A, Akar M, Karaman I, Oner M, Guney B. Clinical outcomes of platelet rich plasma (PRP) as an adjunct to microfracture surgery in osteochondral lesions of the talus. Knee Surg Sports Traumatol Arthroscopy. 2013;23(8):2384–9.
68. Görmeli G, Karakaplan M, Görmeli CA, Sarlkaya B, Elmall N, Ersoy Y. Clinical effects of platelet-rich plasma and hyaluronic acid as an additional therapy for talar osteochondral lesions treated with microfracture surgery: a prospective randomized clinical trial. Foot Ankle Int. 2015;36(8):891–900.
69. Cassano JM, Kennedy JG, Ross KA, Fraser EJ, Goodale MB, Fortier LA. Bone marrow concentrate and platelet-rich plasma differ in cell distribution and interleukin 1 receptor antagonist protein concentration. Knee Surg Sports Traumatol Arthrosc. 2018;26(1):333–42.
70. Fortier LA, Potter HG, Rickey EJ, Schnabel LV, Foo LF, Chong LR, Stokol T, Cheetham J, Nixon AJ. Concentrated bone marrow aspirate improves full-thickness cartilage repair compared with microfracture in the equine model. J Bone Joint Surg Am. 2010;92(10):1927–37.
71. Saw KY, Hussin P, Loke SC, Azam M, Chen HC, Tay YG, Low S, Wallin KL, Ragavanaidu K. Articular cartilage regeneration with autologous marrow aspirate and hyaluronic acid: an experimental study in a goat model. Arthroscopy. 2009;25(12):1391–400.
72. Hannon CP, Ross KA, Murawski CD, Deyer TW, Smyth NA, Hogan MV, Do HT, O'Malley MJ, Kennedy JG. Arthroscopic bone marrow stimulation and concentrated bone marrow aspirate for osteochondral lesions of the talus: a case-control study of functional and magnetic resonance observation of cartilage repair tissue outcomes. Arthroscopy. 2016;32(2):339–7.

Ankle Rehabilitation

31

Andrzej Kępczyński

31.1 Introduction

Rehabilitation of the ankle needs knowledge of the type of surgery procedures to be able to cooperate with surgeon and understand his/her focus [1, 2]. In modern orthopaedic surgery the most important is time. We recommend preoperative physiotherapy to accelerate and optimise the postoperative process. Due to that reason it is extremely important to arrange minimum one appointment with a physiotherapist before the scheduled operation. The surgeon could prior to surgery obtain information from the physiotherapist about:

(a) Functional range of motion during walking, climbing, running etc.
(b) Mobility restrictions of the other joints of the lower limb.
(c) Muscle status of the lower and upper limb i.e. strength, endurance, proprioception.
(d) Ability of the patient to cooperate postoperatively.

It is important to understand today how important it is to make a good preoperative briefing and how that can influence on the finale surgery result. Preoperative communications could help the surgeon to make the best timing for surgery as well as the choice of surgery procedure.

31.2 General Instructions for the Ankle Rehabilitation

For the rehabilitation of the ankle one must plan the milestones of the prospective surgery. Regardless the kind of the surgery the first milestone of the postoperative rehabilitation must be to get painless range of motions.

First milestone:

What is physiologically the mobility of the ankle? The tibiotarsal joint is a hinge joint with one degree of freedom [4]. It allows walking on flat floor. The position of the reference for the ankle is when the foot is perpendicular to the axis of the leg. From that point we measure flexion- 20–30° up and extension 30–50° down. In the end of that mobility the tarsal move occurs. The foot can move about vertical and horizontal, longitudinal axis [4].

Movements of adduction and abduction occur in the vertical plane. Totally these movements are from 35° to 45°.

Longitudinally, the foot can rotate medially- 52° and laterally- 25–30°. That is the physiological range of movements of the foot. During examination it is worth to check and compare mobility of both sides.

Second milestone:

A. Kępczyński (✉)
Physiotherapy, Klinika Ruchu, Warsaw, Poland
e-mail: Andrzej.Kepczynski@klinikaruchu.pl

M. Brittberg, K. Slynarski (eds.), *Lower Extremity Joint Preservation*,
https://doi.org/10.1007/978-3-030-57382-9_31

The second milestone is the active motions produced by the muscles. To achieve that point the physiotherapist should have knowledge about muscle training. One needs to think about muscles like a motor control system and also like part of the proprioception mechanism.

From the very beginning postoperative we have to shape muscle control of the knee, ankle, and foot. Even if the patient has weight bearing restrictions postoperatively, immediately after achieving non-painful passive motion in the joint we manage training of the involved and non-involved muscles. Especially after ankle surgery, isometric contractions are not recommended. We prefer to treat the patient with isotonic exercises. That kind of training will help the patient keep active mobility in acute phase postop [3].

Proprioception training should also be introduced as fast as possible postop. To achieve that point of ankle rehabilitation the most helpful therapy is aqua physiotherapy. One can teach full weight bearing walking under water immediately after healing of the surgical wounds.

Very important in ankle rehabilitation and generally in postoperative rehabilitation is maintaining training with:

1. Non-painful mobility.
2. Non-painful muscle training.

When you follow the above rules, the choice of physiotherapy methods and the physical therapy you use are of secondary importance.

To describe more specific rehabilitation of the ankle a presentation of two rehab protocols after reconstruction of the anterior tibiofibular ligament (ATFL) and arthroscopic anterolateral impingement are shown. These are two very common surgical treatments of the ankle that show differences between accelerated rehabilitation without any restrictions versus rehabilitation with a preoperative phase and the postoperative physiotherapy depending on the remodeling phases of the repair area.

31.2.1 Rehabilitation in Reconstruction of Anterior Talofibular Ligament (ATFL)

31.2.1.1 Preoperative Phase

An average of two weeks of preparing muscle and lower limb before reconstruction is recommended.

In this phase we have two main aims:

1. Preop physio examination for planning a short preoperative physiotherapy individual protocol. Usually the patient with chronic ATFL deficit presents with a protective walk and non-equal side to side weight bearing. Those symptoms produce limitations of the range of motion of the ankle and foot. The second problem usually is weakness and partial atrophy of the quadriceps and gluteus muscle. To increase mobility, we first recommended manual mobilisation of the joints. According to the preoperative examination the patient gets his own set of the stretching and strengthening exercises.
2. Instruction for the postoperative rules. Adjustments of the life style to postoperative conditions. It is time to answer every problematic question about the postoperative period and instruct of how to use the brace and the crutches. That point of the rehabilitation will let patient to know his physiotherapist which will be very helpful when to cooperate especially in early postop phase.

31.2.1.2 Postoperative Phase

Rehabilitation postop starts from day one with strict anaesthesiologist recommendation [6]. The details of the rehabilitation in this phase are described in Table 31.1.

In this phase the best are passive treatments i.e. manual mobilisation of the joint, manual muscle stretching and passive mobility of the range of movement. Home exercises are recommended only for perfectly cooperating patients.

Table 31.1 The rules of the early rehabilitation phase

Early rehabilitation phase (0–4 weeks) Visit for physiotherapy 2–3 times a week and home exercise daily
1. Elevation of the lower limb (most of the time—minimum 6 h a day) 2. Local cryotherapy minimum every 2 h (excluding nights) 3. Lymphatic drainage 4. Partial non-painful weight bearing (20–80% body mass) 5. Passive stretching of the postural muscle of the trunk, hips and knee 6. Active non-resistance exercises flex-ext. in non-painful range 7. Weight relief proprioception exercises in knee ext. and knee flex 8. Leg extensions 9. Leg curl 10. Aquatic rehabilitation in case of unhealed wound
Locomotion—maximum 2 h of holding limb down Orthotic equipment—functional brace (especially at night) and two crutches Walking extra steps up and down
Criteria of the safety passage to next phase: 1. Non-painful full weight bearing in brace 2. Full passive range of motion 3. No symptoms of inflammation and effusion

For the rest, home exercises are forbidden. Manual scar mobilisation earliest 3 weeks postop.

About 4 weeks postop if the patients fulfil the criteria they pass to late rehab phase. Modern physiotherapy is more focused on criteria than time, which determines patient status. We call it traffic lights method.

Late phase is a time when usually the patient does not use any pain killers or anti-inflammatory drugs. Sometimes, especially after progressing from walking to running or two leg jumps to one leg jump, anti-inflammatory treatment can be helpful, which is decided finally by the treating surgeon.

Details of the treatment in this phase are described in Table 31.2.

The last and most difficult phase in rehab in ATFL reconstruction is return-to-sport phase (Table 31.3). Most of the rehabilitation postoperative protocols are time-based. Sport-specific exercises and activities should be introduced as soon as possible i.e. in early rehab phase running between 12–16 week postop is possible when no pain and effusion exist, full range of movement, positive balance and battery test [5]. In this phase, strict cooperation between the trainer and physiotherapist is necessary. The most important is not to accelerate to return to full time activity phase. the trainer should introduce the athlete into the training routine individually looking at his endurance

Table 31.2 Main principles of the late rehabilitation phase

Late rehabilitation phase (4–16 weeks) Visit for physiotherapy ≤8 week postop, three times a week 8–16 week postop, 1–2 times a week
1. Full weight bearing no brace 6 weeks postop 2. Manual therapy if necessary 3. Local cryotherapy if necessary 4. Squats, one leg 6 weeks 5. Strengthening exercises of the cuff and foot using band 6. Gait training 7. Single-leg balance training 8. Bilateral hops 6 weeks 9. Gentle jogging in place 8 weeks 10. Swimming in fins 6 weeks 11. Gentle non-contact sport-specific activities 8 weeks 12. Spinning 8 weeks
Milestones of this phase: 1. No pain and effusion after training 2. Full range of motion 3. Ability to jump one leg

Table 31.3 Return-to-sport phase

Return-to-sport phase ≥16 weeks postop
1. Battery and other combination of tests 2. Evaluate strength, muscle endurance, jumping and running ability 3. Video gait analysis 4. MRI 5. Individually "from the beginner" training with team 6. Cooperaton betwen physio in rehab room and physio on the field—trainer highly recommended until first competition

and skills like the beginner. This is the only way to decrease reinjury risk.

31.2.2 Rehabilitation in Ankle Arthroscopy for Anterolateral Impingement

The second rehabilitation of the ankle that we would like to describe in this chapter is rehabilitation after anterolateral impingement syndrome. This problem is very often recognised like in the beginning of the early degenerative changes in the ankle [7]. Ankle impingement syndrome is initially treated by physical therapy. Ankle impingement syndrome is initially treated only by physical therapy, unfortuantely, it takes a too long time and is unsuccesful especially in profesional dancers [8]. What can be the reason for the late osteoarthritis changes of the ankle? Early osteoarthritis change is very difficult to treat by rehabilitation only. Arthroscopic treatment for anterolateral ankle impingement appears to provide good results with respect to patient satisfaction and with low complication rates [8]. The most important aim of the rehabilitation in ankle arthroscopy for anterolateral impingement is to maintain functional non-painful movement of the ankle and foot. In this case, preoperative physiotherapy usually cannot be done because the patient has a long history of ankle injuries and therapies. Preoperative rehabilitation in this case would be hard to enforce.

We start postoperative phase as soon as possible after arthroscopy to restore mobility and to shorten immobilisation time. Rehabilitation protocol begins from manual mobilisation of the ankle and foot.

In Table 31.4 the early phase of the treatment is described.

The late phase of the rehab in ankle arthroscopy is also return–to-sport phase. The very important part of this protocol is the cooperation link doctor–physiotherapist–trainer. Individually rehab protocol acceleration is allowed at this phase. Also different types of muscle or kind of impingement pain can occure at this phase. It is important to have support from the diagnostic department also. Physiotherapy at field, gym and water physiotherapy can be very helpful to differentiate protocol, especially in professional athletes. We call it sport-specific exercises (Table 31.5).

Table 31.4 Early rehab in ankle arthroscopy

Early rehabilitation phase(0–6 weeks) Visit for physiotherapy 4–5 times a week
1. Manual mobilisation 2. Lymphatic drainage 3. Passive stretching of the muscle of lower limb 4. CPM 3–5 h daily 4 weeks 5. Gentle gait training 6. TENS 7. Local cryotherapy
No brace Two crutches 0–2 weeks postop Anti-oedema tights
Criteria of the safety passage to next phase: 1. Minimum 90% of range of movement compared to non-operated leg 2. No limping 3. No pain during walking 4. Walking up and down the stairs

Table 31.5 Late postop phase and return to sport

Late postop phase 6–16 weeks Visit for physiotherapy two times a week
1. Manual therapy if necessary 2. Local cryotherapy 3. Squats, one leg, two legs 4. Strenghting exercises of the cuff and foot 5. Gentle jogging 6. Single-leg balance training 7. Trampoline exercises 8. Sport-specific exercises
Return to sport: 1. Battery and other combination of tests 2. Evaluate strength, muscle endurance, jumping and running ability 3. Video gait analysis 4. MRI

References

1. Schuh R, Banca E, Willegger M, Hirtler L, Zandieh S, Holinka J, Windhager R. Comparison of Broström technique, suture anchor repair, and tape augmentation for reconstruction of the anterior talofibular ligament. Knee Surg Sports Traumatol Arthrosc. 2016;24(4):1101–7.
2. Kaltenborn FM. Manual mobilization of the extremity joints, volume 1. The extremities. Minneapolis, MN Orthopedic Physical Therapy Products; 1989. p. 168–70.

3. Chaitow L. Muscle energy techniques. London: Pearson Professional Limited; 1996. p. 68–70, 107–109.
4. Kapanji IA. The physiology of the joints. In: The lower limb. 2nd ed. Edinburgh: Churchill Livingstone; 1991. p. 148–50, 166–70.
5. Lunsford BR, Perry J. The standing heel-rise test for ankle plantar flexion: criterion for normal. Phys Ther. 1995;75(8):694–8.
6. Ross KA, Murawski CD. Current concepts review: arthroscopic treatment of anterior ankle impingement. Foot Ankle Surg. 2017;23(1):7–8.
7. Zwiers R, Wiegerinck JI. Arthroscopic treatment for anterior ankle impingement: a systematic review of the current literature. Arthroscopy. 2015;31(8):1585–7.
8. Nihal A, Rose DJ, Trepman E. Arthroscopic treatment of anterior ankle impingement syndrome in dancers. Foot Ankle Int. 2005;26(11):910–2.